Blackwell's Five-Minute Veterinary Consult

Clinical Companion

Blackwell's Five-Minute
Veterinary Consult
Clinical Companion

Small Animal Senior Care

Edited by

Heidi B. Lobprise
Veterinary Dental Specialist
Cibolo Creek Veterinary Hospital
Boerne Texas
USA

WILEY

Published by John Wiley & Sons, Inc., Hoboken, New Jersey.
Published simultaneously in Canada.

Library of Congress Cataloging-in-Publication Data Applied for:

Paperback ISBN: 9781394155774

Cover design: Wiley
Cover image(s): Courtesy of Steve Dale, Courtesy of Mary Gardner, Courtesy of Geneva Kernaghan

Set in 10/12pts Berkeley by Straive, Pondicherry, India

Printed in Singapore
M123346_020425

Dedication

This book is absolutely dedicated to my husband, Joe Kautz, for his patience with my obsession with the book, especially in the past few months. You are my supporter and chauferpa!

I am also adding a dedication to George, who, while not a senior by years, survived many challenges in his 9 years, including systemic histoplasmosis, partial blindness and possible lungworms, and/or lung cancer. He was a constant companion during my writing, sometimes distracting me completely from my work. A week before this book was finished, we went through the process of making euthanasia decisions based on his quality of life and extent of disease. He will forever be in our hearts.

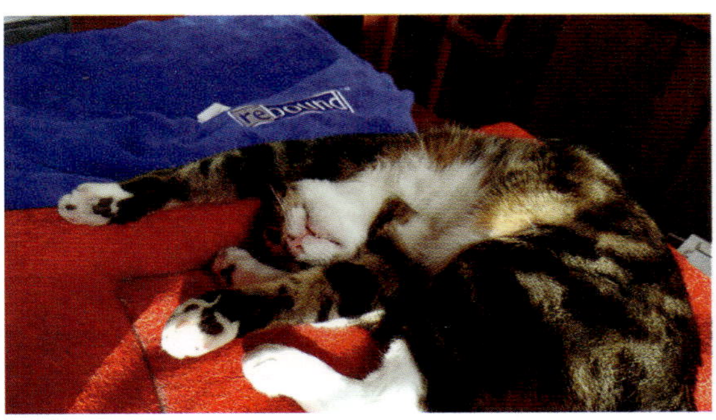

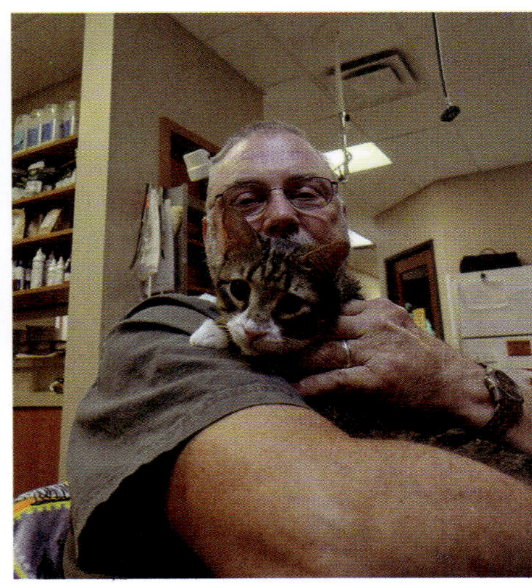

Contents

List of Contributors

Steve Dale, CABC
www.stevedale.tv
www.facebook.com/SteveDalePetWorld/
Instagram: SteveDalesPetWorld
Twitter: SteveDalePets
Chicago, IL, USA

Dr. Jennifer Mathis DVM DAVDC
Board Certified Veterinary Dentist™
Veterinary Medical Acupuncturist
Certified Veterinary Pain Practitioner
https://tooth.vet/

Animal Dentistry Referral Services
Norwalk, Iowa, USA

Preface

You might wonder why a veterinary dentist is writing a book about senior pet care, but as I am reaching my own golden years in semiretirement, I wanted to make and collaborate resources for veterinary professionals that take care of senior pets. I worked for Virbac Animal Health for a few years (beyond just dentistry) and as a "technical manager," I was tasked to help develop key opinion leaders (KOLs) for various fields. I was asked to contact some of the KOLs for senior care, and I realized there wasn't a distinct category. Sure, you can find lectures, articles, and chapters about senior pets pertaining to specific fields, from ophthalmology to internal medicine, anesthesia, and even dentistry, but nothing coalesced around senior care in a comprehensive manner. Back then, veterinary gerontology wasn't even a "thing," with general practitioners being the most well-rounded gerontologists out there.

There were also resources on senior care, including pain management and specific disease therapies, based on product campaigns. These actually provide a good basis of science behind the diseases as well. And certainly, in the hospice, palliative care, and euthanasia realm, there are well-defined guidelines, active associations, and companies such as Lap of Love that provide not only care for patients but education for veterinarian professionals.

There is also now a growing trend with research, particularly in dogs, as they can be better models for aging and therapeutic concepts that translate into human medicine. So as the field of veterinary gerontology grows, I wanted to help bring some of this knowledge together to see what can be done practically for our patients. And once I started—I went down the rabbit hole! From exploring the concepts of immunosenescence and inflammaging to realizing some challenges to serve senior pets could be easily supported by just adding "life stage" and "muscle condition score" fields to practice management systems, it has been a journey.

So as a "senior pet advocate," I hope to be able to continue to bring resources together, many of which are already out there, just scattered a bit. This first edition of the *Five-Minute Veterinary Consultation Clinical Companion: Small Animal Senior Care* has Section 1 to explore aging, senescence, and life expectancy and Section 3 to look at some practice and patient applications, mostly new material, with some help from colleagues. The middle Section 2 is composed of many topics adapted from the seventh edition of the Five-Minute Veterinary Consult, with an effort to focus on those with an indication of prevalence in older pets. Some additional topics may have been passed over, and the entire group of neoplasia had to be left out due to the enormity of that field. I expect this publication to be a flexible entity with the ability to change and grow as our knowledge in this field forever expands.

Thank you for joining me on this journey and let me know what else we can do together.

Sincerely
Heidi B. Lobprise, DVM, DAVDC,
and SPA (senior pet advocate)

Acknowledgments

I thank several people for their assistance in helping me put this book together:

- Steve Dale and Jennifer Mathis for co-contributing to chapters.
- Mary Gardner, Sheliah Robertson, Amy Pike, Amy Farcas, and Gary Oswald for sharing resources that helped build various topics.
- Julie Byron, Joshua Broadwater, Gary Oswald, and Elizabeth Settles for reviewing topics that I had adapted from the seventh edition of Five-Minute Veterinary Consult.

About the Companion Website

This book is accompanied by a companion website:

www.wiley.com/go/lobprise/Senior

This website include:

- Small Animal Senior Care Online Resources Senior Pet Organizations and Research
- Small Animal Senior Care Online Resources for Veterinary Clients
- Small Animal Senior Care Online Resources

Section 1

Senior Care

Chapter 1

Aging and Senescence

BASICS

OVERVIEW

While the adage "Age is not a disease" may be true, the process of aging can be considered one of the most important, and potentially modifiable, causes of disease, disability, and death in adult dogs. (McKenzie) A set of complex but comprehensible processes increase with time that result in a progressive loss of function, a decrease in reserves and recovery capacities, that put the individual at risk for disease and even death. Anticipated, "normal" aging processes need to be distinguished from pathological issues ("non-programmed disruptions of aging")[1] with attempts for coordinated management.

The chronological age of our patients is a major factor, yet it is the individual's response that can greatly influence biological or physiologic age. The ultimate goal is to minimize the impacts of aging changes to maintain health, resilience, and functional capacity for as long as possible (healthspan). Recently, there has been a growing recognition that geroscience approaches in veterinary medicine can have a much greater impact on health and disease burden than traditional biomedical strategies aimed at treating individual diseases in isolation. (Kaeberlein)

Much of the research on aging and associated issues comes from human medicine and laboratory animal data, but there is a growing field of information concerning dogs and even cats. In fact, there is so much literature in this field that this chapter can only present an abbreviated listing of some of the most pertinent facts. When possible, specific dog and cat data is presented.

Terms Defined

- Aging is the decline and deterioration of functional properties at the cellular, tissue, and organ levels. This loss of functional properties yields a loss of homeostasis and decreased adaptability to internal and external stress yielding an increased vulnerability to disease and mortality. (Fedarko)
- Chronological age—actual "calendar" age of the individual
- Biological (genetic) age—how old your cells and tissues are based on physiological parameters—to provide the predicted longevity.
- Lifespan—actual number of years an individual is alive.
- Healthspan—the time an individual is able to maintain good health with a short period of morbidity before death.
- Geroscience refers to research aimed at understanding the mechanisms of biological aging, defining the genetic, epigenetic, and environmental features that determine the rates of aging.[2]

Blackwell's Five-Minute Veterinary Consult Clinical Companion: Small Animal Senior Care, First Edition. Edited by Heidi B. Lobprise.

Companion website: www.wiley.com/go/lobprise/Senior

- Robustness—the ability to maintain optimal physiological function in the face of external stressors.
- Resilience—the ability to return to baseline following stressor disturbance.
- Frailty—a syndrome characterized by the decrease in physiologic reserves, cognitive performance, and dysregulation of multiple body systems with an increased vulnerability to stressors.
- Functional capacity a direct measure of the ability of cells, tissues, and organ systems to operate properly/optimally and is influenced by both genes and environment.
- Senescence—cellular response that blocks further proliferation and alters the cell's phenotype.
- Immunosenescence—the decline in the function of the adaptive immune system that occurs during aging and is associated with thymic involution, alterations in T cell subsets, and reduction in antibody production.
- Inflammaging—the term used to describe the pro-inflammatory state associated with aging.[3]
- Apoptosis—cellular response to remove damaged or aberrant cells through controlled cell death with no inflammatory response.
- Oxidative stress (OS)—the imbalance between free radicals and antioxidants in the body that can cause damage and disease.

ISSUES AND OPTIONS

The "Normal" Aging Process

- Mechanisms of cellular maintenance include:
  - DNA repair
  - synthesis and fidelity surveillance
  - detection and clearance of defective proteins and lipids
  - clearance of defective organelles and cells
  - defense against pathogens and injury
- Main contributors to mammalian aging (Jiminez, Lopez-Otin, Sandor)
  - Genomic instability—damaged with age by mutations, chromosome rearrangement, and increase in copy number variants (CNV)
    - Hinders cell function resulting in cellular senescence, apoptosis, or even malignancy
      - Increased apoptosis can lead to atrophy, or decreased removal of accumulation of senescent cells.
    - Deficiencies in DNA repair
    - Oxidative damage from reactive oxygen species (ROS), free radicals that target DNA, lipids, and protein
      - Oxidative DNA lesions increase with age and with decreased expression of antioxidant enzymes—neurodegeneration
    - Optimal levels of oxidation are needed; they should not be completely irradicated. ROS at low levels are important signaling molecules.
    - Transposable element—transponsons increase with age; can be induced by stressors—heavy metal toxins, genotoxic agents, and nutrition.
    - Assessing when mitochondrial DNA mutations first appear (especially in larger breed dogs), may be helpful in assessing aging and age-related diseases.[4]

- Telomere attrition—the protective portions at the ends of chromosomes that shorten with each cell division in somatic cells (not in germ line cells—they have sufficient telomerase)
    - Limits the number of cycles (Hayflick limit) and correlates with lifespan.
    - May limit the growth of malignant cells but can also contribute to tumorigenesis if chromosomes link end-to-end.
    - Telomeres shorten faster under conditions of chronic inflammation and oxidative stress in humans and animals;[5] even associated with feline chronic kidney disease.[6]
    - Comprehensive lifestyle changes could stabilize telomeres and decrease oxidative stress.
    - Telomeric restriction fragments may vary by dog breed, so this should be considered in evaluation.[7, 8]
- Epigenetic alterations—mechanisms that modulate gene expression and transcription
    - DNA is packed into dense chromatin—heterochromatic or more open euchromatic; their ratio is associated with aging.
    - Methylation of cytosines may block transcription
        - Hyperactive for pro-aging genes but repressing anti-aging genes
    - Regulation by various enzymes working on sirtuin genes—longevity impact
    - Age-related changes—alter mRNA transcriptome: gero-miRNAs (microRNAs) target other longevity miRNAs.
    - Epigenetic regulation may be dog breed specific.[9]
- Proteostasis disruption of proteome (all protein types in a cell)
    - Cell senescence and proteinopathies—accumulation of misfolded proteins
    - Aberrant proteins (altered by glycation) can induce inflammation.
    - Chaperones and protein quality control facilitate appropriate folding of maturing proteins and protect them; these are reduced with aging.
        - Heat-shock proteins (Hsp)—upregulation can extend lifespan in mice
        - Not always protective—can be neurodegenerative
    - Ubiquitin–Proteasome (UPS)—performs selective removal of misfolded and senescent proteins—linked to longevity
    - Autophagy—targets diseased mitochondria and large protein aggregates, fuses with lysosomes and degrades/recycles components
        - If impaired—can be a major factor in aging regulation.
        - Lipofuscin (aging pigment) can accumulate in lysosomes due to oxidation of unsaturated fatty acids. These are insoluble and refractile to cellular removal, compromise organelle function.
- Nutrient-sensing deregulation—nutrients used for cell metabolism, protein synthesis, autophagy
    - TOR—target of rapamycin kinase—determines rates of protein turnover and metabolism
        - Rapamycin—approved immunosuppressant, transplant rejection drug but has severe side effects at medical dosages
        - Increased lifespan seen with a decrease of mammalian mTOR—smaller dosage without side effects
        - Main signaling—insulin and IGF1 signaling pathways
    - FOXO (forkhead box O)—role in tumor suppression and age-related diseases

- Sirtuins and nicotinamide adenine dinucleotide (NAD)-dependent factors.
- AMPK (5′AMP-actived protein kinase)—detects levels of AMP, counteracts IGF1 by inhibiting TOR and activating FOXO3a—neuroprotective role.
- Therapy potential—metformin and acarbose (anti-diabetic medications)—exert anti-aging effect with mild effects at correct dose in dogs.
- The metabolome (the collection of metabolites in a cell or organism) was analyzed in a caloric restriction study on Labradors to help assess metabolic steps that may impact longevity.[10]

- Mitochondrial dysfunction—main source of energy; mitochondrial respiration generates ATP but also ROS
  - Dysfunction is a main driver of neurodegeneration in humans and dogs
    - In a study, antioxidant diet with mitochondrial co-factors (lipoic acid [LA] and carnitine) improved respiration and reduced ROS.[11]
    - Differing study results may be due to baseline nutrition or possible differences across dog breeds.
  - Advanced glycation end-product (AGE) is formed at the end stage of carbohydrate metabolism and can accumulate in long-lived proteins (collagen) with damage to macromolecules, though there is little research in dogs.
    - Oxidative stress may be involved in AGE formation and AGE may induce OS.[12]
  - Altered mitochondrial homeostasis (mihormesis) may benefit from mild stressors to benefit cellular health and longevity as a defense mechanism.
  - Resveratol and metformin might be mild mitochondrial toxins, inducing mihormesis.
  - High genetic variability—may be challenging to target treatment
- Cellular senescence—permanent cell-cycle arrest with phenotypic changes
  - Phenotype—larger cell, senescence-associated Beta-galactosidase, proteases, cell-cycle inhibitors and pro-inflammatory cytokines.[13]
  - Impacted through DNA damage, oncogene expression and supermitogenic signals; cytoskeletal, interferon-related, insulin-like growth factor (IGF)-related, MAP (mitogen-activated protein) kinase, and oxidative stress pathways.
  - Correlates with chronologic age (biomarker)
  - Accumulation in tissue as innate immune system declines with age and less phagocytosis.
  - Produce inflammatory signals, special inflammatory microenvironment around themselves—induce senescence in neighboring cells—bystander effect
- Stem cell exhaustion—tissue renewal depends on tissue-specific stem cells
  - Increase in cell senescence may initially activate stem cells, then they become depleted—accelerates aging
  - Stem cells may also decrease in ability to replicate and differentiate—e.g., in old age anemia.
  - Stem cell therapy potential—especially for neurodegenerative diseases
- Altered intercellular communication and Inflammation
  - Paracrine, endocrine, and neurocrine signaling
  - Growth hormone (GH), insulin/IGF1 (somatotropic axis), supervised by HPA (hypothalamus–pituitary–adrenal) axis and thyroid axis; hormones from digestive and reproductive systems, small molecules from gut bacteria
  - Neuroendocrine signaling—neural aging—a central mechanism

- ◇ BDNF (brain-derived neurotrophic factor) and serotonin affect brain aging; changes due to caloric restriction
- ◇ Hypothalamus—reproductive aging controlled by GnRH (gonadotropin-releasing hormone)
  - Reduction in response to inflammation can aggravate frailty
- ◇ Extracellular vesicles—exosomes and ectosomes
  - Released into blood—transducers of cellular signals and their content
    - ▪ miRNAs—diagnostic and prognostic measures of some diseases
    - ▪ Stem cells of hypothalamus—exosome miRNAs may modulate aging and neurodegeneration
- o Inflammaging and immunosenescence (see inflammaging; see immunosenescence)
- o Microbiome—systemic and immune function can be modulated by bacteria in the gut
  - ◇ Various chemical signals may affect organs (brain) and aging
    - Oral microbiota and inflammation are linked to Alzheimer's disease.
  - ◇ Probiotics and prebiotics that can beneficially alter the biome have been reported to positively influence the aging of the gut and systemic inflammation in people.[14]

Immunosenescence

- ▪ Adaptive immunity declines, low-level, chronic activation of innate immunity systems leads to low-level, chronic pro-inflammatory state
  - Reduced naïve CD8+ T-cells and moderately elevated memory T cells
  - Bone marrow–derived macrophages lose their phagocytic capacity.
  - Altered cytokines can facilitate disease progression
  - Cardiovascular disease, cancer, diabetes mellitus, osteoporosis, rheumatoid arthritis, and cognitive disorders in humans can all be impacted.

Inflammaging

- ▪ Acute inflammation is important for response to stressors
- ▪ Chronic, "sterile," inflammation - pro-inflammatory state, elevated IL-6 levels
  - Cytokines affect growth hormone/IGF-1 (somatotrophic) axis
  - "Sickness behavior"—fatigue, malaise, loss of interest in social, difficulty concentrating, sleep pattern changes.[15]
  - Neuromodulators—depressive disorders
  - Hypothalamic–pituitary–adrenal (HPA) axis hyperactivity—cytokines disturb the negative feedback inhibition of corticosteroids.[16]

The "Appearance" of Aging in Senior Pets

- ▪ As individuals travel through their life stages, the rapid increase in robustness and resilience from birth to maturity levels off during the mature adult stage. Past this mature stage, the physical and functional changes due to the aging process start to become apparent. (See Figure 1.1)
- ▪ There are many changes occurring in the aging pet—appearance and function
  - Phenotypic changes (Figure 1.2)
    - o Fur or coat—graying, thinning, texture; possible decrease in grooming.
    - o Skin—pigmentation, wrinkling, loss of elasticity.

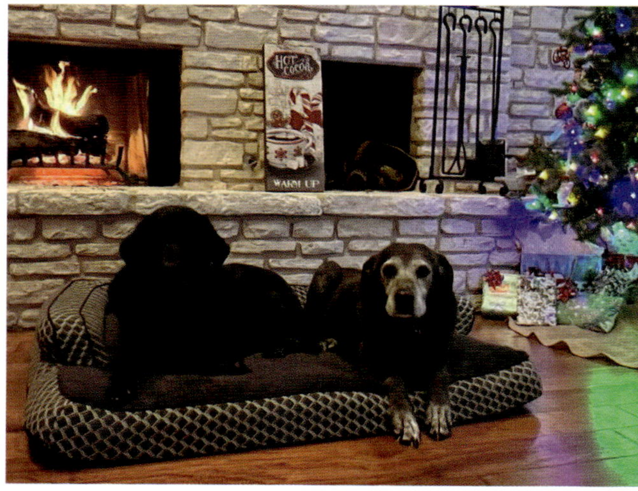

■ **Figure 1.1** The phenotype of aging may occur slowly, but comparing young and old pets, or comparing the older pet to earlier photographs, can make these changes more apparent. Source: With permission of Shannon Strauss.

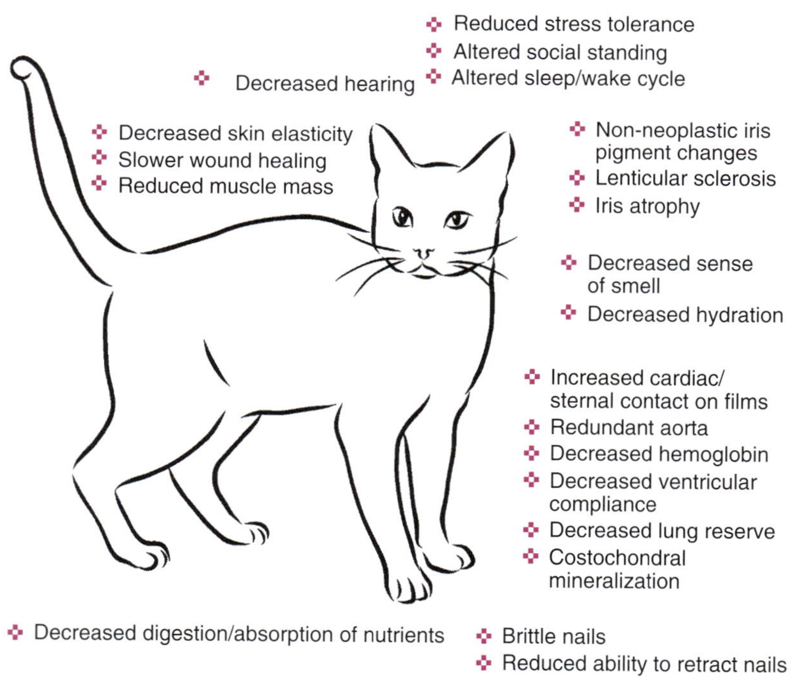

■ **Figure 1.2** Changes associated with aging (and often seen in apparently healthy senior cats). Source: Reprinted from Ray et al.[17].

- Dental disease can be accumulative, but influenced by many factors, not a reliable indicator of age.
- Neoplasia—predisposed to cellular and biochemical changes due to aging factors, but other factors as well.
- Musculoskeletal

    - Muscle mass loss
      - Generalized sarcopenia as a "normal" aging change.[18]
      - Replacement by fat, increase in visceral fat
    - Unintentional weight loss[19]
    - Joint degeneration: other factors may have begun the process, but progressive deterioration
    - Loss of strength and mobility
  - Sensory—auditory, visual, olfactory
  - Organ structure and function
    - Gastrointestinal—
      - Reduced salivary and gastric acid secretion, digestive enzyme function.
      - Intestinal epithelium structure and turnover.
      - GI microbiome (see above)
      - If no specific disease, dogs maintain digestive capacity; protein and fat digestion can decrease in cats.
    - Heart, lungs, kidneys
      - Heart—decreased elasticity and loss of functional capacity
      - Lungs—morphology, elasticity, and functional changes
      - Renal—glomerulosclerosis, interstitial inflammation, and fibrosis; decreased GFR.
    - Endocrine—many changes, not all are well-documented
      - HPA (hypothalamus–pituitary–adrenal) axis – stress responses changed.
      - Thyroid and insulin-like growth factor decline
    - Immune system—see above
  - Behavior
    - Social behavior—also in cognitively unimpaired pets
      - Fearful responses or aggression—rule out pain, physical and sensory disabilities.
    - Activity—less active, less exploratory, sleep more
      - Hard to distinguish between sensory impact and cognition
      - Increase in aimless activity—cognitive, pain, or sleep imbalance
    - Cognitive deficits (see CDS—cognitive dysfunction syndrome)—wide range of changes
    - Elimination issues—house-soiling; of great concern to owners
      - Difficulties in mobility or posturing to eliminate
      - "Lose" their training
    - Vocalization—perceived as a sign of discomfort; pain should be ruled out.
- Changes are highly individualized
- The numbers of "super-seniors"—those living longer than an estimated life expectancy—continues to expand with many pets reaching lifespans that were considered exceptional in the past.[20]

Aging "Clocks"

- Epigenetic clocks
- Some aspects of the genome can change within the course of an individual's lifespan including patterns of DNA methylation, a hallmark of aging.
- Mammalian methylation array—conserved across all species.[21]

- Can predict chronological age and some aspects of biological age.[21]
  - In one study, did not relate well to breed weight or breed lifespan
  - DNAm Average Time to Death assessment predicts average time to death with a positive correlation to breed lifespan and negative correlation to breed weight.
- Useful biomarker in age-extending research and in understanding dog breed differences. [22, 23]
- Clocks based on Frailty[24] (see Frailty)
- The Frailty Index (FI) for humans is a strong predictor of morbidity and mortality
- A study looked at frailty models in mice
  - FRIGHT (Frailty-Inferred Geriatric Health Timeline) clock, a strong predictor of chronological age, not predicting time to mortality
  - AFRAID—Analysis of Frailty and Death—accurately predicts life expectancy and efficacy of intervention
  - Individual frailty items vary in their correlation with age, some items weighted.
  - Able to assess impact of interventions such as administering enalapril and restricting methionine.

Canine Geriatric Syndrome (CGS)

- McKenzie and others have proposed a framework for advancing research in veterinary geroscience.[24]
- "CGS consists of the multiple, interrelated physical, functional, behavioral, and metabolic changes that characterize canine aging as well as the resulting clinical manifestations, including frailty, diminished quality of life, and age-associated disease."
  - Physical changes
  - Clinical disease
  - Functional changes
  - Frailty
  - Metabolic changes
  - Quality of Life and Caregiver burden
- They have also proposed key components of an assessment tool that "would facilitate the development and testing of interventions to prolong health span and lifespan in dogs by directly targeting the biological mechanisms of aging."[6]

Client Communication

- Throughout the lifestages of the pet, it is important to educate the client as to the expected changes that occur within each time frame, and the level of care needed.
  - Providing a continuum of care including preventive care and early detection of specific issues can minimize the impact of aging and disease.
  - Emphasizing that the "geroscience approach" to manage all aspects of the pet's lifestyle (exercise, diet, enrichment, etc.) can have as much of an impact as disease management.
  - It is inevitable that these changes will happen, and we should advocate with the owners to enhance the healthspan of the patient.
- Many impairments can impact comfort, function, and quality of life (QoL) even without specific diseases identified.
  - QoL is often a primary factor in end-of-life (EOL) decisions.
  - Aging impacts both healthspan and lifespan.
  - The human–animal bond can be greatly stressed with ongoing emotional, physical, and financial costs to the owner. Caregiver burden has many aspects and is different for every situation (see Caregiver Burden)

See Also

- Cognitive Dysfunction Syndrome (CDS)
- Frailty
- Immunosenescence
- Inflammaging

Abbreviations

- AFRAID = Analysis of Frailty and Death
- AGE = Advanced glycolation end-product
- AMPK = 5′AMP-actived protein kinase
- ATP = Adenosine triphosphate
- BDNF = brain-derived neurotrophic factor
- CD8 = cytotoxic T-cell lymphocyte with CD8 dimeric co-receptor
- CDS = cognitive dysfunction syndrome
- CNV = copy number variants
- CGS = Canine Geriatric Syndrome
- EOL = end-of-life
- FI = Frailty index
- FRIGHT = Frailty Inferred Geriatric Health Timeline
- FOX = forkhead box O
- GnRH = gonadotropin-releasing hormone
- GFR = glomerular filtration rate
- GH = growth hormone
- HPA = hypothalamus–pituitary–adrenal axis
- Hsp = heat-shock protein
- IGF = insulin growth factor
- IL = interleukin
- LA = lipoic acid
- MAP kinase = mitogen-activated protein kinase
- miRNA = microRNA
- NAD = nicotinamide adenine dinucleotide
- OS = oxidative stress
- QoL = quality of life
- ROS = reactive oxygen species
- TOR = target of rapamycin kinase
- UPS = ubiquitin proteasome

Reading List

Fedarko NS. The biology of aging and frailty. *Clin Geriatr Med* 2011 Feb;27(1):27–37. doi: 10.1016/j.cger.2010.08.006. PMID: 21093720; PMCID: PMC3052959.

Jiménez AG. A revisiting of "the hallmarks of aging" in domestic dogs: current status of the literature. *Geroscience* 2024 Feb;46(1):241–255. doi: 10.1007/s11357-023-00911-5. Epub 2023 Aug 18. PMID: 37594598; PMCID: PMC10828135.

Kaeberlein M, Creevy KE, Promislow DE. The dog aging project: translational geroscience in companion animals. *Mamm Genome* 2016 Aug;27(7–8):279–288. doi: 10.1007/s00335-016-9638-7. Epub 2016 May 3. PMID: 27143112; PMCID: PMC4936929.

López-Otín C, Blasco MA, Partridge L, Serrano M, Kroemer G. The hallmarks of aging. *Cell* 2013 Jun 6;153(6):1194–1217. doi: 10.1016/j.cell.2013.05.039. PMID: 23746838; PMCID: PMC3836174.

McKenzie BA. Comparative veterinary geroscience: mechanism of molecular, cellular, and tissue aging in humans, laboratory animal models, and companion dogs and cats. *Am J Vet Res* 2022 May 8;83(6):ajvr.22.02.0027. doi: 10.2460/ajvr.22.02.0027. PMID: 35524953.

Sándor S, Kubinyi E. Genetic pathways of aging and their relevance in the dog as a natural model of human aging. *Front Genet* 2019 Oct 18;10:948. doi: 10.3389/fgene.2019.00948. PMID: 31681409; PMCID: PMC6813227.

References

1. Lawler DF, Evans RH, Chase K, Ellersieck M, Li Q, Larson BT, Satyaraj E, Heininger K. The aging feline kidney: a model mortality antagonist? *J Feline Med Surg* 2006 Dec;8(6):363–371. doi: 10.1016/j.jfms.2006.06.002. Epub 2006 Nov 7. PMID: 17092751.
2. Kennedy BK, Berger SL, Brunet A et al. Geroscience: linking aging to chronic disease. *Cell* 2014;159:709–713.
3. Day MJ. Ageing, immunosenescence and inflammageing in the dog and cat. *J Comp Pathol* 2010 Jan;142(Suppl 1):S60–S69. doi: 10.1016/j.jcpa.2009.10.011. Epub 2009 Dec 14. PMID: 20005526.
4. Wallace DC. A mitochondrial paradigm of metabolic and degenerative diseases, aging, and cancer: a dawn for evolutionary medicine. *Annu Rev Genet* 2005;39:359–407. doi: 10.1146/annurev.genet.39.110304.095751. PMID: 16285865; PMCID: PMC2821041.
5. Bateson M. Cumulative stress in research animals: telomere attrition as a biomarker in a welfare context? *Bioessays* 2016 Feb;38(2):201–212. doi: 10.1002/bies.201500127. Epub 2015 Dec 8. PMID: 26645576; PMCID: PMC4737400.
6. Quimby J, Erickson A, Mcleland S et al. Renal senescence, telomere shortening and nitrosative stress in feline chronic kidney disease. *Vet Sci* 2021 Dec 8;8(12):314. doi: 10.3390/vetsci8120314. PMID: 34941841; PMCID: PMC8703545.
7. McKevitt TP, Nasir L, Devlin P, Argyle DJ. Telomere lengths in dogs decrease with increasing donor age. *J Nutr* 2002 Jun;132(6 Suppl 2):1604S–1606S. doi: 10.1093/jn/132.6.1604S. PMID: 12042469.
8. Fick LJ, Fick GH, Li Z, Cao E, Bao B, Heffelfinger D, Parker HG, Ostrander EA, Riabowol K. Telomere length correlates with life span of dog breeds. *Cell Rep* 2012 Dec 27;2(6):1530–1536. doi: 10.1016/j.celrep.2012.11.021. PMID: 23260664.
9. Banlaki Z, Cimarelli G, Viranyi Z, Kubinyi E, Sasvari-Szekely M, Ronai Z. DNA methylation patterns of behavior-related gene promoter regions dissect the gray wolf from domestic dog breeds. *Mol Genet Genomics* 2017 Jun;292(3):685–697. doi: 10.1007/s00438-017-1305-5. Epub 2017 Mar 21. PMID: 28321510.
10. Hoffman JM, Kiklevich JV, Klavins K, Valencak TG, Austad SN. Alterations of lipid metabolism with age and weight in companion dogs. *J Gerontol A Biol Sci Med Sci* 2021 Feb 25;76(3):400–405. doi: 10.1093/gerona/glaa186. PMID: 32750116; PMCID: PMC7907484.
11. Head E, Nukala VN, Fenoglio KA, Muggenburg BA, Cotman CW, Sullivan PG. Effects of age, dietary, and behavioral enrichment on brain mitochondria in a canine model of human aging. *Exp Neurol* 2009 Nov;220(1):171–176. doi: 10.1016/j.expneurol.2009.08.014. Epub 2009 Aug 22. PMID: 19703441; PMCID: PMC2761532.
12. Moldogazieva NT, Mokhosoev IM, Mel'nikova TI, Porozov YB, Terentiev AA. Oxidative stress and advanced lipoxidation and glycation end products (ALEs and AGEs) in aging and age-related diseases. *Oxid Med Cell Longev* 2019 Aug 14;2019:3085756. doi: 10.1155/2019/3085756. PMID: 31485289; PMCID: PMC6710759.
13. Muller M. Cellular senescence: molecular mechanisms, in vivo significance, and redox considerations. *Antioxid Redox Signal* 2009;11(1):59–98. PubMed: 18976161.
14. Vaiserman AM, Koliada AK, Marotta F. Gut microbiota: a player in aging and a target for anti-aging intervention. *Ageing Res Rev* 2017 May;35:36–45. doi: 10.1016/j.arr.2017.01.001. Epub 2017 Jan 18. PMID: 28109835.
15. Dantzer R, O'Connor JC, Freund GG, Johnson RW, Kelley KW. From inflammation to sickness and depression: when the immune system subjugates the brain. *Nat Rev Neurosci* 2008 Jan;9(1):46–56. doi: 10.1038/nrn2297. PMID: 18073775; PMCID: PMC2919277.
16. Gaffey AE, Bergeman CS, Clark LA, Wirth MM. Aging and the HPA axis: Stress and resilience in older adults. *Neurosci Biobehav Rev* 2016 Sep;68:928–945. doi: 10.1016/j.neubiorev.2016.05.036.

Epub 2016 Jul 1. PMID: 27377692; PMCID: PMC5621604.McK 8—rapid increase in robustness through maturity.

17. Ray M, Carney HC, Boynton B, Quimby J, Robertson S, St Denis K, Tuzio H, Wright B. 2021 AAFP feline senior care guidelines. *J Feline Med Surg* 2021 Jul;23(7):613–638. doi: 10.1177/1098612X211021538. Erratum in: *J Feline Med Surg* 2021 Oct;23(10):NP4. doi: 10.1177/1098612X211040404. PMID: 34167339; PMCID: PMC10812122.
18. Hutchinson D, Sutherland-Smith J, Watson AL, Freeman LM. Assessment of methods of evaluating sarcopenia in old dogs. *Am J Vet Res* 2012 Nov;73(11):1794–1800. doi: 10.2460/ajvr.73.11.1794. PMID: 23106466.
19. Harper EJ. Changing perspectives on aging and energy requirements: aging, body weight and body composition in humans, dogs and cats. *J Nutr* 1998 Dec;128(12 Suppl):2627S–2631S. doi: 10.1093/jn/128.12.2627S. PMID: 9868223. (25) Harper aging, body weight and body composition 1998 and energy requirements.
20. Cozzi B, Ballarin C, Mantovani R, Rota A. Aging and veterinary care of cats, dogs, and horses through the records of three university veterinary hospitals. *Front Vet Sci* 2017 Feb 14;4:14. doi: 10.3389/fvets.2017.00014. PMID: 28261586; PMCID: PMC5306394.
21. Horvath S, Lu AT, Haghani A et al. DNA methylation clocks for dogs and humans. *Proc Natl Acad Sci USA* 2022;119(21):e2120887119.
22. Wang T, Ma J, Hogan AN et al. Quantitative translation of dog-to-human aging by conserved remodeling of the DNA methylome. *Cell Syst* 2020 Aug 26;11(2):176–185.e6. doi: 10.1016/j.cels.2020.06.006. Epub 2020 Jul 2. PMID: 32619550; PMCID: PMC7484147.
23. Thompson MJ, vonHoldt B, Horvath S, Pellegrini M. An epigenetic aging clock for dogs and wolves. *Aging* 2017 Mar 28;9(3):1055–1068. doi: 10.18632/aging.101211. PMID: 28373601; PMCID: PMC5391218.
24. McKenzie BA, Chen FL, Gruen ME, Olby NJ. Canine geriatric syndrome: a framework for advancing research in veterinary geroscience. *Front Vet Sci* 2022 Apr 21;9:853743. doi: 10.3389/fvets.2022.853743. PMID: 35529834; PMCID: PMC9069128.

Author: Heidi Lobprise

Chapter 2

Frailty

BASICS

OVERVIEW

In human gerontology, the concept of frailty has been the focus of extensive research on how to measure, and potentially manage, the problems it encompasses. Assessing frailty adds to the evaluation of health issues by documenting loss of function or decline that may not be attributable to any particular disease.[1] The development of frailty concepts and parameters in veterinary medicine has just started but has great promise to add to the means of advocating for our patients.

Terms Defined

- Frailty—a syndrome characterized by the decrease in physiologic reserves, cognitive performance, and dysregulation of multiple body systems with an increased vulnerability to stressors.
- Robustness—the ability to maintain optimal physiological function in the face of external stressors.
- Resilience—the ability to return to baseline following stressor disturbance.
- Healthspan—the period of time an individual is able to maintain good health with a short period of morbidity before death.[2]

ISSUES AND OPTIONS

- The decrease in reserves, loss of robustness, and resilience results in increased incidence of disease and decreased ability to heal and return to function.
- Frailty may represent a transition phase between successful aging and disability.[3]
- Delaying the onset of frailty may increase healthspan.[2]
- In the cat, the concept of frailty helps capture a component of the complex conditions that can coalesce in the cat (2021 AAFP Senior Cat Care Guidelines).
- Frailty accounts for wide variability in health outcomes and trajectories among individuals of the same chronological age.[4]
- Frailty scores increase and quality of life (health-related) decreases with age.
  - Large dogs show a faster age-related decline in health-related quality of life.[5]

Frailty-Related Phenotype (FRP) in Humans[6]

- Chronic undernutrition with unintentional weight loss.
- Exhaustion—self-reported.

Blackwell's Five-Minute Veterinary Consult Clinical Companion: Small Animal Senior Care, First Edition. Edited by Heidi B. Lobprise.

Companion website: www.wiley.com/go/lobprise/Senior

- Low physical activity level
  - Measured through a weighted score of number of kilocalories expended per week.
- Poor mobility
  - Assessed as time to walk a distance of 15 feet.
- Weakness
  - Assessed with hand grip strength.

Frailty-Related Phenotype in Dogs—Five FRP Components—Hua (See Table 2.1)

- Weakness—Scored as:
  - No muscle loss
  - Moderate muscle loss vs. muscle atrophy
  - Cachexia
- Exhaustion based on effort tolerance
  - Tolerance present
  - Fatigue-ability
  - Marked breathlessness
- Undernutrition
  - Body Condition Score (BCS)
  - Appetite—unchanged; decreased; increased
  - Hair coat—quality and density of coat
  - Unintentional weight loss of 5% or more
- Poor mobility (See Mobility chapter)
- Gait
  - Normal
  - Lameness or stiffness
  - Ataxia

TABLE 2.1 Dog frailty related phenotype (FRP) assessment with scoring of five components.

Frailty component	Absent	Present
Weakness—muscle mass	Normal muscle mass	Moderate muscle wasting, muscle atropy or cachexia
Exhaustion—effort tolerance	Good tolerance	Fatigability or marked Breathlessness
Low physical activity—perceived activity level	Normal	Moderate or low
Chronic undernutrition		
• Body Condition	Normal	Obese or too thin
• Appetitie	Unchanged	Increased or decreased
• Quality and density of hair	Normal	Sparse hair or alopecia
Poor mobility		
• Gait	Normal	Stiffness, lameness or ataxia
• Joint pain	No signs of pain	Moderate or marked signs of pain

No FRP when 0–1 of components present.
FRP when 2 or more components present.
Source: Adapted from Hua et al.[7]

- Joint pain
    - Normal
    - Moderate pain
    - Marked pain

Frailty Index (FI) in Dogs[8]

- A single continuous variable counting negative health attributes over the life course of an individual
- Questionnaire to address 33 health deficits[9]
    - Each deficit is age-related, adversely related to animal's health and not prone to saturation (not too rare, nor too frequent)
    - Scored either 0 or 1 (absent or present) or 0.0–0.5–1.0—absent, mild, severe
        - Divide sum by 33
    - Deficit accumulation strongly related to mortality
- 401 dogs, age, gender, neuter status, and BCS quantified
    - FI—mean 0.14
        - Young: 0.08
        - Middle-aged: 0.23
        - Old dogs: 0.23 (0–0.61)
    - Essentially a linear relationship
    - Submaximal limit at the 0.7 cut-off point—can be considered as the threshold when the accumulation of deficits becomes incompatible with life
- Moderate accuracy in prediction of short-term mortality; 6 months is a reasonable portion of a dog's lifespan
    - Kaplan–Meier survival curves
    - An increased BCS acted as a protective effect (not age)
        - Hazard ratio (HR) of overweight dogs less than half that of underweight dogs
- FI should be routinely calculated, especially for older patients.
    - Those with FI >0.25 should be treated with particular care and might need more frequent follow-up visits, no matter the age.

Frailty Index in Dogs (FIDo)—The Dog Aging Project (DAP)[1] (See Table 2.2)

- Phenotype model that includes externally apparent components, to be collected by both owners and veterinarians (as compared to Hua's FRP)
- Identifies frail individuals that may be free of diagnosed disease
    - Banzato's FI incorporates diagnostic data and multimorbidity
    - This is a separate assessment tool in the DAP framework
- Compared to Hua—prospectively collected by both owners and vets
- Factors—to be validated by the study to find the components that most accurately reflect conditions
    - Physical condition
        - BCS—body condition score (1–9 scale)
        - Thigh girth deterioration—serial recordings to estimate MCS and sarcopenia
        - Unintentional weight loss
    - Physical activity—dog's interest in activity, vigor of activity, and change in activity patterns
        - Not active/moderately active/very active
        - Average time per day
        - Intensity of activity

TABLE 2.2 The dog aging project FIDo—frailty index for dogs[1]—in development, using 7 domains to assess multiple aspects of a dog's aging changes.

Domain	Factor
Physical condition	Body condition score (BCS) Thigh girth deterioration Unintentional weight loss • Veterinarian-reported • Owner-reported
Physical activity	Customary activity
Mobility	Gait speed • On-leash • Off-leash
Strength	Stair climb
Cognitive performance	Working memory Learned behavior
Mood and social relations	Anxiety/nervousness Social avoidance

- Mobility[10]
    - Time to travel a measured distance on-leash and off-leash—flat surface
    - Off-leash change is usually greater
- Strength
    - Stair climb—timed stair ascent[11]
        - Other tools available, but are expensive and limited availability
- Cognitive task performance—purpose-built at-home
    - Working memory
        - Ability to recall the location of a food item after varying delays or
        - Recall which location still contains a food item (radial array)
    - Learned behavior
- Mood and social relations—assessed by DAP behavioral data CSLB and C-BARQ
    - Anxiety/nervousness
    - Social avoidance

- Canine Social and Learned Behavior (CSLB)—DAP
    - How often does your dog stare blankly at the walls or floor?
    - Compared with 6 months ago, does your dog have difficulty finding food dropped on the floor?
- C-BARQ—Canine Behavioral Assessment and Research Questionnaire—completed annually by DAP participants

JVIM Abstract 2022[12]

- Establishing a Frailty Phenotype for Aging Dogs
    - Nutritional status—poor body condition or appetite
    - Sarcopenia—epaxial muscle atrophy

   - Mobility—owner reported
   - Activity—owner reported
   - Exhaustion—owner-perceived
- Classified as overall frail if they met two or more domains (10 of 51 dogs)
   - Associated with 6-month mortality
- Now being validated in a large prospective study

Frailty Scoring in Cats (2021 AAFP Senior Cat Care Guidelines) (See Table 2.3)

- Phenotype frailty scale in cats[13]—answer yes or no to medical conditions or problems:
   - Unintentional weight loss
   - Weakness
   - Poor endurance, early exhaustion
   - Slowness and low activity
   - Pre-frail—yes to 2 of 4; Frail—yes to 3 or 4 out of 4
- Index frailty scale[14]—answer yes or no to medical conditions or problems:
   - Physiologic deficits
   - Psychological (emotional) deficits
   - Cognitive (task-oriented) deficits
   - Deficits in social function
   - Pre-frail—yes to 2 of 4; Frail—yes to 3 or 4 out of 4

Aging Clocks Based on Frailty[15]

- The Frailty Index (FI) for humans is a strong predictor of morbidity and mortality
- A study looked at frailty models in mice (see Aging and Senescence)
   - FRIGHT (Frailty-Inferred Geriatric Health Timeline) clock, a strong predictor of chronological age, not predicting time to mortality
   - AFRAID—Analysis of Frailty and Death—accurately predicts life expectancy and efficacy of intervention
   - Individual frailty items vary in their correlation with age, some items weighted.
   - Able to assess impact of interventions such as administering enalapril and restricting methionine.

TABLE 2.3 Frailty scales for cats, including the phenotype frailty scale and the index frailty scale

Phenotype frailty scale

Medical conditions/problems present	Yes	No
1. Unintentional weight loss		
2. Weakness		
3. Poor indurance		
4. Slowness and low activity		

Pre-frail: "Yes" to 2 out of 4

Frail: "Yes" to 3 or 4 out of 4

Source: Adapted from Fried et al.[13]

Index frailty scale

Medical conditions/problems present	Yes	No
1. Physiological deficits		
2. Psychological (emotional) deficits		
3. Cognitive (task-oriented) deficits		
4. Deficits in social function		

Pre-frail: "Yes" to 2 out of 4

Frail: "Yes" to 3 or 4 out of 4

Source: Adapted from Mitnitski et al.[14]

APPLICATIONS IN PRACTICE

- Set up protocols for clinic staff to evaluate frailty scales in pets as they reach senior status.
- When signs of frailty are detected, evaluate the patient for potential pathologic causes and intervene where appropriate
- Frailty Prevention Model (2021 AAFP)—three levels of intervention
    - Primary—minimize risk factors and disease onset
        - Wellness, vaccination, parasiticides,
        - Detection of disease in early stages—screening
    - Secondary—delay progression of disease
        - Substaging of renal issues with hypertension and UP/C ratios (proteinuria) persistently over 0.4 (IRIS Guidelines).
        - Implement interventions to keep the senior cat active and self-sufficient can be taken into the home environment.
    - Tertiary—reduce or limit impairments, disabilities, and complications that result from disease
        - Most common level in senior care
- Frailty scores and trends can help assess the quality of life of a patient, help determine optimal treatments, assess risks for anesthesia and surgery, and help assess how close to the end-of-life a pet might be.
    - Anesthetic and surgery risks might be decreased by improving nutritional status and stabilizing organ dysfunction when possible.
- While chronological age cannot be reversed, frailty may be manageable.[1]

Client Communication

- Provide frailty checklists to pet owners to enhance their awareness for early detection of problems.
- Educate them as to the importance of frailty assessment and intervention, even in the absence of identifiable disease.

Examples

- Study of 116 still active guide dogs 8–10 years of age (Hua)
    - Mean “relative age” of 62 years (human equivalent)
    - 8.6% of group had 2 or more FRP components present
    - 4.3% of group had 3 or more FRP components present
        - Predominantly female
        - More: cutaneous nodules, neurological disorders, malignant neoplasia and cardiovascular disorders than the group with 0–1 FRP components.
    - Of the FRP components, low mobility and low physical activity were associated with time to death; chronic undernutrition, weakness and exhaustion were not associated.
- Study of 80 Labrador and Golden Retriever dogs 9 years of age and older[16]
    - Adapted frailty phenotype with five criteria
        - Weakness, slowness, poor endurance, low physical activity, and shrinking
        - Non-frail, pre-frail (1 or 2 criteria), and frail (3 or more criteria) dogs.
        - Time to all-cause death over 5 years of follow-up
        - Median survival times: non-frail (42.5 months), pre-frail (35.4 months), frail (10.5 months)

MISCELLANEOUS

- Aging and senescence
- Mobility
- Weight loss, sarcopenia, and cachexia

Abbreviations

- AAFP = American Association of Feline Practitioners (now known as Feline Veterinary Medical Association or Feline VMA, catvets.org)
- BCS = body condition score
- C-BARQ = canine behavioral assessment and research questionnaire
- CSLB = canine social and learned behavior
- DAP = the Dog Aging Project
- FI = frailty index
- FIDo = frailty index for dogs
- FRP = frailty-related phenotype
- HR = hazard ratio

Internet Resources

Accessed 29 June 2024

2021 AAFP Feline Senior Care Guidelines

- https://journals.sagepub.com/doi/pdf/10.1177/1098612X211021538

IRIS—International Renal Interest Society

- IRIS Kidney—Guidelines (iris-kidney.com)

References

1. Melvin RL, Ruple A, Pearson EB, Olby NJ, Fitzpatrick AL, Creevy KE. A review of frailty instruments in human medicine and proposal of a frailty instrument for dogs. *Front Vet Sci* 2023 Jun 27;10:1139308. doi: 10.3389/fvets.2023.1139308. PMID: 37441560; PMCID: PMC10333704.
2. Larrick JW, Mendelsohn A. Applied healthspan engineering. *Rejuvenation Res* 2010;13:265–280.
3. Cesari M, Prince M, Thiyagarajan JA et al. Frailty: an emerging public health priority. *J Am Med Dir Assoc* 2016;17(3):188–192. doi: 10.1016/j.jamda.2015.12.016.
4. Rockwood K, Song X, MacKnight C, Bergman H, Hogan DB, McDowell I, Mitnitski A. A global clinical measure of fitness and frailty in elderly people. *CMAJ* 2005;173:489–495.
5. Waters DJ. Aging research 2011: exploring the pet dog paradigm. *ILAR J* 2011;52:97–105. (HUA 10).
6. Theou O, Brothers TD, Mitnitski A, et al. Operationalization of frailty using eight commonly used scales and comparison of their ability to predict all-cause mortality. *J Am Geriatr Soc* 2013;61:1537–1551.
7. Hua J, Hoummady S, Muller C et al. Assessment of frailty in aged dogs. *Am J Vet Res* 2016;77:1357–1365.
8. Banzato T, Franzo G, Di Maggio R et al. A frailty index based on clinical data to quantify mortality risk in dogs. *Sci Rep* 2019;9:16749.
9. Searle SD, Mitnitski A, Gahbauer EA, Gill TM, Rockwood K. A standard procedure for creating a frailty index. *BMC Geriatr* 2008;8:24.
10. Gonçalves LCVB, Simões ADGA, Millis DL, De MAJF. Development of a scale to evaluate mobility in dogs. *Cienc Rural* 2016;46:2210–2215. doi: 10.1590/0103-8478cr20160123.
11. Morgan EM, Heseltine JC, Levine GJ, Promislow DEL, Creevy KE. Evaluation of a low-technology system to obtain morphological and mobility trial measurements in dogs and investigation of potential predictors of canine mobility. *Am J Vet Res* 2019;80:670–679. doi: 10.2460/ajvr.80.7.670.

12. Russell K, Fefer G, Mondino A, Olby N. Establishing a frailty phenotype for aging dogs. *Res Abstr JVIM* 2022;36:2382–022.
13. Fried LP, Tangen CM, Walston J, et al. Frailty in older adults: evidence for a phenotype. *J Gerontol A Biol Sci Med Sci* 2001;56:M146–M156.
14. Mitnitski AB, Mogilner AJ and Rockwood K. Accumulation of deficits as a proxy measure of aging. *Sci World J* 2001;1:323–336.
15. Schultz MB, Kane AE, Mitchell SJ, MacArthur MR, Warner E, Vogel DS, Mitchell JR, Howlett SE, Bonkowski MS, Sinclair DA. Age and life expectancy clocks based on machine learning analysis of mouse frailty. *Nat Commun* 2020 Sep 15;11(1):4618. doi: 10.1038/s41467-020-18446-0. Erratum in: *Nat Commun* 2020 Oct 8;11(1):5143. doi: 10.1038/s41467-020-19046-8. PMID: 32934233; PMCID: PMC7492249.
16. Lemaréchal R, Hoummady S, Barthélémy I, Muller C, Hua J, Gilbert C, Desquilbet L. Canine model of human frailty: adaptation of a frailty phenotype in older dogs. *J Gerontol A Biol Sci Med Sci* 2023 Aug 2;78(8):1355–1363. doi: 10.1093/gerona/glad006. PMID: 36617213.

Author: Heidi Lobprise

Chapter 3

Immunosenescence

BASICS

OVERVIEW

In the process of aging, the immune system is deeply affected, with greater impact on the adaptive immune response as compared to the innate immune response. Age-related changes to the immune system are considered the main culprits of co-morbidities and are often associated with declines in life expectancy.[1] While much of the research has been done in other species, increasing studies are correlating these changes in dogs and cats as well.[2]

Terms Defined

- Immunosenescence—the decline in the function of the adaptive immune system that occurs during aging that is associated with thymic involution, alterations in T-cell subsets, and reduction in antibody production.[3]
- Innate immune response—comprises both the anatomical (skin and mucous membranes) and biochemical barriers (antimicrobial proteins, inflammation) and the unspecific cellular response mediated mainly by monocytes, natural killer cells, and dendritic cells.
- Adaptive immune response—provides an antigen-specific response mediated by T and B lymphocytes: B-cells—humoral immunity; T-cells—cellular immunity.
- Immune surveillance system – part of the immune system that identifies cancerous and/or precancerous cells and eliminates them before they can cause harm, crucial in the control of cancer occurrence and progression; tumor immunoediting.[4]

ISSUES AND OPTIONS

Immunosenescence Causes (Castelo-Branco)

- Autoimmune theory: diminished ability to distinguish between "invaders" and normal tissue.
- Immune deficiency theory: immune system no longer able to defend against invaders.
- Immune dysregulation theory: disruption of the regulation between multiple components of the immune process.
- Antagonist pleiotropy: natural selection of genes with short-term benefits through reproductive years (thymic involution in early age).
- Associated factors:
    - Lifelong antigenic stress

Blackwell's Five-Minute Veterinary Consult Clinical Companion: Small Animal Senior Care, First Edition. Edited by Heidi B. Lobprise.

Companion website: www.wiley.com/go/lobprise/Senior

- Filling of the immunologic space
- Accumulation of effector T- and memory cells
- Reduction of naïve T-cells
- Micronutrient inadequacy and metabolic malfunctioning
- Reactivity to self-antigens—risk of triggering autoimmune diseases

Innate Immune System Response

- Ages changes in skin and mucosa
- IgA in saliva—slight decrease
- Dendritic cells—provide the first alert of pathogens and bridge between innate and adaptive immunity responses
    - Diminish in the presence of chronic disease
- Natural killer (NK) cells—cell cytotoxicity or cytotoxins
    - Increase in numbers but not in global cytotoxicity
    - Migration and cytokine secretion may be reduced.
    - Neutrophils—numbers not affected, but ability to remain present at the site of infection is decreased and phagocytic function is reduced.
- Macrophages—tissue resident phagocytic function
    - Reduced production of cytokines
    - Altered expression of molecules that contribute to a poorer T-cell response

Adaptive Immune System Response

- Lymphoid progenitors
    - Hematopoietic stem cells (HSC)—proliferative capacity diminishes
    - Shift toward myeloid progenitors, not lymphoid progenitors.
- B-cells—production of antibodies to a specific antigen
    - Total number of B-cell diminish and a decrease in diversity
        - Decreased naïve B-cells, increased memory B-cells
            - Impaired capacity for response to new antigens
        - Reduced clonal expansion capability of memory B-cells—fewer circulating antibodies to previously known antigen
        - Impaired antibodies that opsonize bacteria for phagocytosis
- T-cells—CD4 or CD8 cell surface expression
    - CD4+—regulatory cells—recognize antigens (Class II MHC—major histocompatibility complex)
    - CD8+—cytotoxic cells—recognize antigens within Class I MHC
        - CD8+ cells are affected to a greater extent in aging.
    - Absolute number decreases with age—especially the naïve subset
        - Impacted by differentiation in the thymus, exported to periphery and mature
    - Functional defects—less capable of producing an adequate response to antigens.
    - Co-stimulatory molecules (CD28, CD27)—expression decreases
- Blunting of anti-inflammatory response to bacterial antigens can complicate sepsis in older individuals.[5]
    - Decreased levels of IL-10 result in more pronounced bacteremia, increased TNF production, and early mortality in mice.
    - Sepsis is characterized by disparity among the inflammatory and anti-inflammatory response.

- Other inflammatory mediators are increased in older people that contribute to chronic inflammation that can impact complications in sepsis and severe sepsis, not necessarily the actual infection.

Thymic Declines[6]

- The age-associated regression of the thymus is linked with immune decline.
- Thymic involution—main mechanism by which naïve T-cell numbers decline with age.
- Dog breed and size variations impact thymic decline.
  - The largest reduction in thymic output occurs between reaching sexual maturity and early middle age.
  - Giant dogs—decline began earlier compared to small breeds.
    - Premature thymic involution might be occurring in short-lived breeds.

Link to Chronic Inflammation

- When adaptive immunity declines, the low-level, chronic activation of innate immunity systems leads to low-level, chronic pro-inflammatory state (See Inflammaging).
  - Cardiovascular disease, cancer, diabetes mellitus, osteoporosis, rheumatoid arthritis, and cognitive disorders in humans.[3]
- Other mechanisms related to age have been proposed to underlie these chronic inflammatory changes are the effects of increased visceral adipose tissue, decline in production of steroid sex hormones, and accumulative oxidative damage.

The Immune System and Cancer[7]

- Three primary roles in the prevention of tumors
  - Eliminate or suppress viral infections that can lead to virus-induced tumors
  - Timely elimination of pathogens and prompt resolution of inflammation to help prevent the establishment of an inflammatory environment conducive to tumorigenesis.
  - Tumor immune surveillance or tumor immune-editing -
    - Elimination—dendritic cells and macrophages present cancer antigens to T-cells; naïve CD8+ cells differentiate into effector T-cells with cytotoxic abilities.
    - Equilibration—the actions of the immune system are sufficient to control tumor progression—until.
    - Escape—when tumor cell variants that can resist, avoid, or suppress the response replicate.
- Immunosenescence is accompanied by a decline in naïve and memory T-cell, impaired proliferation of CD8+ T-cells, and while effector cell subsets have strong cytotoxic potential, they lose cell proliferative capacity.[7]
- Aging can diminish the therapeutic effects of cancer immunotherapies targeting the CD8_ T-cell activation.

Management of Impact on Immunosenescence

- Caloric Restriction[8]
  - Pairs of Labrador Retrievers divided at weaning were placed into two groups, the control group on standard diet and the second group with a caloric restriction (CR) of 75%.
  - In the CR group, age-related declines in the absolute numbers of lymphocytes and T-cells were slowed. These declines were found to be significantly associated with a decreased likelihood of survival in the group fed the standard diet.
  - Additional aspects of aging were impacted by the caloric restriction (see Nutrition)

Client Communication

- With immunosenescence in aging pets, several conservations come to mind:
  - If lifestyle of the pet includes continued exposure to infectious agents, vaccination should continue.
  - Susceptibility to infectious agents and other stressors may be increased.
  - The increased likelihood of tumor formation highlights the need for regular assessment and monitoring.

See Also

- Inflammaging

Abbreviations

- CR = caloric restriction
- HSC = hematopoietic stem cells
- Ig = immunoglobulin
- IL = interleukin
- MHC = major histocompatibility complex
- TNF = tumor necrosis factor

Additional Reading

Castelo-Branco C, Soveral I. The immune system and aging: a review. *Gynecol Endocrinol* 2014 Jan;30(1):16–22. doi: 10.3109/09513590.2013.852531. Epub 2013 Nov 12. PMID: 24219599.

Day MJ. Ageing, immunosenescence and inflammageing in the dog and cat. *J Comp Pathol* 2010 Jan;142 Suppl 1:S60–S69. doi: 10.1016/j.jcpa.2009.10.011. Epub 2009 Dec 14. PMID: 20005526.

References

1. Jiménez AG. A revisiting of "the hallmarks of aging" in domestic dogs: current status of the literature. *Geroscience* 2024 Feb;46(1):241–255. doi: 10.1007/s11357-023-00911-5. Epub 2023 Aug 18. PMID: 37594598; PMCID: PMC10828135.
2. Withers SS, Moore PF, Chang H, Choi JW, McSorley SJ, Kent MS, Monjazeb AM, Canter RJ, Murphy WJ, Sparger EE, Rebhun RB. Multi-color flow cytometry for evaluating age-related changes in memory lymphocyte subsets in dogs. *Dev Comp Immunol* 2018 Oct;87:54–74. doi: 10.1016/j.dci.2018.05.022. Epub 2018 May 31. PMID: 29859828; PMCID: PMC6197816.
3. Fedarko NS. The biology of aging and frailty. *Clin Geriatr Med* 2011 Feb;27(1):27–37. doi: 10.1016/j.cger.2010.08.006. PMID: 21093720; PMCID: PMC3052959.
4. Swann JB, Smyth MJ. Immune surveillance of tumors. *J Clin Invest* 2007 May;117(5):1137–1146. doi: 10.1172/JCI31405. PMID: 17476343; PMCID: PMC1857231.
5. Deitschel SJ, Kerl ME, Chang CH, DeClue AE. Age-associated changes to pathogen-associated molecular pattern-induced inflammatory mediator production in dogs. *J Vet Emerg Crit Care* 2010 Oct;20(5):494–502. doi: 10.1111/j.1476-4431.2010.00565.x. Epub 2010 Sep 28. PMID: 20955300.
6. Holder A, Mella S, Palmer DB, Aspinall R, Catchpole B. An age-associated decline in thymic output differs in dog breeds according to their longevity. *PLoS One* 2016 Nov 8;11(11):e0165968. doi: 10.1371/journal.pone.0165968. PMID: 27824893; PMCID: PMC5100965.
7. Yamauchi A, Yoshimoto S, Kudo A, Takagi S. Negative influence of aging on differentiation and proliferation of CD8+ T-cells in dogs. *Vet Sci* 2023 Aug 25;10(9):541. doi: 10.3390/vetsci10090541. PMID: 37756063; PMCID: PMC10534501.
8. Greeley EH, Spitznagel E, Lawler DF, Kealy RD, Segre M. Modulation of canine immunosenescence by life-long caloric restriction. *Vet Immunol Immunopathol* 2006 Jun 15;111(3–4):287–299. doi: 10.1016/j.vetimm.2006.02.002. Epub 2006 Mar 29. PMID: 16567002.

Author: Heidi Lobprise

Chapter 4

Inflammaging

BASICS

OVERVIEW

In previous topics, an overview of aging processes, including immunosenescence, has been discussed. The effects of immunosenescence, the effects of increased visceral adipose tissue, decline in production of steroid sex hormones, and accumulative oxidative damage are thought to contribute to a state of chronic, low-grade inflammation. This systemic inflammation can have significant effects on all body systems in the aging process.

Terms Defined

- Inflammaging—chronic, sterile, low-grade inflammation that develops with advanced age is the term used to describe this pro-inflammatory state associated with aging.[1]
- Immunosenescence—the decline in the function of the adaptive immune system that occurs during aging that is associated with thymic involution, alterations in T-cell subsets, and reduction in antibody production.

ISSUES AND OPTIONS

Inflammaging

- Acute inflammation is an important response to stressors to return to "normal."
- If that acute inflammation persists, there is upregulation of the process and this can overstimulate the innate immune system and increase oxidative damage, contributing to morbidity and mortality in seniors.[2]
- In humans, this chronic, pro-inflammatory state typically results in elevated IL-6 (interleukin 6), TNF-α (tumor necrosis factor alpha), and CRP (C-reactive protein) levels.
    - Adaptive immunity declines, but low-level, chronic activation of innate immunity lead to this inflammatory state
    - Cytokines can affect growth hormone/IGF-1 (insulin-like growth factor) axis[3]
    - Cytokine-induced "sickness behavior"—fatigue, malaise, loss of interest in social, difficulty concentrating, sleep pattern changes[4]
    - Neuromodulators—depressive disorders—sickness behavior with difficulty concentrating and sleep-pattern disruptions.
    - Hypothalamic–pituitary–adrenal (HPA) axis hyperactivity—cytokines disturb the negative feedback inhibition of corticosteroids[5]

Blackwell's Five-Minute Veterinary Consult Clinical Companion: Small Animal Senior Care,
First Edition. Edited by Heidi B. Lobprise.

Companion website: www.wiley.com/go/lobprise/Senior

- Increased reactive oxygen species (ROS) and a decline in the ability to control oxidative stress can result in pro-inflammatory tissue damage, impacting cellular proteins, lipids, and nucleic acids.[2]
- A decrease in heat-shock proteins (Hsp) that typically help protect cells from oxidative stress can exacerbate the changes.
  - Impaired ability to promote protein re-folding or autophagy, reduce blocking activation of NFκB (nuclear factor kappa B—a transcription factor protein), decreased ability to mount a response to acute stress.
  - In dogs, decreased levels have been linked with cognitive decline and neurodegeneration.[6]
- When nuclear and mitochondrial nucleic acids are damaged by free radicals, oxidative derivatives are formed, the most abundant of these being 8OHdG (8-hydroxy-2-deoxyguanosine) oxidative derivatives produced when nucleic acids are damaged by free radicals.

Inflammaging in Dogs

- Inflammatory mediators
  - In dogs, CRP increases with age, but only at statistically significant levels in the last year of life[1]
    - There was an increase in serum levels of 8OHdG.
    - There was also a significant decrease in baseline Hsp70 unless stressed, at which time the levels increase.
  - It may be that dogs display a smaller increase in inflammation (as indicated by CRP), which would be more difficult to detect, as compared to humans.
  - Other acute-phase proteins, for example, serum amyloid A may be more informative of the inflammatory state in dogs than CRP.[7]
  - In one study, IL-6, IL-8, and TNF-α concentrations all increased with age, and lymphocyte count decreased.[8]
  - In others studies, there was conflicting data:
    - Basal levels of IL-6 were only increased in young dogs with adult dogs having similar concentrations to senior and geriatric dogs.[9]
      - Intact females have the lowest IL-1β concentrations
      - Estrogens may decrease inflammatory pathways overall, in intact females.
    - Stimulated levels of inflammatory mediators measured dermal fibroblasts treated with LPS (lipopolysaccharide), a highly pathogenic toxin.[10]
      - Geriatric dogs had less dramatic increases compared to very young dogs, and this was significantly lower in large breeds.
      - The patterns of inflammation and mediators may be different in dogs compared to other species.
- IgG decreased slightly and IgM increased significantly[1]
- mRNA data suggest an increased macrophage population or increased inflammatory nature in adipose tissue cells (adipocytes) in older dogs.[11]
  - Adipose tissue macrophages have the capacity to produce excessive amounts of pro-inflammatory mediators, though they are usually anti-inflammatory in nature.[12]
- Studies with drugs that have the potential to delay aging or treat frailty (rapamycin, nicotinamide mononucleotide, and mesenchymal stem cells) were shown to reduce levels of inflammatory factors in dogs and impact certain chronic conditions.[13]
- The complex relationship with chronic inflammation, pain, and behavior may contribute to a form of "sickness behavior" in dogs.[14]

Client Communication

- In communicating with, and educating our clients, we need to let them know that while we are making optimal efforts to identify specific diseases and syndromes for their appropriate management, with senior pets, looking at the entire picture is critical.
- Outside of specific diseases, immunosenescence and inflammaging can have a great impact on senior pets and their health.
- While simple, accurate means of detecting chronic inflammation are not widely used, recognizing certain conditions from obesity to osteoarthritis and even dental inflammation can help guide some management strategies.
- Dietary and supplement administration may have some impact, but additional research is still needed.
- Research has started on anti-aging approaches with the dog as a study model. While dogs are used to get the foundations of data for human medicine, this can directly impact our opportunities for advanced opportunities.

See Also

- Immunosenescence

Abbreviations

- 8OHdG = 8-hydroxy-2-deoxyguanosine
- CRP = C-reactive protein
- Hsp = heat-shock proteins
- HPA = Hypothalamic–pituitary–adrenal axis
- IGF-1 = insulin-like growth factor
- IL-6 = interleukin
- LPS = lipopolysaccharide
- NFκB = nuclear factor kappa B
- ROS = reactive oxygen species
- TNF-α = tumor necrosis factor alpha

Additional Reading

Day MJ. Ageing, immunosenescence and inflammageing in the dog and cat. *J Comp Pathol* 2010;142(Suppl 1):S60–S69. doi: 10.1016/j.jcpa.2009.10.011. Epub 2009/12/17. S0021-9975(09)00335-1 [pii]. PMID: 20005526.

References

1. Alexander JE, Colyer A, Haydock RM, Hayek MG, Park J. Understanding how dogs age: longitudinal analysis of markers of inflammation, immune function, and oxidative stress. *J Gerontol A Biol Sci Med Sci* 2018 May 9;73(6):720–728. doi: 10.1093/gerona/glx182. PMID: 29126143.
2. Buzoglu HD, Burus A, Bayazıt Y, Goldberg M. Stem cell and oxidative stress-inflammation cycle. *Curr Stem Cell Res Ther* 2023;18(5):641–652. doi: 10.2174/1574888X17666221012151425. PMID: 36237155.
3. Johnson RW, Arkins S, Dantzer R, Kelley KW. Hormones, lymphohemopoietic cytokines and the neuroimmune axis. *Comp Biochem Physiol A Physiol* 1997 Mar;116(3):183–201. doi: https://doi.org/10.1016/s0300-9629(96)00277-0. PMID: 9102183.
4. Dantzer R, O'Connor JC, Freund GG, Johnson RW, Kelley KW. From inflammation to sickness and depression: when the immune system subjugates the brain. *Nat Rev Neurosci* 2008 Jan;9(1):46–56. doi: 10.1038/nrn2297. PMID: 18073775; PMCID: PMC2919277.
5. Porter RJ, Gallagher P, O'Brien JT. Effects of rapid tryptophan depletion on salivary cortisol in older people recovered from depression, and the healthy elderly. *J Psychopharmacol* 2007 Jan;21(1):71–75. doi: 10.1177/0269881106064341. Epub 2006 Mar 13. PMID: 16533861.NFkB.

6. Romanucci M, Della Salda L. Oxidative stress and protein quality control systems in the aged canine brain as a model for human neurodegenerative disorders. *Oxid Med Cell Longev* 2015;2015:940131. doi: 10.1155/2015/940131. Epub 2015 May 11. PMID: 26078824; PMCID: PMC4442305.ALEX 35.
7. Christensen MB, Langhorn R, Goddard A, Andreasen EB, Moldal E, Tvarijonaviciute A, Kirpensteijn J, Jakobsen S, Persson F, Kjelgaard-Hansen M. Comparison of serum amyloid A and C-reactive protein as diagnostic markers of systemic inflammation in dogs. *Can Vet J* 2014 Feb;55(2):161–168. PMID: 24489396; PMCID: PMC3894877.Jim 2023.
8. Schmid SM, Hoffman JM, Prescott J, Ernst H, Promislow DEL, Dog Aging Project Consortium, Creevy KE. The companion dog as a model for inflammaging: a cross-sectional pilot study. *Geroscience* 2024 Jun 1. doi: 10.1007/s11357-024-01217-w. Epub ahead of print. PMID: 38822125.
9. Jiménez AG. Inflammaging in domestic dogs: basal level concentrations of IL-6, IL-1β, and TNF-α in serum of healthy dogs of different body sizes and ages. *Biogerontology* 2023 Aug;24(4):593–602. doi: 10.1007/s10522-023-10037-y. Epub 2023 May 17. PMID: 37195482.
10. Jimenez AG, Downs CJ, Lalwani S, Cipolli W. Cellular metabolism and IL-6 concentrations during stimulated inflammation in primary fibroblasts from small and large dog breeds as they age. *J Exp Biol* 2021 May 1;224(9):jeb233734. doi: 10.1242/jeb.233734. Epub 2021 May 4. Erratum in: J Exp Biol. 2020 Dec 18:jeb.241992. doi: 10.1242/jeb.241992. PMID: 33257435.
11. Swanson KS, Belsito KR, Vester BM, Schook LB. Adipose tissue gene expression profiles of healthy young adult and geriatric dogs. *Arch Anim Nutr* 2009 Apr;63(2):160–171. doi: 10.1080/17450390902733934. PMID: 19489458.
12. Zeyda M, Farmer D, Todoric J, Aszmann O, Speiser M, Györi G, Zlabinger GJ, Stulnig TM. Human adipose tissue macrophages are of an anti-inflammatory phenotype but capable of excessive pro-inflammatory mediator production. *Int J Obes* 2007 Sep;31(9):1420–1428. doi: 10.1038/sj.ijo.0803632. Epub 2007 Jun 26. PMID: 17593905.
13. Zeng M, Zhou T, Li Z, Li G, Zhang S, Wang L, Huang QG, Li JD, Samarawickrama PN, He Y, Wang GD. Transcriptomic and intervention evidence reveals domestic dogs as a promising model for anti-inflammatory investigation. *Aging Cell* 2024 May;23(5):e14127. doi: 10.1111/acel.14127. Epub 2024 Mar 1. PMID: 38426629; PMCID: PMC11113267.
14. Piotti P, Pierantoni L, Albertini M, Pirrone F. Inflammation and behavior changes in dogs and cats. *Vet Clin North Am Small Anim Pract* 2024 Jan;54(1):1–16. doi: 10.1016/j.cvsm.2023.08.006. Epub 2023 Sep 16. PMID: 37722946.

Author: Heidi Lobprise

Chapter 5

Life Stages, Life Expectancy, and Relative Age

BASICS

OVERVIEW

Throughout the lives of our patients, they pass through distinct cycles of changes, in physical, behavioral, and needs for nutrition, health, and preventive support. A new pet parent gets tremendous amounts of information and care during puppyhood and kittenhood that rolls into a continuum of care for early (young) adult and mature adult phases. As they enter their senior lifestage, their needs in all areas change, and providing enhanced senior care can optimize their health and welfare during their last years.

Terms Defined

- Life Expectancy—refers to the number of years an individual can expect to live, often based on an estimate of the average age that members of a particular group will be when they die.
- Health Span—the expected years to live in good health, without disease, chronic illness, and disability.
- Life Stages—the distinct phases within the individual's life cycle, marked by significant physical, behavioral, and health/preventive needs.
- Senior
  - Dog—AAHA Senior Care Guidelines task force suggests this designation to dogs and cats that are in the last 25% of the predicted life span for their species and breed.
    - AAHA Senior Care Guidelines for dogs and cats
      - Senior is a term used to describe a dog at the end of its life stages, living after its expected lifespan, or one with significant disease.
    - Cat
      - AAFP Life Stage Guidelines defines senior at 10 years and older.
    - Cat PAWS Project
      - Senior—healthy cats 11–14 years of age
      - Super senior—healthy cats over 15 years of age
      - Geriatric—cats with established age-related disease(s).
- Geriatric—is linked to health status (physical and mental), frailty, and functional capacity (in people)
- Relative age—the translation of the chronological age of a dog (or cat) into "human years" to help determine lifestage.

Blackwell's Five-Minute Veterinary Consult Clinical Companion: Small Animal Senior Care, First Edition. Edited by Heidi B. Lobprise.

Companion website: www.wiley.com/go/lobprise/Senior

ISSUES AND OPTIONS

Life Stage

Dogs: 2019 AAHA Canine Life Stage Guidelines

- Puppy: Birth to cessation of rapid growth, 5–9 months, varying with breed and size.
- Young adult: Cessation of rapid growth to completion of physical and social maturation, which occurs in most dogs by 3–4 years of age.
- Mature adult: Completion of physical and social maturation until the last 25% of estimated lifespan (breed and size dependent)
- Senior: The last 25% of estimated lifespan through end of life.
- End of life (EOL): Terminal stage (depends on the specific pathologies)

Cats: 2021 AAHA/AAFP Feline Life Stage Guidelines (see Figure 5.1)

- Kitten: birth up to 1 year
- Young adult: 1–6 years
- Mature adult: 7–10 years
- Senior: >10 years
- End-of-life: variable

Life Expectancy

Cats

- In addition to life stage designation, life expectancy of cats is one of the few areas where they are less frustrating than dogs and less complex.
- There are fewer studies on cats' life expectancy as there are fewer variations
    - Data from >1000 hospitals across 7 years—LE_{birth} (life expectancy at birth) determined:[1] (See Figure 5.2)
        - All cats—11.18 years; mixed breed cats—11.12 years; purebred—11.54 years
        - Female cats—11.68 years; male cats—10.72 years
        - Cat body condition (See Figure 5.3)
            - 3/5–12.18 years
            - 4/5–13.67 years
            - 5/5–12.56 years
    - Data from primary veterinary care clinics[2]
        - All cats—11.74 years; mixed breed cats—11.89 years; purebred—10.41 years
            - Different LE in breeds: Birman 14.42 years; Sphynx 6.68[2] (See Figure 5.4)
        - Female cats—12.51 years; male 11.81 years
        - Early-age mortality—covariates of neuter status and breed
            - Intact cats 4.29 times the odds of death under 3 years of age
            - Purebred had 1.83 higher odds of dying under 3 years of age
    - Nine-point Body Condition Scoring and longevity[3]
        - Australia—at least two clinic visits; maximum BCS (body condition score) of all clinic visits
        - For survival and lifespan, BCS of <5 and 9 were found to be negatively associated.
        - BCS 6—highest survival probability over time and lowest hazard
            - BCS of 7 and 8—hazards not significantly different
        - BCS 3—highest hazard of all-cause mortality
            - Lean body might be related to illness; a risk marker rather than a risk factor
        - Though a BCS of 6–8 may have better survivability, it can still have adverse impacts on health with chronic illnesses and QoL (quality of life).

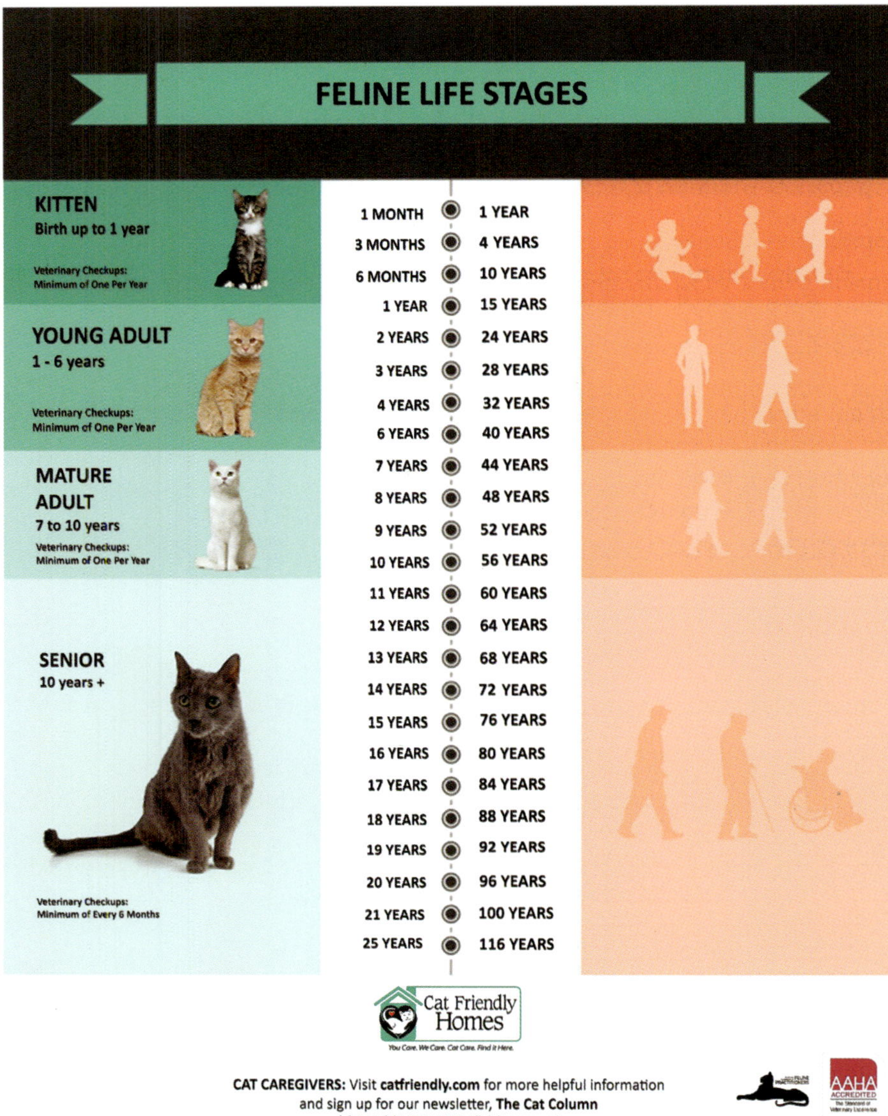

Figure 5.1 Feline life stages. Source: Reproduced with permission of American Association of Feline Practitioners (AAFP).

Dogs

- There are multiple factors that impact longevity and life span in dogs—body size, sex, neutering status, body condition, and breed specifics.
- Over the years, life span has been increasing for the most part.[1]
- Figuring out data from different studies can be challenging for many reasons
  - Time frame of study: life expectancy has been improving.
  - Type of cohort—referral practice or university vs. primary care practice vs. client-response surveys vs. data from insurance companies; mortality data vs. ongoing

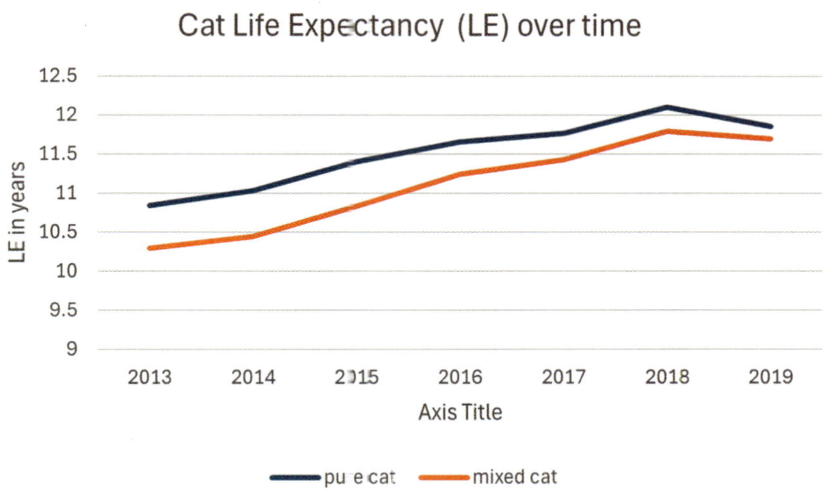

■ **Figure 5.2** The life expectancy (LE) over time of cats (mixed breed and purebred for the years 2013–2019) increasing except in the final year recorded. Source: Adapted from Montoya et al.[1]

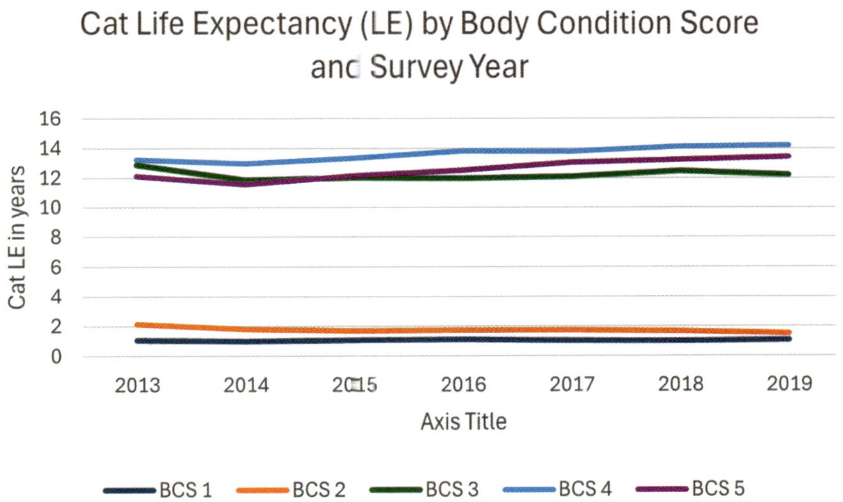

■ **Figure 5.3** Cat life expectancy (LE) by body condition score, showing a decreased life expectancy for cats below optimal body condition. Source: Adapted from Montoya et al.[1]

- Right censored data to exclude outliers.[4]
- Excluding extrinsic causes such as trauma and toxicity

■ Development of life expectancy tables can help estimate the potential mean survival time (MST), beyond just knowing a life expectancy.

Body Size in Dogs

■ In dogs, there is a strong negative correlation between body size and longevity[5] and others, unlike comparisons among different mammals (see Figure 5.5).
- Weight, even more so than height, was a significant predictor of life span.[6]

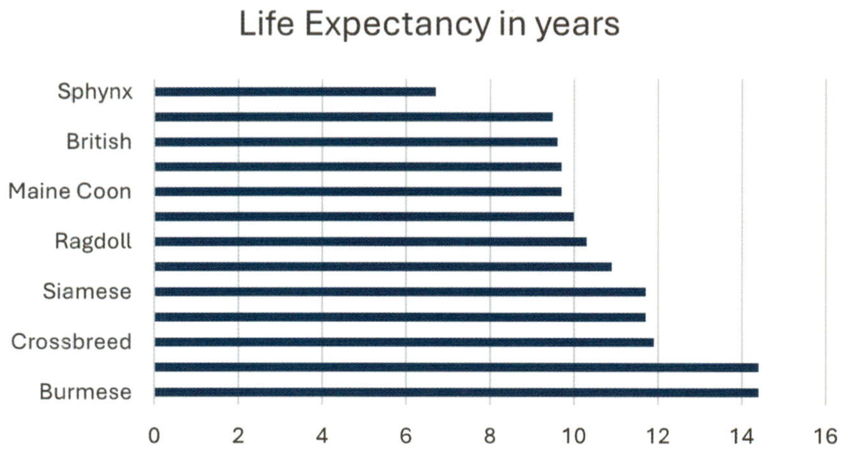

■ **Figure 5.4** Life expectancy for cat breeds. Source: Adapted from Teng et al.[2]

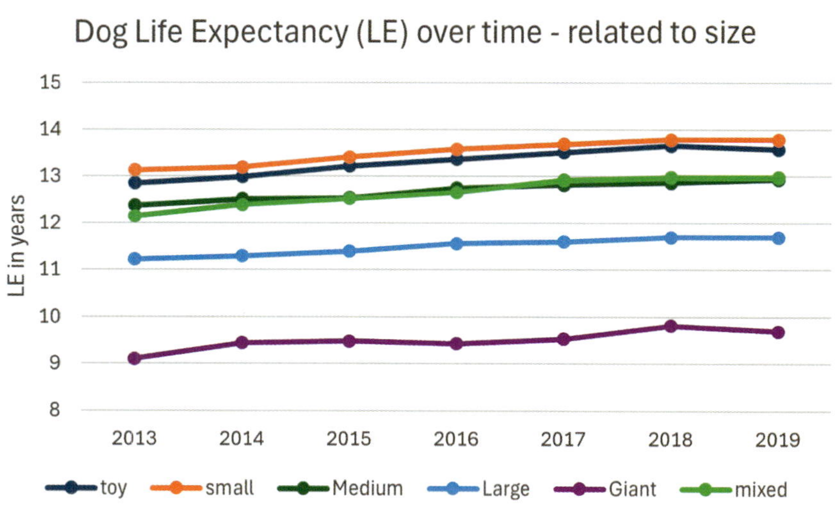

■ **Figure 5.5** Dog life expectancy (LE) over time—related to size, with a gradual increase over the years. Source: Adapted from Montoya et al.[1]

- With marked variation in sizes of dogs, and thus LE, this provides a good opportunity to study the genetic components (translational geroscience).[6]

■ A study sought to investigate if birth mass ratio is key to understanding negative correlation between lifespan and body size.[7]
- Scales negatively with adult size (unlike other mammals)—an index of energy required for growth.
- Although in another study, high-energy expenditure in dogs appears to be positively linked to increased life expectancy—contrary to findings across mammal species but resembling other intra-specific studies.[8]

■ In a study of 39 Labrador retrievers, some with exceptional longevity, it appears that lifelong maintenance of lean body mass and attenuated accumulation of body fat are key factors in longer lifespan.[9]

- Even a lifetime prevalence of malignant tumors increased with increasing dog size class, compared to toy and small dogs.[10]

Sex/Gender and Gonadectomy

- While some studies indicate higher life expectancy in females than males,[1] it is only a small effect on canine longevity, in contrast to humans and most species.[11]
    - Female dogs live longer on average, but there is a sex-by-neutering interaction effect in which neutered females and intact males are the longest lived of their respective sex.[11]
- Gonadectomy effect—most publications agree that there is positive association, but not all.[12]
    - Sterilization was strongly associated with an increase in lifespan—consistent among size classes.[13]
        - Possibly due to the lifespan cost of maintaining reproductive capability
    - Study with data from primary care hospitals:[14]
        - Female/intact—13.77 years
        - Male/intact—14.09 years
        - Male/neutered—14.15 years
        - Female/neutered—14.35 years
        - Data repeated for dogs at least 5 years old
    - Effect of neuter status on longevity of Rottweilers in Australia:[12]
        - Males had a 1.5 year shorter lifespan, females 1 year shorter lifespan.

Body Condition

- Obese dogs significantly lower LE_{birth} than overweight and ideal weight dogs.[1] (See Figure 5.6).
- Median life span shorter in overweight dogs (BCS 3–4/5) compared to normal dogs (BCS 3/5).
    - Greatest different in Yorkshire terriers (12.7 years vs. 16.2 years) and least in German Shepherd dogs (12.1 years vs. 12.5 years).[15]

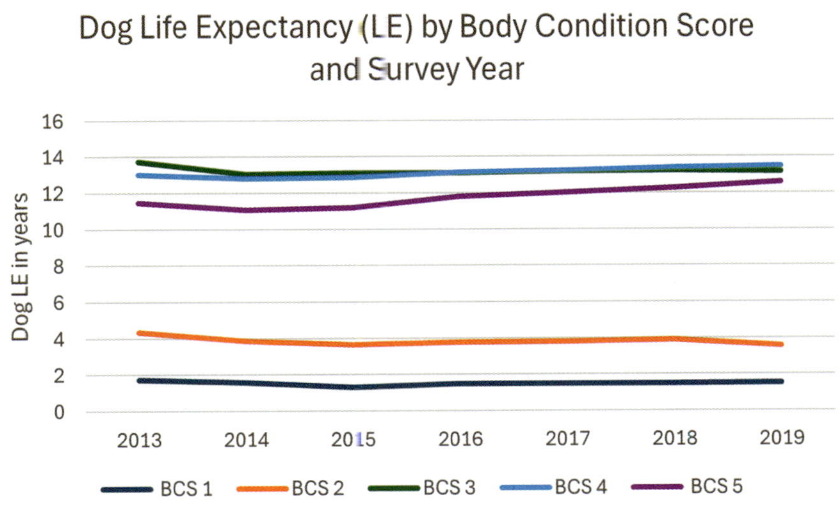

■ **Figure 5.6** Dog life expectancy (LE) by body condition score (BCS) over time. This also shows a decreased life expectancy for dogs below optimal body condition, and a slighter decrease in life expectancy for dogs with a BCS of 5. Source: Adapted from Montoya et al.[1]

Purebred and Mixed Breeds

- Inbreeding depression—when increased homozygosity can unmask recessive deleterious variants or allow the presence of over-dominant loci, the opposite of hybrid vigor.
- Early study showed that within each weight category, median age of death was lower for pure breed dogs.[5]
- In another study, large breeds tended to have higher coefficients of inbreeding than small breeds.[16]
  - But reduced LE is driven more by body size than inbreeding depression.
  - In purebreds, there is a higher baseline hazard and higher absolute rate of aging, lower LE.[16]
- Study assessing survivability among mongrel, cross-bred (with one purebred parent), and purebred dogs:[17]
  - Mongrels—LE 12.761 years mean and lower HR (hazard ratio)
  - Crossbred—LE 11.225 years
  - Purebred—LE 11.085 years
  - Higher morbidity, lower lifespan associated with higher inbreeding coefficients of purebred dogs
  - Crossbred—intermediate inbreeding coefficient.
  - A lower HR and higher survivability in Dogue de Bordeaux is contrary to the trend in larger dogs having a higher morbidity.
    - English bulldog had higher HR, lower survivability.
- Breeds with larger effective population sizes and/or lower inbreeding had median survival times 3–6 months longer than breeds without.[4]
  - No significant difference was shown between purebred and mixed breeds.
  - Mountain ancestral groups—considerably shorter lifespans than other groups by 3.5–4.6 years.[4]

Relative Age

- With all the complexities and varying parameters (and results) concerning longevity in dogs, it is still important to be able to categorize the individual according to appropriate lifestage.
- For the most pertinent communication with clients, this is often best accomplished by translating the actual chronological age of dogs into an age that is relative to human years.
- This is not a linear relationship, so the old rule of "dog's age times 7" is not optimal.
- Numerous age charts and age calculators are available, but few have sufficient data to validate their efforts. As improvements in veterinary care continue, these data may change as life expectancy increases.
- Any of these estimates and calculations are just generalizations, as each individual will have its own aging trajectory.
  - For animals that were adopted as adults, actual chronological age is often unknown and can be estimated at best.
- A classic example of a relative age chart may need to be updated, but it is a good start when helping veterinary teams and clients to assess the dog's relative age and life stage (See Figure 5.7).

Client Communication

- Discussion and client education on senior care should be a continuation of the wellness, preventive and regular diagnostic care you have provided throughout the life of the patient (See Figure 5.8).

Pet's Actual Age	Relative Age of Pet in "Human Years"				
	0-20 pounds	21-50 pounds	51-90 pounds	over 90 pounds	
1 year	7	7	7	9	
2 years	14	15	18	20	
3 years	28	30	32	34	Mature
4 years	32	34	36	38	
5 years	36	37	40	42	
6 years	40	42	45	49	
7 years	44	47	50	56	Senior
8 years	48	51	55	64	
9 years	52	55	61	71	
10 years	56	60	66	78	
11 years	60	65	72	86	Geriatric
12 years	64	69	77	94	
13 years	68	74	82	101	
14 years	72	78	88		
15 years	76	83	93		
16 years	80	87	99		
17 years	84	92	104		
18 years	88	96			
19 years	92				
20 years	96				

Figure 5.7 Relative age of pet in "human years" comparison chart, using the pet's actual age and size. This also assigns a life stage based on the relative age of mature, senior or geriatric. A similar chart can be found on. Source: Adapted from How Old Is My Dog in Human Years? Dog Age Chart (rover.com).

- It may be a tough conversation, like talking about weight loss, as some clients may want to avoid the fact that their pet is getting older, and could be considered "senior"
  - Having the right tools to guide you in this discussion (Life Stage guidelines, relative age chart for dogs) can be placed on your website or displayed on bulletin boards.
  - Training your staff to assess and recognize pets that are seniors can ensure that this communication is heard consistently.

APPLICATION IN PRACTICE

Senior Pet Care

- Based on data from VetSuccess (a veterinary practice metrics analysis company) it is estimated that up to 44% of patients on databases can be classified as "older or aging pets."
- If your practice management system can have customed fields to update, make a "LIFE STAGE" field; this may need to have manual input for each patient, but will allow you to reach a demographic of senior pets that have special needs.
  - Don't forget to update or upgrade a pet's status when they reach the next lifestage designation.
  - Celebrate these "upgrades" on your website or on the clinic social media platform. (Figures 5.9–5.11)

Items to Focus on During Each Life Stage

Observe at home and discuss with your veterinarian

	KITTEN	YOUNG ADULT	MATURE ADULT	SENIOR
Veterinary Checkups	At least once per year (more frequent for cat's with health conditions)			At least every 6 months
At All Ages	• Watch for subtle signs of behavior, illness, pain, and stress • Understand normal feline behaviors and that changes in cat's behavior can be significant • Get your cat comfortable with the carrier • Schedule routine checkups for your cat which can help them long-term • Discuss identification for your cat (microchipping) • Understand scratching is a natural, normal feline behavior; learn about caring for claws • Discuss pet insurance and financial planning options			
Medical History	Common conditions for specific breeds and genetic concerns (if applicable)	Vomiting, hairballs, diarrhea, changes in behavior, and grooming habits	Changes in appetite, hydration, vomiting, diarrhea, vocalization, nighttime activity, mobility, vision, litter box habits, and grooming habits	
Extra Focus During the Checkup	Infectious diseases, genetic findings, and discuss sterilization (spay/neuter)	Heart, lungs, skin, and teeth	• Increased focus on the abdomen, heart, lungs, thyroid, kidneys, eyes, and teeth • Muscle and bone assessment, and thorough pain and arthritis assessment	
Nutrition and Weight Management	Food being fed, amount being fed, frequency of feeding, and food toy/puzzles	Weight gain, obesity risks, play, and exercise	Weight loss and weight gain, type of food being fed to ensure it provides what your senior cat needs, and prescription diets (if needed)	
Behavior and Environment	• Introducing kittens to people and other pets • Petting, brushing, nail trimming, and grooming • Proper play (not using hands or feet as toys to avoid risk of future aggressive behavior) • Becoming comfortable with the carrier, travel, and veterinary visits	• Changes between cats and human-cat interactions • Gentle handling techniques for acceptance of checkups for mouth, ears, and feet	• Adjusting environmental needs as your cat ages • Easy accessibility to the litter box, warm soft bed, and food/water • Watching closely for subtle behavior changes	
	• Number and location of resources (litter box, food, water, sleeping areas) • Housing (indoor/outdoor/partial outdoor access), hunting activity, and others in the home • Housemate cats and their usual interactions • Changes in behavior, problematic or unwanted behaviors, and use of positive reinforcement • Environmental needs (toys, scratching posts, resting places, play)			
Litter Box	• Litter box setup, location, litter type, cleaning, and litter preference • Normal toileting behavior	Review and adjust litter box size and location to accommodate growth	• Litter box location to avoid stairs • Review and adjust litter box size, location, and cleaning regimens as necessary	
	• Toileting habits, stool appearance, and litter ball size • Urination or defecation outside the litter box • Differences between toileting and marking (territory) behaviors • Litter box management (number of boxes, size, location, litter type, cleaning)			
Oral Health	Getting used to mouth handling and brushing/wiping of teeth	Specific dental food type (if needed)	Changes in appearance to your cat's mouth, if your cat appears to be in pain when eating, or if your cat is not eating or chewing	
	Dental examination, dental disease, preventive care, and home care with brushing/wiping of teeth			
Parasite Control	• Risks of parasites for cats regardless of indoor/outdoor status • Risks of exposure based on lifestyle, geographic location, and travel • Year round treatment for the prevention of heartworms, fleas, ticks, and intestinal parasites (regardless of indoor/outdoor status) • Zoonotic risks (diseases passed between animals and people)			

Figure 5.8 Items to focus on during each life stage—a chart to help client discussion on the continuum of care needed throughout a cat's life stages. Source: Reproduced with permission from the American Association of Feline Practitioners (AAFP). 2021 AAHA/AAFP Feline Life Stage Guidelines. www.catvets.com/life-stage.

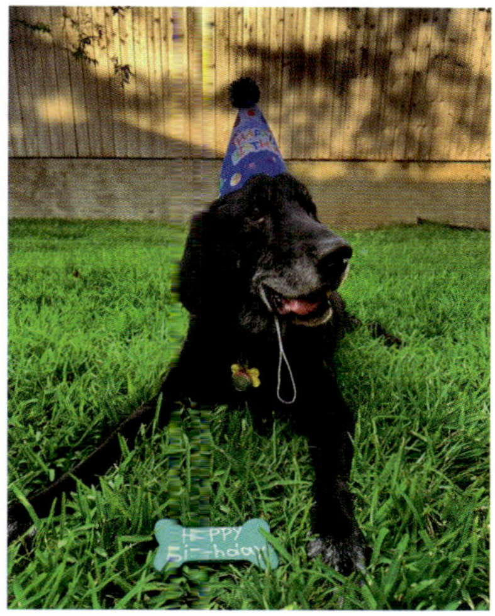

■ **Figure 5.9** Celebrate your senior patients, especially on their birthdays, on your website or with social media posts. Source: With permission of Jennie Kernaghan

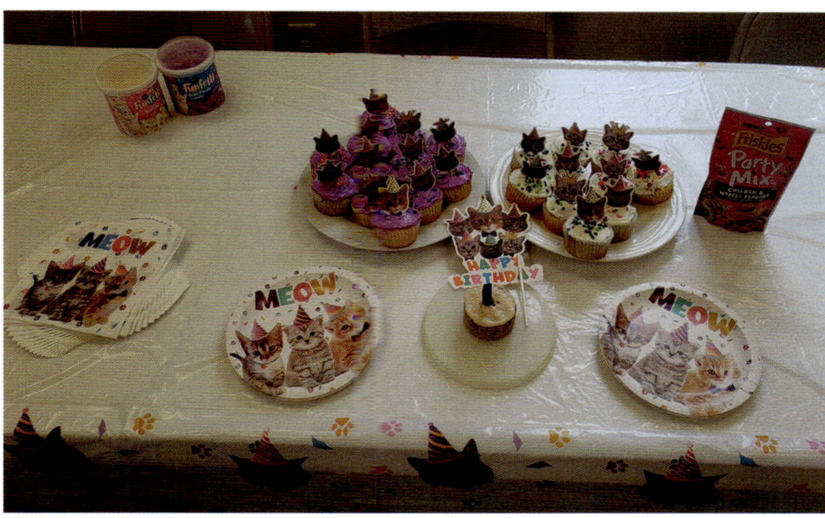

■ **Figure 5.10** You can even celebrate your clinic pets. Our clinic celebrated Tony's 11th birthday, upgrading him to senior status. This gave an opportunity to discuss senior care needs with the entire team.

- Beyond just having resources for "life expectancy," be familiar with how to utilize Life Expectancy Tables. These provide estimations of how many years may be left in a pet's life based on their current age. (See Table 5.1)

Abbreviations

- BCS = body condition score
- HR = hazard ratio
- LE_{birth} = life expectancy at birth
- MST = mean survival time
- QoL = quality of life

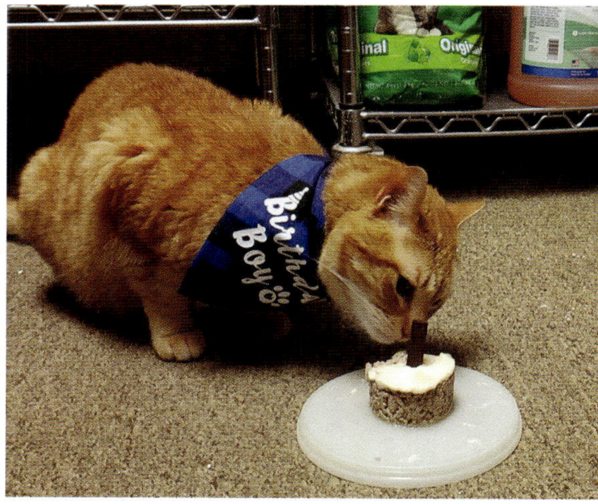

■ **Figure 5.11** Tony appreciated the cat cupcake!

TABLE 5.1 Life expectancy table: to help estimate the potential mean survival time (MST) of mixed breed and purebred cats (how many years may be left, based on their current age.

Current age (years)	LE at time—mixed breeds	LE at time—purebred cats
10–11	5.51	5.58
11–12	4.87	4.97
12–13	4.29	4.34
13–14	3.72	3.72
14–15	3.20	2.76
15–16	2.73	2.45
16–17	2.32	2.12
17–18	1.92	1.62
18–19	1.63	1.52
19–10	1.41	1.35
20+	1.31	1.22

Source: Adapted from Montoya et al.[1]

Internet Resources

Accessed 29 June 2024

- 2023 AAHA Senior Care Guidelines JAAHA7343_proof.pdf
- Life Stage Guidelines|American Association of Feline Practitioners (catvets.com)

Additional Reading

Creevy KE, Grady J, Little SE, Moore GE, Strickler BG, Thompson S, Webb JA. AAHA canine life stage guidelines. *J Am Anim Hosp Assoc* 2019 Nov/Dec;55(6):267–290. doi: 10.5326/JAAHA-MS-6999. PMID: 31622127.

Quimby J, Gowland S, Carney HC, DePorter T, Plummer P, Westropp J. AAHA/AAFP feline life stage guidelines. *J Feline Med Surg* 2021 Mar;23(3):211–233. doi: 10.1177/1098612X21993657. Erratum in: *J Feline Med Surg* 2021 Aug;23(8):NP3. doi: 10.1177/1098612X211024041. PMID: 33627003; PMCID: PMC10812130.

References

1. Montoya M, Morrison JA, Arrignon F, Spofford N, Charles H, Hours MA, Biourge V. Life expectancy tables for dogs and cats derived from clinical data. *Front Vet Sci* 2023 Feb 21;10:1082102. doi: 10.3389/fvets.2023.1082102. PMID: 36896289; PMCID: PMC9989186.
2. Teng KT, Brodbelt DC, Church DB, O'Neill DG. Life tables of annual life expectancy and risk factors for mortality in cats in the UK. *J Feline Med Surg* 2024 May;26(5):1098612X241234556. doi: 10.1177/1098612X241234556. PMID: 38714312.
3. Teng KT, McGreevy PD, Toribio JL, Raubenheimer D, Kendall K, Dhand NK. Strong associations of nine-point body condition scoring with survival and lifespan in cats. *J Feline Med Surg* 2018 Dec;20(12):1110–1118. doi: 10.1177/1098612X17752198. Epub 2018 Feb 2. PMID: 29393723; PMCID: PMC11104206.
4. Urfer SR, Kaeberlein M, Promislow DEL, Creevy KE. Lifespan of companion dogs seen in three independent primary care veterinary clinics in the United States. *Canine Med Genet* 2020 Jun 16;7:7. doi: 10.1186/s40575-020-00086-8. PMID: 32835231; PMCID: PMC7386164.
5. Patronek GJ, Waters DJ, Glickman LT. Comparative longevity of pet dogs and humans: implications for gerontology research. *J Gerontol A Biol Sci Med Sci* 1997 May;52(3):B171–B178. doi: 10.1093/gerona/52a.3.b171. PMID: 9158552.
6. Greer KA, Canterberry SC, Murphy KE. Statistical analysis regarding the effects of height and weight on life span of the domestic dog. *Res Vet Sci* 2007 Apr;82(2):208–214. doi: 10.1016/j.rvsc.2006.06.005. Epub 2006 Aug 21. PMID: 16919689.
7. Fan R, Olbricht G, Baker X, Hou C. Birth mass is the key to understanding the negative correlation between lifespan and body size in dogs. *Aging* 2016 Dec 8;8(12):3209–3222. doi: 10.18632/aging.101081. PMID: 27956710; PMCID: PMC5270664.
8. Speakman JR, van Acker A, Harper EJ. Age-related changes in the metabolism and body composition of three dog breeds and their relationship to life expectancy. *Aging Cell* 2003 Oct;2(5):265–275. doi: 10.1046/j.1474-9728.2003.00061.x. PMID: 14570234.
9. Adams VJ, Watson P, Carmichael S, Gerry S, Penell J, Morgan DM. Exceptional longevity and potential determinants of successful ageing in a cohort of 39 Labrador retrievers: results of a prospective longitudinal study. *Acta Vet Scand* 2016 May 11;58(1):29. doi: 10.1186/s13028-016-0206-7. PMID: 27169845; PMCID: PMC4863359.
10. Schwartz SM, Urfer SR, White M, Megquier K, Shrager S, Dog Aging Project Consortium, Ruple A. Lifetime prevalence of malignant and benign tumours in companion dogs: cross-sectional analysis of dog aging project baseline survey. *Vet Comp Oncol* 2022 Dec;20(4):797–804. doi: 10.1111/vco.12839. Epub 2022 Jun 2. PMID: 35574975; PMCID: PMC10089278.
11. Hoffman JM, O'Neill DG, Creevy KE, Austad SN. Do female dogs age differently than male dogs? *J Gerontol A Biol Sci Med Sci* 2018 Jan 16;73(2):150–156. doi: 10.1093/gerona/glx061. PMID: 28472238; PMCID: PMC5861885.
12. Joonè CJ, Konovalov DA. The effect of neuter status on longevity in the Rottweiler dog. *Sci Rep* 2023 Oct 19;13(1):17845. doi: 10.1038/s41598-023-45128-w. PMID: 37857755; PMCID: PMC10587138.
13. Hoffman JM, Creevy KE, Promislow DE. Reproductive capability is associated with lifespan and cause of death in companion dogs. *PLoS One* 2013 Apr 17;8(4):e61082. doi: 10.1371/journal.pone.0061082. PMID: 23613790; PMCID: PMC3629191.
14. Urfer SR, Wang M, Yang M, Lund EM, Lefebvre SL. Risk factors associated with lifespan in pet dogs evaluated in primary care veterinary hospitals. *J Am Anim Hosp Assoc* 2019 May/Jun;55(3):130–137. doi: 10.5326/JAAHA-MS-6763. Epub 2019 Mar 14. PMID: 30870610.
15. Salt C, Morris PJ, Wilson D, Lund EM, German AJ. Association between life span and body condition in neutered client-owned dogs. *J Vet Intern Med* 2019 Jan;33(1):89–99. doi: 10.1111/jvim.15367. Epub 2018 Dec 11. PMID: 30548336; PMCID: PMC6335446.

16. Yordy J, Kraus C, Hayward JJ, White ME, Shannon LM, Creevy KE, Promislow DEL, Boyko AR. Body size, inbreeding, and lifespan in domestic dogs. *Conserv Genet* 2020 Feb;21(1):137–148. doi: 10.1007/s10592-019-01240-x. Epub 2019 Dec 5. PMID: 32607099; PMCID: PMC7326369.
17. Mata F, Mata A. Investigating the relationship between inbreeding and life expectancy in dogs: mongrels live longer than pure breeds. *PeerJ* 2023 Jul 19;11:e15718. doi: 10.7717/peerj.15718. PMID: 37483958; PMCID: PMC10362839.

Author: Heidi Lobprise

Section 2

Disease/Systems

Behavior

Chapter 6

Cognitive Disorders

BASICS

DEFINITION

Syndrome associated with brain aging. Leads to alterations in awareness, decreased responsiveness to stimuli, deficits in learning and memory, agitation, and anxiety. Subtle signs seen in early stages of cognitive decline may include alterations in activity, social interactions, and increasing anxiety.

PATHOPHYSIOLOGY

- Neuronal loss, decreased frontal lobe volume, increased ventricular volume, and neurotoxic deposits including lipofuscin and beta-amyloid.
- Toxic free radicals (reactive oxygen species) increase with age because of illness and stressors, age-related decline in mitochondrial efficiency, and decreased clearance mechanisms.
- Unclear which changes are associated with the clinical signs; possible correlation between cognitive decline, amount of beta-amyloid in the cerebral cortex, and increases in toxic free radicals.
- Compromised cerebral vascular blood flow and infarcts may be contributory.
- Neurotransmission is compromised; may be a decline in catecholamine and cholinergic transmission.

SYSTEMS AFFECTED

- Behavioral.
- Nervous.

GENETICS

Unknown; may be genetic factors contributing to beta-amyloid deposition and the age at which it begins to accumulate.

INCIDENCE/PREVALENCE

- Clinical signs of cognitive dysfunction syndrome (CDS) have been reported to arise in 41–68% (or higher) of dogs over 14.
- Overall prevalence in dogs over 10 estimated as at least 14.2%.

Blackwell's Five-Minute Veterinary Consult Clinical Companion: Small Animal Senior Care, First Edition. Edited by Heidi B. Lobprise.

Companion website: www.wiley.com/go/lobprise/Senior

- Clinical signs reported to arise in 50% of cats over 15.
- Prevalence in cats over 10 estimated at 35%.
- Progressive—over 6 months, 24% of dogs with mild signs progressed to moderate and 42% with no impairment progressed to mild.

SIGNALMENT

Species

Dogs and cats.

Mean Age and Range

- Increased prevalence with increasing age.
- Neuropsychological testing in dogs and cats has identified a decline in memory and learning as early as 6–8 years of age.
- Initial signs may not be noticed by pet owners, except perhaps in dogs trained to perform more specialized tasks (e.g., guide and hearing dogs, drug detection, agility).
    - Larger dogs not affected at earlier ages—limited cognitive decline in larger breeds with a shortened senior period (truncation theory).[1]
    - Smaller dogs, dolichocephalic breeds and purebred dogs had a higher CCD risk prevalence[2]

SIGNS

Historical Findings

- Clinical signs have been categorized using the acronym DISHAA for dogs (Figure 6.1).
    - Disorientation, including getting lost in familiar environments, confusion, inability to navigate through familiar routes (e.g., goes to hinge side of door), dropping food and not retrieving.
    - Interactions with humans or other animals may be altered (irritability, decreased interest in play/affection, or increased attention seeking).
    - Sleep–wake cycle alterations including night waking, vocalization, and/or increased sleep during the day.
    - Housetraining and other previously learned behaviors might deteriorate.
    - Activity may be altered—including a decline in activity level, exploration, and self-care; however, as the condition progresses, activity may increase with signs of restlessness, pacing, aimless wandering, vocalization, or excessive licking.
    - Anxiety and agitation.
- For cats, the acronym VISHDAAL has been used:
    - V—inappropriate vocalization; owners may feel this is primarily due to disorientation or is attention seeking, but often stressful
    - I—altered social interaction
        - Increased affection toward owner may be reported.[3]
    - S—change in sleep pattern
    - H—house soiling
    - D—disorientation—spatial and temporal
    - A—change in activity
    - A—anxiety
    - L—learning and memory deficits

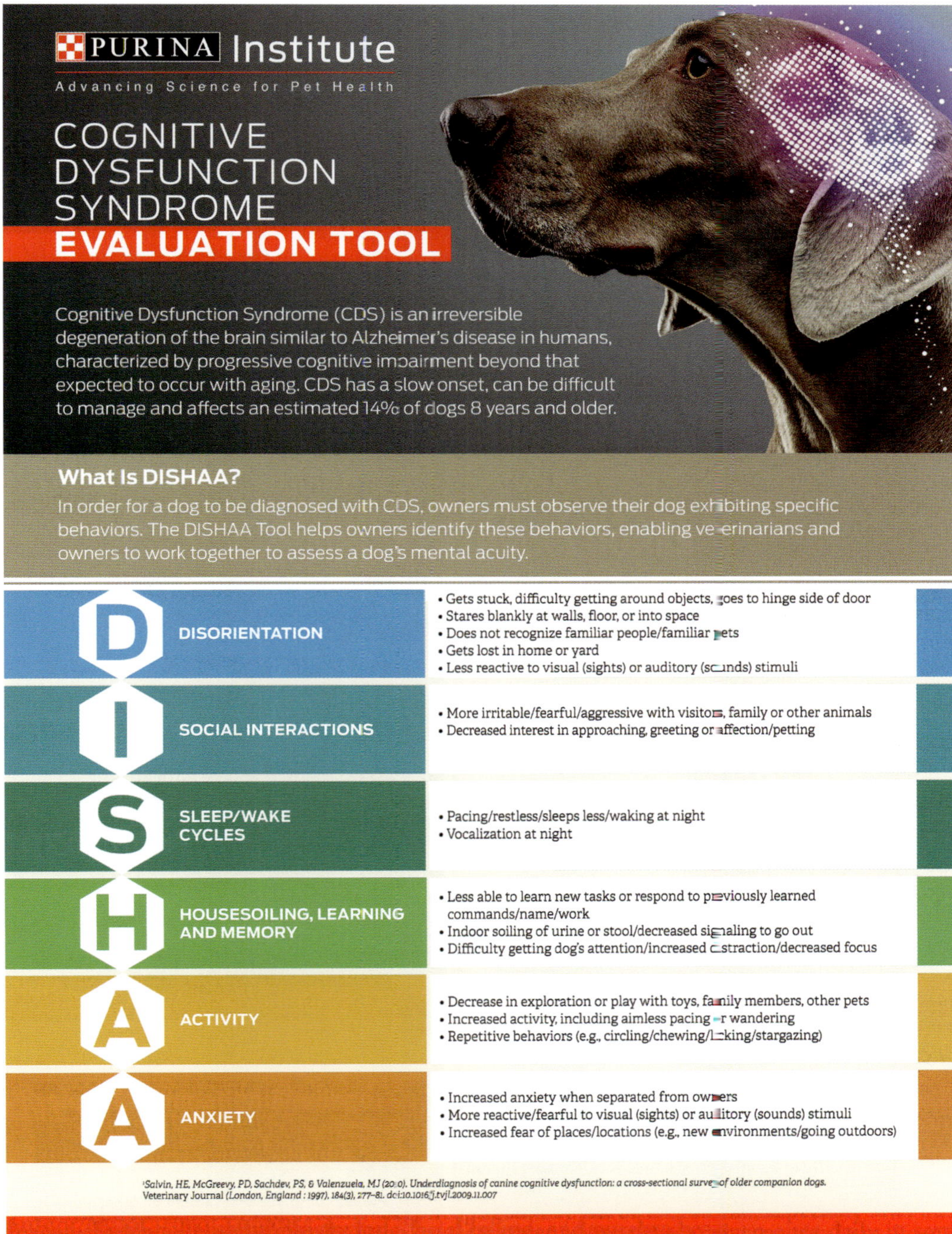

Figure 6.1 Cognitive dysfunction syndrome evaluation tool. Source: Nestlé Purina/https://www.purinainstitute.com/sites/default/files/2021-04/DISHAA-Assessment-Tool.pdf/last accessed on 06 August 2024.

PURINA Institute

Advancing Science for Pet Health

COGNITIVE DYSFUNCTION SYNDROME
ASSESSMENT TOOL

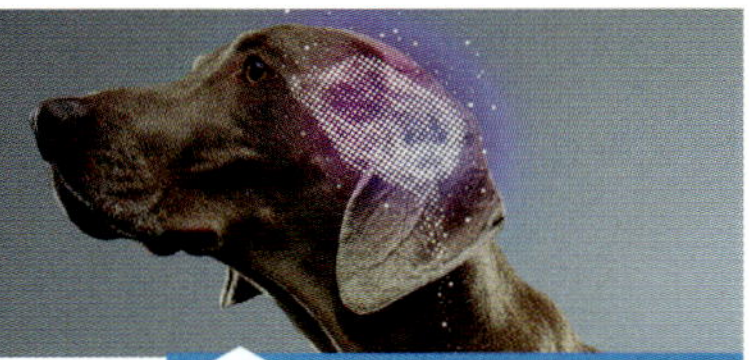

Cognitive Dysfunction Syndrome (CDS) is an irreversible degeneration of the brain similar to Alzheimer's disease in humans, characterized by progressive cognitive impairment beyond that expected to occur with aging. CDS has a slow onset, can be difficult to manage and affects an estimated 14% of dogs 8 years and older.

- **D** DISORIENTATION
- **I** SOCIAL INTERACTIONS
- **S** SLEEP/WAKE CYCLES
- **H** HOUSESOILING, LEARNING AND MEMORY
- **A** ACTIVITY
- **A** ANXIETY

What is DISHAA?

DISHAA is a tool to help you and your veterinarian assess the mental acuity of your dog, and for your veterinarian to potentially diagnose Cognitive Dysfunction Syndrome (CDS).

Date: ____________

Owner's name: ____________ Pet's name: ____________

Age: ____________ Gender: ☐ Male ☐ Female Neutered/Spayed: ☐ No ☐ Yes

Breed: ____________ Weight: ____________

BCS (Body Condition Score 1-9): ____________ Current Diet: ____________

Medications and Dosage Frequency: ____________

Please complete this canine senior pet cognitive assessment. If you've noticed changes in multiple behavioral categories, be sure to talk to your veterinarian today about the health of your pet's aging brain.

BEHAVIORAL SIGNS Identify signs that have arisen or progressed since 8 years of age and older. **Score as 0=none, 1=mild, 2=moderate, 3=severe**	**Score**
DISORIENTATION	
Gets stuck, difficulty getting around objects, goes to hinge side of door	
Stares blankly at walls, floor, or into space	
Does not recognize familiar people/familiar pets	
Gets lost in home or yard	
Less reactive to visual (sights) or auditory (sounds) stimuli	

Please complete assessment on other side.

■ **Figure 6.1** (Continued)

PURINA Institute
Advancing Science for Pet Health

COGNITIVE DYSFUNCTION SYNDROME
ASSESSMENT TOOL
CONTINUED

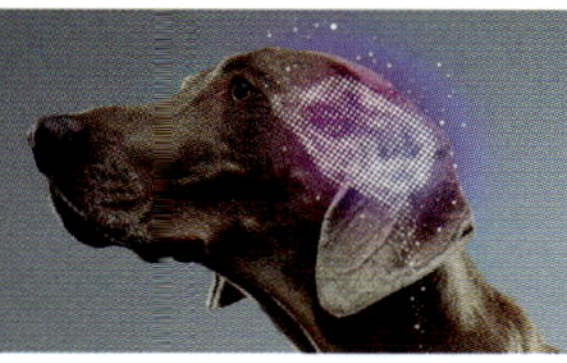

BEHAVIORAL SIGNS

Identify signs that have arisen or progressed since 8 years of age and older.
Score as 0=none, 1=mild, 2=moderate, 3=severe

	Score
SOCIAL INTERACTIONS	
More irritable/fearful/aggressive with visitors, family or other animals	
Decreased interest in approaching, greeting or affection/petting	
SLEEP/WAKE CYCLES	
Pacing/restless/sleeps less/waking at night	
Vocalization at night	
HOUSESOILING, LEARNING AND MEMORY	
Less able to learn new tasks or respond to previously learned commands/name/work	
Indoor soiling of urine ___ or stool ___ /decreased signaling to go out	
Difficulty getting dog's attention/increased distraction/decreased focus	
ACTIVITY	
Decrease in exploration or play with toys, family members, other pets	
Increased activity including aimless pacing or wandering	
Repetitive behaviors, e.g., circling ___ chewing ___ licking ___ stargazing ___	
ANXIETY	
Increased anxiety when separated from owners	
More reactive/fearful to visual (sights) or auditory (sounds) stimuli	
Increased fear of places/locations (e.g., new environments/going outdoors)	
TOTAL (BE SURE TO CARRY OVER THE SCORES FROM FRONT SIDE OF SHEET)	

Once this form is completed, your veterinarian will determine the cause of these signs through a physical examination and recommended diagnostic tests. However, even if your senior pet is experiencing multiple health issues associated with aging, there may be some degree of CDS.

A score of 4-15 is consistent with mild, 16-33 is moderate, and >33 is severe CDS.

Assessment was created by: Dr. Gary Landsberg, DVM, DACVB, DECAWBM, Vice President, Veterinary Affairs CanCog Technologies; to aid in diagnosing Canine Cognitive Dysfunction Syndrome.

Figure 6.1 (Continued)

Physical Examination

- No specific abnormalities associated with cognitive dysfunction.
- Other age-related medical disorders might be noted.

CAUSES

- Exact cause is unknown and animals are variably affected.
- Environmental factors may contribute to age-related degeneration.
- May be predisposing genetic factors.
- Diet, enrichment, and stress management may be in part preventive.

RISK FACTORS

- Chronic oxidative stress and chronic low-grade inflammation.
- Conditions that affect cerebral vascular blood supply (e.g., systemic hypertension, anemia).
- Deficiency in docosahexaenoic acid (DHA), B6, B12, and folic acid, high homocysteine, low-quality diets.

  Quality sleep is essential for homeostasis; time of clearance of amyloid beta through glymphatic system.
    - Sleep disruption can be a consequence of CDS but can also contribute to the disease in a vicious cycle.[4]

DIAGNOSIS

DIFFERENTIAL DIAGNOSIS

- Any medical condition that affects the pet's mental attitude or behavior must be ruled out.

  More signs associated with musculoskeletal and neurological problems, including pain and sensory decline.[5]
- Pain (e.g., arthritis, dental disease) can lead to increased irritability, anxiety, and altered response to stimuli.
- If mobility is affected, the pet may be less able to avoid fearful stimuli and less able to access its elimination area.
- Impaired sight or hearing might lead to decreased responsiveness or increased reactivity to stimuli.
- Difficulty finding dropped food could be an indicator of decreased olfaction.
- Diseases of the urinary or gastrointestinal tract can cause house-soiling.
- Organ failure, tumors, immune diseases, and endocrinopathies can also affect behavior.
- Diseases that affect the CNS or its circulation can affect behavior.

CBC/BIOCHEMICAL/URINALYSIS

Normal with CDS, but concurrent disease processes common in aged dogs.

OTHER LABORATORY TESTS

Normal with CDS.

IMAGING

- Used to rule out primary organic/structural cause.
- Most important when there are abnormalities on the neurologic examination or when the onset is sudden; less likely to be of diagnostic value if signs are slowly progressive in the absence of other neurologic findings.

DIAGNOSTIC PROCEDURES

- Diagnosis is based on identifying clinical signs on screening questionnaire, e.g., DISHAA (Pan et al.), VISHDAAL (Sordo et al.), CADEs (Madari et al.), and CCDR (Salvin et al.), ruling out possible medical causes.
- Early and mild signs not likely to be reported; therefore, veterinarians must ask (e.g., with screening questionnaire).
- Endoscopy, radiography, ultrasound, and other specialized diagnostic procedures may be necessary to rule out other causes of the clinical signs.
- Further ophthalmic and neurologic assessment if indicated to rule out visual or auditory deficits and neurologic disease.
- Therapeutic trial might be considered to rule out and treat other potential causes of the signs, e.g., pain.

PATHOLOGIC FINDINGS

Loss of frontal and temporal lobe volume, neuronal loss, meningeal calcification, microhemorrhage and infarcts, beta-amyloid deposition and hyperphosphorylated tau.

TREATMENT

NURSING CARE

Support and home care by pet owners.

ACTIVITY

- Maintain exercise, play, reward-based training, work, feeding enrichment (e.g., food-filled toys), and daily routines that are appropriate for the pet's age and health.
- Maintaining mental stimulation and physical activity have been shown to reduce or slow progression of cognitive decline.

  In cats with significant CDS, any changes could be stressful.[6]

DIET

- Diet should be fed that meets and prioritizes medical and cognitive health care needs.
- For dogs, diet supplemented with antioxidants including vitamins E and C, selenium, beta carotene, and flavonoids and carotenoids, omega-3 fatty acids, and carnitine and alpha lipoic acid (for mitochondrial health) has been shown to improve memory, learning ability, and clinical signs of cognitive dysfunction (Hills Prescription Diet b/d).
    - Cellular antioxidants—vitamins E, C, fruits and vegetables
    - Mitochondrial co-factors (lipoid acid and carnitine)—decreased ROS (reactive oxygen species) production and increased NADH-linked (nicotinamide adenine dinucleotide + hydrogen) respiration.[7]
    - Any formulations for cats should not include alpha lipoic acid that can be toxic.[6]
- As cerebral glucose metabolism declines with increasing age in dogs, a diet supplemented with 5.5% medium-chain triglyceride (MCT) oil to provide ketone bodies as an alternative source of energy for aging neurons has been demonstrated to improve cognitive function in middle-aged and senior dogs (e.g., Purina ProPlan Bright Mind 7+®).
- A brain support blend containing arginine (to enhance nitrous oxide synthesis), antioxidants including vitamins C, E, and selenium; B vitamins; and omega-3 fatty acids has been demonstrated to improve cognitive function in laboratory studies in senior dogs and middle-aged cats (Pan).
- A combination of the brain support blend and 6.5% MCT supplementation has been demonstrated to improve clinical signs of cognitive dysfunction in dogs (Purina Pro Plan Veterinary Diets NC NeuroCare®).
- For dogs—supplements containing phosphatidylserine (Senilife, CEVA Animal Health and Activait, VetPlus), *S*-adenosyl-L-methioninetosylate disulfate (SAMe; Novifit, Virbac Animal Health), and apoaequorin have demonstrated some evidence of efficacy.
- For cats—SAMe and diets containing fish oil, arginine, B vitamins, and antioxidants have demonstrated beneficial effects.

CLIENT EDUCATION

- Lifelong therapy is required, and concurrent medications may be necessary if the pet has multiple problems.
- Any changes in the pet's health or behavior should be reported immediately, as this may be due to cognitive dysfunction or new health problems.
- Considering the pet's health and cognitive status, the owner must be advised on any limitations on what might be achieved.
- Signs are generally progressive; treatment is aimed at slowing the progression of the disease, not cure.

MEDICATIONS

DRUG(S) OF CHOICE

Dogs

- Selegiline—monoamine oxidase (MAO) B inhibitor, may contribute to improved catecholamine transmission, decrease in free radicals, and neuroprotective effect; 0.5–1 mg/kg PO q24h in the morning and maintained if effective; reevaluate clinical signs for improvement after 1–2 months; side effects might include occasional gastrointestinal upset and restlessness, and repetitive behavior at higher doses.

- Propentofylline—not licensed in North America but is licensed in other countries; xanthine derivative; purported to inhibit platelet aggregation and thrombus formation, make the red cells more pliable, and increase blood flow; may increase oxygen supply to CNS without increasing glucose demand; 3–5 mg/kg PO q12h.
- Nicergoline—alpha-adrenergic antagonist that may improve cognitive function through vasodilatory effects on cerebral circulation 0.25–0.5 mg/kg PO q24h.

Cats

- No therapeutic agents licensed for treatment of CDS.
- Selegiline (0.5–1 mg/kg PO q24h), propentofylline (1/4 of 50 mg tablet PO q24h), and nicergoline (0.25–0.5 mg/kg PO q24h) have been used off-label in cats, with anecdotal evidence of effect.

CONTRAINDICATIONS

- Selegiline should not be used concurrently with MAO inhibitors such as amitraz, narcotics, alpha-adrenergic agents such as phenylpropanolamine or ephedrine, or selective serotonin reuptake inhibitors (e.g. fluoxetine) or tricyclic antidepressants (e.g., clomipramine).
- A 2-week washout is suggested following most tricyclic antidepressants and up to 5 weeks following fluoxetine before starting selegiline.

Cats should not receive supplements with alpha lipoic acid.

PRECAUTIONS

- Choose medications that are least sedating and least anticholinergic.
- Potential drug interactions must be considered with concurrent use of drugs and over-the-counter medications.

ALTERNATIVE DRUG(S)

- Consider potential benefits vs. risks including contraindications, side effects, off-label use, and evidence of effect.
- Anti-inflammatory medications and natural supplements such as gingko biloba and curcumin might be considered based on preliminary work in other species.
- Medication used in humans for Alzheimer's disease to enhance cholinergic transmission might be useful, but doses and pharmacokinetics in dogs have not been determined; side effects might include nausea, vomiting, diarrhea, and sleep–wake disturbances.
- For anxiety, agitation, apathy, and night waking consider adjunctive therapeutics including buspirone or fluoxetine for ongoing use, or trazodone, benzodiazepines, and alpha-2 agonists for as needed use.

Evaluate all medication and supplement combinations for serotonin effects.

- Natural supplements including pheromones, melatonin, valerian, l-theanine, alpha-casozepine, γ-aminobutyric acid (GABA), magnolia and phellodendron (Solliquin®), or Souroubea (Zentrol®) might help to reduce signs related to anxiety and night-time waking.

FOLLOW-UP

PATIENT MONITORING

- If a drug or diet for CDS is dispensed, therapeutic response should be evaluated after 30–60 days and the dose adjusted or treatment changed if there is insufficient improvement.
- If the pet is stable, twice-yearly checkups are recommended unless new problems arise before reassessment is due.

PREVENTION/AVOIDANCE

- Providing an enriched environment, ongoing training, and physical activity that is appropriate and practical for the pet's age and health may help to prevent or delay the onset of cognitive decline.
- Early CDS dietary intervention may address risk factors and slow the progression of disease.

EXPECTED COURSE AND PROGNOSIS

Diet and medication may improve signs and slow progression in most cases; however, with increasing age, CDS may progress and other concurrent health problems will ultimately arise.

MISCELLANEOUS

Synonyms

- Age-related cognitive and affective disorders, involutional depression, dysthymia.
- Dementia.
- Senility.

Abbreviations

- CDS = cognitive dysfunction syndrome
- DHA = docosahexaenoic acid.
- GABA = γ-aminobutyric acid.
- MAO = monoamine oxidase.
- MCT = medium-chain triglyceride.
- SAMe = *S*-adenosyl-L-methionine-tosylate disulfate.

Internet resources

Accessed 29 June 2024
https://www.purinainstitute.com/sites/default/files/2021-04/DISHAA-Assessment-Tool.pdf

Suggested Reading

Landsberg GM, Madari A, Zilka N (eds). *Canine and Feline Dementia: Molecular Basis, Diagnostics, and Therapy*. Cham: Springer, 2017.

Madari A, Farbakova J, Katina S, et al. Assessment of severity and progression of canine cognitive dysfunction syndrome using the Canine Dementia Scale (CADES). *Appl Anim Behav Sci* 2015;17:138–145.

Pan Y, Landsberg G, Mougeot I, et al. Efficacy of a therapeutic diet on dogs with signs of cognitive dysfunction syndrome (CDS): a prospective double blinded placebo controlled clinical trial. *Front Nutr* 2018. doi: 10.3389/fnut.2018.00127.

Pan Y, Araujo JA, Burrows J, et al. Cognitive enhancement in middleaged and old cats with dietary supplementation with a nutrient blend containing fish oil, B vitamins, antioxidants, and arginine. *Br J Nutr* 2013;110(1):40–49.

Salvin HE, McGreevy PD, Sachdev PS, et al. The canine cognitive dysfunction rating scale (CCDR): a data-driven and ecologically relevant assessment tool. *Vet J* 2011;188:331–336.

Sordo L, Gunn-Moore DA. Cognitive dysfunction in cats: update on neuropathological and behavioural changes plus clinical management. *Vet Rec* 2021 Jan;188(1):e3. doi: 10.1002/vetr.3. Epub 2021 Jan 12. PMID: 34651755.

References

1. Watowich MM, MacLean EL, Hare B, Call J, Kaminski J, Miklósi Á, Snyder-Mackler N. Age influences domestic dog cognitive performance independent of average breed lifespan. *Anim Cogn* 2020 Jul;23(4):795–805. doi: 10.1007/s10071-020-01385-0. Epub 2020 Apr 30. PMID: 32356029; PMCID: PMC7384235.
2. Turcsán B, Kubinyi E. Differential behavioral aging trajectories according to body size, expected lifespan, and head shape in dogs. *Geroscience* 2024 Apr;46(2):1731–1754. doi: 10.1007/s11357-023-00945-9. Epub 2023 Sep 23. PMID: 37740[illegible]0; PMCID: PMC10828231.
3. Sordo L, Breheny C, Halls V, Cotter A, Tørnqvist-Johnsen C, Caney SMA, Gunn-Moore DA. Prevalence of disease and age-related behavioural changes in cats: past and present. *Vet Sci* 2020 Jul 6;7(3):85. doi: 10.3390/vetsci7030085. PMID: 32640581; PMCID: PMC7557453.
4. Mondino A, Catanzariti M, Mateos DM, Khan M, Ludwig C, Kis A, Gruen ME, Olby NJ. Sleep and cognition in aging dogs. A polysomnographic study. *Front Vet Sci* 2023 Apr 28;10:1151266. doi: 10.3389/fvets.2023.1151266. PMID 37187924; PMCID: PMC10175583.
5. Wrightson R, Albertini M, Pirrone F, McPeake E, Piotti P. The relationship between signs of medical conditions and cognitive decline in senior dogs. Animals 2023 Jul 5;13(13):2203. doi: 10.3390/ani13132203. PMID: 37443999; PMCID: PMC10340034.
6. Gunn-Moore D, Moffat K, Christie LA, Head E. Cognitive dysfunction and the neurobiology of ageing in cats. *J Small Anim Pract* 2007 Oct;48(10):546–553. doi: 10.1111/j.1748-5827.2007.00386.x. Epub 2007 Jul 6. PMID: 17617164.
7. Head E, Nukala VN, Fenoglio KA, Muggenburg BA, Cotman CW, Sullivan PG. Effects of age, dietary, and behavioral enrichment on brain mitochondria in a canine model of human aging. *Exp Neurol* 2009 Nov;220(1):171–176. doi: 10.1016/j.expneurol.2009.08.014. Epub 2009 Aug 22. PMID: 19703441; PMCID: PMC2761532.

Author/editor: Heidi Lobprise
Topic adapted from Five Minute Veterinary Consultation, 7th edition, 2021
Original Topic: Cognitive Dysfunction Syndrome/Canine Cognitive Dysfunction (CCD)

Authors: Gary M. Landsberg and Sagi Denenberg
Consulting Editor: Gary M. Landsberg

Chapter 7

Excessive Vocalization

BASICS

DEFINITION

- Vocalization that is uncontrollable, excessive, at inappropriate times of day or night (night-time waking), or that disrupts owners, neighbors, or other animals.

PATHOPHYSIOLOGY

- Cats are crepuscular, so early morning waking may be normal.
- May be due to medical conditions that cause anxiety, discomfort, irritability, or altered sleep–wake cycles.
- Hearing decline may be associated with increased vocalization.
- Cognitive dysfunction syndrome (CDS) can lead to sleep disturbances, anxiety, and excessive vocalization.
- Night waking may be due to a change in schedule, environment, or activity, especially in senior pets that are more sensitive to change.

SYSTEMS AFFECTED

- Behavioral.

SIGNALMENT

Species

Dog and cat.

Mean Age and Range

- Senior pets may be more prone to vocalization and night waking due to underlying medical conditions.

SIGNS

Historical Findings

- Sleeping pattern altered—does not fall asleep at bedtime, awakens during the night, or sleeps more during the day.

Blackwell's Five-Minute Veterinary Consult Clinical Companion: Small Animal Senior Care, First Edition. Edited by Heidi B. Lobprise.

Companion website: www.wiley.com/go/lobprise/Senior

- Pets with CDS may pace, wander aimlessly, have decreased interest in social interactions, be less responsive to stimuli, and increasingly anxious.
- Additional signs related to medical causes.

Physical Examination Findings

Signs associated with underlying medical issues.

CAUSES

- Vocalization and night waking—medical: gastrointestinal, metabolic (renal, hepatic), urogenital, CNS disorders, CDS, hypertension, hyperadrenocorticism or hypothyroidism (dog), hyperthyroidism (cat), pain, sensory decline.
- Night waking and vocalization
    - Normal crepuscular rhythm—cat.
    - Changes in routine and/or environment—insufficient enrichment/scheduling.
    - Owner inadvertently reinforces – increased anxiety when punished

RISK FACTORS

- Increasing age.
- Changes in schedule or environment.

DIAGNOSIS

DIFFERENTIAL DIAGNOSIS

Sleep disorders.

CBC/BIOCHEMISTRY/URINALYSIS

To determine if underlying medical cause.

OTHER LABORATORY TESTS

- T_4 and blood pressure—senior cats
- Rule out hypothyroidism and hyperadrenocorticism in dogs.

IMAGING

To rule out medical/neurologic if indicated.

DIAGNOSTIC PROCEDURES

- Behavioral diagnosis based on history; observation of pet, owner, and their interactions; video if available.
- Intraocular pressure.
- Brainstem auditory-evoked response (BAER) if indicated to rule out auditory decline.

TREATMENT

APPROPRIATE HEALTH CARE

If any medical issues.

NURSING CARE

If any medical issues.

ACTIVITY

Ensure behavioral needs (e.g., social interactions, exercise, elimination, routine, and mental stimulation) are adequately met each day.

DIET

- Feed from toys to encourage normal hunting and scavenging behaviors.
- Timed feeders and multiple small meals.

CLIENT EDUCATION

Individualize for the pet, home, and problem.

Behavior Modification

- Provide a quiet and calm environment for security, rest, and sleep.
- Owner anxiety, verbal reprimands, and punishment may increase anxiety and potentiate barking.
- Interrupting vocalization by directing into an alternative behavior may help to achieve quiet, which can then be reinforced; however, aversive techniques may increase anxiety.

Environmental Modification

Modify environment to avoid or minimize exposure to stimuli that incite vocalization or wake the pet, e.g., covered crate, quiet room, thunder cap, classical music, white noise, or fan.

SURGICAL CONSIDERATIONS

N/A

MEDICATIONS

DRUG(S) OF CHOICE

- Short term or as needed for situations of anxiety or for inducing sleep.
- Benzodiazepines—dog: clonazepam 0.05–0.25 mg/kg, diazepam 0.5–2.2 mg/kg; cat: oxazepam 0.2–0.5 mg/kg, alprazolam 0.125–0.25 mg/cat, clonazepam 0.02–0.2 mg/kg.
- Trazodone—dog: 5–10 mg/kg; cat: 25–50 mg/cat.

- Gabapentin—dog: 20–30 mg/kg; cat: 50–100 mg/cat.
- Melatonin—dog: 3–6 mg and cat: 1.5–12 mg.
- For ongoing therapy for chronic anxiety or compulsive disorders—clomipramine (tricyclic antidepressant [TCA]): dog: 1–3 mg/kg PO q12h, cat: 0.5–1 mg/kg PO q24h; fluoxetine or paroxetine (selective serotonin reuptake inhibitors [SSRIs]): dog: 1–2 mg/kg PO q24h, cat: 0.5–1.5 mg/kg PO q24h.
- Natural products that might be used adjunctively for anxiety—Adaptil®, Feliway®, l-theanine, alpha-casozepine, Harmonease®, *S*-adenosyl-L-methionine-tosylate disulfate (SAMe), or aromatherapy (lavender).
- For CDS—selegiline and cognitive supplements (see Cognitive Dysfunction Syndrome).

CONTRAINDICATIONS

Review contraindications and side effects for each drug used.

PRECAUTIONS

- Caution with drugs that might sedate in elderly pets.
- Monitor for undesirable behavioral effects.
- Avoid anticholinergic drugs in pets with CDS.

POSSIBLE INTERACTIONS

Do not use SSRIs and TCAs together with monoamine oxide (MAO) inhibitors such as selegiline and amitraz, and use cautiously or avoid with buspirone and tramadol.

ALTERNATIVE DRUG(S)

- Concurrent sedation with acepromazine 0.5–2.2 mg/kg might be considered, but it is not anxiolytic and may increase noise sensitivity and vocalization.
- For a less sedating anxiolytic consider buspirone at 0.5–1 mg/kg (dogs: q8–12h; cats: q12h).
- Analgesics for pain control.

FOLLOW-UP

PATIENT MONITORING

Modify the program based on response to therapy.

PREVENTION/AVOIDANCE

Train calm and settle on cue (sit, down, go to mat).

POSSIBLE COMPLICATIONS

- Night-time waking can lead to fatigue, increased irritability, and possibly aggression.
- Both night waking and vocalization can be particularly distressing to the pet owner's health and wellbeing and greatly weaken the bond.

EXPECTED COURSE AND PROGNOSIS

- Variable—based on diagnosis, environment, pet, and owner expectations.
- Most can be improved over time, but might not be eliminated.

MISCELLANEOUS

Associated Conditions

CDS

Age-Related Factors

Increased anxiety and night waking more common in senior pets.

Synonyms

Sleep disturbances.

See Also

- Cognitive Disorders

Abbreviations

- BAER = brainstem auditory-evoked response
- CDS = cognitive dysfunction syndrome.
- MAO = monoamine oxide.
- SAMe = *S*-adenosyl-L-methionine-tosylate disulfate.
- SSRI = selective serotonin reuptake inhibitor.
- TCA = tricyclic antidepressant.

Suggested Reading

Landsberg GM, DePorter T, Araujo JA. Management of anxiety, sleeplessness and cognitive dysfunction in the senior pet. *Vet Clin North Am Small Anim Pract* 2011;41(3):565–590.

Horwitz DF (ed.). *Blackwell's Five-Minute Veterinary Consult Clinical Companion: Canine and Feline Behavior*, 2nd edn. Hoboken, NJ: Wiley, 2018; pp. 885–894.

Author/editor: Heidi Lobprise
Topic adapted from Five Minute Veterinary Consultation, 7th edition, 2021
Original Topic: Excessive Vocalization and Waking at Night—Dogs and Cats

Authors: Sagi Denenberg and Gary M. Landsberg
Consulting Editor: Gary M. Landsberg

Chapter 8

Housesoiling

BASICS

DEFINITION

Urination and/or defecation, in locations that owners consider inappropriate.

PATHOPHYSIOLOGY

- Anxiety.
- Cognitive dysfunction.

SYSTEMS AFFECTED

Behavioral—shelter relinquishment, euthanasia, or rehoming.

INCIDENCE/PREVALENCE

- Approximately 15% in general population, specific senior/geriatric data not available
- Housesoiling is a common reason to see a veterinary behaviorist.

SIGNALMENT

Species

Dog

Mean Age and Range

- Housesoiling is a common complaint from owners of elderly dogs.

SIGNS

General Comments

- Inappropriate elimination is the most common individual reason for shelter relinquishment.
- Housesoiling can be associated with medical problems.

Blackwell's Five-Minute Veterinary Consult Clinical Companion: Small Animal Senior Care,
First Edition. Edited by Heidi B. Lobprise.

Companion website: www.wiley.com/go/lobprise/senior

Historical Findings

- History of urination and/or defecation in inappropriate areas.
- May be associated with signs of other behavioral disorders (such as separation anxiety)
- May be associated a change in behavior—cognitive issues of forgetting where to go
- May be associated with mobility issues—unable to make it through a "doggy door" due to osteoarthritis

Physical Examination Findings

- If examination findings and laboratory results are normal, housesoiling is more likely due to a behavioral cause.
- There may have been an inciting medical cause that has been resolved, but the animal continues to eliminate inappropriately.

CAUSES

Canine inappropriate elimination can be due to a primary behavioral problem or secondary to/concurrent with a medical disorder. Medical causes should be ruled out if a previously house-trained dog begins to soil.

Behavioral

- Separation anxiety.
- Cognitive dysfunction syndrome.

Medical Causes

Degenerative

- Osteoarthritis.
- Renal failure.
- Neuromuscular.

Metabolic/Endocrine

- Incontinence.
- Diabetes mellitus.
- Diabetes insipidus.
- Hepatic insufficiency.
- Hyperadrenocorticism.
- Hypoadrenocorticism.
- Neurologic.

Neoplastic

- Genitourinary neoplasia.
- Neurologic.
- Other neoplastic diseases causing weakness.

Infectious/Inflammatory

- Urinary tract infection or inflammation.
- Crystalluria with cystitis.
- Inflammatory bowel disorder.
- Pancreatic disease.
- Intestinal parasites.

RISK FACTORS

- Concurrent behavioral problem, such as separation anxiety or cognitive dysfunction.

DIAGNOSIS

DIFFERENTIAL DIAGNOSIS

Differentiate behavioral causes of inappropriate elimination from medical causes (see Causes) with a proper workup.

CBC/BIOCHEMISTRY/URINALYSIS

Indicated to rule out medical causes.

DIAGNOSTIC PROCEDURES

- Complete behavioral and medical history, including household layout and locations soiled.
- Videorecording when the owner is present to view household interactions with the dog.
- Journal to monitor potential causal factors, as well as to monitor improvement of the problem.
- Videorecording when the owner is gone from the home to rule in/out separation anxiety or other anxiety disorders.

TREATMENT

APPROPRIATE HEALTH CARE

Appropriate measures to assure continued good health of the dog.

ACTIVITY

- Take dog outside often on a schedule to ensure enough access to eliminate outside, or provide acceptable access to the outside, e.g., via a dog door if the dog is trained properly; monitor posturing during defecation to make sure discomfort/osteoarthritis does not cause them to interrupt elimination

DIET

- If the dog is inappropriately eliminating stool, feeding scheduled meals may help to maintain the dog on a schedule of elimination.
- Feeding a diet of higher caloric density may help decrease the urge to defecate as frequently.
- Water should not be withheld.

CLIENT EDUCATION

General Comments

- Counsel the owner as to the cause(s) of the inappropriate elimination, as well as potential long-term management of the problem.
- Treat underlying/contributing medical problems.
- Treat other underlying/contributing behavioral problems.
- Counsel owners not to use punishment-based or aversive training methods—punishment creates fear, anxiety, and stress, which can increase housesoiling.
- Clean the soiled areas with an enzymatic cleaner to help eliminate any odor that may attract the dog to eliminate there again; if the soiled object is a piece of clothing or other smaller cloth object, such as a throw rug, wash it.
- Change the significance of the soiled area, such as by feeding the dog in the area.

MEDICATIONS

DRUG(S) OF CHOICE

- Selective serotonin reuptake inhibitors (SSRIs), tricyclic antidepressants (TCAs)/anti-anxiety medications, or other anti-anxiety medications may be helpful, especially with underlying anxiety—SSRI: fluoxetine at 1–2 mg/kg PO q24h; TCA: clomipramine at 1–3 mg/kg PO q12h.
- For SSRIs and TCAs, the full onset of action can be 4–6 weeks after initiation of treatment; inform owners of time required for response to be noted.
- Side effects of SSRIs and TCAs can include nausea, vomiting, diarrhea, and lethargy.
- Additional side effects of TCAs can include potentiation of seizure activity.

CONTRAINDICATIONS

- Medication without concurrent behavior modification.
- Tricyclic antianxiety medications are contraindicated in seizures and cardiac disease, and may interfere with thyroid medications.

PRECAUTIONS

Based on drug chosen.

POSSIBLE INTERACTIONS

Do not use an SSRI and TCA together or in conjunction with a monoamine oxidase (MAO) inhibitor or opioid.

ALTERNATIVE DRUG(S)

Pheromones, or supplements containing alpha-casozepine, L-theanine, or a calming probiotic may help to decrease anxiety.

FOLLOW-UP

PATIENT MONITORING

Monitor with owner by follow-up visits or telephone calls. The owner should keep a journal of incidents, inciting factors, and treatments instituted to have an objective view of improvement.

PREVENTION/AVOIDANCE

- Monitor for signs and treat any underlying medical condition. • Treat any underlying behavioral condition.

POSSIBLE COMPLICATIONS

Recurrence if owner relapses in treatment, perhaps pet relinquishment.

EXPECTED COURSE AND PROGNOSIS

- Prognosis for any behavioral problem is highly dependent on an owner's ability and willingness to follow guidance—the following estimations of prognosis are based on the owner's ability and commitment to follow instructions.
- Some animals with a medical cause of inappropriate elimination will still eliminate inappropriately after the medical cause has been treated due to learning (e.g., self-reinforcing, new location preferences).

MISCELLANEOUS

Age-Related Factors

- Cognitive dysfunction becomes more likely as the dog ages.

See Also

- Cognitive Disorders
- Environmental Enrichment and Adjustment
- Mobility in Senior Pets

Abbreviations

- MAO = monoamine oxidase.
- SSRI = selected serotonin reuptake inhibitor.
- TCA = tricyclic antidepressant.

Internet Resources

Accessed 29 June 2024

- https://www.dacvb.org
- https://avsab.org

Suggested Reading

Col R, Day C, Phillips CJC. An epidemiological analysis of dog behavior problems presented to an Australian behavior clinic, with associated risk factors. *J Vet Behav* 2016;15:1–11.

Horwitz D (ed.). *Blackwell's Five-Minute Veterinary Consult Clinical Companion: Canine and Feline Behavior*, 2nd edn. Ames, IA: Wiley-Blackwell, 2018; pp. 655–667.

Horwitz DF, Ciribassi J, Dale S (eds). *Decoding Your Dog: The Ultimate Experts Explain Common Dog Behaviors and Reveal How to Prevent or Change Unwanted Ones*. Boston, MA: Houghton Mifflin Harcourt, 2014.

Landsberg G, Hunthausen W, Ackerman L. *Handbook of Behavior Problems of the Dog and Cat*, 3rd edn. Philadelphia, PA: Saunders, 2012.

Author/editor: Heidi Lobprise
Topic adapted from Five Minute Veterinary Consultation, 7th edition, 2021
Original Topic: Housesoiling

Author: Melissa J. Bain
Consulting Editor: Gary M. Landsberg

Cardiovascular

Chapter 9

Aortic Thromboembolism

BASICS

DEFINITION

Embolization of a thrombus (blood clot) that is lodged within the aorta or peripheral artery, causing severe ischemia to the tissues served by that arterial segment.

PATHOPHYSIOLOGY

- Commonly associated with heart disease in cats and dogs; can also occur in association with other hypercoagulable conditions such as protein losing enteropathy or nephropathy.

SYSTEMS AFFECTED

- Cardiovascular—most affected cats have advanced heart disease and left heart failure.
- Nervous/musculoskeletal—severe ischemia to muscles and nerves served by segment of occluded aorta causes variable pain and paresis. Gait abnormality or paralysis results in leg or legs involved.

GENETICS

HCM, a common associated disease, is likely heritable. Additionally, a family of domestic shorthair cats with remodeled HCM who all died of ATE has been reported.

INCIDENCE/PREVALENCE

- In a recent observation study of over 1000 asymptomatic cats with HCM, nearly 12% developed ATE within 10 years after initial diagnosis. In two previous smaller case series of cats with clinical and preclinical HCM, 12–16% presented with signs of ATE; only 11–25% of cats had evidence of previously known heart disease.
- Rare in dogs.

Blackwell's Five-Minute Veterinary Consult Clinical Companion: Small Animal Senior Care, First Edition. Edited by Heidi B. Lobprise.

Companion website: www.wiley.com/go/lobprise/Senior

SIGNALMENT

Species

Cat, rarely dog.

Breed Predilections

Mixed-breed cats most commonly affected. Abyssians, Birmans, and ragdolls over-represented in one study. In dogs, no breed predilection identified in United States; European study suggested cavalier King Charles spaniels may be overrepresented.

Mean Age and Range

Age range—1–20 years. Median age—approximately 8–9 years (cats); 8–10 years (dogs).

Predominant Sex

Cats—males > females (2 : 1). Dogs—no sex predilection in United States; European study suggested male predilection.

SIGNS

Presence of 5 "Ps" is helpful to remember classic clinical signs associated with ATE—Pain, Paralysis or Paresis, Pulselessness, Pallor, and Poikilothermic (cold).

Historical Findings

- Acute-onset paralysis and pain—most common in cats. Vocalization and anxiety also common.
- Lameness or gait abnormality, typically of several weeks' duration, more common in dogs.
- Tachypnea or respiratory distress common in cats.
- About 15% of cats may vomit prior to ATE.

Physical Examination Findings

- Usually paraparesis or paralysis of rear legs with signs of lower motor neuron injury. Less commonly, monoparesis of a front leg. In dogs, majority are paretic and ambulatory.
- Absent or diminished femoral pulses.
- Pain upon palpation of legs.
- Gastrocnemius muscle often becomes firm several hours after embolization.
- Cyanotic or pale nail beds and foot pads.
- Tachypnea/dyspnea and hypothermia are common in cats.
- Since commonly associated with heart disease in cats, cardiac murmur, arrhythmias, or gallop sound may be present.

CAUSES

- Cardiomyopathy (all types).
- Hyperthyroidism.
- Neoplasia.
- Sepsis (dogs).
- Hyperadrenocorticism (dogs).
- Protein-losing nephropathy and enteropathy (dogs).

RISK FACTORS

- In cats, cardiomyopathy, male sex, and gallop sound on exam are risk factors. Echocardiographic risk factors include enlarged left atrium, decreased left atrial function and left atrial appendage velocity, presence of spontaneous echocardiographic contrast (smoke) or left atrial thrombus, and restrictive left ventricular filling pattern.
- In dogs, hypercoagulable conditions, such as neoplasia, sepsis, endocarditis, protein-losing nephropathies/enteropathies, and hyperadrenocorticism, are risk factors.

DIAGNOSIS

DIFFERENTIAL DIAGNOSIS

Hind limb paresis secondary to spinal neoplasia, trauma, myelitis, fibrocartilaginous infarction, or intervertebral disc protrusion. These conditions resulting in spinal cord injury present with signs of upper motor neuron disease, whereas ATE patients present with signs of lower motor neuron disease.

CBC/BIOCHEMISTRY/URINALYSIS

- High creatine kinase due to muscle injury.
- Higher blood lactate and lower blood glucose in affected limbs compared to normal limbs.
- High aspartate aminotransferase and alanine aminotransferase due to muscle and liver injury.
- Stress hyperglycemia.
- High blood urea nitrogen and creatinine due to low cardiac output and possible renal emboli.
- Electrolyte derangements, due to low output and muscle damage, such as hypocalcemia, hyponatremia, hyperphosphatemia, and hyperkalemia, are not uncommon.
- Nonspecific CBC and urinalysis changes.

OTHER LABORATORY TESTS

Routinely available coagulation profiles typically do not reveal significant abnormalities because hypercoagulability results from hyperaggregable platelets. In dogs, thromboelastography may suggest hypercoagulable state with clot strength (increased maximum amplitude) or shortened clotting time (decreased R).

IMAGING

Radiography

- Cardiomegaly is common in cats.
- Pulmonary edema and/or pleural effusion in approximately 50% of cats.
- Rarely, a mass is seen in the lungs, suggestive of neoplasia.

Echocardiography

- In cats, changes consistent with cardiomyopathy. HCM is most common, followed by restrictive or unclassified cardiomyopathy, and then dilated cardiomyopathy.

- Most cases have severe left atrial enlargement (i.e., left-atrial-to-aortic ratio of ≥2). Decreased left atrial function (fractional shortening) and decreased left atrial appendage velocity (<0.2 m/s).
- Left atrial thrombus or spontaneous echocardiographic contrast (smoke) may be seen.

Abdominal Ultrasonography

- May be able to identify the thrombus and visualize lack of blood flow in the caudal aorta.
- Typically unnecessary to reach a diagnosis in cats, but often needed to reach a diagnosis in dogs.

DIAGNOSTIC PROCEDURES

ECG

- Sinus rhythm and sinus tachycardia most common. Less common rhythms include atrial fibrillation, ventricular arrhythmias, supraventricular arrhythmias, and sinus bradycardia.
- Left ventricular enlargement pattern and left ventricular conduction disturbances (left anterior fascicular block) are common.

Doppler Blood Pressure

No or diminished audible blood flow in affected limbs.

TREATMENT

APPROPRIATE HEALTH CARE

Initially, cats with ATE should be treated as inpatients, as many have concurrent congestive heart failure (CHF) and require injectable drugs, in addition to being in considerable pain and distress.

NURSING CARE

- Fluid therapy is cautiously used, as most cats have advanced myocardial disease. If in CHF, IV fluids may not be necessary.
- Supplemental oxygen or thoracocentesis may be beneficial if in CHF.
- Initially, minimally handle affected legs. However, as reperfusion occurs, physical therapy (passive extension and flexion) may speed full recovery.
- Do not perform venipuncture on affected legs.
- Animals may have difficulty posturing to urinate and may need bladder expression to prevent overdistention or urine scald.

ACTIVITY

Restrict activity and stress.

DIET

Initially, most cats are anorexic; tempt with any type of diet to keep them eating and avoid hepatic lipidosis.

CLIENT EDUCATION

- Short- and long-term prognosis is poor in both dogs and cats.
- Many cats do not survive their initial episode of ATE; if they survive, the cat will often reembolize or die of CHF within a few months to 1 year. Most cats that survive an initial episode will be on some type of anticoagulant and heart failure medications that may require frequent reevaluation and an indoor lifestyle.
- Most cats that survive an initial episode will recover complete function to the legs; however, if ischemia is severe and prolonged, sloughing of parts of the distal extremities or persistent neurologic deficits may result. In one study, approximately 15% of cats had permanent neuromuscular abnormalities after surviving the initial ATE.
- Prognosis in dogs is generally poor but may be better in dogs presenting with chronic (vs. acute) lameness and dogs treated appropriately with warfarin.

SURGICAL CONSIDERATIONS

- Surgical embolectomy typically not recommended, since patients are high risk due to severe heart disease.
- Rheolytic thrombectomy has been used with limited success in a small number of cats with ATE.

MEDICATIONS

DRUG(S) OF CHOICE

Medical management focuses on (1) the thrombus, (2) analgesia, and (3) heart failure treatments (if needed).

Management of Thrombus

- Thrombolytic therapy (e.g., tissue plasminogen activator [TPA]) is used extensively in humans and infrequently in animals. These drugs are expensive and carry a significant risk for bleeding complications; to date, improved treatment efficacy is unproven and thus they are rarely used in general practice. TPA is theorized to be more beneficial if given early, ideally within the first few hours of the ATE.
- Unfractionated heparin is the preferred anticoagulant in general practice for initial management of feline ATE. Heparin has no effect on the established clot; however, it prevents further activation of the coagulation cascade. In either cat or dog, use an initial dose of 100–200 units/kg IV and then 200–300 units/kg SC q8h. Alternatively, heparin can be continued as a constant rate infusion, at a dose of 25–35 units/kg/h. Some advocate titrating the dose to prolong the activated partial thromboplastin time (APTT) approximately twofold.
- Clopidogrel is an antiplatelet aggregation drug. A loading dose may be chosen for treatment of an acute ATE. The loading dose in the cat is 75 mg/cat PO once, and then a maintenance dose of 18.75 mg/cat (one-fourth of a 75 mg tablet) PO q24h. The loading dose in the dog is approximately 10 mg/kg once, and then a maintenance dose of 1 mg/kg q24h. Compared to aspirin, clopidogrel was superior in preventing reembolization, resulting in improved survival times in cats that had survived an ATE. The combination of unfractionated heparin and clopidogrel is commonly used for the management of ATE in cats

Other Options

- Aspirin is theoretically beneficial during and after an ATE event due to its antiplatelet effects. The dose in cats is an 81 mg tablet PO q48–72h. Vomiting and diarrhea are not uncommon. Some specialists advocate a mini dose of 5 mg/cat q72h. Antithrombotic dose recommendations for dogs range from 0.5 to 2 mg/kg q24h. Always give aspirin with food.
- Warfarin, a vitamin K antagonist, is the anticoagulant most widely used in humans and has been proposed for prevention of reembolization in cats surviving an initial episode. The initial dose is 0.25–0.5 mg/cat PO q24h, or 0.05–0.2 mg/kg PO q24h in the dog. Overlap with heparin therapy for 3 days. The dose is then adjusted to prolong the prothrombin time (PT) approximately twice its baseline value, or to attain an international normalized ratio (INR) of 2–3. Long-term management with warfarin can be challenging because of frequent monitoring and dose adjustments in addition to bleeding complications. In one study, dogs treated appropriately with warfarin had a better clinical outcome.
- • Low-molecular-weight heparin (LMWH) has recently been proposed for the long-term prevention of feline ATE. LMWH has a more predictable relationship between dose and response than warfarin and does not need monitoring or dose adjustments. It also has a lower risk of bleeding complications. The main disadvantages are high drug cost and the injectable route of administration. The two LMWHs that have been used in feline ATE are dalteparin (100–150 units/kg SC q8–24h) and enoxaparin (1 mg/kg SC q12–24h). The best dose is unknown. LMWH is usually started q24h due to cost. Some studies suggest q6h dosing is necessary for stable blood levels, but may increase bleeding risk. LMWH can be used as an adjunctive anticoagulant combined with clopidogrel.
- Rivaroxaban, a newer anticoagulant drug, is an inhibitor of activated clotting factor X and prothrombinase activity that has shown promise for treatment and prevention of arterial thromboembolism in both dogs and cats. Rivaroxaban has a more predictable anticoagulant effect than warfarin and does not require any monitoring or dose adjustments. The cat dose is 1.25 mg/cat PO q24h. The dose recommended in dogs is 0.5–1 mg/kg PO q24h. The main disadvantage of rivaroxaban is its high cost at the time of this writing. However, it has the advantage of a shorter half-time than clopidogrel if there is a need to discontinue the medication because of a bleeding complication or need to perform an invasive procedure. A clinical trial is currently ongoing to compare rivaroxaban and clopidogrel in cats that have survived an ATE.

Analgesics

- Buprenorphine in the cat is a useful and widely available drug for analgesia and sedation at a dose of 5–20 μg/kg IV, SC, or in cheek pouch q6–8h. For stronger analgesia, use fentanyl or hydromorphone. Butorphanol, while a good sedative, does not provide sufficient analgesia.
- Acepromazine may be cautiously used for its sedative and vasodilatory properties at a dose of 0.01–0.02 mg SC q8–12h. However, vasodilatory effects are mixed, and therefore results are often variable.

PRECAUTIONS

- Anticoagulant therapy with heparin, warfarin, or thrombolytics may cause bleeding complications.
- Avoid a nonselective beta blocker such as propranolol as it may enhance peripheral vasoconstriction.

POSSIBLE INTERACTIONS

Warfarin may interact with other drugs, which may enhance its anticoagulant effects.

FOLLOW-UP

PATIENT MONITORING

- ECG monitoring while cat in hospital is helpful to detect reperfusion injury and hyperkalemia-related ECG changes. Look for loss of P-waves and widening of QRS complexes.
- Monitoring electrolytes and renal parameters periodically may be helpful to optimize management of cardiac disease.
- Examine legs frequently to assess clinical response. Initially, APTT should be performed once daily to titrate heparin dose.
- If warfarin used, PT or INR is measured approximately 3 days after initiation of therapy and then weekly until desired anticoagulant effect reached. Thereafter, measure 3–4 times yearly or when drug regimen is altered.

PREVENTION/AVOIDANCE

Because of high rate of reembolization, prevention with either clopidogrel aspirin, warfarin, or LMWH is strongly recommended.

POSSIBLE COMPLICATIONS

- Bleeding with anticoagulant therapy.
- Permanent neurologic deficits or muscular abnormalities in hind limbs may arise with prolonged ischemia.
- Recurrent CHF or sudden death.
- Reperfusion injury and death usually associated with hyperkalemic arrhythmias.

EXPECTED COURSE AND PROGNOSIS

- Expected course is days to weeks for full recovery of function to legs.
- Prognosis both short and long term, is poor in cats.
- In two large studies, ~60% of cats were euthanized or died during initial thromboembolic episode. Long-term prognosis varies between 2 months and several years; however, average is a few months with treatment. Predictors of poorer prognosis include hypothermia (<99 °F) and CHF. One study demonstrated median survival time of 77 days in cats with CHF and 223 days in cats without CHF. Predictors of better prognosis include normothermia, single leg affected, and presence of motor function on initial exam.
- In dogs, the disease is rare and prognosis in general is also poor. One study suggested a better prognosis if the dog had chronic clinical signs and if treated with warfarin.
- Recurrence of ATE is common.

MISCELLANEOUS

Abbreviations

- APTT = activated partial thromboplastin time
- ATE = aortic thromboembolism.
- CHF = congestive heart failure.
- HCM = hypertrophic cardiomyopathy.
- INR = international normalized ratio.
- LMWH = low-molecular-weight heparin.
- PT = prothrombin time.
- TPA = tissue plasminogen activator.

Suggested Reading

Luis Fuentes V. Arterial thromboembolism: risks, realities and a rational first-line approach. *J Feline Med Surg* 2012;14(7):459–470.

Winter RL, Sedacca CD, Adams A, Orton EC. Aortic thrombosis in dogs: presentation, therapy, and outcome in 26 cases. *J Vet Cardiol* 2012;14:333–342.

Author/editor: Heidi Lobprise
Thanks to: Gary Oswald for review
Topic adapted from Five Minute Veterinary Consultation, 7th edition, 2021
Original Topic: Aortic Thromboembolism

Author: Teresa C. DeFrancesco
Consulting Editor: Michael Aherne

Chapter 10

Arrhythmias

BASICS

DEFINITION

- Irregular heartbeat/rate due to electrical conductions abnormalities of the heart
  - Sick Sinus Syndrome—a disorder of impulse formation within, and conduction out of, the sinus node;
  - Atrioventricular block, second degree—Mobitz Type II (AV Block II Mobitz II)—refers to failure of one or more P waves, but not all P waves, to be conducted; when one or more P waves are blocked without a preceding progressive delay in AV transmission.
    - AV block, second degree—Mobitz Type I—PR interval becomes progressively longer prior to the appearance of a P wave that is not followed by a QRS complex; usually results from conduction delay within the AV node itself. Generally not pathologic or hemodynamically significant. (see Miscellaneous)
  - Atrioventricular block, complete (third degree)—All atrial impulses are blocked at the atrioventricular (AV) junction; atria and ventricles beat independently. A secondary "escape" pacemaker site (junctional or ventricular) stimulates the ventricles.
    - Atrial rate normal.
    - Idioventricular escape rhythm slow.
  - Many other arrhythmias can impact animals of all ages; these have been selected due to their impact in older dogs and cats. See Miscellaneous for additional information.

ECG Features

- SSS—inappropriate sinus bradycardia, sinus pauses, slow ectopic atrial rhythm or alternating periods of sinus bradyarrhythmias and supraventricular tachycardia (SVT); P waves and QRS complexes usually normal though P waves may be abnormal or absent.
- AV Block II—Mobitz II
  - One or more P waves not followed by a QRS complex; PR interval is constant but may be either normal or consistently prolonged.
  - Ventricular rate—usually slow.
  - Fixed ratio of P waves to QRS complexes may occur (e.g., 2 : 1, 3 : 1, 4 : 1 AV block).
  - High-grade (advanced) second-degree AV block is characterized by two or more consecutively blocked P waves.
  - In second-degree AV block with a 2 : 1 conduction ratio or higher, it is impossible to observe prolongation of the PR interval before the block, so a designation of Mobitz type I vs. II is not appropriate.

Blackwell's Five-Minute Veterinary Consult Clinical Companion: Small Animal Senior Care,
First Edition. Edited by Heidi B. Lobprise.

Companion website: www.wiley.com/go/lobprise/Senior

- QRS complexes may appear normal, but may also be wide or have an abnormal morphology due to aberrant intraventricular conduction or ventricular enlargement.
- Abnormally wide QRS complexes may indicate serious, extensive cardiac disease.

■ AV Block III—
- Ventricular rate slower than atrial rate (more P waves than QRS complexes)—ventricular escape rhythm (idioventricular) usually <40 bpm; junctional escape rhythm (idiojunctional) 40–60 bpm in dogs and 60–100 bpm in cats.
- P waves—usually normal configuration.
- QRS complex—wide and bizarre when pacemaker located in the ventricle, or in the lower AV junction in a patient with bundle branch block; normal when escape pacemaker in the lower AV junction (above the bifurcation of the bundle of His) in a patient without bundle branch block.
- No conduction between the atria and the ventricles; P waves have no constant relationship with QRS complexes; P–P and R–R intervals relatively constant (except for a sinus arrhythmia).

PATHOPHYSIOLOGY

■ SSS—ECG changes may precede signs resulting from failure of subsidiary pacemakers to generate escape rhythms if sinus node fails; transient decreases in organ perfusion (cerebral and skeletal muscle); rarely CHF develops

■ AV Block II—Mobitz II
- Rare in healthy animals.
- May be hemodynamically important when ventricular rate is abnormally slow.
- May progress to complete AV block, particularly when accompanied by wide QRS complexes.
- Typically this type of AV block results from conduction delay within the AV node itself (rather than delay in another segment of the AV conducting system) that is characterized by normal or prolonged AH intervals, with intermittent block between A and H deflections on a His bundle electrogram.

■ AV Block III
- Slow ventricular escape rhythms (<40 bpm) result in low cardiac output and eventual heart failure, often when animal is excited or exercised, since demand for greater cardiac output is not satisfied. As the heart fails, signs increase with mild activity.

SYSTEMS AFFECTED

Cardiovascular

GENETICS

■ SSS

■ AV Block II Mobitz II - may be... (with indent)

■ AV block III

SIGNALMENT

Species

Dog and cat.

Breed Predilections

- SSS—Miniature schnauzers, cocker spaniel, dachshund, and WHWT
- AV Block II—Mobitz II—American cocker spaniel, pug dachshund, Airedale terrier, Doberman pinscher
- AV Block III—
  - Cocker spaniel—can have idiopathic fibrosis.
  - Pug and Doberman pinscher—can have associated sudden death, AV conduction defects, and bundle of His lesions.

Mean Age and Range

- SSS—most dogs >6 years of age (mature)
- AV Block II, Mobitz II—generally occurs in older animals
- AV Block III—Geriatric animals, except congenital heart disease patients. Median age for cats—14 years.

Predominant Sex

- AV Block III and SSS—female dogs
- AV Block II Mobitz II—n/a

SIGNS

Historical Findings

- SSS
  - Clinical signs vary from asymptomatic to weakness, syncope, collapse, and/or seizures.
  - Sudden death is infrequent.
- AV Block II Mobitz II
  - Presenting complaint may be syncope, collapse, weakness, or lethargy.
  - Some animals are asymptomatic.
  - Animals may show signs of the underlying disease process if present.
- AV Block III
  - Exercise intolerance.
  - Weakness or syncope.
  - Occasionally, congestive heart failure (CHF).

Physical Examination Findings

- SSS
  - Heart rate may be abnormally rapid or abnormally slow.
  - Pauses may be noted.
  - Some patients appear normal.
- AV Block II, Mobitz II
  - ±Weakness.
  - Bradycardia common with intermittent pauses in the cardiac rhythm.
  - An S4 may be audible in lieu of the normally expected heart sounds (i.e., S1, S2) when the block occurs.
  - If associated with digoxin intoxication, there may be vomiting, anorexia, and diarrhea.
  - May be other abnormalities reflecting the underlying etiology.
- AV Block III

- Bradycardia.
- Variable third and fourth heart sounds.
- Variation in intensity of first heart sounds.
- Signs of CHF possible.
- Intermittent "cannon" A waves in jugular venous pulses.
- Often bounding arterial pulses.

CAUSES AND RISK FACTORS

- SSS
  - Idiopathic.
  - Familial in miniature schnauzers.
  - Metastatic disease.
  - Ischemic disease.
- AV Block II Mobitz II
  - Heritable in pugs.
  - Enhanced vagal stimulation from noncardiac diseases.
  - Degenerative change within the cardiac conduction system—replacement of AV nodal cells and/or Purkinje fibers by fibrotic and adipose tissue in old cats and dogs.
  - Pharmacologic agents (e.g., digoxin, β-adrenergic antagonists, calcium channel blocking agents, propafenone, α_2-adrenergic agonists, muscarinic cholinergic agonists, or severe procainamide or quinidine toxicity).
  - Infiltrative myocardial disorders (neoplasia, amyloid).
  - Endocarditis (particularly involving the aortic valve), myocarditis, cardiomyopathy in cats
- AV Block III
  - Isolated congenital defect.
  - Idiopathic fibrosis.
  - Infiltrative cardiomyopathy (amyloidosis or neoplasia).
  - Hypertrophic cardiomyopathy in cats.
  - Digitalis toxicity.
  - Hyperthyroidism in cats.
  - Myocarditis.
  - Endocarditis.
  - Electrolyte disorder.
  - Myocardial infarction.
  - Other congenital heart defects.
  - Lyme disease.
  - Chagas disease.

DIAGNOSIS

DIFFERENTIAL DIAGNOSIS

- SSS
  - Healthy dogs may exhibit sinus bradycardia (rate as low as 30 beats/min) and sinus pauses (as long as 3.5 seconds) normally during sleep.

- Bradycardia and sinus arrest due to normal or enhanced vagal tone.
- Drug-induced (digitalis, α-adrenergic antagonists, α_2-adrenergic agonists, calcium channel antagonists, cimetidine, opioids).
- Seizures or syncope due to noncardiac disease.
- Atrial standstill secondary to hyperkalemia or atrial disease.
- Weakness due to neurologic, musculoskeletal, or metabolic disease.

■ AV Block II Mobitz II
- High-grade (advanced) form must be distinguished from complete AV block.
- Nonconducted P waves arising from refractoriness of the conduction system during supraventricular tachycardias must be differentiated from pathologic conduction block.

■ AV Block III
- Advanced second-degree AV block.
- Atrial standstill.
- Accelerated idioventricular rhythm.

CBC/BIOCHEMISTRY/URINALYSIS

■ SSS—normal

■ AV Block II Mobitz II
- Serum electrolytes—hypokalemia and hyperkalemia may predispose to AV.
- Conduction disturbances.
- Leukocytosis—may be noted with bacterial endocarditis or myocarditis.
- Electrolyte abnormalities (e.g., severe hypokalemia, hyperkalemia, or hypercalcemia) may predispose to AV block.

■ AV Block III
- Abnormal serum electrolytes (e.g., hyperkalemia, hypokalemia) possible.
- High white blood cell count with left shift in animals with bacterial endocarditis.

OTHER LABORATORY TESTS

■ AV Block II Mobitz II
- Serum digoxin concentration—may be high.
- High thyroxine (T_4) in cats—if associated with hyperthyroidism.
- High arterial blood pressure—if associated with hypertensive heart disease.
- Positive *Borrelia*, *Rickettsia*, or *Trypanosoma cruzi* titers—if associated with one of these infectious agents.
- Blood cultures may be positive in patients with vegetative endocarditis.

■ AV Block III
- High serum digoxin concentration if AV block due to digoxin toxicity.
- Lyme titer and accompanying clinical signs if AV block due to Lyme disease.

IMAGING

■ SSS—Breeds predisposed to SSS are also predisposed to degenerative valvular disease; echocardiography may be used to confirm presence of significant valvular disease when heart murmur is present.

■ AV Block II Mobitz II—Echocardiographic examination may reveal structural heart disease (e.g., endocarditis, neoplasia, or cardiomyopathy).

- AV Block III—Echocardiography and Doppler ultrasound to assess cardiac structure and function.

DIAGNOSTIC PROCEDURES

- SSS
    - Atropine response testing—indicated in dogs with sinus bradycardia, sinus arrest, and sinoatrial exit block. Administer atropine 0.04 mg/kg IM and evaluate the ECG 20–30 minutes later. A normal (positive) response is >50% increase in heart rate with abolishment of pauses; dogs with SSS generally have no response or an incomplete response to atropine.
    - Electrophysiologic testing of sinus node recovery time and sinoatrial conduction time.
    - 24-hour ambulatory ECG (Holter) or event recording to correlate clinical signs with arrhythmia.
- AV Block II Mobitz II
    - Atropine response test—administer
    - 0.04 mg/kg atropine IM and repeat ECG in 20–30 minutes; may be used to determine whether AV block is due to high vagal tone.
    - Electrophysiologic testing is generally unnecessary, but can be done to confirm this type of AV block if surface ECG findings are equivocal.
- AV Block III
    - Electrocardiography.
    - His bundle electrogram to determine the site of the AV block is possible.
    - Long-term (Holter) ambulatory recording if AV block is intermittent.

PATHOLOGIC FINDINGS

- SSS—vary with cause
- AV Block II Mobitz II—Old animals with degenerative change of the conduction system may have focal mineralization of the interventricular septal crest visible grossly; chondroid metaplasia of the central fibrous body and increased fibrous connective tissue in the AV bundle is noted histopathologically.
- AV Block III—Degeneration or fibrosis of the AV node and its bundle branches, associated with endocardial and myocardial fibrosis and organized endomyocarditis.

TREATMENT

APPROPRIATE HEALTH CARE

- SSS
    - Hospitalization rarely necessary except for electrophysiologic testing or pacemaker implantation.
    - Do not treat asymptomatic animals.
- AV Block II—Mobitz II
    - Treatment—may be unnecessary if heart rate maintains adequate cardiac output.

- Positive dromotropic interventions are indicated for symptomatic patients.
- Treat or remove underlying cause(s).

- AV Block III
  - Temporary or permanent cardiac pacemaker—only effective treatment in symptomatic patients.
  - Carefully monitor asymptomatic patients without a pacemaker for development of clinical signs.

NURSING CARE

- AV Block III—Cage rest prior to pacemaker implantation; when the pulse generator is implanted into a subcutaneous pocket, a nonconstricting bandage is placed around the ventral neck or abdomen for 3–5 days to prevent seroma formation or pacemaker movement.

ACTIVITY

- SSS—avoid vigorous exercise and stressful situations
- AV Block II Mobitz II—cage rest advised for symptomatic patients
- AV Block III—Restrict if symptomatic.

DIET

- AV Block III and SSS: No modifications unless required to manage underlying condition (e.g., low-salt diet).

CLIENT EDUCATION

- SSS—owner should be aware that medical management is often ineffective
- AV Block II Mobitz II
  - Need to seek and specifically treat underlying cause.
  - Pharmacologic agents may not be effective long term
- AV Block III
  - Temporary or permanent cardiac pacemaker—only effective treatment in symptomatic patients.
  - Asymptomatic patients without a pacemaker—must be carefully monitored for development of clinical signs.

SURGICAL CONSIDERATIONS

- SSS
  - Permanent artificial pacemaker necessary for dogs failing to respond to medical treatment and those exhibiting unacceptable medication side effects.
  - Permanent artificial pacemaker usually required for dogs with bradycardia–tachycardia syndrome.
  - Transvenous placement of a pacing lead in the right atrium or auricle may successfully abolish the sinus pauses.
- AV Block II Mobitz II—Permanent pacemaker may be required for long-term management of symptomatic patients.

- AV Block III
  - Most patients—at high anesthetic cardiopulmonary risk; usually paced preoperatively with a temporary external pacemaker system.
  - The small size of cats makes pacemaker implantation more difficult than in dogs.

MEDICATIONS

DRUG(S) OF CHOICE

- SSS
  - Do not treat asymptomatic animals.
  - Symptomatic dogs are grouped into those showing primarily bradycardia, sinus arrest, and/or sinoatrial exit block and those with supraventricular tachycardia followed by sinus arrest.
  - Atropine-responsive symptomatic dogs with bradycardia or sinus arrest—anticholinergic agents (propantheline: small dogs, 3.75–7.5 mg PO q8–12h; medium dogs, 15 mg PO q8h; large dogs, 30 mg PO q8h; hyoscyamine: 3–6 µg/kg q8h).
  - Dogs with bradycardia and sinus arrest—may try theophylline (Theo-Dur) 20 mg/kg PO q12h, terbutaline 0.2 mg/kg PO q8–12h, or hydralazine 1–2 mg/kg PO q8–12h if anticholinergic drugs are ineffective (avoid hydralazine if patient is hypotensive).
  - Dogs with bradycardia–tachycardia whose clinical signs are due to tachycardia or tachycardia-induced sinus arrest—can give digoxin 5 µg/kg PO q12h or atenolol 0.5–1 mg/kg PO q12–24h in attempt to suppress the SVT (monitor closely for exacerbation of bradycardia).
  - Therapy for tachycardias should only be considered, once pacing is established to avoid worsening of bradyarrhythmias.
- AV Block II Mobitz II
  - Atropine (0.02–0.04 mg/kg IV/IM) or glycopyrrolate (5–10 µg/kg IV/IM) may be used short term if positive atropine response.
  - Chronic anticholinergic therapy (propantheline 0.5–2 mg/kg PO q8–12h or hyoscyamine 3–6 µg/kg q8h)—indicated for symptomatic patients if improved AV conduction with atropine response test.
  - Isoproterenol (0.04–0.09 µg/kg/min IV to effect) or dopamine (2–5 µg/kg/min IV to effect) may be administered in acute, life-threatening situations to enhance AV conduction and/or accelerate an escape focus
- AV Block III
  - Treatment with drugs—usually of no value. Traditionally used to treat complete AV block: atropine, isoproterenol, corticosteroids, and dobutamine.
  - Intravenous isoproterenol infusion may help increase the rate of the ventricular escape rhythm to stabilize hemodynamics.
  - If CHF—diuretic and vasodilator therapy may be needed before pacemaker implantation.

CONTRAINDICATIONS

- SSS
  - Avoid drugs that may worsen sinus node dysfunction (e.g., β-adrenergic antagonists, calcium-channel-blocking agents, phenothiazines, class I and III antiarrhythmic agents, opioids, cimetidine, α_2-adrenergic agonists).
- AV Block Mobitz II

- Drugs with vagomimetic action (e.g., digoxin, bethanechol, physostigmine, pilocarpine) may potentiate block.
- Avoid drugs likely to impair impulse conduction further or depress a ventricular escape focus (e.g., procainamide, quinidine, lidocaine, calcium-channel-blocking agents, β-adrenergic blocking agents).

■ AV Block III
- Avoid digoxin, xylazine, acepromazine, beta blockers (e.g., propranolol and atenolol), and calcium channel blockers (e.g., verapamil and diltiazem); ventricular antiarrhythmic agents are dangerous because they suppress lower escape foci.

PRECAUTIONS

■ SSS
- Attempts to manage bradycardia–tachycardia syndrome medically without prior pacemaker implantation carry significant risk because drugs used to control SVT may worsen the bradyarrhythmias and vice versa.
- Adverse effects of anticholinergic medication (constipation, difficulty voiding, keratoconjunctivitis sicca, emesis, anxiety) occur commonly.

■ AV Block II Mobitz II
- Hypokalemia—increases sensitivity to vagal tone and may potentiate AV conduction delay.

■ AV Block III
- Vasodilators—may cause hypotension in animals with complete AV block; monitor closely if used, especially prior to pacemaker implantation.

FOLLOW-UP

PATIENT MONITORING

■ SSS
- ECG in asymptomatic patients—to detect progression of disease.
- ECG in patients treated medically or with pacemaker implantation.

■ AV Block II Mobitz II—periodic ECG because of risk of progression to complete (third degree) AV Block

■ AV Block III
- Monitor—pacemaker function with serial electrocardiograms.
- Radiographs—following pacemaker implantation, to confirm the position of the lead and generator.

POSSIBLE COMPLICATIONS

■ SSS
- Rarely, reduced cerebral or renal perfusion results in chronic renal dysfunction or CNS damage.
- Presence of significant valvular disease has implications for type of permanent pacing mode selected.

■ AV Block Mobitz II—Prolonged bradycardia may cause secondary congestive heart failure or inadequate renal perfusion.

- AV Block III—Pulse generators—pacemaker replacement necessary if battery becomes depleted, pulse generator malfunction occurs, or exit block develops; pacemaker leads can become dislodged and infected.

EXPECTED COURSE AND PROGNOSIS

- SSS
  - Good, following pacemaker implantation in animals without congestive heart failure.
  - Medical management—often ineffective; initial beneficial effects often not sustained.
- AV Block II Mobitz II—variable, depends on cause. If degenerative disease of the cardiac conduction system, often progresses to complete (third-degree) AV block.
- AV Block III
  - Poor long-term prognosis if no cardiac pacemaker implanted, especially when the animal has clinical signs. Cats can sometimes survive >1 year without a permanent pacemaker.

MISCELLANEOUS

Atrial Premature Complexes

- Premature atrial complexes or beats (APC) that originate outside the sinoatrial node and disrupt the normal sinus rhythm for 1 or more beats.
- May be normal finding in aged dogs; atrial enlargement secondary to chronic mitral valvular insufficiency—small, older dogs; cats with HCM
- Can presage more serious rhythm disturbances

AV Block Second-Degree Mobitz Type I

- in 64% of healthy adult dogs and 100% of healthy puppies 8–12 weeks of age as a manifestation of high vagal tone.
- May be normal unless signs of more generalized myocardial disease or noncardiac disease are present.
- Rarely noted in old dogs with degenerative conduction system disease (e.g., upper airway disease, cervical and thoracic masses, gastrointestinal disorders, and high intraocular pressure).
- Atropine response test—administer 0.04 mg/kg atropine IM and repeat ECG in 20–30 minutes; may be used to determine whether AV block is due to vagal tone; resolution of AV block with atropine supports vagal cause.

Synonyms—SSS

- Bradycardia–tachycardia syndrome.
- Sinus node dysfunction.
- Tachycardia–bradycardia syndrome.

Abbreviations

- AV = atrioventricular
- CHF = congestive heart failure.
- ECG = electrocardiogram.
- SSS = sick sinus syndrome.
- SVT = supraventricular tachycardia
- T4 = thyroxine

Suggested Reading

Kellum HB, Stepien RL. Third-degree atrioventricular block in 21 cats (1997–2004). *J Vet Intern Med* 2006;20:97–103.

Kraus MS, Gelzer ARM. Treatment of cardia arrhythmias and conduction disturbances. In: Smith FWK, Tilley LP, Oyama M, Sleeper M (eds) *Manual of Canine and Feline Cardiology*, 5th edn. St. Louis, MO: Saunders Elsevier, 2016; pp. 313–329.

Santilli R, Moise NS, Pariaut R, Perego M. *Electrocardiography of the Dog and Cat: Diagnosis of Arrhythmias*, 2nd edn. Milan: Edra, 2018.

Schrope DP, Kelch WJ. Signalment, clinical signs, and prognostic indicators associated with high-grade second or third-degree atrioventricular block in dogs: 124 cases (January 1, 1997–December 31, 1997). *J Am Vet Med Assoc* 2006;228:1710–1717.

Tilley LP, Smith FWK Jr. Electrocardiography. In: Smith FWK, Tilley LP, Oyama M, Sleeper M (eds) *Manual of Canine and Feline Cardiology*, 5th edn. St. Louis, MO: Saunders Elsevier, 2016; pp. 49–76.

Willis R, Oliveira P, Mavropoulou A. *Guide to Canine and Feline Electrocardiography*. Ames, IA: Wiley-Blackwell, 2018.

Author/editor: Heidi Lobprise
Topic adapted from Five Minute Veterinary Consultation, 7th edition, 2021
Original Topics: Arrthymia

Author: Larry P. Tilley
Consulting Editor: Michael Aherne

Chapter 11

Congestive Heart Failure (CHF)

BASICS

DEFINITION

Failure of the heart to advance blood at a sufficient rate to meet the metabolic needs of the patient: *Right-sided CHF*—fails to prevent blood from pooling within the systemic venous circulation. *Left-sided CHF*—fails to prevent blood from pooling within the pulmonary venous circulation.

PATHOPHYSIOLOGY

Right-sided CHF

- High hydrostatic pressure leads to leakage of fluid from venous circulation into the pleural and peritoneal space and potentially into the pericardium and interstitium of peripheral tissue.
- When fluid leakage exceeds ability of lymphatics to drain the affected areas, pleural effusion, ascites, pericardial effusion, and peripheral edema develop.

Left-sided CHF

- High hydrostatic pulmonary venous pressure causes leakage of fluid from pulmonary venous circulation into pulmonary interstitium and alveoli; when fluid leakage exceeds ability of lymphatics to drain affected areas, pulmonary edema develops.
- Low cardiac output causes lethargy, exercise intolerance, syncope, and prerenal azotemia.

SYSTEMS AFFECTED

Right sided: All systems can be affected by either poor delivery of blood or the effects of passive congestion from backup of venous blood.
Left sided: All systems can be affected by poor perfusion: Respiratory—increased rate and effort because of elevated pulmonary venous pressures/edema; Cardiovascular.

GENETICS

Right sided: Some congenital cardiac defects have a genetic basis in certain breeds.

- Arrhythmogenic right ventricular cardiomyopathy (ARVC) appears to have a genetic basis in boxers and possibly some cats.

Left sided: Some congenital heart defects, cardiomyopathies, and valvular heart disease have genetic basis in some breeds.

Blackwell's Five-Minute Veterinary Consult Clinical Companion: Small Animal Senior Care, First Edition. Edited by Heidi B. Lobprise.

Companion website: www.wiley.com/go/lobprise/Senior

INCIDENCE/PREVALENCE

Common in both.

SIGNALMENT

Both right and left-sided CHF.

Species

Dog and cat.

Breed Predilections, Mean Age and Range, Predominant Sex

Varies with cause.

SIGNS

General Comments

Right and left sided: Signs vary with underlying cause and between species.

Right sided

- Pleural effusion without ascites and hepatomegaly is rare in dogs with right-sided congestive heart failure (R-CHF).
- Ascites without pleural effusion is rare in cats with R-CHF.
- Small-volume pericardial effusion without tamponade is relatively common in cats with R-CHF.
- Interstitial peripheral edema is a rare manifestation of R-CHF in both species.

Historical Findings

Right sided

- Weakness.
- Lethargy.
- Exercise intolerance.
- Abdominal distension.
- Dyspnea, tachypnea.

Left sided

- Weakness, lethargy, exercise intolerance.
- Coughing (dogs with large left atria, concurrent tracheobronchial disease, or such severe edema that large airways affected) and dyspnea (increased respiratory rate and effort); respiratory signs often worsen at night and may require assuming standing, sternal, or "elbows abducted" position (orthopnea).
- Cats rarely cough from heart failure; coughing should prompt search for primary airway disease.

Physical Examination Findings

Right sided

- Jugular venous distention.
- Hepatojugular reflux.
- Jugular pulse in some animals.
- Hepatomegaly.

- Ascites common in dogs and rare in cats with R-CHF.
- Possible regurgitant murmur in tricuspid valve region or ejection murmur at left heart base (pulmonic stenosis).
- Muffled heart sounds if animal has pleural or pericardial effusion.
- Weak femoral pulses.
- Rapid, shallow respiration if animal has pleural effusion or severe ascites
- Peripheral edema (infrequent).

Left sided

- Tachypnea and dyspnea.
- Coughing, often soft in conjunction with tachypnea (dogs).
- Pulmonary crackles and wheezes.
- Pale/gray/cyanotic mucous membranes.
- Prolonged capillary refill time.
- Possible murmur or gallop.
- Weak femoral pulses.

CAUSES

Myocardial (Pump) Failure

Right ventricle

- Idiopathic dilated cardiomyopathy (DCM).
- ARVC.
- Hypertrophic cardiomyopathy (cats).
- Restrictive cardiomyopathy (cats).
- Trypanosomiasis.
- Doxorubicin cardiotoxicity.
- Chronic hyperthyroidism.

Left ventricle

- Dilated cardiomyopathy (DCM)/diet-induced DCM.
- Trypanosomiasis (rare).
- Doxorubicin cardiotoxicity (dogs).
- Hypothyroidism (rare).
- Hyperthyroidism (rarely causes pump failure; more commonly causes high output failure).
- Tachycardia-induced cardiomyopathy (caused by persistent pathologic supraventricular or ventricular tachyarrhythmia).

Volume Overload

Right ventricle

- Chronic atrioventricular (AV) valve (mitral ± tricuspid) insufficiency due to myxomatous valvular degeneration.
- Tricuspid valve dysplasia.
- Large atrial septal defect.

Left heart

- Degenerative mitral valve disease (dogs).
- Mitral valve dysplasia (cats and dogs).
- Patent ductus arteriosus (dogs).

- Ventricular septal defect, especially if complicated by aortic valve insufficiency.
- Aortic valve insufficiency secondary to endocarditis (dogs).
- Chronic, severe anemia.
- Inadvertent high-volume fluid administration.
- Steroid administration (cats, often with previously asymptomatic underlying hypertrophic cardiomyopathy [HCM]).

Pressure Overload

Right ventricle

- Heartworm disease.
- Chronic obstructive pulmonary disease with pulmonary hypertension.
- Pulmonary thromboembolism.
- Pulmonic stenosis.
- Tetralogy of Fallot.
- Right ventricular tumors.
- Heart base tumors (occasionally, compression of the pulmonary artery).
- Primary pulmonary hypertension.

Left heart

- Systemic hypertension (uncommon cause of heart failure in animals).
- Subaortic stenosis.
- Aortic coarctation (rare; Airedale predisposed).
- Left ventricular tumors (rare).

Impediment to Filling

Right ventricle

- Pericardial effusion (tamponade).
- Constrictive/restrictive pericarditis.
- Right atrial or caval masses.
- Tricuspid stenosis.
- Cor triatriatum dexter.

Left ventricle

- Restrictive cardiomyopathy (rare in dogs, more common in cats).
- Pulmonary vein stenosis (rare).
- HCM.
- Left atrial masses (e.g., tumor or thrombus).
- Mitral stenosis (rare).
- Cor triatriatum sinister (cats, rare).

Rhythm Disturbances

Right sided

- Bradycardia, generally complete AV block.
- Tachyarrhythmias, generally sustained supraventricular tachycardia.

Left sided

- Bradyarrhythmia (high-grade atrioventricular block).
- Tachyarrhythmia (e.g., atrial fibrillation, sustained supraventricular tachycardia, ventricular tachycardia).

RISK FACTORS

Right sided

- No heartworm prophylaxis.
- Offspring of animal with right-sided congenital cardiac defect.
- Conditions that augment demand for cardiac output (e.g., hyperthyroidism, anemia, pregnancy).

Left sided

- Bradyarrhythmia (high-grade atrioventricular block).
- Tachyarrhythmia (e.g., atrial fibrillation, sustained supraventricular tachycardia, ventricular tachycardia).

DIAGNOSIS

DIFFERENTIAL DIAGNOSIS

Right sided

- Must differentiate from other causes of pleural effusion and ascites.
- Animals with ascites or pleural effusion due to heart failure should have jugular venous distension.

Left sided

- Must differentiate from other causes of coughing, dyspnea, and weakness.

CBC/BIOCHEMISTRY/URINALYSIS

Right sided

- CBC usually normal; animals with heartworm disease may have eosinophilia.
- Mild-to-moderately high alanine aminotransferase, aspartate aminotransferase, and alkaline phosphatase due to passive liver congestion; bilirubin generally normal.
- Prerenal azotemia in some animals.

Left sided

- CBC usually normal; may be stress leukogram.
- Mild-to-moderate liver enzyme elevation; bilirubin generally normal.
- Prerenal azotemia in some animals.

OTHER LABORATORY TESTS

Right sided

- Heartworm test may be positive.
- NT-proBNP concentrations higher in animals with cardiac causes of fluid accumulation.

Left sided

- Thyroid disorders may be detected.
- Serum NT-proBNP and cardiac troponin I concentrations higher in animals with left-sided congestive heart failure (L-CHF) than in normal animals.

IMAGING

Thoracic Radiography

Right sided

- Right cardiomegaly in some animals.
- Dilated caudal vena cava (diameter greater than the length of the vertebra directly above the heart).
- Pleural effusion (especially cats).
- Hepatosplenomegaly and possible ascites (especially dogs).

Left sided

- Left heart and pulmonary veins enlarged.
- Pulmonary edema, often hilar, especially involving right caudal lung lobe in acute edema of dog, but may be patchy, especially in cats; acute pulmonary edema may begin in right caudal lung lobe.

Echocardiography

Right sided

- Findings vary with underlying cause; especially useful for documenting congenital defect, cardiac mass, and pericardial effusion.
- Abdominal ultrasound reveals hepatomegaly with hepatic vein dilation, flow reversal in the hepatic veins (Doppler), and possibly ascites.

Left sided

- Findings vary markedly with cause but left atrial enlargement relatively consistent finding in cardiogenic pulmonary edema.
- Diagnostic test of choice for documenting congenital defects, cardiac masses, and pericardial effusion.

DIAGNOSTIC PROCEDURES

ECG Findings

Right sided

- Small (<1 mV) QRS complexes in all frontal axis leads if pericardial or pleural effusion.
- Electrical alternans or elevated ST segment with pericardial effusion
- Evidence of right cardiomegaly (e.g., tall [>0.4 mV] P waves in lead II, deep S waves in leads I, II, aVF, and right axis deviation).
- Atrial or ventricular arrhythmias.
- ECG may be normal.

Left sided

- Atrial or ventricular arrhythmias.
- Evidence of left cardiomegaly (e.g., wide P waves, tall and wide QRS complexes, and left axis orientation).
- May be normal.

Abdominocentesis—Right Sided

Analysis of ascitic fluid in patients with R-CHF generally reveals modified transudate with total protein >2.5 mg/dL.

Thoracentesis—Right Sided

- Cats with pleural effusion associated with R-CHF may have transudate, modified transudate, or chylous effusion.
- Dogs with pleural effusion and R-CHF may have transudate or modified transudate.

Central Venous Pressure—Right Sided

Central venous pressure is high (>9 cmH_2O) or rises dramatically to that level and remains elevated for more than 1h following a fluid bolus (e.g., 5–10 mL/kg IV).

PATHOLOGIC FINDINGS

Right sided
- Cardiac findings vary with disease.
- Hepatomegaly in animals with centrolobular necrosis (chronic condition).

Left sided
- Cardiac findings vary with disease.

TREATMENT

APPROPRIATE HEALTH CARE

Right sided
- Most animals treated as outpatients unless dyspneic or collapsed (e.g., significant pleural or pericardial effusion).

Left sided
- Usually treat as outpatient unless dyspneic or severely hypotensive.
- Identify and correct underlying cause whenever possible.
- Minimize handling of critically dyspneic animals—stress can kill!

NURSING CARE

Right sided: Thoracentesis and abdominocentesis may be required periodically for patients no longer responsive to medical management or those with severe dyspnea due to pleural effusion or ascites.
Left sided: Oxygen supplementation and postural support in dyspneic patients.

ACTIVITY

Right sided: Restrict activity.
Left sided: Restrict activity when dyspneic or tachypneic.

DIET

Right sided: Restrict sodium moderately; severe sodium restriction indicated for animals with advanced disease.
Left sided: Initiate moderately sodium-restricted diet with adequate protein and calories. Severe sodium restriction indicated with advanced disease.

CLIENT EDUCATION

Right sided

- With few exceptions (e.g., in heartworm disease, arrhythmias, hyperthyroidism, and idiopathic pericardial effusion), R-CHF is not curable.
- Most patients improve with initial treatment but often have recurrent failure.

Left sided

- With few exceptions (e.g., animals with thyroid disorders, anemia, arrhythmias, nutritionally responsive heart disease, congenital heart disease), L-CHF is not curable.

SURGICAL CONSIDERATIONS

Right sided

- Surgical intervention or balloon valvuloplasty is indicated to treat certain congenital defects such as pulmonic stenosis or cor triatriatum dexter, and Amplatz occluder placement for morphologically appropriate atrial septal defects.
- Pericardiocentesis or pericardectomy for pericardial effusion.
- Removal of heartworms from the heart via the jugular vein in dogs with caval syndrome.

Left sided

- Surgical intervention, coil embolization, Amplatz occluder placement, or balloon valvuloplasty may benefit selected patients with some forms of congenital and acquired valvular heart disease; response to these interventions varies.
- Pericardiocentesis in animals with pericardial effusion.

MEDICATIONS

DRUG(S) OF CHOICE

Drugs should be administered only after a definitive diagnosis is made.

Diuretics

Right sided

- Furosemide (1–2 mg/kg q8–24h) or another loop diuretic is the initial diuretic of choice; diuretics are indicated to remove excess fluid accumulation.
- Torsemide (0.2–0.8 mg/kg q24h) may be a useful substitute for furosemide in animals requiring a daily furosemide dose in excess of 12 mg/kg.
- Spironolactone (2 mg/kg PO q12–24h) increases survival in humans with heart failure; use in combination with furosemide.

Left sided

- Furosemide (1–2 mg/kg q8–24h) or other loop diuretic is initial diuretic of choice; diuretics indicated to reduce preload and remove pulmonary edema; critically dyspneic animals often require high doses (2–4 mg/kg) IV to stabilize, dose can be repeated in 1 hour if animal still severely dyspneic; IV bolus of 0.66 mg/kg followed by CRI of 0.66–1 mg/kg/h for 1–4 hours causes greater diuresis than equal dose divided into two IV boluses given 4 hours apart; once edema resolves, taper to lowest effective dose.

- Spironolactone (0.5–2 mg/kg PO q12–24h) increases survival in humans with CHF and is in clinical trials in dogs; use in combination with furosemide.
- Thiazide diuretics can be added to furosemide and spironolactone in refractory heart failure cases.
- Torsemide (0.2–0.8 mg/kg q24h) may be useful as substitute for furosemide in animals requiring daily furosemide dosing in excess of 12 mg/kg, and it may be more effective than furosemide at delaying death due to cardiac disease in dogs with CHF secondary to degenerative valve disease.

Vasodilators

Right sided

- Angiotensin-converting enzyme (ACE) inhibitors such as enalapril (0.5 mg/kg q12–24h) or benazepril (0.25–0.5 mg/kg q24h) are helpful when CHF is secondary to DCM or chronic AV valve insufficiency.
- Sildenafil (0.5–1 mg/kg PO q12h up to 2–3 mg/kg q8h) may be beneficial for pulmonary hypertension.

Venodilators

Left sided

- Nitroglycerin ointment (one-fourth inch/5 kg q6–8h) causes venodilation, lowering left atrial filling pressures.
- Used for acute stabilization of patients with severe pulmonary edema and dyspnea, but uncertain benefit.

Pimobendan

Right sided

- Calcium sensitizer that acts as an inodilator, causing arterial vasodilation and increasing myocardial contractility.
- Especially useful in myocardial failure.
- Dose—0.25–0.3 mg/kg PO q12h.

Left sided—positive inotropes

- Pimobendan (0.25–0.3 mg/kg PO q12h) is a calcium channel sensitizer that dilates arteries and increases myocardial contractility; first-line agent in treating DCM or CHF due to degenerative valve disease efficacy in cats with CHF is not known, but possibly beneficial.
- Dobutamine (dogs: 2.5–10 µg/kg/min; cats: 0.5–5 µg/kg/min) is a potent positive inotropic agent that may provide valuable short-term support of a heart failure patient with poor cardiac contractility.
- Positive inotropes in general are potentially arrhythmogenic—monitor carefully.

Digoxin

Right sided

- Digoxin (dogs: 0.22 mg/m^2 q12h; cats: 0.01 mg/kg q48h) is used in animals with myocardial failure (e.g., DCM) and atrial fibrillation.
- Digoxin indicated in animals with refractory CHF that have supraventricular arrhythmias.

Left sided: Treat arrhythmias if clinically indicated.

CONTRAINDICATIONS

Right sided

- Avoid diuretics in patients with pericardial effusion/tamponade.
- Avoid vasodilators in patients with pericardial effusion or fixed outflow obstructions.

Left sided

- Avoid vasodilators in patients with pericardial effusion or fixed outflow obstruction.

PRECAUTIONS

Right and left sided

- ACE inhibitors and arterial dilators must be used with caution in patients with possible outflow obstructions.
- Pulmonary hypertension, hypothyroidism, and hypoxia increase risk for digoxin toxicity; hyperthyroidism diminishes effects of digoxin.
- ACE inhibitors and digoxin—use cautiously with renal disease.
- Dobutamine—use cautiously in cats.
- Spironolactone—may cause facial pruritis in cats.

POSSIBLE INTERACTIONS

Right sided

- Combination of high-dose diuretics and ACE inhibitors may alter renal perfusion and cause azotemia.
- Combination diuretic therapy promotes risk of dehydration and electrolyte disturbances.

Left sided

- ACE inhibitors and arterial dilators must be used with caution in patients with possible outflow obstruction.
- Pulmonary hypertension, hypothyroidism, and hypoxia increase risk for digoxin toxicity; hyperthyroidism diminishes effects of digoxin.
- ACE inhibitors and digoxin—use cautiously in patients with renal disease.
- Dobutamine—use cautiously in cats.
- Spironolactone—may cause facial pruritis in cats.

ALTERNATIVE DRUG(S)

Right sided

- Patients unresponsive to furosemide, spironolactone, vasodilator, pimobendan, and digoxin (if indicated) may benefit from triple diuretic therapy by adding a thiazide diuretic, or substitution of torsemide for furosemide, generally at 0.1–0.2 mg of torsemide for each 1 mg of furosemide previously administered.
- Potassium and magnesium supplementation if deficiency documented; use potassium supplements cautiously in animals receiving ACE inhibitors or spironolactone.
- Treat arrhythmias if clinically indicated.
- Taurine supplementation in cats with DCM and dogs with DCM and taurine deficiency.
- Carnitine supplementation may help some dogs with DCM (e.g., cocker spaniels and boxers).

Left sided

- **Arterial dilators**: Hydralazine (0.5–2 mg/kg PO q12h; 0.5 mg/kg PO to start when added to ACE inhibitor) or amlodipine (0.05–0.2 mg/kg PO q24h) can be substituted for ACE inhibitor in patients that do not tolerate the drug or have advanced renal failure; monitor for hypotension and tachycardia; can be cautiously added to ACE inhibitor in animals with refractory L-CHF.
- Nitroprusside (1–10 µg/kg/min) is potent arterial dilator usually reserved for short-term support of patients with life-threatening edema.
- Digoxin (dogs: 0.22 mg/m^2 q12h; cats: 0.01 mg/kg q48h) is used in animals with atrial fibrillation and myocardial failure (e.g., DCM); commonly used in combination with diltiazem to control rate of atrial fibrillation.
- Digoxin is also indicated to treat dogs with refractory heart failure from either myocardial failure or volume loads; however, its use as a primary agent in myocardial failure has been replaced by pimobendan.
- **Calcium channel blockers:** Diltiazem (0.5–1.5 mg/kg PO q8h) is frequently used in L-CHF patients for rate control in animals with supraventricular arrhythmias.
- **Beta blockers:** Atenolol and metoprolol are sometimes used for rate control in animals with supraventricular tachycardia, hypertrophic cardiomyopathy, and hyperthyroidism.
    - Used alone or with a class 1 antiarrhythmic drug for control of ventricular arrhythmias; these drugs depress contractility (negative inotropes), so use cautiously in patients with myocardial failure or active signs of CHF.
    - On basis of human studies, may enhance survival in animals with idiopathic DCM; treatment is best initiated under guidance of a cardiologist, starting with very low dosage and gradually increasing; carvedilol is sometimes used for this purpose, starting at 0.1 mg/kg q24h and titrating to 0.5 mg/kg q12h.

Nutritional supplements

- Potassium and magnesium supplementation if deficiency is documented; use potassium supplements cautiously in animals receiving ACE inhibitor or spironolactone.
- Taurine supplementation in cats with DCM and dogs with DCM and taurine deficiency (e.g., American cocker spaniels)
- L-carnitine supplementation may help some dogs with DCM.
- Coenzyme Q_{10} is of potential value based on results in humans with DCM.
- Ensure animal receiving a nutritionally balanced diet (see Cardiomyopathy, Nutritional).

FOLLOW-UP

PATIENT MONITORING

Right sided

- Monitor renal status, electrolytes, hydration, respiratory rate and effort, bodyweight, and abdominal girth (dogs).
- If azotemia develops, reduce diuretic dosage; if azotemia persists and the animal is also on an ACE inhibitor, reduce or discontinue this drug; if azotemia develops, reduce digoxin dosage to avoid toxicity.
- Monitor ECG periodically to detect arrhythmias.
- Monitor digoxin concentrations—normal value 0.5–1.5 ng/mL for serum sample obtained 8–10 hours after dose is administered.

Left sided

- Monitor resting respiratory rate and effort, appetite, renal status, electrolytes, hydration, heart rate, bodyweight.
- If azotemia develops, reduce diuretic dose; if azotemia persists and animal is also on ACE inhibitor, reduce or discontinue ACE inhibitor; use digoxin with caution if azotemic.
- Monitor ECG if arrhythmias suspected.
- Check digoxin concentration (0.5–1.5 ng/mL, 8–10 hours post dose).

LEFT-SIDED PREVENTION/AVOIDANCE

- Minimize stress, exercise, and sodium intake in patients with heart disease.
- Pimobendan delays onset of CHF in Doberman pinschers, and in dogs with hemodynamically significant myxomatous mitral valve regurgitation; prescribing an ACE inhibitor with pimobendan early in course of heart disease in patients with DCM may slow progression of heart disease and delay onset of CHF; role of ACE inhibitors in asymptomatic animals with mitral valve disease remains controversial.

POSSIBLE COMPLICATIONS

Right sided

- Pulmonary thromboembolism.
- Arrhythmias.
- Electrolyte imbalances.
- Digoxin toxicity.
- Azotemia and renal failure.

Left sided

- Syncope.
- Aortic thromboembolism (cats).
- Arrhythmias.
- Electrolyte imbalances.
- Digoxin toxicity.
- Azotemia and renal failure.

EXPECTED COURSE AND PROGNOSIS

Right sided: Prognosis varies with underlying cause.
Left sided: Prognosis varies with underlying cause; cats and dogs that survive initial episode of pulmonary edema and can be reliably medicated often survive months to more than a year with good quality of life. Animals with reversible causes of L-CHF may recover to normal lives.

MISCELLANEOUS

Age-Related Factors

Both right and left

- Congenital causes seen in young animals.
- Degenerative heart conditions and neoplasia generally seen in old animals.

See Also

MMVD

Abbreviations

- ACE = angiotensin-converting enzyme
- ARVC = arrhythmogenic right ventricular cardiomyopathy.
- AV = atrioventricular.
- DCM = dilated cardiomyopathy.
- R-CHF = right-sided congestive heart failure.
- HCM = hypertrophic cardiomyopathy.
- L-CHF = left-sided congestive heart failure.
- MMVD = myxomatous mitral valve disease

Author/editor: Heidi Lobprise
Thanks to: Gary Oswald for review
Topic adapted from Five Minute Veterinary Consultation, 7th edition, 2021
Original Topic: Congestive Heart Failure—Right and Left sided

Authors: Francis W.K. Smith, Jr. and Bruce W. Keene
Consulting Editor: Michael Aherne

Chapter 12

Dilated Cardiomyopathy

BASICS

DEFINITION

- Dilated cardiomyopathy (DCM) is a disease of the heart muscle characterized by systolic myocardial failure and a dilated, volume-overloaded heart that leads to signs of congestive heart failure (CHF) or low cardiac output.
- Before 1987, DCM in cats was secondary as a result of taurine deficiency. Primary idiopathic DCM is now an uncommon cause of heart disease in cats.
- IN dogs, left-sided CHF signs predominate; severe right-sided disease can occur; diastolic dysfunction with restrictive physiology is a negative predictor of survival.

SYSTEMS AFFECTED

- Cardiovascular, renal (poor perfusion), respiratory (pulmonary edema), pleural effusion in cats
- Musculoskeletal – in cats, complication with aortic thromboembolism (ATE), which causes acute paraparesis or monoparesis.

GENETICS

Cats

- No definitive mutation has been identified in the cat to date

Dogs

- Genetic cause or heritable susceptibility strongly suspected in most breeds and documented in some (Portuguese water dog, boxer, and Doberman pinscher) with variable forms of inheritance.
- A genetic test is available for striatin in boxer dogs and Doberman pinscher (NCSU DCM 1—pyruvate dehydrogenase kinase; NCSU DCM 2—titin).
- Doberman pinschers with both mutations have an earlier onset of clinical disease with a predisposition to sudden death; boxers homozygous for the mutation are more likely to develop the DCM phenotype.

Blackwell's Five-Minute Veterinary Consult Clinical Companion: Small Animal Senior Care,
First Edition. Edited by Heidi B. Lobprise.

Companion website: www.wiley.com/go/lobprise/Senior

INCIDENCE/PREVALENCE

Cats

- Idiopathic feline DCM is relatively uncommon now that taurine is adequately supplemented in cat foods.

Dogs

- Estimated at 0.5–1.1% in predisposed breeds; Chagas' cardiomyopathy US Gulf Coast and Central and South America

SIGNALMENT

Cat

- Mean age and range: 9 years (5–13 years); no breed or sex predilections

Dog

- Breed predilections
    - Doberman pinscher, boxer.
    - Giant breeds—Scottish deerhound, Irish wolfhound, Great Dane, St. Bernard, Newfoundland.
    - Cocker spaniel, Portuguese water dog (juvenile).
- Mean age and range: 4–10 years.
- Predominant sex: Males > females in most but not all breeds (minor predisposition).

SIGNS

Historical Findings

Cats

- Signs related to low cardiac output—anorexia, weakness, depression.
- Signs related to CHF—dyspnea, tachypnea (rarely diagnosed prior to onset of clinical signs)
- Signs related to ATE—sudden-onset pain and paraparesis.

Dogs

- Respiratory—tachypnea, dyspnea, coughing.
- Weight loss (lean muscle mass), weakness, lethargy, anorexia.
- Abdominal distention.
- Syncope, usually associated with arrhythmias (atrial fibrillation; ventricular tachycardia).
- Some are asymptomatic (preclinical DCM) well described in specific breeds.
- Echocardiographic parameters with cardiac biomarkers (NT-proBNP; cardiac troponin I [cTnI]) may help identify dogs with preclinical DCM.

Physical Examination Findings

Cats

- Heart rate can be fast, normal, or slow; Soft systolic heart murmur; Weak left cardiac impulse; Gallop sound; Possible arrhythmia.
- Hypothermia. prolonged capillary refill time.
- Tachypnea; Quiet lung sounds (pleural effusion); Crackles (pulmonary edema).
- Ascites.
- Hypokinetic femoral pulses.
- Possibly, posterior paresis and pain as a result of ATE.

Dogs

- May be completely normal with preclinical DCM.
- Weakness, possibly cardiogenic shock.
- Hypokinetic femoral pulse from low cardiac output.
- Pulse deficits with atrial fibrillation, ventricular or supraventricular premature contractions, and paroxysmal ventricular tachycardia.
- Jugular pulses from tricuspid regurgitation, arrhythmias, or right-sided CHF.
- Breath sounds—muffled with pleural effusion, crackles with pulmonary edema.
- S3 or summation gallop sounds.
- Mitral and/or tricuspid regurgitation murmurs are common but usually focal and soft.
- Auscultatory evidence of cardiac arrhythmia is common.
- Slow capillary refill time, infrequent cyanosis.
- Hepatomegaly with or without ascites.

CAUSES

Cats

- Unknown for idiopathic DCM, although a genetic predisposition in some families of cats. Taurine deficiency was a common cause of secondary myocardial failure before 1987.

Dogs

- Majority of cases represent familial abnormalities of structural, energetic or contractile cardiac proteins, some of which have been identified.
- Nutritional deficiencies (taurine and/or carnitine) have been documented in several breeds including golden retriever, boxer, Newfoundland, and cocker spaniel; diet-associated DCM, which may be associated with taurine deficiency, commonly secondary to boutique, exotic-ingredient, or grain-free (BEG) diets, is increasing recognized and potentially reversible.
- Viral, protozoal, and immune-mediated mechanisms have been proposed but not proven.
- Doxorubicin toxicity.
- Hypothyroidism and persistent tachyarrhythmias (sometimes associated with congenital tricuspid valve malformation) may cause reversible myocardial failure.
- Chagas—*Trypanosoma cruzi* infections.

DIAGNOSIS

CBC/BIOCHEMISTRY/URINALYSIS

Cats

- Many cats will have prerenal azotemia related to low cardiac output.

Dogs

- Routine hematologic tests and urinalysis are usually normal unless altered by severe reductions in cardiac output or severe elevations in venous pressures (e.g., prerenal azotemia, high alanine aminotransferase, hyponatremia), therapy for heart failure (e.g., hyponatremia, hypokalemia, hypochloremia, azotemia, and metabolic alkalosis from diuresis), or concurrent disease.

OTHER LABORATORY TESTS

Cats

- Ensure that thyroid concentrations are normal.
- Plasma taurine less than 40 nmol/L or whole blood taurine less than 250 nmol/L, are subnormal; assays are performed at a limited number of institutions and require special handling.
- Cardiac biomarkers: plasma amine terminal B-type natriuretic peptide (NT-proBNP) and cardiac troponin I (cTnI).

Dogs

- Cardiac biomarkers including NT-proBNP and cTnI are elevated in both the preclinical and clinical stages of the disease.

IMAGING

Radiography

Cats

- Radiography often shows pleural effusion or pulmonary edema.
- Generalized cardiomegaly.

Dogs

- Typically normal in the preclinical phase.
- Generalized cardiomegaly and signs of CHF are common.
- Left ventricular (LV) enlargement and left atrial enlargement in early cases.
- In some, the degree of cardiomegaly less than expected for the severity signs.
- Pleural effusion, hepatomegaly, ascites.

Echocardiography—Diagnostic Modality of Choice

Cats

- Thin ventricular walls, enlarged left ventricular end-systolic and end-diastolic dimensions, left atrial enlargement, and low fractional shortening.
- Pleural and pericardial effusion may be visualized.
- Spontaneous echocardiographic contrast or a thrombus may be visualized.

Dogs

- LV dilation often precedes overt reductions in indices of systolic function.
- Ventricular and atrial dilation.
- Myocardial systolic function indices may be reduced (fractional shortening [FS%]), ejection fraction, area shortening, and mitral annular motion by tissue Doppler imaging.
- Spectral Doppler—decreased velocity and/or acceleration of trans-aortic flow as well as mitral regurgitation and/or tricuspid regurgitation.
- Doppler evidence of restrictive LV filling is associated with decreased survival.

DIAGNOSTIC PROCEDURES

ECG

Cats

- ECG may be normal or may show left atrial or ventricular enlargement patterns.
- Both ventricular and supraventricular arrhythmias can be seen.

Dogs

- Sinus rhythm or sinus tachycardia with isolated atrial or ventricular premature complexes.
- Atrial fibrillation and ventricular tachycardia (paroxysmal or sustained) are very common in Doberman pinschers.
- Boxers commonly have isolated ventricular arrhythmias without evidence of functional or anatomic heart disease.
- Prolonged QRS (>0.06 second), possible increased voltages (R >3 mV lead II), suggesting LV enlargement.
- May have "sloppy" R wave descent with ST-T coving, suggesting myocardial disease or LV ischemia.
- May have low voltages (pleural or pericardial effusion, concurrent hypothyroidism).

Pleural Effusion Analysis—Cats

- Pleural effusion typically is a modified transudate with total protein <4 g/dL and nucleated cell counts of less than 2500/mL; chylous effusion may also be present.
- Analysis of the pleural effusion is important to rule out other causes of pleural effusion such as pyothorax, infectious peritonitis, or lymphosarcoma.

PATHOLOGIC FINDINGS

Cats

- Heart: body ratio is increased, all four chambers dilated ventricular walls thin, valve anatomy normal
- Histopathology shows myocytolysis and myocardial fibrosis.

Dogs

- Dilation of all chambers with or without thinning of chamber walls.
- Slightly thickened endocardium with pale areas within myocardium (necrosis, fibrosis).
- Two histologically distinct forms—fatty infiltration: degenerative type seen in boxers and Doberman pinschers; and attenuated wavy fiber type: seen in many giant-, large-, and medium-sized breeds, including some boxers and Doberman pinschers.

TREATMENT

APPROPRIATE HEALTH CARE

Cats

Usually present in CHF and should be treated as inpatients, typically in an intensive care setting until more stable.

Dogs

Most therapy can be administered on an outpatient basis unless severely affected.

NURSING CARE

Cats:

- Thoracocentesis is often utilized for both therapeutic and diagnostic purposes.
- Supplemental oxygen therapy is beneficial for cats in CHF to decrease the work of breathing.
- If hypothermic, cautious external heat (incubator or heating water pad) is recommended.

ACTIVITY

Cats

- Indoors only after hospital discharge to reduce stress. Let cat dictate its own activity.

Dogs

- Allow the dog to choose its own level of activity

DIET

Cats

- Tempt their appetite with many types of food if anoretic. Eventually, a low-sodium diet is recommended.

Dogs

- Maintaining adequate caloric intake is paramount.
- Goal—reduce dietary sodium intake to <12–15 mg/kg/day; as severe restriction may affect appetite
- Best to use commercially prepared diets.

CLIENT EDUCATION

Cats

- Some cats will need chronic intermittent thoracocentesis to manage significant accumulations of pleural effusion despite medical therapy.

Dogs

- Emphasize potential signs associated with progression of disease and adverse side effects of medication.
- Monitoring sleeping respiratory rate often gives insight into impending decompensation.

MEDICATIONS

DRUG(S) OF CHOICE

Cats

- Furosemide to manage pulmonary edema and pleural effusion: 1–4 mg/kg q8–12h, parenterally then oral. Long-term use the lowest effective dose of furosemide.
- Pimobendan at 0.1–0.3 mg/kg PO q12h. Not currently licensed for use in cats, several recent publications have demonstrated its safety in cats and possibly a beneficial effect.
- Taurine supplementation initially in all cats with DCM at 250 mg PO q12h, until diagnostic testing or lack of response to taurine is demonstrated.
- Nitroglycerin (2% ointment) one-fourth to one-half inch applied topically with diuretics in the acute management of severe CHF to further reduce preload. Nitroglycerin will lower the dose of furosemide and is particularly useful in patients with hypothermia or dehydration.
- Enalapril or benazepril, at a dose of 0.25–0.5 mg/kg PO q24h, to reduce afterload and preload when oral medication possible and clinically stable. (If creatinine <2.5 mg/dL.)
- Digoxin optional at 0.03 mg/cat (one-fourth of a 0.125 mg tablet) or 0.01 mg/kg PO q48h. Can be given with pimobendane, but possible side-effects and pill burden of multiple medications.

- Dobutamine - extremely low dosages 0.25–5 μg/kg/min IV CRI if severe signs of CHF and low cardiac output. ECG monitoring is recommended.
- Clopidogrel (antithrombotic for ATE) at 18.75 mg (one-fourth of a 75 mg tablet) PO q24h. Options of aspirin 81 mg PO q72h (with food) or low-molecular-weight heparin (e.g., dalteparin 100–150 units/kg SC q8–24h or enoxaparin 1 mg/kg SC q12–24h).
- Antiarrhythmic drugs for significant supraventricular tachycardia or rapid atrial fibrillation: diltiazem at 7.5 mg/cat PO q8h or a sustained-release (Cardizem CD® at 10 mg/kg PO q24h or Dilacor XR® 30 mg/cat [or 1/2 of an inner 60 mg tablet] PO q12h). Injectable form if PO not possible (0.05–0.1 mg/kg slow IV, repeated PRN up to 0.25 mg/kg). If rapid and sustained ventricular tachycardia, lidocaine slow IV 0.2–0.5 mg/kg (repeat once or twice max) or sotalol PO 2 mg/kg q12h is recommended.
- Beta blockers, for supraventricular and ventricular arrhythmias. Use cautiously, as they acutely decrease contractility and could worsen CHF. Recommended atenolol dose ranges from 3.125 to 6.25 mg PO q12–24h. Start low and titrate up based on heart rate and clinical signs.

Dogs

Preclinical Disease

- Early intervention with pimobendan monotherapy substantially changes the course of preclinical disease in Doberman pinschers, not proven in other breeds. Early use of ACE minimal to no benefit.

Initial Stabilization—Dogs

- Manage hypoxemia and body temperature.
- If pulmonary edema—furosemide (1–4 mg/kg IM/IV, then 1–2 mg/kg q6–12h for first 1–3 days), or CRI 1–2 mg/kg/h (author's preference).
- 2% topical nitroglycerin for first 24–48 hours for severe pulmonary edema—apply 1–2 inches q8h (beware of hypotension in both patients and staff).
- If significant pleural effusion—drain each hemithorax.
- If severe heart failure and cardiogenic shock—dobutamine may be indicated (5–15 μg/kg/min infused for 24–72 hours; titrate up); may exacerbate arrhythmias in hypoxic dogs; oral pimobendan (see dosing below) may have important acute (2–4 hours) hemodynamic benefit as well; IV pimobendan (0.15 mg/kg) is available in select countries.
- If paroxysmal ventricular tachycardia is present—administer lidocaine slowly in 2 mg/kg boluses (up to 8 mg/kg total over 30 minutes) to convert to sinus rhythm; follow with lidocaine infusion (50–100 μg/kg/min).
- If lidocaine is ineffective—administer procainamide slowly at dose of 2–5 mg/kg (up to 15 mg/kg) IV to convert to sinus rhythm; follow with 25–50 μg/kg/min CRI (beware of proarrhythmia and infrequently hypotension).

Maintenance Therapy—Dogs

- ACE inhibitors (enalapril, benazepril, lisinopril) are considered cornerstone of therapy for DCM. Monitor renal function if used with diuretics.
- Enalapril (0.25–0.5 mg/kg PO q12h), benazepril (0.5 mg/kg PO q12–24h), or lisinopril (0.5 mg/kg PO q 12–24h) should be initiated early in the therapeutic regimen.
- Furosemide (1–4 mg/kg PO q8–12h) is used to control signs of congestion.
- Torsemide (0.1–0.4 mg/kg PO q8–12h), an alternative to furosemide, particularly in later-stage disease.
- Spironolactone (1–2 mg/kg PO q12h) survival benefit by blocking aldosterone; higher doses can be used for refractory heart failure (2–4 mg/kg PO q12h).
- Hydrochlorthiazide (1–2 mg/kg PO q12h) as a third diuretic.

- Beta blockers; cautiously if tolerated, may improve myocardial function; carvedilol (0.25–1.25 mg/kg PO q12h—start low then titrate up over 6 weeks). Use in clinical DCM patients can result in rapid and profound clinical deterioration.
- Pimobendan (0.25–0.3 mg/kg PO q12h) improves functional heart failure class and in Doberman pinschers increases survival time; 0.5 mg/kg PO q8h in refractory cases.
- American cocker spaniels with DCM respond favorably to taurine and L-carnitine supplementation, with additional cardiac medications.
- Other vasodilators, including hydralazine and amlodipine, may be used instead of or in addition to ACE inhibitors (beware of hypotension).
- Role of co-enzyme Q10, fish oil, and arginine remains to be determined.

Arrhythmias

- In atrial fibrillation, decrease ventricular rate response (does not convert a-fib to sinus rhythm) with chronic administration of extended-release diltiazem (Dilacor®) 2–7 mg/kg PO q12h, or atenolol 0.75–1.5 mg/kg PO q12h (never start in patient with active CHF), occasionally combined with digitalis at dose of 0.005 mg/kg PO q12h; therapeutic drug monitoring recommended when administering digoxin; avoid in severe uncontrolled paroxysmal ventricular tachycardia, if renal function compromised or hypokalemic.
- Quinidine, amiodarone, and diltiazem may increase serum digoxin levels and predispose to digitalis intoxication.
- Renal dysfunction, hypothyroidism, and hypokalemia predispose to digitalis intoxication.
- Therapeutic goal is obtaining resting ventricular rate of 100–140 bpm.
- Amiodarone (10–15 mg/kg PO q24h for 7–10 days followed by 5–10 mg/kg PO q24h) may either control ventricular response rate or in some cases result in conversion to normal sinus rhythm.
- Chronic oral therapy for ventricular tachycardia includes sotalol (1–2 mg/kg PO q12h), mexiletine (5–10 mg/kg PO q8h), or amiodarone (5–10 mg/kg PO q24h).
- Mexiletine can be combined with sotalol if necessary.

FOLLOW-UP

PATIENT MONITORING

Cats

- Within 1 week—repeat blood pressure, diagnostic imaging (either a thoracic radiograph or focused thoracic ultrasound for fluid assessment), and chemistry panel.
- Home resting respiratory rate monitoring.
- Periodically monitor electrolyte and renal parameters. Periodically monitor for CHF fluid accumulation with diagnostic imaging.
- Digoxin serum blood concentrations—measure in 10–14 days (0.5–1.5 ng/dL 8–12 hours post-pill).
- 2–3 months: repeat echocardiogram in 2–3 months after initiating taurine supplementation; dramatic clinical response should be seen within 2 weeks cat has taurine-responsive DCM.

Dogs

- Serial clinical examinations, thoracic radiographs, blood pressure measurements, routine serum biochemical evaluations (including electrolytes), and electrocardiography are most helpful.
- Repeat echocardiography is rarely informative or indicated.
- Serial evaluation of serum digoxin levels (therapeutic range: 0.5–1 ng/mL) taken 6–8 hours post-pill and serum biochemistries may help prevent iatrogenic problems.

PREVENTION/AVOIDANCE

Cats

- Ensure that cats eat a high-protein diet with sufficient dietary taurine. No vegetarian diets.

POSSIBLE COMPLICATIONS

Cats

- ATE is the most feared complication of any feline myocardial disease.

Dogs

- Sudden death due most commonly to arrhythmias.
- Iatrogenic problems associated with medical management (see above).

EXPECTED COURSE AND PROGNOSIS

Cats

- Poor prognosis despite intensive therapy. If not taurine responsive, survival is usually weeks to months.
- CHF can be medically refractory and recurrent despite appropriate medical therapy.
- Repeated thoracocentesis may be necessary.

Dogs

- Always fatal unless associated with nutritional deficiencies.
- Death usually occurs 6–24 months following diagnosis.
- Dobermans typically have worst prognosis; however, with addition of pimobendan, survival following identification in *preclinical* phase averages over 700 days.
- Atrial fibrillation, paroxysmal ventricular tachycardia, Doppler evidence of restrictive LV filling, markedly decreased FS%, homozygosity for known mutations (boxer), or presence of multiple mutations (Doberman pinschers) are believed to be markers for shortened survival and increased risk for sudden arrhythmogenic death.

MISCELLANEOUS

Associated Conditions

Cats

- CHF.
- ATE.
- Pleural effusion.
- Cardiac arrhythmias.

Dogs

- Prevalence increases with age

See Also

- Aortic Thromboembolism.
- Congestive Heart Failure

Abbreviations

- ACE = angiotensin-converting enzyme
- ATE = aortic thromboembolism.
- AV = atrioventricular.
- BEG = boutique, exotic-ingredient, or grain free.
- CHF = congestive heart failure.
- cTnI = cardiac troponin I.
- DCM = dilated cardiomyopathy.
- FS% = percent fractional shortening.
- LV = left ventricular.

INTERNET RESOURCES

Accessed 29 June 2024
https://cardiaceducationgroup.org

Suggested Reading

Ferasin L, Sturgess CP, Cannon MJ, et al. Feline idiopathic cardiomyopathy: a retrospective study of 106 cats (1994–2001). *J Feline Med Surg* 2003; 5:151–159.

Hambrook LE, Bennett PF. Effect of pimobendan on the clinical outcome and survival of cats with non-taurine responsive dilated cardiomyopathy. *J Feline Med Surg* 2012; 14:233–239.

Kittleson MD. Feline myocardial disease. In: Ettinger SJ, Feldman EC (eds) *Textbook of Veterinary Internal Medicine*, 6th edn. St. Louis, MO: Elsevier, 2005; pp. 1082–1103.

Lawler DF, Templeton AJ, Monti KL. Evidence of genetic involvement in feline dilated cardiomyopathy. *J Vet Intern Med* 1993;7:383–387.

Pion PD, Kittleson MD, Rogers QR, et al. Myocardial failure in cats associated with low plasma taurine: a reversible cardiomyopathy. *Science* 1987;237:764–768.

Author/editor: Heidi Lobprise
Topic adapted from Five Minute Veterinary Consultation, 7th edition, 2021
Original Topic: Dilated Cardiomyopathy—Cat and Dilated Cardiomyopathy—Dog

Author: Teresa C. DeFrancesco (cat)

Author: Matthew W. Miller (dog)
Consulting Editor: Michael Aherne

Chapter 13

Hypertension, Systemic Arterial

BASICS

DEFINITION

Sustained increase in arterial blood pressure, systolic BP (SBP) ≥160 mmHg during multiple measurements.

Usually occurs in association with a clinical disease or treatment known to cause HT that overwhelm or interfere with normal homeostatic mechanisms or vascular responsiveness; categorized as secondary (Figure 13.1).

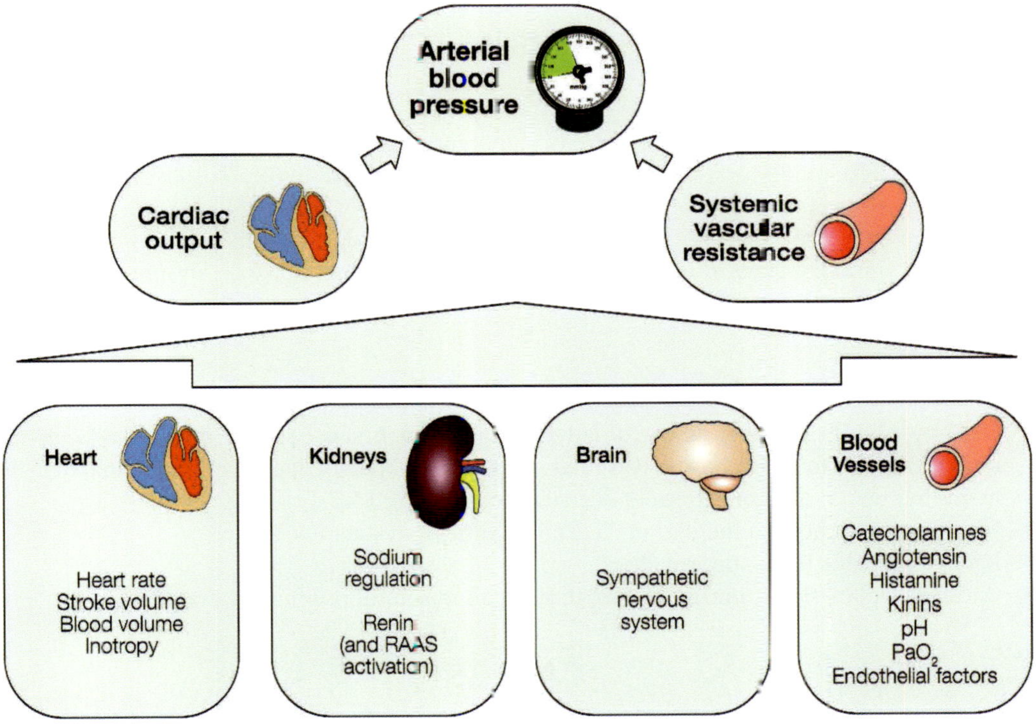

Figure 13.1 Overview of some of the important mechanisms involved in the regulation of blood pressure. RAAS = renin–angiotensin–aldosterone system. Source: Reproduced from Sage Publications, Ltd: Taylor, SS, et al. ISFM Consensus Guidelines on the Diagnosis and Management of Hypertension in Cats. *Journal of Feline Medicine and Surgery* (2017) 19, 288–303; DOI: 10.1177/1098612X17693500. © ISFM and AAFP.

Blackwell's Five-Minute Veterinary Consult Clinical Companion: Small Animal Senior Care, First Edition. Edited by Heidi B. Lobprise.

Companion website: www.wiley.com/go/lobprise/Senior

Chronic, sustained BP increases may cause injury to several organs, referred to as target organ damage (TOD).

INCIDENCE/PREVALENCE

- Reported prevalence in HT-associated diseases—chronic kidney disease (CKD), 9–93% (dogs) and 19–65% (cats); diabetes mellitus, 24–67% (dogs) and 0–15% (cats); hyperadrenocorticism, 20–80% (dogs); hyperthyroidism, 5–25% (cats); pheochromocytoma, 43–86% (dogs).

SIGNALMENT

Species

Dog and cat.

Mean Age and Range

- Usually older animals; median age: 13–15 years (cats).

SIGNS

Historical Findings

- Signs attributable to underlying disease (e.g., polyuria/polydipsia, anorexia, vomiting, weight loss with CKD; hindlimb weakness, cervical ventroflexion with hyperaldosteronism).
- Acute-onset or progressive blindness (retinal; neurological).
- Altered mental state, lethargy, seizures (generalized or focal), or ataxia.
- Rarely, respiratory signs due to congestive heart failure (CHF), e.g., dyspnea/orthopnea (cats/dogs), cough (dogs).
- Epistaxis (rare).

Physical Examination Findings

- Ocular—blindness, mydriasis, exudative retinal detachment, retinal hemorrhage/edema, retinal vascular tortuosity or perivascular edema, vitreal hemorrhage, bullous retinal detachment, hyphema, glaucoma, retinal degeneration (Figure 13.2).
- Neurologic—abnormal mentation, central blindness, nystagmus, ataxia.
- Renal—palpable renal abnormalities.
- Cardiovascular—heart murmur, arrhythmia, gallop sound, pulmonary crackles.

CAUSES

Idiopathic

Subclinical CKD thought to contribute in some cases.

Secondary Hypertension

- CKD.
- Acute kidney injury (AKI).
- Hyperadrenocorticism.
- Hyperthyroidism.
- Diabetes mellitus.
- Pheochromocytoma.

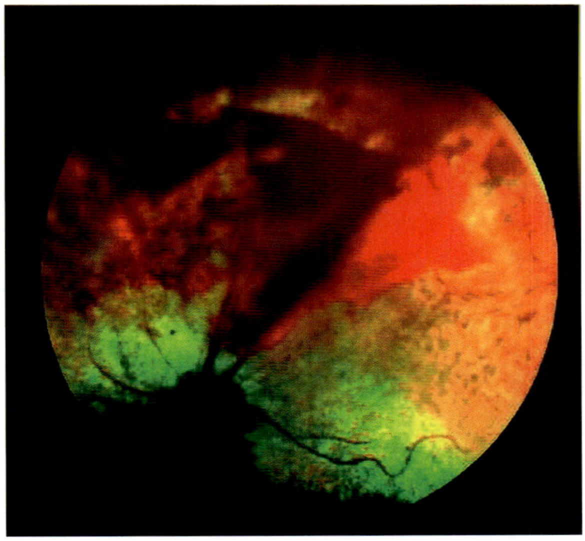

Figure 13.2 SBP 182 mmHg. Left eye. Dorsal to the optic nerve head is substantial fresh vitreal hemorrhage. There are also some areas of retinal thinning and laterally there is retinal degeneration. Source: Taylor et al. (2017)/Sage Publications.

- Primary hyperaldosteronism.
- Hypothyroidism.
- Polycythemia.
- Drug-related—glucocorticoids (uncommon), mineralocorticoids (high dosages), erythropoietin/darbepoetin, phenylpropanolamine, phenylephrine, ephedrine, toceranib phosphate.
- Intoxicants—cocaine, methamphetamine/amphetamine, 5-hydroxytryptophan.

RISK FACTORS

Renal disease or endocrinopathy.

DIAGNOSIS

DIFFERENTIAL DIAGNOSIS

Differential signs—differentiate from other causes of acute-onset blindness, central neurologic signs, CHF, or epistaxis, depending on presenting signs and clinical findings.

CBC/BIOCHEMISTRY/URINALYSIS

- Packed cell volume may be decreased (CKD) or mildly increased (hyperthyroidism).
- CBC may reveal stress leukogram and/or thrombocytosis (hyperadrenocorticism).
- May note azotemia, hyperphosphatemia, hyperkalemia (AKI, CKD); hyperglycemia (diabetes mellitus); increased serum alkaline phosphatase (hyperadrenocorticism); increased serum alanine aminotransferase (hyperthyroidism); hypokalemia (hyperaldosteronism).
- Urinalysis may reveal low urine specific gravity, proteinuria, hematuria, pyuria, bactiuria (AKI, CKD, hyperadrenocorticism); glucosuria (diabetes mellitus).

OTHER LABORATORY TESTS

- Assessment of glomerular filtration rate may detect early renal dysfunction.
- Urinary protein: creatinine ratio may disclose proteinuria.
- Serum total T_4 concentration, T_3 suppression test to evaluate for hyperthyroidism (cats).
- Serum T_3, T_4, free T_3, free T_4, and thyroid-stimulating hormone concentrations; T_3 and T_4 autoantibodies to evaluate for hypothyroidism (dogs).
- Screening tests for hyperadrenocorticism in dogs with other suggestive findings.
- Plasma aldosterone concentration if primary hyperaldosteronism suspected (cats).
- Plasma and urinary catecholamine concentrations if pheochromocytoma suspected.

IMAGING

- Abdominal ultrasonography to evaluate kidneys, liver, and adrenal glands.
- Echocardiography to evaluate for cardiac TOD—may be normal or disclose left ventricular concentric and/or eccentric hypertrophy, diastolic dysfunction, left atrial enlargement.
- CT or MRI if cerebral hemorrhage, hyperadrenocorticism suspected.
- Thyroid scintigraphy to evaluate hyperthyroidism.

DIAGNOSTIC PROCEDURES

- Diagnosis requires documentation of persistently (i.e., during ≥2 sessions, performed on different days) high SBP, using reliable direct or indirect measurement methods.
- Methods should be standardized to avoid inaccuracies caused by common technical errors.
- Substantial effort should be made to minimize patient stress to reduce risk of falsely diagnosing "true" HT in patient with situational HT.

Direct (Invasive) BP Measurement Methods

- Gold standard—involve catheterization or needle puncture of peripheral artery.
- Reserved for monitoring under anesthesia or during emergency management of severe HT.

Indirect (Noninvasive) BP Measurement Methods

- More clinically useful than direct methods for outpatient setting.
- Utilize devices that rely on Doppler ultrasonography or oscillometry.
- Require placement of inflatable cuff to temporarily occlude arterial blood flow in extremity by applying external, compressive force (Figure 13.3).

Ancillary Diagnostics

Fundoscopic examination to evaluate for retinal lesions.

TREATMENT

Treatment Guidelines for Dogs and Cats

- General goal to reverse/limit ongoing TOD and prevent future TOD.
- If identified, treatment of underlying disease may resolve HT.

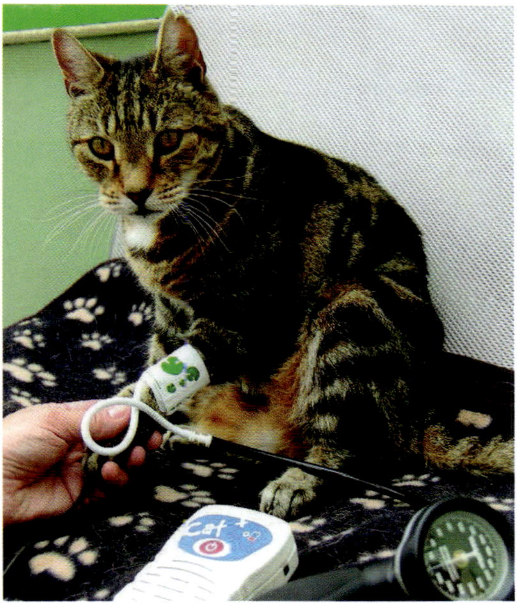

■ **Figure 13.3** Positioning of the cuff for blood pressure measurement. Forelimb (a) and tail (b) for Doppler measurement; tail (c) for measurement by high-definition oscillometry. Source: Taylor et al. (2017)/Sage Publications.

- Antihypertensive therapy indicated in dogs and cats with:
  - SBP ≥160 mmHg on two or more occasions for which situational hypertension considered unlikely.
  - SBP ≥160 mmHg on single occasion if clear evidence of ongoing neurologic or ocular TOD.
- Animals without evidence of TOD and mildly increased SBP (140–159 mmHg, "prehypertensive"), or suspected situational HT, should not be treated.
- Therapeutic targets—ideally, normotension (SBP 120–140 mmHg); SBP <160 mmHg at minimum.
- Gradual (i.e., over several weeks) reduction in BP should be targeted.
- HT considered an emergency if severe neurologic or ocular TOD is present; in these cases, goal is to cautiously reduce SBP to approximately 160 mmHg over 3–6 hours and to <140 mmHg over 1–2 days, with continuous/frequent BP monitoring.

APPROPRIATE HEALTH CARE

Usually managed on outpatient basis. Inpatient care may be necessary depending on underlying condition and severity of target organ damage.

ACTIVITY

No restrictions.

DIET

- Dietary sodium restriction is controversial.
- Avoid high sodium intake.

CLIENT EDUCATION

- Unless underlying cause is curable or controllable, patient is likely to require lifelong antihypertensive therapy.
- HT may persist or develop even with control of underlying disease (e.g., hyperthyroidism).
- Multiple agents and periodic dosage adjustments may be required for adequate control of HT.
- Frequent monitoring necessary until adequate BP control is achieved.

SURGICAL CONSIDERATIONS

May be indicated for pheochromocytoma, primary hyperaldosteronism, hyperthyroidism, and some forms of hyperadrenocorticism.

MEDICATIONS

DRUG(S) OF CHOICE

- Depend on underlying disease (e.g., adrenergic antagonists preferred in patients with pheochromocytoma, aldosterone antagonists in those with primary aldosteronism).
- Cats—amlodipine or telmisartan first line for SBP 160–200 mmHg; amlodipine first line if SBP >200 mmHg or ocular/neurologic TOD; angiotensin-converting enzyme (ACE) inhibitor or telmisartan may be added if proteinuria or poor control with amlodipine alone.
- Dogs—ACE inhibitor or angiotensin receptor blocker (ARB) first line; amlodipine coadministered as first line if SBP >200 mmHg or added if SBP 160–200 mmHg and poor control with ACE inhibitor or ARB.
- In hypertensive emergency (HT with severe ocular or neurologic TOD), parenteral hydralazine, sodium nitroprusside, or fenoldopam can be used; continuous direct BP monitoring is necessary in these cases.

Dihydropyridine Calcium Channel Blocker

Amlodipine—dogs: 0.1–0.5 mg/kg PO q24h; cats: 0.625–1.25 mg/cat PO q24h (consider 1.25 mg/cat if SBP >200 mmHg; may be increased to 2.5 mg/cat if necessary).

ACE Inhibitor

Enalapril or benazepril—dogs: 0.5–1.0 mg/kg PO q12h; cats: 0.5 mg/kg PO q12–24h.

ARB

Telmisartan—dogs: 1.0 mg/kg PO q24h; cats: 2.0 mg/kg PO q 24h; in United States labeled to start with 1.5 mg/kg PO BID protocol for 2 weeks and then adjust to 2.0 mg/kg q24h.

Direct-Acting Vasodilator

Hydralazine—dogs: 0.5 mg/kg PO q12h, stepwise increase to 3 mg/kg PO q12h if needed; cats: 2.5 mg/cat q12–24h.

Alpha-Adrenergic Receptor Antagonist

Phenoxybenzamine—dogs: 0.25 mg/kg PO q8–12h; cats: 2.5 mg/cat PO q8–12h.

Aldosterone Antagonist

Spironolactone—dogs and cats: 1.0–2.0 mg/kg PO q12h.

CONTRAINDICATIONS

Decrease or discontinue vasoconstricting drugs (e.g., phenylpropanolamine).

PRECAUTIONS

- Abrupt BP reduction and hypotension (SBP <120 mmHg) should be avoided; use of rapidly acting drugs or combinations of vasodilators increases this risk.
- Direct arteriolar vasodilators and IV antihypertensives may cause reflex tachycardia.
- Discontinue antihypertensives 48 hours prior to general anesthesia

POSSIBLE INTERACTIONS

- Use of antihypertensives in combination increases risk of hypotension.
- Hyperkalemia may result from coadministration of any combination of ACE inhibitor, ARB, and spironolactone.

ALTERNATIVE DRUG(S)

For Hypertensive Emergency

- Sodium nitroprusside (inorganic nitrate)—dogs and cats: 0.5–5 µg/kg/min IV, start low and increase by increments of 0.1–0.5 µg/kg/min to effect.
- Hydralazine (direct arteriolar vasodilator)—dogs: 0.5–2 mg/kg SC/IM q8–12h *or* 0.1–0.5 mg/kg IV q2–8h, CRI 1.5–5.0 µg/kg/min; cats: 1.0–2.5 mg/cat SC.
- Fenoldopam (dopamine-1 antagonist)—dogs and cats: 0.1–1.6 µg/kg/min; start low, increase by increments of 0.1 µg/kg/min to effect.

FOLLOW-UP

PATIENT MONITORING

- BP and manifestations of ocular or neurologic TOD should be checked weekly (or every 1–3 days if severe TOD) until normotension (SBP 120–140 mmHg) achieved (ideally), or SBP <160 mmHg (at minimum).

- Periodic monitoring of laboratory tests to evaluate for side effects of medications and clinical response (e.g., proteinuria, hematuria, anemia, thrombocytopenia, potassium balance, sodium balance, azotemia).

POSSIBLE COMPLICATIONS

- Progression of underlying renal disease.
- Retinopathy, choroidopathy.
- Encephalopathy, cerebral vascular accident.
- CHF (uncommon), aortic aneurysm/dissection/rupture (rare).
- Gingival hyperplasia may develop with amlodipine treatment in dogs.
- Facial dermatitis/excoriation may develop with spironolactone treatment in cats (uncommon).

EXPECTED COURSE AND PROGNOSIS

- Treatment of systemic hypertension may reverse or slow progression of TOD.
- Rapid and complete improvement of neurologic signs (usually within 24–48 hours) is expected with adequate BP control.
- Improvement/resolution of visual deficits may take weeks with BP control; most blind eyes do not regain normal vision.

MISCELLANEOUS

Associated Conditions and Age-Related Factors

- CKD.
- Endocrinopathies—hyperthyroidism and hyperadrenocorticism

See Also

- Diabetes Mellitus—Cats and Dogs
- Diabetes Mellitus Without Complication—Dogs.
- Hyperadrenocorticism (Cushing's Syndrome)—Dogs.
- Hyperthyroidism.

Abbreviations

- ACE = angiotensin-converting enzyme
- AKI = acute kidney injury.
- ARB = angiotensin receptor blocker.
- CHF = congestive heart failure.
- CKD = chronic kidney disease.
- HT = systemic arterial hypertension.
- SBP = systolic arterial blood pressure.
- TOD = target organ damage.

Internet Resources

Accessed 29 June 2024
https://icatcare.org/vets/guidelines/hypertension-cats

Suggested Reading

Acierno MJ, Brown S, Coleman AE, et al. ACVIM consensus statement: guidelines for the identification, evaluation, and management of systemic hypertension in dogs and cats. *J Vet Intern Med* 2018;32(6):1803–1822.

Carter J. Hypertensive ocular disease in cats: a guide to fundic lesions to facilitate early diagnosis. *J Feline Med Surg* 2019;21:35–45.

Jepson RE, Feline systemic hypertension: classification and pathogenesis. *J Feline Med Surg* 2011;13(1):25–34.

Taylor SS, Sparkes AH, Briscoe K, et al. ISFM consensus guidelines on the diagnosis and management of hypertension in cats. *J Feline Med Surg* 2017;19(3):288–303.

Taylor, SS, et al. ISFM Consensus Guidelines on the Diagnosis and Management of Hypertension in Cats. *Journal of Feline Medicine and Surgery* (2017) 19, 288–303; DOI: 10.1177/1098612X17693500. © ISFM and AAFP.

Author/editor: Heidi Lobprise
Topic adapted from Five Minute Veterinary Consultation, 7th edition. 2021
Original Topic: Hypertension—Systemic Arterial

Author: Amanda E. Coleman
Reference: (figures 13.1 and 13.3)

Chapter 14

Myxomatous Mitral Valve Disease

BASICS

DEFINITION

Myxomatous mitral valve disease (MMVD) is progressive degeneration that most commonly affects the mitral valve, though any valve can be involved.

PATHOPHYSIOLOGY (COMPLETE SECTION AVAILABLE IN ONLINE RESOURCES)

- Pathologic weakened and disorganized valvular connective tissue, in which the valve leaflets become thickened and elongated.
- Degenerative changes in chordae tendineae contribute to valve flattening and prolapse.
- Insufficient systolic coaptation of the leaflets, leading to backward regurgitation of blood from the ventricle into the atrium.
- Severity of mitral regurgitation depends on severity of valve lesions.
- Compensatory cardiac dilation and eccentric hypertrophy, increased force of contraction, increased heart rate, increased pulmonary lymphatic drainage, fluid retention, and neuro-hormonal modulation of cardiovascular function.
- Eventually may not be compensated, leading to reduced cardiac output and increased venous pressures, leading to pulmonary edema if left-sided congestive heart failure (CHF) and ascites if right-sided CHF.
- Acute cardiac tamponade may result from atrial tear.

SYSTEMS AFFECTED

- Cardiovascular
- Hepatobiliary—passive congestion at advanced stages.
- Renal/urologic—prerenal azotemia at advanced stages.
- Respiratory—if edema and/or pulmonary hypertension (PH) develops.

GENETICS

Possible genetically determined dystrophic process initiates valve degeneration. Age of onset—polygenetic threshold trait (i.e., multiple genes and a certain threshold has to be reached before

Blackwell's Five-Minute Veterinary Consult Clinical Companion: Small Animal Senior Care, First Edition. Edited by Heidi B. Lobprise.

Companion website: www.wiley.com/go/lobprise/Senior

the disease develops): sire and dam with early onset of MMVD likely have offspring that have an early onset of the disease. A combination of dogs with late onset will give offspring that manifest the disease at old age or never.

INCIDENCE/PREVALENCE

The most common cardiac disease in dogs. Common in old dogs, less common in young dogs. MMVD highest prevalence is in small-to-medium-sized dog breeds. The prevalence reaches >90% in some affected dog breeds >10 years.

SIGNALMENT

Species

Dogs; extremely rare in cats.

Breed Predilections

Typically small breeds (<20 kg, but may be encountered in larger dogs), such as cavalier King Charles spaniel (CKCS), Chihuahua, miniature schnauzer, Maltese terrier, Pomeranian, cocker spaniel, Pekingese, poodle, and others.

Mean Age and Range

Murmur may be detected from 2 years of age with a peak incidence for detection at 6–8 years in widely affected breeds such as the CKCS. Onset of CHF from 8–12 years.

Predominant Sex

Males develop the disease at a younger age than females, which means higher prevalence at a given age in males,

SIGNS

Signs depend on the stage of disease. The descriptions here align with the grading system described in the American College of Veterinary Internal Medicine (ACVIM) consensus statement on MMVD.[1]

Clinically Healthy Patients but at a Higher Risk of Developing the Disease (ACVIM Stage A)

No abnormal findings.

Dogs Diagnosed with the Disease but with No Overt Clinical Signs (ACVIM Stage B) 1 and 2

- Systolic click (early stage).
- Systolic murmur best heard over the mitral or tricuspid areas.
- Murmurs may range from soft low-intensity to loud holosystolic.
- With progression, murmurs typically get louder and radiate more widely.
- Initially, patients have no obvious radiographic or echocardiographic changes in cardiac chamber size or have mild cardiomegaly and do not meet the so-called "EPIC trial criteria"

(see ACVIM stage B1). Stage B2 is defined as dogs with cardiac enlargement meeting EPIC trial criteria, i.e., presenting a moderate or loud intensity murmur (≥3/6), VHS >10.5, body-weight normalized left ventricular end-diastolic diameter (LVIDDn) ≥1,7, and a left atrial-to-aortic root ratio (LA/Ao) ≥1.6.

Dogs with Overt Clinical Signs of CHF or with Clinical Signs Stabilized by CHF Therapy (ACVIM Stages C and D)

- Usually a loud holosystolic heart murmur.
- Tachypnea/dyspnea/orthopnea if decompensated CHF.
- Tachycardia and loss of respiratory sinus arrhythmia if decompensated CHF.
- Arrhythmia, such as supraventricular premature beats, ventricular premature beats, or atrial fibrillation, may be present.
- Respiratory crackles if decompensated CHF.
- Weak femoral pulse, prolonged capillary refill time and pale mucous membranes in low output failure.
- Pink froth, i.e., pulmonary edema, may be evident in the nares and oropharynx in severe decompensated CHF.
- Ascites if right-sided CHF (caused by myxomatous tricuspid lesions and/or pulmonary hypertension [PH]).

DIAGNOSIS

DIFFERENTIAL DIAGNOSIS

- Bacterial endocarditis (see below).
- Congenital heart disease.
- Dilated cardiomyopathy.
- Chronic airway or interstitial lung disease.
- Pneumonia.
- Pulmonary embolism.
- Pulmonary neoplasia.
- Heartworm disease.

CBC/BIOCHEMISTRY/URINALYSIS

- CBC/biochemistry usually unremarkable unless severe disease and ongoing CHF therapy.
- Prerenal azotemia secondary to impaired renal perfusion; high urine specific gravity unless complicated by underlying kidney disease or recent/ongoing diuretics.
- High liver enzyme activity in many patients with right-sided CHF.

OTHER LABORATORY TESTS

- Natriuretic peptides—often unremarkable unless moderate-to-severe disease.
- Serum troponin I—unremarkable unless severe disease.

IMAGING

Radiography

- Heart size ranges from normal to left-sided or generalized cardiomegaly.
- LA enlargement is usually the earliest finding.
- LV may be enlarged.
- Left-sided CHF—pulmonary congestion; increased interstitial pattern ± alveolar pattern with air bronchograms. Initially, congestion and edema are perihilar, but all lungfields may eventually show changes.

Echocardiography

- Thickened and distorted mitral valve leaflets.
- Elongated and ruptured chordae tendineae, causing mitral valve prolapse.
- Normal-to-severely dilated atrium (uni- or bilateral).
- LV may be dilated and is hyperdynamic if regurgitant flow is significant and myocardial function intact; as LV becomes more grossly distended, it may become normo- or, uncommonly, hypodynamic because of myocardial failure.
- Pericardial effusion (usually mild) may be present in severe disease.
- Doppler studies show a jet of regurgitation into the atrium.
- Doppler evaluation for the presence of PH should be routinely performed.

DIAGNOSTIC PROCEDURES

- Arterial/venous blood gases can be used to quantify hypoxemia and monitor treatment response.
- Systemic blood pressure should be monitored; especially patients receiving diuretics and other cardiovascular drugs to check for hypotension; hypertension is not associated with the disease, but if concurrent can exacerbate the disease.

Electrocardiographic Findings

- Sinus tachycardia common in patients with CHF.
- May show evidence of LA enlargement (P mitrale) or LV enlargement (tall and wide R waves).
- Supraventricular, or ventricular arrhythmias may develop in severe disease.

PATHOLOGIC FINDINGS (COMPLETE SECTION AVAILABLE IN ONLINE RESOURCES)

TREATMENT

APPROPRIATE HEALTH CARE

Dogs with preclinical MMVD can be managed at home with scheduled rechecks to identify dogs that meet EPIC trial criteria for initiation of pimobendan. Some dogs with mild-to-moderate signs of CHF may be managed at home, whereas dogs with more severe signs should be hospitalized initially for intensive CHF therapy.

NURSING CARE

Oxygen therapy as needed for hypoxemic dogs with moderate-to-severe CHF. Dogs receiving diuretics must be given the opportunity to urinate. Dyspnea-associated anxiety should be treated. Carefully monitor blood pressure and respiratory response to narcotics and tranquilizers in the setting of acute decompensated CHF. Butorphanol 0.2–0.25 mg/kg IM or IV is commonly used for sedation, but combinations of buprenorphine 0.0075–0.01 mg/kg and acepromazine 0.01–0.03 mg/kg IV, IM, or SQ can also be used.

ACTIVITY

- Exercise restriction for symptomatic patients in acute decompensated CHF.
- Exercise recommended for stable CHF patients on medical therapy, but avoid strenuous exercise.

DIET

- Prevent cardiac cachexia by ensuring adequate calorie intake.
- Avoid high-sodium diets.

CLIENT EDUCATION

- Discuss the progressive nature of the disease.
- Mild disease severity is suggestive of a long period without clinical signs; moderate-to-severe disease indicates a shorter period until signs of CHF may develop.
- If a breeder, inform about the disease genetics and impact for future breeding.
- Pimobendan therapy prolongs preclinical period and survival times in dogs meeting the EPIC criteria.
- Appropriate level of exercise, but at the same time maintain quality of life.
- Common signs of CHF listed earlier.
- How to medicate (if indicated)—information about consistent dosing and that diuretic doses should be adjusted in consultation with the veterinarian.
- Possible adverse side reactions of medications.
- How to monitor resting and/or sleeping respiratory rates (RRR) at home, and at which rate new contact with the clinician should be initiated.
- Diet (if indicated)—emphasize importance of avoiding cardiac cachexia by paying close attention to appetite and using an appropriate diet. Salt loads should be avoided.

SURGICAL CONSIDERATIONS

Surgical valve repair can be performed at a few sites in the world.

MEDICATIONS

DRUG(S) OF CHOICE

Recommended treatment depends on disease stage; these recommendations follow the guidelines set by the consensus statement developed by the ACVIM.

Patients Without Overt Clinical Signs (ACVIM Stage B)

- If no cardiomegaly, no treatment currently recommended.
- Pimobendan 0.25–0.3 mg/kg q12h PO prolongs preclinical period (by a median of approximately 15 months) and survival in Stage B2 dogs.
- Administering angiotensin-converting enzyme inhibitors (ACEIs) to Stage B patients has been shown to be ineffective in two clinical trials.

Patients Showing Overt Clinical Signs (ACVIM Stages C and D)

Acute Decompensated CHF

- Furosemide IV, SC, IM, or PO; dose is dependent on severity of CHF:
  - Mild-to-moderate CHF: 2–4 mg/kg q8–24h.
  - Severe or fulminant CHF: 4–8 mg/kg q2–6h, preferably IV, IM, or SC.
  - Monitor outcome of treatment by respiratory rate and general clinical status.
  - Dose can often be reduced once the patient is stabilized.
- Oxygen supplementation and cage rest to patients with significant dyspnea: 40% in O_2 cage (can intermittently go as high as 100%) up to 24 hours; nasal O_2 may be used in large-breed dogs, 50–100 mL/kg/min through humidifier.
- Pimobendan 0.25–0.3 mg/kg q12h PO. In many countries outside of the United States, IV pimobendan is available and used as an initial single-dose treatment before oral medication.
- Additional options in severe fulminant CHF:
  - Nitroglycerin: ointment (one-fourth inch/5 kg up to 2 inches percutaneously), sublingual spray (one puff/10 kg) or injectable (1–5 µg/kg/min CRI).
  - Arterial vasodilator to decrease afterload rapidly, e.g., hydralazine 0.5 mg/kg q12h (titrate up to 2 mg/kg if necessary) or sodium nitroprusside 1–10 µg/kg/min (expensive drug and difficult to obtain). Both drugs require blood pressure monitoring and should be considered only in hospitalized dogs under care of a specialist.
  - Dobutamine—dogs: 1–10 µg/kg/min; cats: 1–5 µg/kg/min.
- Antiarrhythmics—as needed.
- Severe ascites may require abdominocentesis.

Chronic CHF (Typically Treated as an Outpatient)

- Exact composition of medical therapy depends on disease severity and clinical signs. All dogs with CHF require life-long treatment with a diuretic, such as furosemide:
  - Mild-to-moderate CHF: 1 mg/kg q12h to 2 mg/kg q8h PO.
  - Moderate-to-severe CHF: 2–3 mg/kg q12h or higher.
- Pimobendan at 0.25–0.3 mg/kg q12h PO.
- ACEI (e.g., enalapril, benazepril, ramipril)—dose and frequency depend on ACEI used, e.g., enalapril 0.5 mg/kg q12–24h; benazepril 0.25–0.5 mg/kg q24h.
- Spironolactone 2 mg/kg q12–24h PO and/or hydrochlorothiazide at 2–4 mg/kg q12h PO.
- Digoxin 0.22 mg/m^2 q12h PO, or lower.
- Antiarrhythmics—as needed.
- Sildenafil 1–2 mg/kg q8–12h if PH present.

PRECAUTIONS

- Use digoxin, diuretics, and ACEIs cautiously in patients with renal disease.
- Beta blockers are negative inotropes and may have an acute adverse effect on myocardial function and clinical status.

POSSIBLE INTERACTIONS

- Furosemide potentiates the effects of ACEIs, spironolactone, or thiazides.
- Use nonsteroidal anti-inflammatory drugs cautiously in patients receiving furosemide or ACEIs.

ALTERNATIVE DRUG(S)

- Diuretics—add thiazide and/or spironolactone in refractory animals.
- Torsemide—administered at approximately 1/10th of the furosemide dose, or 0.1–0.6 mg/kg once to twice daily is an alternative to furosemide.
- Vasodilators—isosorbide dinitrate can be used in place of nitroglycerin ointment in patients requiring long-term nitrate administration.

FOLLOW-UP

PATIENT MONITORING

- Frequency of rechecks depends on stage of MMVD and severity of CHF (if present).
- Dogs without signs of CHF:
    - Mild-to-moderate disease—perform echocardiography when a murmur is first detected and every 6–12 months (interval depends on findings of previous echocardiogram) thereafter to document progressive cardiomegaly. Baseline radiographs may be useful.
    - Owners are instructed to regularly measure respiratory rates at home during rest or sleep and contact the veterinarian should rates be consistently higher than 30 breaths/minute.
- Dogs with signs of CHF:
    - Once acute CHF has been successfully treated, dogs can be treated at home.
    - Follow-up with owner, by phone or email, should be conducted after 1–3 days at home, to monitor for maintained treatment effect. A change in the furosemide dose (partly based on respiratory rates during sleep or deep rest and amount of side effects of the treatment initiated) may be performed.
    - Reexamine after 1–2 weeks (check for signs of decompensated CHF, dehydration, electrolyte imbalance, renal dysfunction, and presence of complications) or sooner if treatment response is unsatisfactory.
    - Thereafter once every 3–6 months if the patient is stable on the medications. More severe cases may require more frequent monitoring.
- Monitor BUN and creatinine especially when high doses of diuretics and ACEIs are used.
- Monitor potassium, especially if combinations of spironolactone, ACEIs, and digoxin are used.

POSSIBLE COMPLICATIONS

- Preclinical patients may develop acute CHF.
- Recurrent decompensated CHF in patients stabilized by medical therapy.
- PH.
- Biventricular CHF in dogs with initial left-sided CHF.

- Mild pleural and/or pericardial effusion. Arrhythmia.
- Rupture of major chordae tendineae, leading to a flail valve leaflet and acute decompensation.
- Atrial tear leading to acquired atrial septal defect or cardiac tamponade.

EXPECTED COURSE AND PROGNOSIS

Valve lesions are progressive in nature and myocardial function may worsen, requiring increased drug dosages. Long-term prognosis depends on response to therapy and stage of heart disease.

MISCELLANEOUS

Synonyms

- Chronic valvular disease (CVD).
- Chronic mitral valve disease.
- Degenerative valvular disease.
- Degenerative mitral valve disease (DMVD).
- Degenerative valve disease.

See Also

- Congestive Heart Failure

Abbreviations

- ACEI = angiotensin-converting enzyme inhibitor.
- ACVIM = American College of Veterinary Internal Medicine.
- CHF = congestive heart failure.
- LA = left atrium.
- LV = left ventricle.
- MMVD = myxomatous mitral valve disease.
- PH = pulmonary hypertension.
- RRR = resting respiration rate

Internet Resources (and References)

Accessed 29 June 2024

ACVIM consensus guidelines for the diagnosis and treatment of myxomatous mitral valve disease in dogs—Keene, 2019, *Journal of Veterinary Internal Medicine*, Wiley Online Library.

Reference

1. Keene BW, Atkins CE, Bonagura JD, et al. ACVIM consensus guidelines for the diagnosis and treatment of myxomatous mitral valve disease. *J Vet Intern Med* 2019;33(3):1127–1140.

Author/editor: Heidi Lobprise
Topic adapted from Five Minute Veterinary Consultation, 7th edition. 2021
Original Topic: Myxomatous Mitral Valve Disease

Authors: Ingrid Ljungvall and Jens Häggström
Consulting Editor: Michael Aherne

Dentistry

Chapter 15

Feline Alveolar Osteitis

OVERVIEW

Thickening of bone over the jugum of tooth roots due to inflammation. Alveolar osteitis most commonly occurs over the maxillary canine tooth roots of middle-aged and older cats (sometimes also called buttressing). This process appears to be secondary to periodontal inflammation. Tooth resorption and extrusion (supereruption) may also be seen in affected teeth. Feline alveolar osteitis should be distinguished from benign alveolar bone expansion (also called buccal bone expansion), which is devoid of inflammation.

SIGNALMENT

Although alveolar osteitis can occur in dogs, it is far more common in cats.

There are no established breed or sex predilections, and no established genetic basis.

Middle-aged and older cats are most commonly affected.kay

SIGNS

History

- Owner may report thickening or bulging over the maxillary canine teeth roots, usually bilateral, but can be unilateral (see Figure 15.1).
- Evidence of oral pain is not often noted by pet owners.
    - Discomfort may occur with mobile teeth.
    - Discomfort may occur when extruded maxillary canine teeth contact the lower lip or the opposing canine, resulting in an acquired malocclusion.

Clinical Findings

- Bulging of alveolar bone on the buccal surface of the root; variable degree of gingival inflammation.
- Patient may have abnormal periodontal pocket depths on probing (normal sulcus depth for cats is 0–1 mm); patients often exhibit vertical bone loss with infrabony pockets (see Figures 15.2–15.4).
- Patients may exhibit extrusion (supereruption) of one or more teeth; extended tooth length may cause trauma to lower lip or malocclusion with opposing mandibular canine tooth.
- May progress to tooth mobility and acquired dental malocclusion due to contact between maxillary and mandibular canine teeth.

Blackwell's Five-Minute Veterinary Consult Clinical Companion: Small Animal Senior Care, First Edition. Edited by Heidi B. Lobprise.

Companion website: www.wiley.com/go/lobprise/Senior

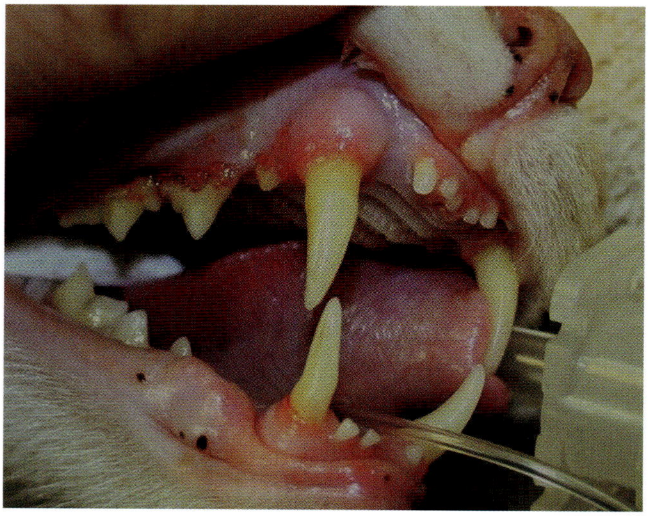

■ **Figure 15.1** Feline Alveolar Osteitis with bulging over the maxillary canine teeth roots and root exposure due to extrusion or super-eruption of the tooth. Source: With permission of Heidi Lobprise.

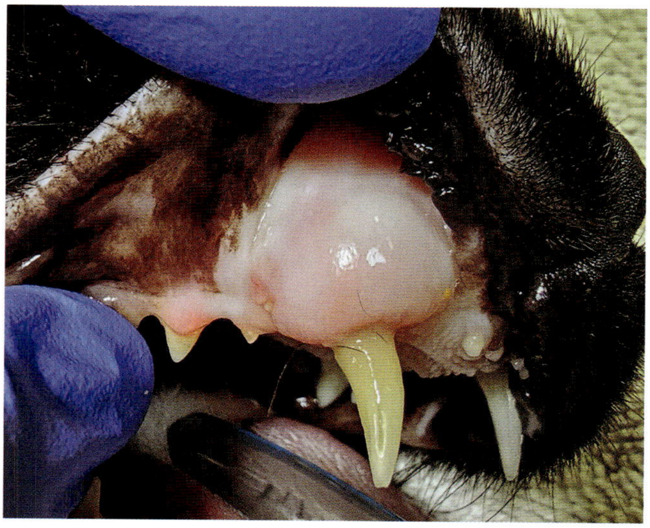

■ **Figure 15.2** Feline Alveolar Osteitis with extensive swelling/bulging of the buccal alveolar bone and inflammation.

CAUSES AND RISK FACTORS

Cause is unknown, but buttressing in humans is considered to be an attempt by the body to stabilize a diseased tooth. Cats that are prone to periodontal disease may be at a higher risk for developing alveolar osteitis.

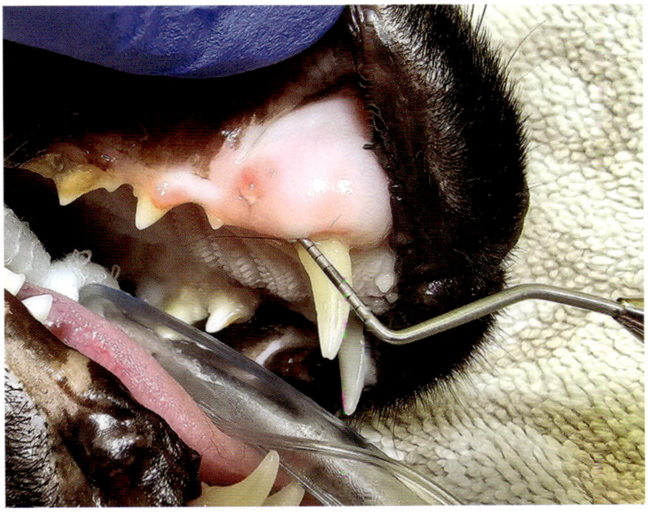

■ **Figure 15.3** A deep periodontal pocket is present on the buccal surface of the tooth, with indication of a periodontal abscess draining tract or parulis at the distal aspect.

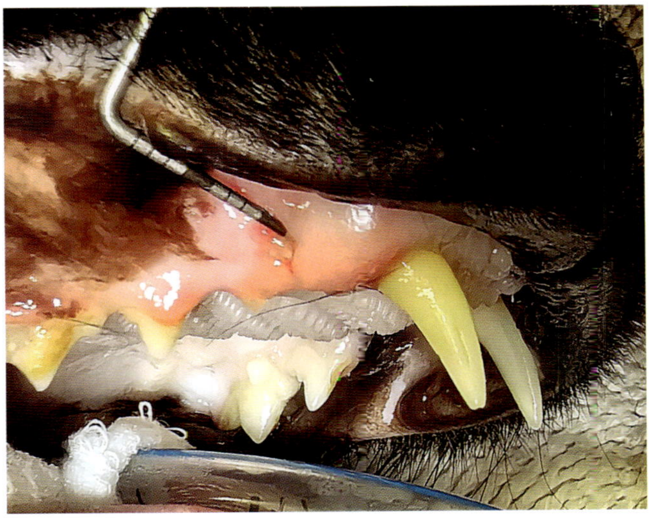

■ **Figure 15.4** A periodontal probe enters the parulis opening, connecting with the periodontal pocket. With this much periodontal disease, extraction is the treatment of choice.

DIAGNOSIS

DIFFERENTIAL DIAGNOSIS

Alveolar bone expansion, also known as buccal bone expansion, is an enlargement of alveolar bone that looks similar to alveolar osteitis. However, when biopsied, alveolar bone expansion may show no signs of inflammation.

CBC/BIOCHEMISTRY/URINALYSIS

No specific abnormalities seen related to alveolar osteitis.

IMAGING

Intraoral dental radiographs typically show evidence of vertical periodontal bone loss along the long axis of the root on the palatal and buccal surface of the root. The expanded bone may be less dense than normal adjacent alveolar bone.

DIAGNOSTIC PROCEDURES

- Appropriate preanesthetic diagnostics when indicated prior to procedure.
- Complete oral examination with periodontal probing—assess for periodontal pockets, gingival bleeding, or tooth mobility; pay particular attention to probing depth of palatal surface of maxillary canine teeth.
- Intraoral radiographs under anesthesia—assess extent of osseous changes; assess root stability, attachment loss, and evidence of tooth resorption.
- Consider biopsy if bone changes are unilateral or if aggressive osseous changes are seen on dental radiographs.

TREATMENT

- If mild periodontal changes are present (moderate pocket depth, no tooth mobility, minimal extrusion, no oronasal fistulation), a professional ultrasonic dental cleaning with root planing and subgingival curettage ± placement of periodontal pocket antimicrobial treatment ± osseous surgery.
- If extensive periodontal disease is present (deep periodontal pocket, tooth mobility, extensive extrusion, patient discomfort, oronasal fistula), consider extraction. Buccal-attached gingiva may be very thin, making it difficult to elevate a gingival flap. Ostectomy/osteoplasty of buccal alveolar bulge is necessary after raising the gingival flap and prior to closure. Biopsy of buccal alveolar bone can be accomplished with rongeurs once a mucogingival flap has been elevated. Gently elevate palatal mucosal edge to facilitate closure.

MEDICATIONS

DRUG(S) OF CHOICE

Appropriate antimicrobials and pain medications when indicated.

FOLLOW-UP

PATIENT MONITORING

Recheck patient at 2 weeks postoperatively, with regular reevaluations depending on what treatment was chosen.

PREVENTION/AVOIDANCE

No known methods of prevention.

POSSIBLE COMPLICATIONS

Complications include those that may occur when extracting teeth (perforation of mucogingival flap, dehiscence, iatrogenic oronasal fistula, etc.).

EXPECTED COURSE AND PROGNOSIS

Good with appropriate treatment, unless neoplasia is diagnosed with biopsy.

Suggested Reading

Beebe DE, Gengler WR. Osseous surgery to augment treatment of chronic periodontitis of canine teeth in a cat. *J Vet Dent* 2007;24(1):30–38.

Author/editor: Heidi Lobprise
Topic adapted from Five Minute Veterinary Consultation, 7th edition, 2021
Original Topic: Feline Alveolar Osteitis

Author: John R. Lewis
Consulting Editor: Heidi B. Lobprise

Chapter 16

Pathologic Mandibular Fractures

BASICS

DEFINITION

Fractures of the mandible(s) precipitated by periodontal loss of bone and osteomyelitis that weakens the mandible and places it at risk for fracture with trauma, even mild trauma.

SIGNALMENT

Species

Dog, smaller individuals.

SIGNS

- Vary greatly according to the location, type, extent, cause, and underlying risk factors resulting in the injury.
- Facial deformity, malocclusion, oral or bleeding, and inability to properly close the jaw are common signs.

PHYSICAL EXAMINATION

- Many pathologic mandibular fractures occur in the region of the mandibular first molar, where periodontal bone loss can greatly compromise the strength of the bone. (Figure 16.1)
- Some fractures may also occur near the mandibular canines, or at the mandibular symphysis where bone loss is common in small, older dogs.
    - Note: many smaller dogs, especially older ones, may already display slight mobility in the mandibular symphysis; this should always be evaluated and recorded before any procedures (extractions) in the region.

CAUSES

- Injury or trauma in a dog with periodontal bone loss of the mandible.
    - Dog fight injury
    - Jumping off bed and hitting jaw.

Blackwell's Five-Minute Veterinary Consult Clinical Companion: Small Animal Senior Care, First Edition. Edited by Heidi B. Lobprise.

Companion website: www.wiley.com/go/lobprise/Senior

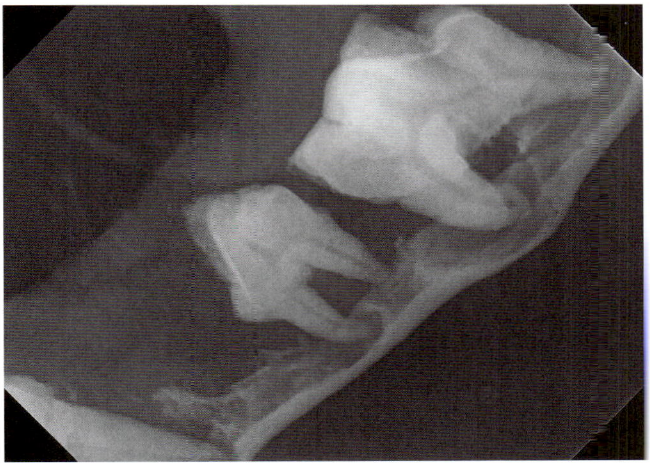

■ **Figure 16.1** When there is extensive periodontal bone loss of the mandible, as shown in this dental radiograph, even a small traumatic event can cause a pathologic fracture of the jaw.

RISK FACTORS

- Oral infections (e.g., periodontal disease, osteomyelitis), neoplasia, or certain metabolic diseases (e.g., hypoparathyroidism)—may result in weaker jaws that are more prone to injury.
- Traumatic injury affecting the jaws or teeth.
    - Periodontal disease increases in older dogs; potential bone healing capabilities may be decreased in these patients
    - Concurrent systemic disease must be managed in many of these patients (cardiac, renal, etc.)

DIAGNOSIS

A thorough and complete physical examination is very important in traumatic jaw injuries as many unseen or multiple injuries and complications are possible.

DIFFERENTIAL DIAGNOSIS

- Temporomandibular joint (TMJ) conditions—see Temporomandibular Joint Disorders.
- Tooth subluxation or luxation (i.e., interference with jaw closure).
- Endodontic disease (e.g., tooth abscess).
- Foreign body lodged in or near the oral cavity.
- Maxillary or mandibular nerve injury or disease.
- Masticatory muscle myositis.
- Neoplasia.

CBC/BIOCHEMISTRY/URINALYSIS

As required—to assess and treat shock from initial injury; to assess animal prior to surgery.

IMAGING

Radiography—intraoral and extraoral; CT and MRI.

DIAGNOSTIC PROCEDURES

- Oral examination.
- Neurologic examination.
- Biopsy for histopathology, if indicated.
- Bacterial culture and sensitivity, if indicated.

TREATMENT

APPROPRIATE HEALTH CARE

- While there are many types of treatment for various classes of fractures including interdental wiring/splints, internal fixation (wires, plates) and external fixation, the site of a pathologic fracture often has insufficient healthy bone strength to allow for proper reduction, fixation, stabilization, and adequate healing (Figures 16.2–16.4)
- Extensive surgical techniques with autologous rib bone implants and mini-plates can help reconstruct the mandibular fracture. Healing capabilities of the patient need to be considered, as well as length of time under anesthesia.
- Comorbidities should also be considered as fracture repair generally takes long anesthetic times.
- For some patient, a palliative rostral mandibulectomy may be the treatment of choice: removing that portion of the mandible rostral to the fracture site—to the mandibular symphysis.
    - This can also be done bilaterally if necessary.

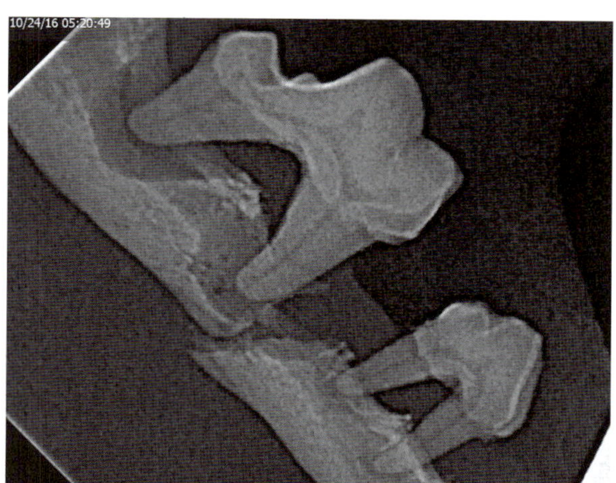

Figure 16.2 Significant bone loss of the right mandible with mandibular fracture.

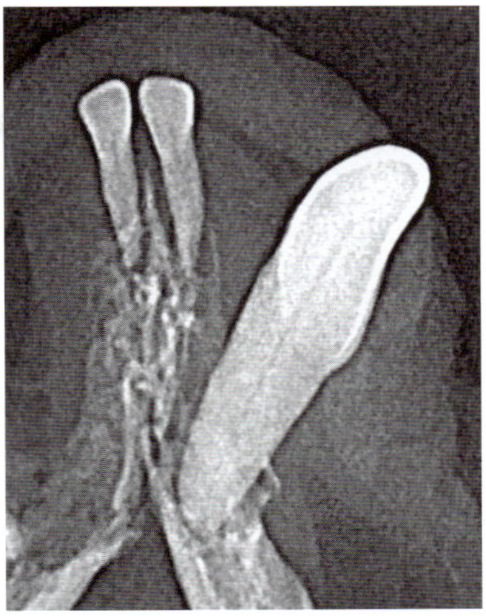

■ **Figure 16.3** Significant bone loss of the rostral mandibular symphysis and possible right canine alveolar fracture.

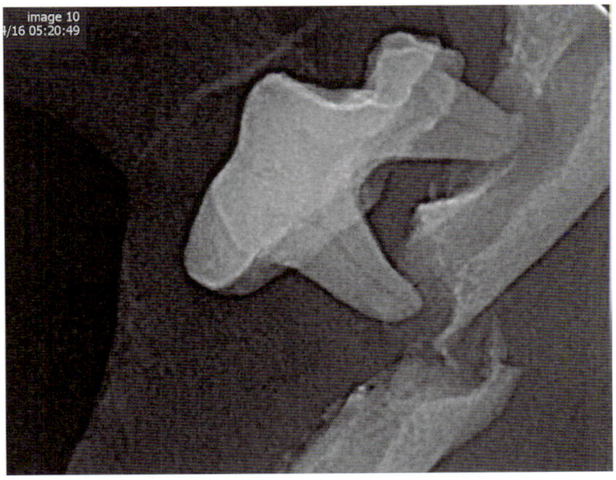

■ **Figure 16.4** With a bilateral mandibular fracture and compromised bone at the left mandibular first molar, this patient may be a candidate for bilateral rostral mandibulectomy.

Procedure

- Administer an inferior alveolar (caudal mandibular) nerve block: bilaterally if necessary.
- Fully evaluate the fracture visually, with palpation and radiographically.
- Determine if the tooth just distal to the fracture also needs extraction.
- Evaluate the mandibular symphysis
- Extensive bone loss at the fracture sites as well as symphyseal bone loss or instability at the mandibular canine can help you decided to perform this procedure.

■ Incise soft tissue
- Buccally – just apical to the attached gingiva (mucosa is easier to elevate), from the fracture site to midline symphysis (Figure 16.5)
- Lingually – just apical to gingival margin – from fracture to symphysis (Figures 16.6 and 16.7)
- Bluntly dissect away soft tissue
  - Ligate the middle mental foramina neurovascular bundle.

■ Separate the mandible at the symphysis from the opposite side.

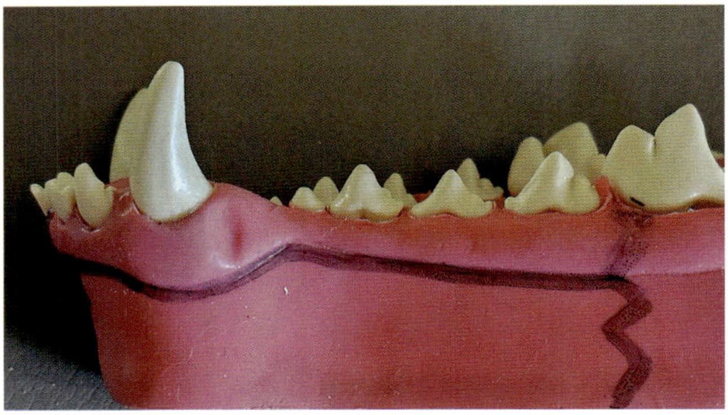

■ **Figure 16.5** Marks on dental model illustrating partial rostral mandibulectomy for palliative management of a pathologic fracture of the left mandible. From the site of the fracture, on the buccal aspect, an incision is made just ventral to the attached gingiva, extending rostrally to mandibular symphyseal midline.

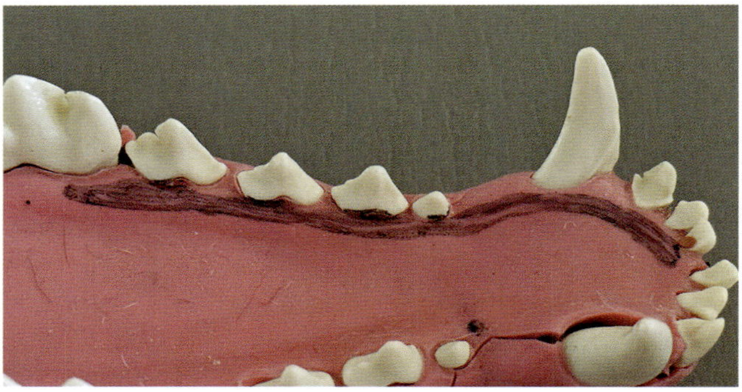

■ **Figure 16.6** From the site of the fracture, on the lingual aspect, an incision is made just ventral to the gingival margin, extending rostrally to mandibular symphyseal midline.

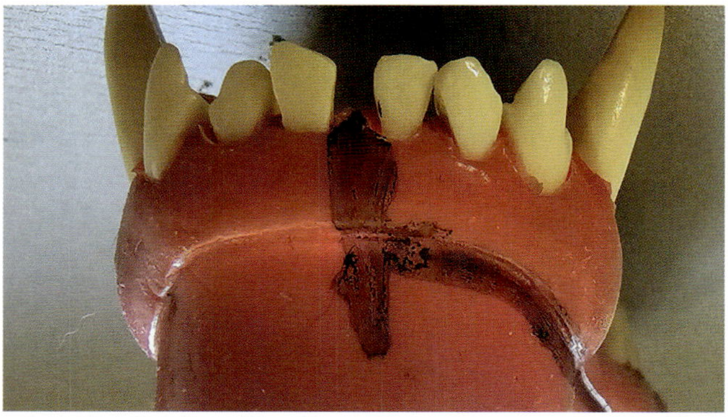

■ **Figure 16.7** The two incisions are joined at the rostral mandibular symphysis with soft-tissue reflection to expose the bone and separate

- Grasp the rostral aspect of the mandibular fragment and continue to bluntly dissect soft tissue and muscles, but don't separate from distal fragment. (See Figure 16.3) (Placeholder)
- If still intact, identify the mandibular canal neurovascular bundle and ligate it; incise the bundal rostral to the ligature; remove the rostral mandibular fragment.
  - Extract distal tooth or roots as needed
  - Alveoloplasty of the distal fragment
  - Close with absorbable suture (poliglecaprone 4-0).

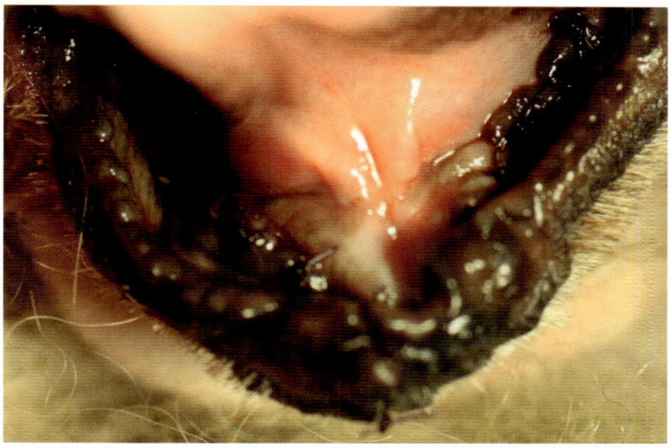

■ **Figure 16.8** After a bilateral rostral mandibulectomy, cheiloplasty with removing a rostral wedge of lip/chin tissue can result in a more cosmetic result.

- Bilateral rostral mandibulectomy: if both sides are fractured and compromised, this procedure can be done bilaterally.
- There will be extra or redundant tissue of the lips that will hang down, unsupported, so a cheiloplasty will be required. (Figure 16.8)
    - A single, larger wedge can be done rostrally at mid-line.
    - Two smaller wedges done bilaterally can help keep the structure of the rostral lip, but is more complicated.

Homecare

- Especially with a bilateral procedure, let the owner know that the tongue will likely hang out; if it gets too desiccated, regular moistening may be needed.
- With a unilateral procedure, the opposite jaw may drift to the side of the mandibulectomy. In this author's experience, most pets adjusted well. Rarely was intervention necessary (stabilization or extracting the opposite lower canine)
- Diet—soft food or gruel may be required during healing. Raising the food and water bowls to a platform that is shoulder-height can help; feed on an easily cleaned surface.

MEDICATIONS

DRUG(S) OF CHOICE

Pain Management

- Local anesthesia—intraoral local blocks; regional nerve blocks: mental n., mandibular n., infraorbital n., and maxillary n.
- Injectables—hydromorphone, buprenorphine, fentanyl, CRI, certain drug combinations.
- Transdermal patches—fentanyl.
- Oral—nonsteroidal anti-inflammatory drugs (NSAIDs); gabapentin, tramadol, hydrocodone.

Antibiotics

Limit usage to cases with suspected osteomyelitis; bacterial culture and sensitivity should be performed to prescribe appropriate drug.

FOLLOW-UP

PATIENT MONITORING

- Physical—recheck in 2 weeks
- Most patients have other teeth with extensive periodontal disease that also need treatment/extraction. This is often staged 2–4 weeks after the mandibulectomy to reduce anesthetic time at the first procedure.

POSSIBLE COMPLICATIONS

- Malocclusion; mandibular drift.
- Neurologic defects.
- Facial pain syndrome.
- Impaired mastication.
- Temporary weight loss.

EXPECTED COURSE AND PROGNOSIS

- Generally good.

MISCELLANEOUS

Abbreviations

- MMF = maxillomandibular fixation
- NSAID = nonsteroidal anti-inflammatory drug.
- TMJ = temporomandibular joint.

Internet Resources

Accessed 29 June 2024
https://avdc.org/avdc-nomenclature/

Suggested Reading

Taney K, Smithson CW. Oral surgery—fracture and trauma repair. In: Lobprise HB, Dodd JR (eds) *Wigg's Veterinary Dentistry: Principles and Practice*, 2nd edn. Hoboken, NJ: John Wiley & Sons, 2019; pp. 265–288.

Author/editor: Heidi Lobprise
Topic adapted from Five Minute Veterinary Consultation, 7th edition, 2021
Original Topic: Obesity

Author: Maxillary and Mandibular Fractures Kendall Taney
Consulting Editor: Heidi B. Lobprise

Chapter 17

Periodontal Disease

BASICS

DEFINITION

Inflammation and destruction of the periodontium (i.e., gingiva, cementum, periodontal ligament, and alveolar bone) secondary to the subgingival biofilm of bacteria.

PATHOPHYSIOLOGY

A pellicle of salivary glycoproteins adheres to the clean tooth and first colonizing Gram-positive aerobic bacteria attach; the plaque biofilm is created. The supragingival plaque biofilm matures and influences the development of the subgingival biofilm. The constituents of the biofilm progress to Gram-negative anaerobic, motile, and spirochete bacteria. Bacterial byproducts and proteolytic enzymes with the host inflammatory response cause destruction of the periodontium, resulting in the loss of attachment for the tooth. The biofilm forms within days. Calculus is the mineralization of plaque. It is rough, acts a surface area for more plaque development, and can be mechanically irritating to the tissues.

SYSTEMS AFFECTED

Gastrointestinal—oral cavity/dentition (primary); systemic inflammation/distant organ changes.

INCIDENCE/PREVALENCE

Common—estimated to be around 85%.

SIGNALMENT

Species

Dog and cat.

Breed Predilections

Toy, brachycephalic, sighthounds, long-facial haired, and purebred cats.

Blackwell's Five-Minute Veterinary Consult Clinical Companion: Small Animal Senior Care, First Edition. Edited by Heidi B. Lobprise.

Companion website: www.wiley.com/go/lobprise/Senior

Mean Age and Range

- Can begin as juvenile disease and progresses through life.
- Studies show incidence/prevalence increases with increased age

SIGNS

Historical Findings

Hidden/no clinical signs to halitosis, head shyness, oral bleeding, dropping food, reluctance to chew, pawing at the mouth, exaggerated jaw movements, face rubbing, maxillofacial swellings, ptyalism, sneezing, and nasal discharge.

Physical Examination Findings

- Conscious examination—inflammation of the gingiva, plaque and/or calculus, root exposure, furcation exposure, mobile teeth, parulides, disproportionate plaque and calculus distribution, oral discharge, maxillofacial swellings, and mandibular lymphadenopathy. The conscious examination significantly underestimates the presence and severity of PD, and therefore an anesthetized examination with periodontal probing and intraoral radiographs is required for complete assessment.
- Anesthetized examination—the degree of severity of periodontal disease relates to a single tooth.
- American Veterinary Dental College (AVDC) nomenclature:
    - Normal (PD 0)—clinically normal; no gingival inflammation or periodontitis clinically evident.
    - Stage 1 (PD 1)—gingivitis only without attachment loss. The height and architecture of the alveolar margin are normal (Figure 17.1).
    - Stage 2 (PD 2)—early periodontitis; less than 25% of attachment loss, or at most, there is a Stage 1 furcation involvement in multirooted teeth.
    - Stage 3 (PD 3)—moderate periodontitis; 25–50% of attachment loss, and/or there is a Stage 2 furcation involvement in multirooted teeth (Figure 17.2).
    - Stage 4 (PD 4)—advanced periodontitis; more than 50% of attachment loss or there is a Stage 3 furcation involvement in multirooted teeth (Figure 17.3).
        - Furcation indices subjectively measure when the periodontal probe extends less than halfway between the roots (F1), extends greater than halfway (F2), or

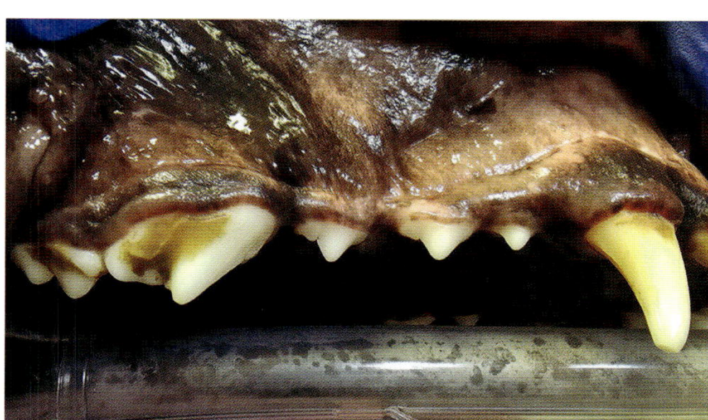

Figure 17.1 Stage 1 periodontal disease may have inflammation of the gingival margin, but there is no loss of attachment.

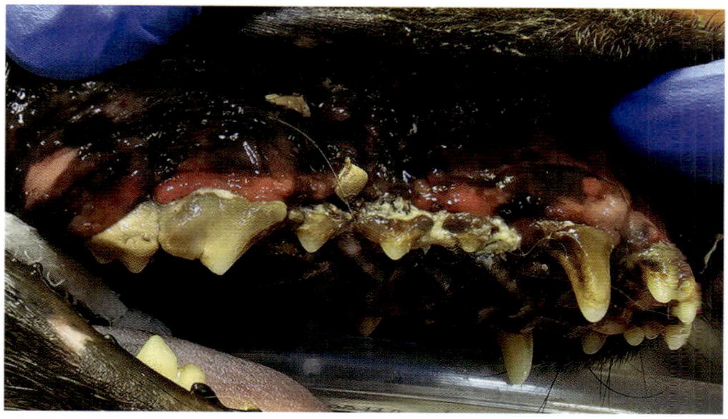

■ **Figure 17.2** This patient has significant plaque and calculus with significant gingival inflammation, indicating there is some level of attachment loss (gingiva and bone). Until radiographs are taken and probing depths are measured, full assessment of the level of periodontal disease cannot be made.

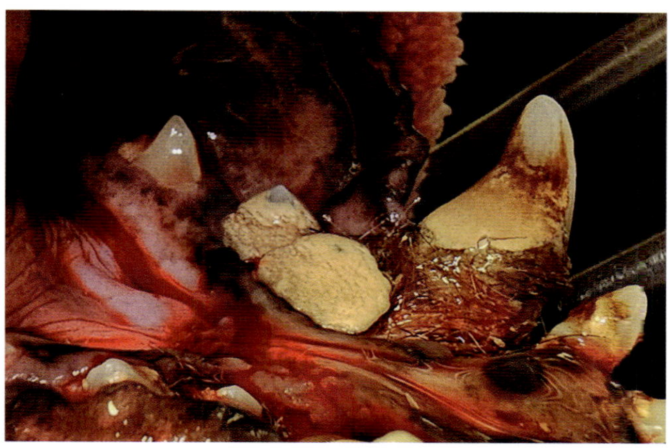

■ **Figure 17.3** The extensive calculus and gingival recession is a good indication that stage 4 periodontal disease is present in this patient.

through and through from one side of the furcation and out the other under the crown (F3).

- Periodontal attachment loss is measured by probing of the clinical attachment level and radiographic determination of the distance of the alveolar margin from the tooth's cementoenamel junction relative to the length of the root.

CAUSES

Bacterial plaque biofilm and associated host inflammatory response.

RISK FACTORS

Lack of daily preventive home care and professional veterinary dental care, signalment, systemic health (e.g., immunosuppression from pharmaceuticals or metabolic disease), inappropriate chewing behavior, malocclusions, crowding of dentition, oral foreign bodies.

DIAGNOSIS

DIFFERENTIAL DIAGNOSIS

- Oral neoplasia
- Drug-associated gingival enlargement (e.g., cyclosporine, amlodipine),
- Oral autoimmune inflammatory conditions,
- Viral ulcerative gingivitis/mucositis (e.g., calicivirus),
- Oral trauma and foreign bodies, rare fungal.

CBC/BIOCHEMISTRY/URINALYSIS

Overall systemic/metabolic health status and for preparation for anesthesia.

IMAGING

- Intraoral radiography—required diagnostic instrument to assess attachment loss, to include marginal bone loss, loss of the lamina dura, widening of the periodontal ligament space, horizontal and vertical bone loss, inflammatory resorption of the tooth root surface, furcation bone loss, combined patterns of bone loss.
  - Horizontal bone loss is a pattern where the cortical and alveolar bone surrounding the tooth and adjacent teeth are lost at a similar rate; the periodontal pocket is above the bone (i.e., suprabony pocket) (Figure 17.4).
  - Vertical bone loss is a pattern where there is bone loss around a tooth root where the adjacent supporting bone remains more coronal; the periodontal pocket is within the bone (i.e., infra(intra) bony pocket) (Figure 17.5).
    - Vertical bone loss at the mandibular first molar is often a factor in pathologic mandibular fractures. (See Pathologic Mandibular Fractures)

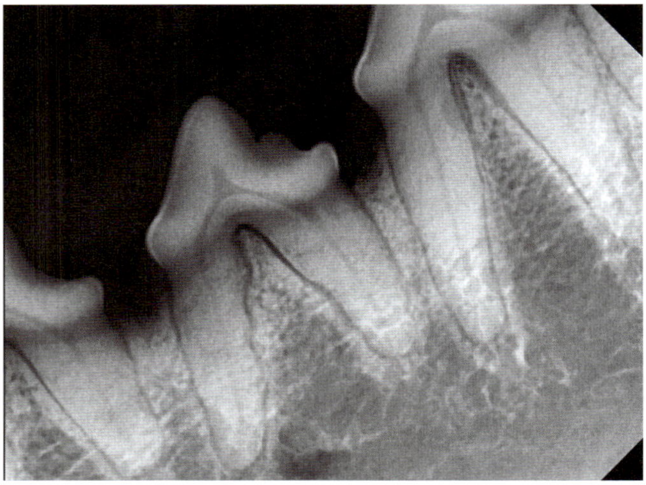

■ **Figure 17.4** Intraoral radiographs are essential to assess both the extent and pattern of bone loss. There is a pattern of horizontal bone loss across these left mandibular premolars.

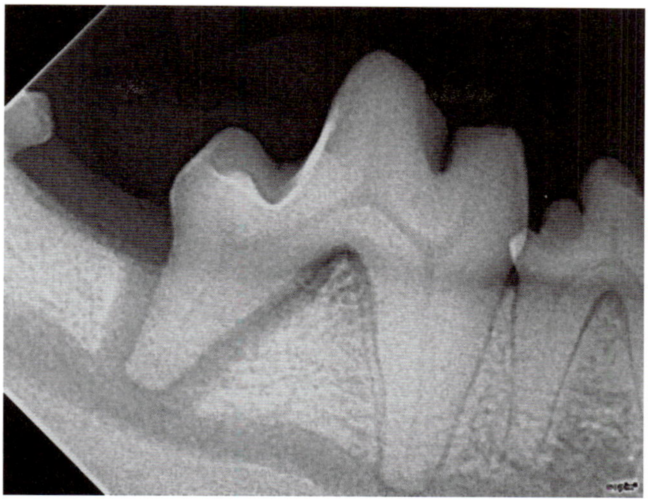

■ **Figure 17.5** There is a vertical bone loss pattern down the mesial root of 409 in this radiograph. The extension of bone loss to the apex indicates that periodontal pathogens have likely entered the pulp chamber through the apex, necessitating extraction.

- Osteopermeative patterns mimicking neoplasia can be present in severe cases.
  - Osteitis secondary to the inflammation may result in paradoxical proliferation of bone.
- Cone-beam CT has been reported to be of additional valuable in assessing periodontal attachment loss in brachycephalic breeds.

DIAGNOSTIC PROCEDURES

- Periodontal probing—the distance between free gingival margin and apical extent of the sulcus or pocket; probing depths <3 mm in dogs and <1 mm in cats are considered normal gingival sulcus; variations based on the range of breed sizes in dogs.
- Measurement of root exposure, furcation exposures, and tooth mobility are recorded.
- Clinical probing information and intraoral radiographic assessment are used to assign periodontal score to each tooth (PD0–PD4).

TREATMENT

APPROPRIATE HEALTH CARE

- Prevention of PD with daily home care and annual preventive cleaning, starting in first 1–2 years of life; oral examinations and periodontal treatments before excessive attachment loss.
- Daily home care prevention should begin in the first year of life. Daily tooth brushing is the best daily home care prevention.
- Annual or semi-annual evaluations and periodontal cleanings/“prophylaxis” and treatment based on the patient signalment and progressive PD stage status.
- Client communication and education throughout all patient life stages.

NURSING CARE

Acute-on-chronic periodontal abscessation—nonsteroidal anti-inflammatory medications, if not contraindicated; analgesia and appropriate antibiotic selection pending scheduling for anesthesia, assessment, and treatment.

DIET

Dental diets with fiber arrangements and/or added dental products added for patients without other dietary restrictions, or needs, and who have teeth remaining to chew.

CLIENT EDUCATION

Daily home care, the necessity of general anesthesia, and the lifelong prevention, management, and treatment of PD.

SURGICAL CONSIDERATIONS

- Remove the plaque biofilm and calculus, eliminate periodontal pocket(s), prevent further attachment loss, extract hopelessly compromised teeth, address contributing dental factors, and treat oral/dental pain. Individualized general anesthetic management.
- Periodontal surgery including, but not limited to, gingivectomy/gingivoplasty, periceutical treatment, closed root planing, open root planing, periodontal flaps, osseous resective surgery, osseous additive surgery including bone augmentation and guided tissue regeneration. Plans are based on PD stage, tooth/teeth involved, overall systemic health of the patient, ability for home care, ability to have further follow-up treatments and anesthetic procedures, and overall financial aspects for the client with the goal to have a pain- and infection-free oral cavity.

MEDICATIONS

DRUG(S) OF CHOICE

Systemic use of antimicrobials is *not* indicated in the treatment of PD without surgical attention to the underlying cause. Clindamycin, amoxicillin/clavulanic acid, and doxycycline may be chosen to augment periodontal surgical treatment. Metronidazole may be selected based on clinical findings and patient history.

CONTRAINDICATIONS

- Immunosuppressive drugs in untreated PD can cause acute-on-chronic exacerbations.
- Chronic use of bisphosphonates should be avoided unless the oral cavity and dentition have all active infection and inflammation treated.

PRECAUTIONS

Prolonged/increased dosages of immunosuppressive medications may contribute to acute on chronic exacerbations.

POSSIBLE INTERACTIONS

Oral chlorhexidine and oral fluoride inactivate with simultaneous use.

FOLLOW-UP

PATIENT MONITORING

The diagnosed PD stage guides the recheck interval; evaluation every 3–12 months.

PREVENTION/AVOIDANCE

- Daily tooth brushing with pet toothpaste mechanically removes the supragingival plaque biofilm.
- Oral 0.1–0.12% chlorhexidine products target oral bacteria involved in the plaque biofilm.
- Dental diets, dental chews, barriers sealants, dental wipes, dental enzyme systems, dental gels, and water additives can be a part of a dental home care program based on individual patient and client needs.
- The Veterinary Oral Health Council can help guide selection of pet dental products.

EXPECTED COURSE AND PROGNOSIS

Due to the multifactorial aspect of PD and individual patient response, the expected course and prognosis can be variable, but predicable with appropriate treatment.

MISCELLANEOUS

Age-Related Factors

- Progresses with age; adult-onset periodontitis is most common; juvenile and aggressive forms of periodontitis occur.
- The chronic presence of periodontal inflammation and infection, particularly when not managed effectively, can impact systemic inflammation and inflammaging (see Inflammaging).
    - Minimizing the effects of chronic inflammation from the oral cavity is a distinct way to impact systemic inflammation. Patients that have been treated (often with multiple extractions) often have significant improvement in overall health and quality of life, in this author's experience. Owners claim they are "like a new dog"!
- The benefits of optimal oral and dental care in most cases outweigh the potential risks of general anesthesia, with appropriate patient assessment, stabilization and customized pain and anesthetic protocols (see Anesthesia for Senior Pets).
- If significant disease and extended anesthetic times are anticipated for complete dental care, it is appropriate to consider staging the procedures. For the first procedure, perform a complete dental cleaning, take full mouth radiographs, and extract loose teeth. For the second procedure (2–4 weeks later), finish the remaining oral surgery and extractions.

See Also

- Inflammaging
- Anesthesia for Senior Pets

Abbreviations

- AVDC = American Veterinary Dental College
- PD = periodontal disease.

Internet Resources

Accessed 29 June 2024

- https://avdc.org/avdc-nomenclature/
- http://www.vohc.org

Suggested Reading

Lobprise H, Stepaniuk K. Oral surgery—periodontal surgery. In: Lobprise H, Dodd JR (eds) 'Wiggs' *Veterinary Dentistry—Principles and Practice*, 2nd edn. Hoboken, NJ: Wiley-Blackwell, 2019; pp. 193–228.

Author/editor: Heidi Lobprise
Topic adapted from Five Minute Veterinary Consultation, 7th edition, 2021
Original Topic: Periodontal Disease

Author: Kevin S. Stepaniuk
Consulting Editor: Heidi B. Lobprise

Dermatology

Chapter 18

Dermatoses, Neoplastic

BASICS

DEFINITION

- Neoplastic proliferation of cells derived from the skin or migrating to the skin.
- Epidermal tumors from keratinocytes, melanocytes, Merkel cells, and Langerhans cells, and epitheliotropic lymphoma.
- Adnexal tumors from hair follicles, sebaceous glands, and sweat glands.
- Dermal and subcutaneous skin tumors include those of mesenchymal origin and tumors of round cell origin.

PATHOPHYSIOLOGY

- Ultraviolet light promotes tumor development by damaging DNA and suppressing the immune system.
- Many viruses promote tumor growth through stimulating cell proliferation and/or suppressing the immune system.
- Reports of specific cutaneous neoplasia associated with medications and/or vaccinations.

INCIDENCE/PREVALENCE

- The combined incidence rate for skin tumors has been reported as (0.728%) for dogs and 84/100,000 for cats.
- The skin is the most common site of occurrence of neoplasia in the dog (30% of total tumors) and the second most common site in the cat (20% of total tumors).
- Canine skin tumors are approximately 55% mesenchymal, 40% epithelial, and 5% melanocytic.
- The most common for dogs are lipoma, sebaceous gland adenoma, mast cell tumor, papilloma, and histiocytoma.
- Feline skin tumors are approximately 50% epithelial, 48% mesenchymal, and 2% melanocytic.
- The most common in cats are basal cell tumor, squamous cell carcinoma, mast cell tumor, and fibrosarcoma.
- Skin tumors in cats are more frequently malignant; skin tumors in dogs are more frequently benign.

Blackwell's Five-Minute Veterinary Consult Clinical Companion: Small Animal Senior Care, First Edition. Edited by Heidi B. Lobprise.

Companion website: www.wiley.com/go/lobprise/Senior

GEOGRAPHIC DISTRIBUTION

Geographic regions near the equator, with high altitude, or with sand or other reflective surfaces, have a higher incidence of solar-induced neoplastic dermatoses.

SIGNALMENT

Species

Dogs and cats.

Breed Predilections

- Canine breeds with the highest overall incidence of skin tumors include boxer, Scottish terrier, bullmastiff, basset hound, Weimaraner, Kerry blue terrier, and Norwegian elkhound.
- Feline breeds with the highest overall incidence of skin tumors include Siamese and Persian.
    - Squamous cell carcinoma—no predisposed breed reported.
    - Mast cell tumor—Siamese.
    - Fibrosarcoma—no predisposed breed reported.

Mean Age and Range

- The median age for cutaneous neoplasia is 10.5 years in dogs and 12 years in cats.
- The peak age period for cutaneous neoplasia in dogs and cats is 6–14 years.

Predominant Sex

- Females have a higher incidence of tumors in dogs (56%).
- Males have a higher incidence of tumors in cats (56%).

SIGNS

General Comments

Most common clinical sign is a cutaneous or subcutaneous nodule; some tumors have an ulcerated surface; others may result in excessive scaling or in the formation of cutaneous plaques.

Historical Findings

- Tumors are most often slow growing; the owner may find them during petting, bathing, or grooming of the pet.
- Tumors may be rapidly growing and appear (or increase in size) quickly (e.g., histiocytoma).

Physical Examination Findings

- Nodules—cutaneous or subcutaneous.
- Cutaneous ulcers.
- Excessive scaling.
- Cutaneous papillomas.
- Cutaneous plaques.

CAUSES

- Genetic (gene mutations).
- Environmental (e.g., ultraviolet light, radiation exposure).

- Viruses (e.g., papillomaviruses, feline leukemia virus, feline immunodeficiency virus).
- Toxins (e.g., tars).
- Drugs (e.g., immunosuppressive agents, chemotherapeutic agents).
- Epidermal neoplasms:
  - Keratinocytes—papillomas, squamous cell carcinoma, basal cell carcinoma, basosquamous carcinoma.
  - Melanocytes—melanoma.
  - Merkel cells—Merkel cell carcinoma.
  - Langerhans cells—histiocytoma and malignant histiocytosis.
  - Epitheliotropic lymphoma—T lymphocytes.
- Adnexal neoplasms:
  - Hair follicles—trichofolliculoma, trichoepithelioma, infundibular keratinizing acanthoma, tricholemmoma, pilomatrixoma, trichoblastoma.
  - Sebaceous glands—sebaceous adenoma, sebaceous epithelioma, sebaceous adenocarcinoma, perianal gland epithelioma, perianal gland carcinoma.
  - Sweat glands—apocrine cystadenoma, apocrine secretory adenoma/adenocarcinoma, apocrine ductal adenoma/carcinoma, eccrine carcinoma.
- Dermal and subcutaneous neoplasms:
  - Mesenchymal origin—soft-tissue sarcoma: fibroma/fibrosarcoma, myxoma/myxosarcoma, hemangiopericytoma, lymphangioma/lymphangiosarcoma, hemangioma/hemangiosarcoma, lipoma/liposarcoma, neurofibrosarcoma, leiomyoma/leiomyosarcoma, synovioma/synovial sarcoma, rhabdomyoma/rhabdomyosarcoma.
  - Round cell origin—transmissible venereal tumor, mast cell tumor, plasmacytoma, lymphoma, histocytoma, and histocytic tumors.
- Secondary or metastatic skin tumors result from the metastasis of primary neoplasms in other organs to the skin.

RISK FACTORS

- Hair coat color and length (e.g., hairless breeds, white hair coat, lightly pigmented skin—increased risk for squamous cell carcinoma).
- Age (e.g., young animals highest risk for viral infections, older animals at highest risk for environment-associated neoplasia).
- Sunlight exposure (e.g., dogs and cats that sunbathe or spend time outdoors on reflective surfaces have higher risk of ultraviolet light–induced skin tumors).
- Genetics—certain breeds have higher risk of developing specific types of tumors (see above and Suggested Reading).

DIAGNOSIS

DIFFERENTIAL DIAGNOSIS

- Cyst.
- Abscess.
- Inflammatory nodule/granuloma/plaque—sterile granulomatous and pyogranulomatous disease, sterile panniculitis, fungal infection, mycobacterial infection, foreign body.
- Trauma/self-induced skin ulceration.
- Hamartoma/nevus.

CBC/BIOCHEMISTRY/URINALYSIS

N/A

OTHER LABORATORY TESTS

- Cytology (fine-needle aspirate or impression smear).
- Regional lymph node aspirate (for staging).

IMAGING

Thoracic radiographs and abdominal ultrasonography useful for staging (evaluate for metastatic disease or underlying primary neoplasia).

DIAGNOSTIC PROCEDURES

- Cytology.
- Biopsy with histopathologic examination.
- Immunohistochemistry (useful in confirming certain types of tumors).

PATHOLOGIC FINDINGS

Varies with tumor type; see specific tumors for additional information.

TREATMENT

APPROPRIATE HEALTH CARE

- Varies with tumor type.
- Observation is appropriate for some benign tumors.
- Surgical excision, cryosurgery, radiation therapy, and/or tumor-specific chemotherapy or immunotherapy may be curative or palliative.

NURSING CARE

- Varies with tumor type and location.
- Traumatized tumors may become secondarily infected.

ACTIVITY

Varies with tumor type and location.

DIET

Diets high in omega-3 fatty acids, arginine, and protein may be beneficial in boosting the immune response and preventing cancer-associated cachexia.

CLIENT EDUCATION

Varies with tumor type and location.

SURGICAL CONSIDERATIONS

- Vary with tumor type and location—wide margins may be needed to prevent reoccurrence of infiltrative tumors.
- Pretreatment with antihistamines appropriate when excising mast cell tumors.

MEDICATIONS

DRUG(S) OF CHOICE

Vary with tumor type—chemotherapy protocols are useful in some cases.

CONTRAINDICATIONS

Vary with tumor type and presence of concurrent disease.

PRECAUTIONS, POSSIBLE INTERACTIONS, AND ALTERNATIVE DRUG(S)

Vary with tumor type and location.

FOLLOW-UP

PATIENT MONITORING, POSSIBLE COMPLICATIONS, EXPECTED COURSE AND PROGNOSIS

Varies with tumor type and location.

PREVENTION/AVOIDANCE

- Varies with tumor type and location.
- Minimize exposure to ultraviolet light to help prevent some types of tumors.

MISCELLANEOUS

Associated Conditions and Age-Related Factors

Vary with tumor type and location.

See Also (in Blackwell's Five-Minute Veterinary Consult, Canine and Feline, 7th ed)

- Adenocarcinoma, Skin (Sweat Gland, Sebaceous).
- Basal Cell Tumor.
- Fibrosarcoma, Bone.
- Lipoma, Infiltrative.
- Malignant Fibrous Histiocytoma.
- Mast Cell Tumors.
- Papillomatosis.
- Squamous Cell Carcinoma, Skin.

Internet Resources

Accessed 29 June 2024

- http://www.vetcancersociety.org

Suggested Reading

Campbell KL (ed.). *Small Animal Dermatology Secrets*. Philadelphia, PA: Hanley & Belfus, 2004; pp. 385–453.

Goldschmidt MH, Shofer FS. *Skin Tumors of the Dog and Cat*. Oxford: Butterworth Heinemann, 1992.

Gross TL, Ihrke PJ, Walder EJ, et al. *Skin Diseases of the Dog and Cat: Clinical and Histopathologic Diagnosis*, 2nd edn. Oxford: Blackwell, 2005; pp. 561–893.

Martin PD, Argyle DJ. Advances in the management of skin cancer. *Vet Dermatol* 2013;24:173–180.

Miller WH, Griffin CE, Campbell KL (eds). *Muller & Kirk's Small Animal Dermatology*, 7th edn. Philadelphia, PA: Elsevier, 2013; pp. 774–843.

Shearer D, Dobson J. An approach to nodules and draining sinuses. In: Foster A, Foil C (eds) *BSAVA Manual of Small Animal Dermatology*, 2nd edn. Gloucester: BSAVA, 2003; pp. 55–65.

Author/editor: Heidi Lobprise
Topic adapted from Five Minute Veterinary Consultation, 7th edition, 2021
Original Topic: Dermatoses—Neoplastic

Author: Karen L. Campbell
Consulting Editor: Alexander H. Werner Resnick

Chapter 19

Lupus Erythematosus, Cutaneous (Discoid)—Generalized

BASICS

OVERVIEW

- Considered to be a relatively benign variant of systemic lupus erythematosus (SLE).
- Divided into facial discoid lupus erythematosus (FDLE) and generalized DLE (GDLE).
- FDLE is one of the most common immune-mediated skin diseases in dogs.
- FDLE predominantly involves the nasal planum, face, and ears.
- GDLE—lesions progress beyond the head.

SIGNALMENT

- Dogs and cats.
- Very uncommon in cats.
- FDLE—collie, German shepherd dog, Siberian husky, Shetland sheepdog, Alaskan Malamute, chow chow, and their crosses.
- GDLE—German shepherd dog and Chinese crested (predominantly).
- FDLE—no age predilection; GDLE—older dogs.

SIGNS

FDLE

- Initial depigmentation of nasal planum and/or lips progresses to erosions and ulcerations.
- Loss of normal “cobblestone” architecture of the nasal planum.
- Tissue loss and scarring can occur.
- Chronic lesions are fragile and may easily bleed; severe hemorrhage associated with arteriole damage.
- May involve pinnae and periocular region.

GDLE

- Lesion behind the neck and/or on mucocutaneous junctions.
- Initial lesion—annular hyperpigmented plaques with adherent crust, follicular plugging, and central alopecia.
- Advanced lesions—reticulated patterns of hyperpigmentation or hypertrophic scars.

Blackwell's Five-Minute Veterinary Consult Clinical Companion: Small Animal Senior Care, First Edition. Edited by Heidi B. Lobprise.

Companion website: www.wiley.com/go/lobprise/Senior

CAUSES AND RISK FACTORS

- Actinic radiation may alter antigenic nature of keratinocytes.
- Seasonal and geographic exacerbation.

DIAGNOSIS

DIFFERENTIAL DIAGNOSIS

Major Considerations

- Other immune-mediated diseases (pemphigus foliaceus, pemphigus erythematosus, SLE, ischemic dermatitis, vasculitis).
- Drug reaction.
- Dermatomyositis.
- Nasal dermatophytosis.
- Mucocutaneous pyoderma.
- Insect bite hypersensitivity.

Other (Rare) Considerations

- Contact allergy.
- Zinc-responsive dermatosis.
- Trauma.
- Superficial necrolytic dermatitis.
- Epitheliotropic lymphoma.
- Squamous cell carcinoma.

CBC/BIOCHEMISTRY/URINALYSIS

Normal unless due to an underlying cause.

OTHER LABORATORY TESTS

Antinuclear antibody (ANA), LE preparation, and Coombs' tests—usually normal or negative except in SLE.

DIAGNOSTIC PROCEDURES

- Biopsy and histopathology will differentiate DLE from most other disorders; may be complicated by untreated mucocutaneous pyoderma.
- Biopsy early lesions—depigmented areas, mild erosions, or mildly crusted lesions.

PATHOLOGIC FINDINGS

Interface-lichenoid dermatitis with prominent basal cell apoptosis, varying degrees of epidermal atrophy, and pigment incontinence;. chronic lesions may include scarring.

TREATMENT

- FDLE—good prognosis; may be disfiguring.
- GDLE—guarded prognosis; depends on response to therapy.
- Avoid sunlight/apply sunblock.

MEDICATIONS

DRUG(S) OF CHOICE

- Topical therapy (FDLE):
  - Glucocorticosteroids—potent fluorinated product initially; less potent product later if possible (q24h for 14 days; then q48–72h).
  - Tacrolimus ointment (0.1%) q12–24h initially then taper to q24–72h once in remission.
  - Use a soft muzzle for 10 minutes after applying topical therapy to prevent medication removal by the patient.
- Systemic therapy (GDLE; severe FDLE):
  - Tetracycline and niacinamide—250 mg each PO q8h for dogs <10 kg; 500 mg PO q8h for larger dogs (alternatives include doxycycline 10 mg/kg PO q24h and minocycline 5 mg/kg PO q12h).
  - Prednisolone—2–4 mg/kg/day either solely or in combination with azathioprine 2 mg/kg PO q48h; taper prednisone to 0.5–1 mg/kg PO q48h for long-term maintenance.
  - Cyclosporine—5–10 mg/kg PO q24h as alternative immunosuppressive therapy.
- Systemic antibiotic treatment for 3–4 weeks prior to systemic immunosuppressive therapy to differentiate from mucocutaneous pyoderma.
- Vitamin E—10–20 IU/kg PO q12h may help reduce inflammation and protect the skin.
- Hydroxychloroquine—5 mg/kg q24h; antimalarial drug that has been used in human cases.

FOLLOW-UP

PATIENT MONITORING

- Recheck 4 weeks after initiating treatment to evaluate for clinical response.
- CBC and biochemistry—every 12 months (topical therapy); every 3–6 months (systemic therapy).
- Azathioprine—CBC and platelet counts every 2 weeks for the first month, then every 3–6 months.

PREVENTION/AVOIDANCE

Affected animals should avoid UV light exposure.

POSSIBLE COMPLICATIONS

- Scarring.
- Secondary pyoderma.

- Hemorrhage.
- Disfigurement.

EXPECTED COURSE AND PROGNOSIS

- FDLE—progressive but not usually life-threatening if left untreated.
- With proper treatment, expect remission in majority of cases.
- GDLE—prognosis is more guarded.

MISCELLANEOUS

Abbreviations

- ANA = antinuclear antibody
- FDLE = facial discoid lupus erythematosus.
- GDLE = generalized discoid lupus erythematosus.
- LE = lupus erythematosus.
- SLE = systemic lupus erythematosus.

Suggested Reading

Banovic F. Canine cutaneous lupus erythematosus: newly discovered variants. *Vet Clin Small Anim* 2019;49:37–45.

Thierry O, Linder KE, Banovic F. Cutaneous lupus erythematosus in the dogs: a comprehensive review. *BMC Vet Res* 2018;14:132.

Author/editor: Heidi Lobprise
Topic adapted from Five Minute Veterinary Consultation, 7th edition, 2021
Original Topic: Lupus Erythemaotis, Cutaneous (Discoid)—Generalized

Author: Dawn E. Logas
Consulting Editor: Alexander H. Werner Resnick

Chapter 20

Nasal Dermatoses—Canine

BASICS

DEFINITION

Pathologic condition of the nasal skin involving either the haired portion (bridge of the nose/dorsal muzzle) or non-haired portion (nasal planum).

SIGNALMENT

- Epitheliotropic lymphoma—older dogs (also squamous cell carcinoma and basal cell carcinoma)
- Senile idiopathic nasal hyperkeratosis—cocker spaniel, Boston terrier, bulldogs.
- Other nasal conditions – not specific to older patients, but may be present in seniors
- Eosinophilic folliculitis and furunculosis (often insect trigger; also seen in adult patients).
- Autoimmune diseases: discoid lupus erythematosus (DLE)—collie, Shetland sheepdog, German shepherd dog.
- DLE may occur more often in females. Other bullous diseases not confined to older patients
- Dermal arteritis of the nasal philtrum—Saint Bernard and other large breeds.
- Nasal solar dermatosis—lightly pigmented breeds.
- Seasonal nasal hypopigmentation—Labrador retriever, golden retriever, Siberian husky, Bernese mountain dog.
- Mucocutaneous pyoderma – German shepherd dog.
- Contact dermatitis—irritant or hypersensitivity; plastic dish dermatitis, topical drug hypersensitivity (neomycin).

SIGNS

- Hyperkeratosis.
- Depigmentation.
- Erythema.
- Erosion/ulceration.
- Vesicles/pustules.
- Crusts.
- Scarring.
- Alopecia.
- Nodules/plaques.

Blackwell's Five-Minute Veterinary Consult Clinical Companion: Small Animal Senior Care, First Edition. Edited by Heidi B. Lobprise.

Companion website: www.wiley.com/go/lobprise/Senior

RISK FACTORS

- Rooting behavior—pyoderma, dermatophytosis.
- Sun exposure—nasal solar dermatitis, DLE, SLE, PE.
- Poorly pigmented nose—nasal solar dermatitis, squamous cell carcinoma.
- Immunosuppression—demodicosis, pyoderma, dermatophytosis.
- Insect exposure—mosquito-bite dermatitis, eosinophilic folliculitis and furunculosis.

DIAGNOSIS

DIFFERENTIAL DIAGNOSIS

Nasal Solar Dermatitis

- Lesions—confined to nose; precipitated by heavy sunlight exposure.
- Begins in poorly pigmented skin at junction of nasal planum and dorsal muzzle.
- Lightly pigmented eyelid margins may also be affected.

DLE

- Primarily affects nasal area.
- May affect mucocutaneous margins of the lips and eyelids.
- Exacerbated by sunlight.
- Dermatitis often preceded by depigmentation.
- Biopsy—interface dermatitis with pigmentary incontinence.

Contact Dermatitis: Plastic (or Rubber) Dish Dermatitis

- Depigmentation and erythema of anterior nasal planum and lips.
- No ulceration or crusting.
- Uncommon; overly suspected—lesions more often due to trauma from roughened bowl edges. Similar symptoms seen with trauma from rubber toys.

Eosinophilic Folliculitis and Furunculosis

- Rapid progression from popular papular/nodular pattern to ulcers and plaques.
- Highly pruritic.
- Acute reaction to insect or arthropod bite and stings.

Mucocutaneous Pyoderma

Crusting and fissures on mucocutaneous junctions of lateral aspects of the nares, lips, and perioral skin.

Mosquito Bite Hypersensitivity

- Seasonal pruritic dermatitis.
- Erythema, papules, crusts affecting face and nasal planum, occasionally lesions on pinnae and feet.
- Biopsy—eosinophilic inflammation, collagen necrosis around the hair follicles.
- Idiopathic nasal hyperkeratosis—dry, horny growths of keratin localized to nasal planum; may or may not be associated with digital hyperkeratosis, possibly associated with senility.
- Other diseases—differentiate by history or biopsy (i.e., neoplastic cell infiltrate).

CBC/BIOCHEMISTRY/URINALYSIS

- Usually normal.

DIAGNOSTIC PROCEDURES

- Skin scrapings and cultures (bacteria, fungal)
- Neoplasia—cytology or biopsy.

TREATMENT

- Reduce exposure to sunlight—DLE, nasal solar dermatitis, squamous cell carcinoma.
- Discourage rooting behavior—pyoderma, dermatophytosis.
- Protection from insects (mosquito-bite dermatitis; eosinophilic folliculitis furunculosis).
- Warm soaks—aid removal of exudate and crusts.
- Replace plastic or rubber dish and avoid contact with topical drug or other agent causing hypersensitivity reaction.

MEDICATIONS

DRUG(S) OF CHOICE

- Nasal solar dermatitis—topical corticosteroids; antibiotics for secondary infection; sunscreens; firocoxib.
- DLE and PE—topical corticosteroids or tacrolimus 0.1% (Protopic); cyclosporine (Atopica); tetracycline and niacinamide; oral therapy (as for PF) if temporarily needed in severe cases.
- Neoplasia—surgical excision; chemotherapy; radiation therapy.
- Idiopathic nasal hyperkeratosis—topical antibiotic-corticosteroid cream, topical keratolytic and humectant; topical tacrolimus; soybean oil balm.

FOLLOW-UP

PATIENT MONITORING

Varies with specific disease and treatment prescribed.

MISCELLANEOUS

Abbreviations

- DLE = discoid lupus erythematosus

Suggested Reading

Harvey RG, Haar G. *Ear, Nose and Throat Diseases of the Dog and Cat*. Boca Raton, FL: CRC Press, 2017; pp. 225–288.

Helton Rhodes KA, Werner A. *Blackwell's Five Minute Veterinary Consult: Clinical Companion; Small Animal Dermatology*, 2nd edn. Chichester: Wiley-Blackwell, 2011.

Author/editor: Heidi Lobprise
Topic adapted from Five Minute Veterinary Consultation, 7th edition, 2021
Original Topic: Nasal Dermatoses—Canine

Author: Clarissa P. Souza
Consulting Editor: Alexander H. Werner Resnick

Chapter 21

Panniculitis/Steatitis

BASICS

OVERVIEW

Inflammation of the subcutaneous fat tissue.

SYSTEMS AFFECTED

Skin/exocrine.

SIGNALMENT

Species

Steatitis—predominantly cats but can occur in dogs with concurrent diseases.

Mean Age and Range

- Panniculitis—any age.
- Steatitis—young-to-middle-aged cats; older dogs.

SIGNS

- Uncommon in dogs and cats.
- Single or multiple subcutaneous nodules or draining tracts.
- May be painful and fluctuant to firm.
- Nodules—few millimeters to several centimeters in diameter.
- Involved fat may necrose.
- Exudate—usually a small amount of oily discharge; yellow-brown to bloody.
- Multiple lesions (dogs and cats)—systemic signs common (e.g., anorexia, pyrexia, lethargy, and depression).

CAUSES AND RISK FACTORS

- Infectious—bacterial, fungal (deep mycosis or dermatophyte), opportunistic mycobacteria, *Nocardia*, viral.
- Immune-mediated—lupus panniculitis, erythema nodosum, vasculitis, or drug reaction.

Blackwell's Five-Minute Veterinary Consult Clinical Companion: Small Animal Senior Care, First Edition. Edited by Heidi B. Lobprise.

Companion website: www.wiley.com/go/lobprise/Senior

- Idiopathic—sterile nodular panniculitis, thromboembolism, sterile pyogranulomatous dermatitis and panniculitis.
- Trauma.
- Neoplastic—multicentric mast cell tumors, cutaneous lymphoma, pancreatic carcinoma.
- Foreign bodies.
- Post-injection—corticosteroids, vaccines, other subcutaneous injections.
- Nutritional—vitamin E deficiency in cats, oily fish-based diet (steatitis).

DIAGNOSIS

DIFFERENTIAL DIAGNOSIS

Infectious

- More common than sterile/immune-mediated panniculitis.
- Deep pyoderma.
- Feline infectious peritonitis.

Cutaneous Cyst

- Usually nonpainful, noninflamed.
- Well demarcated.

Lipoma

- Soft; usually well demarcated.
- No inflammation or draining tracts.
- Usually solitary.

Mast Cell Tumors/Epitheliotropic Lymphoma

- Multifocal.
- Often erythematous.
- Variable presentations.

Sterile Nodular Panniculitis

Diagnosis made by ruling out other causes of panniculitis.

CBC/BIOCHEMISTRY/URINALYSIS

- Panniculitis—no abnormalities.
- Steatitis and panniculitis (occasional)—moderate-to-severe neutrophilia with mild eosinophilia; mild-to-moderate leukocytosis; mild nonregenerative anemia; hypoalbuminemia and proteinuria; possible hypocalcemia.

OTHER LABORATORY TESTS

- Antinuclear antibody—lupus panniculitis.
- Serum protein electrophoresis.

- Serum lipase/amylase levels.
- Feline leukemia virus/feline immunodeficiency virus.

IMAGING

Abdominal ultrasound:

- Panniculitis—pancreatitis may be a contributing factor.
- Steatitis—may see mottled subcutaneous, inguinal, or falciform fat; loss of contrast in abdominal cavity.

DIAGNOSTIC PROCEDURES

- Aspirates and impression smears:
  - Pyoderma—numerous neutrophils and variable numbers of mononuclear cells and bacteria.
  - Fungal infections—fungal organisms and variable numbers of mononuclear cells may be noted.
- Blastomycosis—urine antigen testing.
- Bacterial culture and susceptibility testing (tissue)—identify primary or secondary bacterial infection.
- Fungal and opportunistic mycobacteria culture (tissue).
- Biopsy with negative cultures for diagnosis of sterile nodular panniculitis.
- Special stains of histopathologic samples—may help identify causative agent.

PATHOLOGIC FINDINGS

- Surgical excisional biopsies—more accurate than punch biopsy specimens in most cases.
- Panniculitis—lobular or diffuse infiltrate (granulomatous, pyogranulomatous, suppurative, eosinophilic, necrotizing, or fibrosing) of panniculus; may identify if vasculitis present.
- Steatitis—lumpy, granular fat, normal to yellowish-orange coloration of body fat.

TREATMENT

DIET

Steatitis—remove fish products from diet; feed nutritionally complete, balanced, commercially prepared food; may require parenteral feeding (e.g., PEG tube, esophagostomy feeding tube).

MEDICATIONS

DRUG(S) OF CHOICE

Positive culture results require appropriate antibacterial, antifungal, or antimycobacterial treatment.

Sterile Nodular Panniculitis

- Systemic treatment with corticosteroids; prednisolone 2.2 mg/kg daily in dogs or 4.4 mg/kg daily in cats: taper based on response: may require low dose to maintain remission.

- Azathioprine (dogs: 1 mg/kg PO daily initially)—used with corticosteroids if insufficient response.
- Oral vitamin E 200 IU q12h <10 kg, 400 IU q12h >10 kg.
- Cyclosporine beneficial in some dogs (initially 5 mg/kg q24h for 4–8 weeks, then tapered).

Steatitis

Oral vitamin E 200 IU q12h <10 kg, 400 IU q12h >10 kg; corticosteroids at an anti-inflammatory dosage; S-adenosylmethionine PO on an empty stomach.

FOLLOW-UP

- Depends on underlying etiology type and duration of treatment.
- Monitor CBC, platelet count, chemistry profile, and urinalysis/urine bacterial culture and sensitivity if immunosuppressive agents or long-term corticosteroids prescribed.

MISCELLANEOUS

Associated Conditions

- Pancreatic carcinoma.
- Chylous ascites.
- Peritonitis.

Abbreviations

- PEG tube = percutaneous endoscopically placed gastrostomy tube

Suggested Reading

Helton Rhodes KA, Werner A. *Blackwell's Five-Minute Veterinary Consult: Clinical Companion: Small Animal Dermatology*, 3rd edn. Hoboken, NJ: Wiley-Blackwell, 2018.

Author/editor: Heidi Lobprise
Topic adapted from Five Minute Veterinary Consultation, 7th edition, 2021
Original Topic: Panniculitis/Steatitis

Author: Karen A. Kuhl
Consulting Editor: Alexander H. Werner Resnick

Chapter 22

Skin Fragility Syndrome, Feline

BASICS

OVERVIEW

- A disorder of multifactorial causes characterized by extremely fragile skin.
- Tends to occur in old cats that may have concurrent hyperadrenocorticism, diabetes mellitus, excessive use of megestrol acetate or other progesterone compounds, or as a paraneoplastic syndrome.
- A small number of cats have no biochemical alterations.

SYSTEMS AFFECTED

- Skin/exocrine.
- Endocrine/metabolic.

SIGNALMENT

- Naturally occurring disease tends to be recognized in old cats.
- Iatrogenic cases have no age predilection.
- No breed or sex predilection.

SIGNS

Historical Findings

- Gradual onset of clinical signs.
- Progressive alopecia (not always present).
- Often associated with weight loss, lusterless coat, poor appetite, and lack of energy.

Physical Examination Findings

- Skin becomes markedly thin and tears with normal handling.
- Skin rarely bleeds upon tearing.
- Multiple lacerations (both old and new) may be noted on close examination.
- Partial-to-complete alopecia of the truncal region may be noted.
- Sometimes associated with "rat tail," pinnal folding, pot-belly appearance.
- Differentiated from cutaneous asthenia by lack of hyperextensibility.

Blackwell's Five-Minute Veterinary Consult Clinical Companion: Small Animal Senior Care, First Edition. Edited by Heidi B. Lobprise.

Companion website: www.wiley.com/go/lobprise/Senior

CAUSES AND RISK FACTORS

- Hyperadrenocorticism—pituitary- or adrenal-dependent.
- Iatrogenic—secondary-to-excessive corticosteroid or progesterone drug administration.
- Diabetes mellitus—rare, unless associated with hyperadrenocorticism.
- Possibly idiopathic or paraneoplastic syndrome.

DIAGNOSIS

DIFFERENTIAL DIAGNOSIS

- Cutaneous asthenia.
- Feline paraneoplastic syndrome—pancreatic neoplasia, hepatic lipidosis, cholangiocarcinoma.

CBC/BIOCHEMISTRY/URINALYSIS

- Little diagnostic significance in most cases.
- Approximately 80% of cats with hyperadrenocorticism have concurrent diabetes mellitus (hyperglycemia, glucosuria).

OTHER LABORATORY TESTS

- Adrenocorticotropic hormone (ACTH)-stimulation test—70% of cats with hyperadrenocorticism have an exaggerated response.
- Low-dose dexamethasone-suppression test—15–20% of normal cats may fail to decrease cortisol levels; typically unsuppressed with hyperadrenocorticism and nonadrenal illness.
- High-dose dexamethasone-suppression test—normal cats show decreases in cortisol concentrations; typically decreased with nonadrenal illnesses; considered by many clinicians to be the best screening test for hyperadrenocorticism; unreliable for discriminating between adrenal tumors and pituitary-dependent causes of hyperadrenocorticism, because both conditions fail to show suppression.
- Endogenous ACTH levels—normal range for most labs is 20–100 pg/mL.

IMAGING

- Abdominal ultrasonography—adrenal masses are often small until end-stage disease; cholangiocarcinoma and hepatic lipidosis have been reported.
- CT and MRI—small pituitary tumors may be difficult to visualize; MRI may be more successful.

PATHOLOGIC FINDINGS

Histopathology—suggestive, not diagnostic; epidermis and dermis are thin; attenuated collagen fibers are evident.

TREATMENT

- Underlying metabolic disease should be ruled out.
- Many patients are debilitated and require supportive care.
- Surgical correction of the lacerations—difficult because the tissue cannot withstand pressure from sutures.
- Protect skin—clothing; reduce activities that can traumatize the skin; remove sharp edges from the environment; prevent damage from interaction with other animals.
- Discontinue exogenous corticosteroids if administered.
- Hyperadrenocorticism—adrenalectomy is the preferred treatment.
- Cobalt-60 radiation therapy—variable success in the treatment of pituitary tumors.

MEDICATIONS

DRUG(S) OF CHOICE

- Medical management—may be useful for preparing patient for surgery and for minimizing postoperative complications (e.g., infections and poor wound healing).
- No known effective medical therapy for feline hyperadrenocorticism.
- Mitotane (1,1-(*o,p′*-dichlorodiphenyl)-2,2-dichloroethane [*o,p′*-DDD]) 12.5–50 mg/kg PO q12h; response has been equivocal; side effects include anorexia, vomiting, and diarrhea.
- Metyrapone 65 mg/kg PO q12h; clinical improvement noted more often with this drug than the others.

CONTRAINDICATIONS/POSSIBLE INTERACTIONS

Hyperadrenocorticism—closely monitor diabetic cats; adjust insulin to prevent hypoglycemia when the cortisol levels fall.

FOLLOW-UP

Patients are often quite debilitated, making any form of treatment risky; close monitoring is required in all cases.

MISCELLANEOUS

See Also

- Frailty

Abbreviations

- ACTH = adrenocorticotropic hormone

Suggested Reading

Gross TL, Ihrke PJ, Walder EJ. *Veterinary Dermatopathology*. Philadelphia, PA: Mosby, 1992.

Little SE. *August's Consultations in Feline Internal Medicine*, Volume 7. Philadelphia, PA: Saunders, 2016.

Vogelnest LJ. Skin as a marker of general feline health: cutaneous manifestations of systemic disease. *J Feline Med Surg* 2017;19(9):948–960.

Author/editor: Heidi Lobprise
Topic adapted from Five Minute Veterinary Consultation, 7th edition, 2021
Original Topic: Skin Fragility Syndrome—Cats

Author: Guillermina Manigot
Consulting Editor: Alexander H. Werner Resnick

Endocrinology

Chapter 23

Diabetes Mellitus—Cats and Dogs

BASICS

DEFINITION

- Disorder of carbohydrate, fat, and protein metabolism caused by an absolute or relative insulin deficiency, resulting in the hallmark abnormality of persistent hyperglycemia.

Cats

- The most common form in cats resembles Type II or non-insulin-dependent diabetes mellitus (DM) of humans.

Dogs

- Fasting hyperglycemia of sufficient magnitude to result in characteristic clinical signs including weight loss with normal or increased appetite, polydipsia (PD), and polyuria (PU) caused by glucosuria.
- Canine diabetes mellitus (DM) is often characterized by loss of insulin-secreting ability through presumed immune-mediated destruction of pancreatic beta cells.
- May develop as result of combination of relative insulin-deficient state with concurrent peripheral insulin resistance.

PATHOPHYSIOLOGY

Cats

- Insulin resistance impairs the ability of tissues (especially muscle, adipose tissue, and liver) to use carbohydrates, fats, and proteins.
- Impaired systemic glucose utilization with ongoing hepatic gluconeogenesis causes persistent hyperglycemia; directly impairs insulin secretion by reducing functional beta cell mass ("glucose toxicity").
- Initial beta cell dysfunction progresses to irreversible failure of insulin production as reactive oxidative species, inflammatory cytokines, and amyloid deposition perpetuate beta cell injury and loss.

Dogs

- Absolute or relative insulin deficiency results in accelerated tissue catabolism, impaired ability to maintain carbohydrate, lipid, and protein homeostasis, as well as insulin resistance.
- Reduced insulin-secreting ability, peripheral insulin resistance, and continued hepatic gluconeogenesis result in persistent hyperglycemia of sufficient severity to overload renal tubular glucose resorption; leading to glucosuria, osmotic diuresis, PU accompanied by compensatory PD.

Blackwell's Five-Minute Veterinary Consult Clinical Companion: Small Animal Senior Care, First Edition. Edited by Heidi B. Lobprise.

Companion website: www.wiley.com/go/lobprise/Senior

- Loss of insulin-dependent glucose-mediated hypothalamic satiation signaling results in polyphagia.
- Decreased insulin-dependent utilization of glucose results in catabolic protein breakdown with weight loss and increased lipid mobilization (hyperlipidemia, hepatic lipidosis, production of ketoacids).
- Accumulation of large amounts of ketone bodies leads to metabolic acidosis (see Diabetes Mellitus With Ketoacidosis).

SYSTEMS AFFECTED

- Endocrine/metabolic—electrolyte depletion, metabolic acidosis.
- Hepatobiliary—chronic pancreatitis, hepatic lipidosis.
- Neuromuscular—muscle wasting, peripheral neuropathy (cats)
- Renal/urologic—osmotic diuresis with compensatory polydipsia (PD); urinary tract infection.

GENETICS

Genetic susceptibility suspected in certain breeds (e.g., European Burmese cats) and certain dog breeds over- and under-represented

INCIDENCE/PREVALENCE

Cats
- Reported at between ~1 : 250 (0.4%) to ~1 : 100 (1.2%) cats.

Dogs
- Prevalence varies between 1 : 400 and 1 : 500 (0.25–0.2%).
- Onset has seasonal incidence; more animals diagnosed in autumn and winter.

SIGNALMENT

Breed Predilections

Cats
- Breeds with possible increased susceptibility include Burmese (Europe, Australia, and New Zealand), Maine Coon, Russian Blue, Siamese, and Norwegian Forest cats.

Dogs
- Samoyed, Tibetan terrier, Cairn terrier, golden retriever (United States only) overrepresented.
- Keeshond, poodle, dachshund, miniature schnauzer, beagle may have increased predisposition.
- Boxer, German shepherd, golden retriever (UK only) underrepresented.

Mean Age and Range

Cats: Over 80% of cases are 7 years or older at diagnosis; range: 1–19 years.
Dogs: Mean ~8 years; range: 4–14 years (excluding rare juvenile form).

Predominant Sex

Cats: Males are overrepresented, but common in both sexes.
Dogs: Female

SIGNS

Historical Findings

Cats

- Obesity often present prior to diagnosis.
- Polyuria (PU)/PD, polyphagia, weight loss, generalized muscle wasting, poor coat quality.
- Signs suggesting a complication—anorexia, lethargy, depression, vomiting, jaundice.
- Physical exam: Hepatomegaly, dehydration, plantigrade stance (diabetic neuropathy).

Dogs

- PU/PD, polyphagia with weight loss.
- Hepatomegaly.
- Cataracts common finding—approximately 80% of dogs with DM for >12 months will have cataracts regardless of level of control.
- Lethargy, depression, inappetence, anorexia, and vomiting may occur in animals with ketoacidosis.

CAUSES

Cats

- Genetic susceptibility.
- Islet amyloid deposition.
- Pancreatitis.
- Diseases causing insulin resistance (e.g., hyperadrenocorticism and acromegaly).
- Drugs (e.g., glucocorticoids and progestogens).
- Hypersomatotropism—growth-hormone-induced insulin resistance (GH-induced IR)

Dogs

- Immune-mediated isletitis.
- Disorders that predispose to secondary immune-mediated isletitis—pancreatitis, viral illness.

RISK FACTORS

Cats

- Obesity.
- Advanced age.

Dogs

- Diestrus.
- Genetic susceptibility.
- Use of glucocorticoids or progestins.

DIAGNOSIS

DIFFERENTIAL DIAGNOSIS

Cats

- Stress hyperglycemia—no PU/PD or weight loss; blood glucose concentration normal if sample taken when cat is not stressed; normal fructosamine concentration.

Cats and Dogs

- Renal glucosuria—absence of hyperglycemia; usually does not cause PU/PD or weight loss.

CBC/BIOCHEMISTRY/URINALYSIS

Cats

- Mild normocytic, normochromic anemia possible.
- Glucose >150 mg/dL.
    - BG ≥270 mg/kL with signs of hyperglycemia or crisis and at least one of the following:
        - Increased serum glycated protein concentrations; glycosuria on more than one occasion (home collection at least 2 days after any stressful events.
    - BG between 130 and 270 mg/dL and at least two of the above parameters including signs/crisis.
- High alkaline phosphatase (ALP), alanine aminotransferase (ALT), and aspartate aminotransferase (AST) activities.
- Hypercholesterolemia, hyperbilirubinemia, and hypertriglyceridemia.
- Total CO_2 or HCO_3 low with ketoacidosis or severe dehydration.
- Glucosuria, ketonuria uncommon in uncomplicated DM.
- Isosthenuria, proteinuria.

Dogs

- Hemogram usually normal.
- Glucose >200 mg/dL, possible ketonemia.
- High serum alkaline phosphatase (ALP) and alanine aminotransferase (ALT) enzyme activities, generally with greater proportionate increase in ALP.
- Hypercholesterolemia, lipemia.
- Electrolyte alterations vary; hypokalemia and hypophosphatemia may be present.
- Total CO_2 or HCO_3 will be low with ketoacidosis or severe dehydration.
- Glucosuria, ketonuria in some dogs.
- Urinary specific gravity variable depending on degree of glucosuria.

OTHER LABORATORY TESTS

Cats

- Fructosamine >350 µmol/L—confirms persistence of hyperglycemia.
- Feline pancreas-specific lipase >3.50 µg/L—identifies presence of pancreatitis.
- Urine culture—positive in 10–15% of newly diagnosed DM.

Dogs

- Anion gap—high in patients with ketoacidosis.
- Glycated proteins—fructosamine or glycosylated hemoglobin: directly related to blood glucose concentration over lifespan of protein in circulation (10–20 days for fructosamine, 4–8 weeks for hemoglobin).
    - Can be modified by changes in albumin or hemoglobin concentrations; accelerated albumin turnover will lower fructosamine level.
    - For ongoing management of relatively stable diabetic patients; fructosamine concentration in upper third of reference range reflects excellent diabetic control; concentration in lower third is more suggestive of overzealous diabetic control and possible increased risk of hypoglycemia.

- Plasma insulin concentrations not particularly helpful—while low insulin concentration suggests insulin deficiency, may be reflection of reversible islet exhaustion (persistent hyperglycemia can impair insulin secretory activity, even if functional beta cells present).

IMAGING

Cats
- Thoracic and abdominal radiography—to evaluate comorbidities (e.g., neoplasia, cystic or renal calculi, emphysematous cystitis, or cholecystitis).
- Abdominal ultrasonography—in selected patients, particularly those with jaundice, to evaluate for hepatic lipidosis, cholangiohepatitis, and pancreatitis.

Dogs
- Radiography—useful to look for comorbidities (e.g., cystic or renal calculi, emphysematous cystitis, cholecystitis, pancreatitis).
- Ultrasonography—indicated in selected patients, particularly those with jaundice, to evaluate for presence of obstructive hepatopathy or pancreatitis.

DIAGNOSTIC PROCEDURES—CATS AND DOGS

Liver fine-needle aspiration—if concern for hepatic lipidosis (cats), hepatopathy (dogs).

PATHOLOGIC FINDINGS

Cats
- Usually no gross necropsy changes; pancreatic weight may be increased.
- Histopathology—normal, more likely to reveal islet amyloidosis, vacuolar or hydropic degeneration of the islets of Langerhans; lymphoplasmacytic pancreatic infiltration rare in cats.

Dogs
- Necropsy findings—hepatomegaly with significant hepatic lipid accumulation.
- Histopathologic findings generally reveal dramatic reduction in size and number of pancreatic islets with relatively normal exocrine tissue architecture.

TREATMENT

APPROPRIATE HEALTH CARE

Cats
- Compensated cats can be managed as outpatients if they are alert, hydrated, and eating and drinking without vomiting.
- For decompensated patients, see Diabetes Mellitus With Ketoacidosis.

Dogs
- Compensated dogs generally alert, well hydrated, eating and drinking without vomiting, and can be managed as outpatients.
- For management of decompensated patients, see Diabetes Mellitus With Ketoacidosis.

NURSING CARE

Cats: Fluid therapy—in decompensated patients.

ACTIVITY

Cats: Strenuous activity may lower insulin requirements; consistent daily activity level is helpful.

DIET

Cats: Ultra-low-carbohydrate (<12% metabolizable energy) and high protein (>40% metabolizable energy) canned diets may improve glycemic control, and increase the likelihood of diabetic remission in newly diagnosed diabetic cats.

CLIENT EDUCATION

Cats

- Maintain a consistent daily feeding and medication schedule, home glucose monitoring, signs of hypoglycemia and what to do, and when to seek veterinary assistance.
- Chart pertinent daily information about the pet, such as any home-obtained glucose readings or patterns of exhibited clinical signs (e.g., PU/PD or appetite).

Dogs

- Diet should be calorically and constitutively consistent; appropriate for ideal bodyweight (~60kcal/kg) and eaten reliably and quickly
- Obese diabetic dogs—feed restricted caloric intake to ensure ideal bodyweight achieved within 2–4 months using high-fiber, low-calorie food; high-fiber diet may improve patient satiety but has no role in improving diabetic control.
- Ideally glucose-lowering effects of insulin should match glucose-raising effects of the meal.
    - Most insulins act maximally 2–4 hours after SC administration, and most food absorbed within 1h of consumption; improved glycemic control if fed 60–90 minutes *after* q12h insulin dosing.
    - Animals that "graze" throughout day can be fed dry food ad libitum and given two small meals of canned food as above.
    - If insulin can only be administered once daily, feed total daily caloric intake in two or three meals within first 6–8 hours after insulin dosing.
- While snacks should generally be avoided, small treats given at time of injection to positively reinforce owner–patient interaction should be encouraged.
- Discuss daily feeding and medication schedule, home monitoring, signs of hypoglycemia and what to do, and when to call or visit veterinarian.
- Chart pertinent information about pet (daily water consumption, weekly bodyweight, current insulin dose, and amount of food consumed).

SURGICAL CONSIDERATIONS—CATS AND DOGS

Intact females should have ovariohysterectomy when stable; progesterone secreted during diestrus makes management of DM difficult.

MEDICATIONS

DRUG(S) OF CHOICE

Cats

- Insulin is treatment of choice and should be initiated at 1–2 units per cat SC q12h; based on routine monitoring, some cats may eventually be reduced to once-daily dosing.
- Two U-40 insulin formulations are FDA-approved for use in cats—protamine zinc (PZI) and porcine zinc lente insulin suspension.
- Most consensus recommendations support the use of PZI or glargine (U-100) as first-choice insulin therapy for cats.

Dogs

- Insulin—almost always required
    - Vetsulin® (porcine-origin lente) 0.75 units/kg SC q12h initial dose. *Note*: U-40 insulin—must use with U-40 insulin syringe; availability may be limited.
    - Humulin N—intermediate-acting, human insulin; 0.75 units/kg SC q12h initial dose.
    - Novolin N—intermediate-acting, human insulin; 0.75 units/kg SC q12h initial dose.
    - PZI Vet® (intermediate-to-longer-acting protamine zinc human insulin) rarely used in dogs; *note*: U-40 insulin—must use with U-40 syringe.
    - Detemir insulin—longer-acting, synthetic insulin; part of reason for its delayed release is because bound to albumin; unlike insulins mentioned above, starting dose should be considerably lower: 0.1 unit/kg SC q12h initial dose.
    - Glargine insulin—longer-acting, synthetic insulin; 0.75 units/kg SC q12h initial dose.
- Species of origin of insulin may affect pharmacokinetics; canine and porcine insulin have identical amino acid sequence; hence, Vetsulin does not produce significant insulin antibody response, whereas most other commercially available insulins do; however, no evidence of the development of insulin antibodies has any clinical significance.

PRECAUTIONS

Cats

- Glucocorticoids, megestrol acetate, and progesterone cause insulin resistance. If steroid therapy is necessary, use oral methylprednisolone. Avoid injectable steroids.

Dogs

- Glucocorticoids, megestrol acetate, and progesterone cause insulin resistance.
- Hyperosmotic agents (e.g., mannitol and radiographic contrast agents) should be avoided if patient is already hyperosmolar from hyperglycemia.

POSSIBLE INTERACTIONS

- Drugs that may increase insulin sensitivity—angiotensin-converting enzyme inhibitors, sulfonamides, tetracycline, beta blockers, monoamine oxidase inhibitors, salicylates.
- Drugs that increase insulin resistance—glucocorticoids, estrogen supplements, furosemide, thiazide diuretics, and calcium channel blockers.
- Always consult a new medication's product insert.

ALTERNATIVE DRUG(S)

Cats

- Oral sulfonylureas (e.g., glipizide)—only when insulin therapy is not possible. Initial dose of 2.5 mg PO q12h with monitoring; if not controlled after 2 weeks, dose of 5 mg PO q12h may be tried; however, response is seen in <40% of cats and often not sustained long term. Potential side effects are hypoglycemia, hepatic enzyme alterations, icterus, and vomiting.
- Acarbose—an alpha-glucosidase inhibitor used to limit intestinal glucose absorption. Often used in combination with diet and insulin at a starting dose of 12.5 mg PO q12h; diarrhea is most common side effect.
- Drugs warranting further study for utility in managing feline DM include once-weekly injected glucagon-like peptide 1 analogues and oral renal tubular transporter inhibitors.
- Medications are now available for treating early cases of feline through inhibition of sodium-glucose cotransporter 2 (SGLT2). These lower blood sugar by increasing urine excretion of glucose and results in effective glycemic control. The two forms are bexagliflozin 15 mg once-daily tablet and velagliflozin 1 mg/kg daily liquid.

Dogs

- Oral hypoglycemic agents are generally not recommended.

FOLLOW-UP

PATIENT MONITORING

Cats

- Owner-assessed clinical signs (PU/PD, appetite, attitude) and bodyweight—if signs are normal and weight stable to increasing, disease is likely to be regulated.
- Glucose curves—ideally generated by the owner at home. Perform 5–14 days after starting insulin or after any dose adjustments until controlled, then again at 1 month, and every 3–6 months thereafter.
- Fructosamine—maintain <400 µmol/L. Recheck monthly during initial regulation, then every 3–6 months as part of routine monitoring visits.
- Urinary monitoring—useful for identifying ketones in chronically unregulated patients or persistently negative glucose in cats likely entering remission.
- Flash glucose monitoring system (FreeStyle Libre®)—24-hour glucose monitoring system that measures blood glucose BG every 5 minutes for up to 14 days. Anecdotal evidence suggests the device is not 100% accurate, but helpful in assessing BG trends in cats in which a BG curve is not possible.

Dogs

- Regular evaluation every 3–4 months if animal is stable and clinical signs are controlled, or more frequently if control is poor or variable.
    - Clinical signs—degree of PU/PD, appetite, and bodyweight; if within acceptable limits, disease likely well regulated; consider using standardized clinical scoring system to consistently evaluate clinical phenotype.
    - Glycated proteins—fructosamine or glycosylated hemoglobin; see above.
    - Glucose curve—to assess insulin effectiveness, duration of action, nadir and potential rebound hyperglycemia; attempt to minimize stress of hospitalization and multiple blood draws; used when establishing initial control, changing insulin type, dose, or frequency, or problem solving for difficult diabetic; duration of curve ideally matches dosing interval

(12 or 24 hours)—identify nadir (low) and glucose level at time of dosing; establish effective insulin dose (decline to 100–200 mg/dL) for appropriate duration (majority of 12- or 24-hour dosing interval) with nadir >80 and <150 mg/dL; in dogs average glucose levels for 12-hour period overnight are lower than during daylight period.

- Home glucose monitoring using serial blood glucose estimations or real-time measures using SC glucose monitoring devices—requires owner commitment, compliance, and competence; most useful as early indicator of need for reduction in dose in patients with well-controlled clinical signs; should never be used by owner to make independent adjustment of insulin dose; owner-measured urine glucose levels not particularly useful.

PREVENTION/AVOIDANCE

Cats

- Prevent or correct obesity; avoid unnecessary use of glucocorticoids or megestrol acetate.

Dogs

- Neuter females; avoid unnecessary use of megestrol acetate.
- No evidence exists to suggest obesity increases risk of DM in neutered dogs.

POSSIBLE COMPLICATIONS

Cats

- Seizure, blindness, or coma with insulin overdose.
- Diabetic ketoacidosis or hyperglycemic hyperosmolar syndrome.

Dogs

- Cataracts can occur even with good glycemic control.
- Weakness, especially with exercise; seizures or coma may occur with insulin overdose.

EXPECTED COURSE AND PROGNOSIS

Cats

- Prognosis with treatment and monitoring is good; most animals have a normal lifespan.
- Some cats may recover insulin-secreting ability ("diabetic remission"), typically if glycemic control is achieved within 6 months of diagnosis; however, relapse is common (~30%).
- Reported remission rates vary greatly (0–100%); however, studies surveying general practitioners have suggested ~25–30% is reasonable expectation.

Dogs

- Dogs generally have permanent disease unless affected during estrus cycle, where neutering may resolve diabetes for a period.
- Prognosis with twice-daily insulin treatment and feeding aligned with insulin's maximum effects is good.

MISCELLANEOUS

Associated Conditions

Cats

- Urinary tract infection,
- Chronic pancreatitis.
- Clinical diabetic polyneuropathy—more common in cat than dog

- Affects peripheral motor, sensory, autonomic, and/or cranial nerves, in any combination.
- Can be secondary to insulinoma-associated hypoglycemia—middle-aged to older animals.
- Findings—owner reports non-neurologic clinical signs associated with weakness.
- Physical examination: paresthesia—feline diabetic neuropathy, sensory neuropathies.
- Management (DM): monitor food intake; in cats, feed a low-carbohydrate, high-protein diet; diabetic neuropathy often reversible with treatment.
- Expected Course and Prognosis: fair-to-good prognosis with successful treatment of primary metabolic abnormality; insulinomas have high recurrence rate.

Dogs

- Urinary tract infection.
- Cataracts.

Note: management of chronic inflammatory conditions, such as periodontal disease and even obesity can help in stabilizing glycemic control.

Abbreviations

- ALP = alkaline phosphatase
- ALT = alanine aminotransferase.
- AST = aspartate aminotransferase.
- BG = blood glucose.
- DM = diabetes mellitus.
- PU/PD = polyuria and polydipsia.
- PZI = protamine zinc insulin.

Internet Resources

Accessed 29 June 2024
2018 AAHA Diabetes Management Guidelines for Dogs and Cats
JAAHADiaGuidelines_proof.pdf
AAFP Diabetes Tool-Kit
Diabetes Educational Toolkit|American Association of Feline Practitioners (catvets.com)

Suggested Reading

Behrend E, Holford A, Lathan P, et al. 2018 AAHA diabetes management guidelines for dogs and cats. *J Am Anim Hosp Assoc* 2018;54:1–21.

Sparkes A, Cannon M, Church D, et al. ISFM consensus guidelines on the practical management of diabetes mellitus in cats. *J Feline Med Surg* 2015;17:235–250.

Author/editor: Heidi Lobprise
Topic adapted from Five Minute Veterinary Consultation, 7th edition, 2021
Original Topic: Diabetes Mellitus without Complications—Cat and Dog

Author: Andrew C. Bugbee—Cats

Author: David B. Church—Dogs
Consulting Editor: Patty A. Lathan

Chapter 24

Diabetes Mellitus With Hyperosmolar Hyperglycemic State

BASICS

DEFINITION

- The hyperosmolar hyperglycemic state (HHS) is a complicated form of diabetes mellitus (DM) characterized by severe hyperglycemia and dehydration that produces a marked elevation in serum osmolarity. Unlike diabetic ketoacidosis (DKA), ketone production and metabolic acidosis are not major features of HHS.
- Specific guidelines for HHS diagnosis are lacking in dogs and cats, but serum effective osmolarity >320 mOsm/L, glucose concentration >600 mg/dL, and bicarbonate concentration >18 mEq/L, along with minimal ketonuria, are criteria in humans.

PATHOPHYSIOLOGY

- Hyperglycemia is due to insulin deficiency from DM; insulinopenia reduces tissue glucose utilization and increases hepatic glucose production, leading to increased extracellular glucose concentrations; the magnitude of hyperglycemia in HHS is usually greater than in DKA.
- Hyperosmolarity develops secondary to hyperglycemia and is exacerbated by dehydration and reduced extracellular fluid volume; the contribution of glucose to total plasma osmolarity is significant in HHS.
- Dehydration and volume deficit are typically severe and are caused by several factors, including reduced water intake and volume losses via gastrointestinal and renal systems.
- Reduced plasma volume decreases glomerular filtration rate and urine production, leading to azotemia; in HHS, severe volume contraction with reduced urinary glucose excretion results in severe hyperglycemia and plasma hyperosmolarity.
- Hyperketonemia and ketonuria are not major features of HHS; lactic acidosis secondary to volume depletion, tissue hypoperfusion, and impaired glucose metabolism is the major cause of acidosis in patients with HHS.

SYSTEMS AFFECTED

- Endocrine.
- Renal/urologic—prerenal azotemia due to decreased extracellular fluid volume; urine production usually maintained by glucose-induced diuresis unless volume deficit is severe or acute kidney injury is present.

Blackwell's Five-Minute Veterinary Consult Clinical Companion: Small Animal Senior Care, First Edition. Edited by Heidi B. Lobprise.

Companion website: www.wiley.com/go/lobprise/Senior

- Cardiovascular—hypovolemia; metabolic acidosis and electrolyte abnormalities may contribute to hypotension and poor myocardial contractility.
- Nervous—hyperosmolarity promotes intracellular dehydration and neuronal dysfunction.

SIGNALMENT

Species

Dog and cat (more frequent).

Mean Age and Range

Most common in middle-aged dogs (mean: 9 years) and cats (mean: 12 years).

SIGNS

Historical Findings

- All patients have DM.
- Some patients have concurrent chronic illness.
- Signs caused by DM—may not be appreciated after HHS onset:
    - Polydipsia.
    - Polyuria.
    - Polyphagia.
    - Weight loss.
- Signs caused by HHS:
    - Weakness/lethargy.
    - Vomiting.
    - Reduced appetite.
    - Neurologic complaints—abnormal responsiveness, coma.

Physical Examination Findings

- Findings associated with dehydration and hypovolemia:
    - Decreased skin turgor.
    - Prolonged capillary refill time.
    - Reduced pulse pressure.
    - Tachycardia.
    - Hypothermia.
- Findings associated with hyperosmolarity:
    - Lethargy, depressed mentation, stupor, or coma.
    - Seizure.
- Findings associated with DM:
    - Low body condition score.
    - Cataracts (dogs).

CAUSES

- Develops in patients with DM and severe dehydration/volume loss.
- Reduced water intake may precede onset of HHS.
- Comorbid conditions common.

RISK FACTORS

Risk for HHS may be higher in diabetic animals with concurrent disorders, including heart disease, renal insufficiency, hyperadrenocorticism, acute pancreatitis, and neoplasia.

DIAGNOSIS

DIFFERENTIAL DIAGNOSIS

- DM—may be uncomplicated to complicated, including DKA and HHS; all have similar clinical signs and laboratory findings, but can be subcategorized based on magnitude of hyperglycemia and hyperketonemia.
- Hypernatremia—severe hypernatremia produces CNS signs similar to HHS, but with sodium as major osmole; polyuria and polydipsia may be present, particularly if hypernatremia develops secondary to diabetes insipidus.
- Hyperosmolarity of any cause—may produce similar CNS abnormalities; toxins (e.g., ethylene glycol or alcohol) or CNS lesions (e.g., causing adipsia) may cause hyperosmolarity.
- CNS disease—primary CNS disorders may produce clinical signs of HHS; marked fluid deficits are not expected.
- Myxedema coma—manifestation of severe hypothyroidism with similar clinical signs without hyperosmolarity or hyperglycemia; low total thyroxine and elevated thyroid-stimulating hormone present.

CBC/BIOCHEMISTRY/URINALYSIS

- Hyperglycemia—blood glucose concentration frequently exceeds 600 mg/dL and severe hyperglycemia (1500–2000+ mg/dL) exists in some patients.
- Azotemia—elevated blood urea nitrogen (BUN) and serum creatinine concentrations are common, usually prerenal, but renal azotemia occurs in some patients.
- Sodium—hypo- or hypernatremia may be observed; hyperosmolarity is most severe with concurrent hyperglycemia and hypernatremia.
- Potassium—hypokalemia is common; hyperkalemia is associated with acute kidney injury or reduced urine output.
- Acidosis—metabolic acidosis is less severe than DKA; hypobicarbonemia and hyperlactatemia occur secondary to hypovolemia or renal failure.
- Glucosuria—present; mild ketonuria possible.
- Urine-specific gravity (USG) variable; may be misleading due to glucosuria, which increases USG.

OTHER LABORATORY TESTS

- Blood and urine osmolarity—serum osmolarity >320 mosm/L consistent with HHS; urine osmolality elevated due to glucosuria.
- Serum osmolarity can be estimated from routine serum chemistry results: $2([Na^+] + [K^+]) + [BUN]/2.8 + [Glucose]/18$; if results are in IU, equation is modified: $2([Na^+] + [K^+]) + [BUN] + [Glucose]$.

PATHOLOGIC FINDINGS

- Pancreas—consistent with DM: islet atrophy and loss (dogs and cats) and islet amyloid (cats).
- Brain—changes not specific for HHS; evidence of CNS edema.

TREATMENT

APPROPRIATE HEALTH CARE

Life-threatening medical emergency requiring inpatient treatment. After HHS resolution, patients require treatment and follow-up for DM.

NURSING CARE

- Correction of fluid deficits—major treatment goal, begin prior to insulin replacement; IV fluid replacement indicated for ill patients; enteral water can assist with free water replacement in patients that tolerate oral intake.
- Fluid type and rate depend on patient's hydration and volume status and magnitude of metabolic derangements; fluid deficit is estimated using the equation: %volume depletion * body weight (kg) = fluid deficit (L).
- Hypo- and normonatremic patients—isotonic crystalloid solution is appropriate for initial volume replacement; replacement of volume deficit should occur over 12–24 hours; patients with hypotension or shock due to hypovolemia should receive fluid bolus of 20–25% of estimated blood volume (dog: 80 mL/kg; cat: 50 mL/kg), which can be repeated until blood pressure is adequate; once blood pressure is restored, the remaining deficit is replaced over 12–24 hours.
- Hypernatremic patients—hypernatremia implies a free water deficit and its occurrence with hyperglycemia in HHS may result in life-threatening hyperosmolarity; isotonic (0.9%) saline solution appropriate for initial volume replacement in hypernatremic patients with hypovolemic hypotension; if hypernatremia persists after blood pressure and urine output are restored, use of hypotonic (0.45%) saline solution indicated to replace free water and reduce sodium, unless oral water intake possible; recommended that serum sodium concentration reduction should not exceed 12 mEq/day (see Hypernatremia).
- Electrolyte replacement—potassium deficiency is expected and should be replaced unless hyperkalemia is present; dosage based on magnitude of hypokalemia; potassium replacement by IV infusion should not exceed 0.5 mEq K^+/kg/h and fluids with supplemented K^+ should be avoided during rapid volume infusion; supplementation of other electrolytes (e.g., magnesium, phosphorus) may also be necessary.
- Glucose supplementation—some protocols recommend using dextrose infusion to prevent hypoglycemia during insulin therapy; 2.5–5% dextrose CRI used as needed to maintain blood glucose concentrations between 150 and 250 mg/dL.

CLIENT EDUCATION

- Patients frequently have a serious concurrent disorder(s) that affects prognosis.
- Permanent DM is expected and survivors will require lifelong treatment for DM.

MEDICATIONS

DRUG(S) OF CHOICE

- CRI of regular insulin is recommended for initial glucose control; insulin therapy should be started 2–6 hours after starting fluid therapy, so initial decrease in serum glucose is not extreme.
- CRI preparation—regular insulin at 2.2 U/kg/24 h (some protocols recommend 1.1 U/kg/24 h dose in cats) added to 250 mL of 0.9% NaCl; prior to beginning CRI 50 mL of solution should pass through plastic administration tubing and be discarded (insulin binds to some plastics); CRI started at 5 mL/h (cat) or 10 mL/h (dog) and infusion rate adjusted as needed to reduce hyperglycemia at desired rate and maintain target glucose concentration.
- Once HHS is resolved and patient stable, discontinue insulin CRI and transition to longer-acting insulin to be used for chronic DM management.

PRECAUTIONS

- Brain edema may occur when hyperosmolarity is corrected too rapidly; patients with edema develop worsening neurologic status during treatment; minimizing rapid decreases in glucose and sodium during treatment lowers edema risk.
- Insulin administration can result in hypokalemia; electrolytes should be monitored frequently (q4–6h) until stable.

ALTERNATIVE DRUG(S)

- Ultrashort-acting insulins (insulin aspart or insulin lispro) may be substituted for regular insulin in CRI protocols.
- Protocol for intermittent IM use of regular insulin (when CRI not available)—0.2 U/kg IM initially, followed by 0.1 U/kg IM q1h until glucose <250 mg/dL; subsequent doses 0.5–1.0 U/kg IM q4–6h to maintain glucose concentration between 150 and 250 mg/dL.

FOLLOW-UP

PATIENT MONITORING

- Volume and hydration status—monitor heart rate, pulse quality, capillary refill time, blood pressure, bodyweight, and urine output.
- Blood glucose—monitor q1–2h to guide insulin therapy; aim for gradual reduction of serum glucose (50–100 mg/dL/h) to 150–250 mg/dL without hypoglycemia.
- Monitor serum Na^+ and K^+ concentrations, especially during correction of hypernatremia or K^+ supplementation; magnesium and phosphorus should be monitored, especially after start of insulin therapy.
- After stabilization, long-term monitoring appropriate for DM is indicated.

PREVENTION/AVOIDANCE

- Adequate insulin therapy and monitoring of glycemia in patients with DM may reduce risk of HHS.
- Early recognition and effective treatment of new-onset DM may reduce risk of DKA or HHS.

POSSIBLE COMPLICATIONS

- Hypoglycemia or electrolyte disturbances may develop during treatment.
- Severe neurologic signs, including coma and death, may occur.
- Dehydration and shock can precipitate acute kidney injury.
- Death due to shock or coma may occur in untreated animals.

EXPECTED COURSE AND PROGNOSIS

- Hydration and blood pressure should improve within a few hours of initiating fluid therapy and resolve over 12–24 hours; hyperglycemia is corrected over 6–12 hours once insulin therapy started.
- Electrolyte derangements must be managed to avoid osmotic complications secondary to sodium fluctuations, and to avoid hypo-/hyperkalemia, hypophosphatemia, or hypomagnesemia.
- Depending on patient response, prognosis is guarded; worse if severe neurologic compromise or renal failure is present.

MISCELLANEOUS

Associated Conditions

- DKA and HHS have significant overlap in clinical signs and laboratory abnormalities.
- Patients with HHS should be evaluated for concurrent conditions (cardiac or renal failure, pancreatitis, neoplasia, etc.).

Synonyms

- Diabetic coma.
- Hyperosmolar nonketotic syndrome.

See Also

- Diabetes Mellitus With Ketoacidosis.
- Diabetes Mellitus—Dogs and Cats

Abbreviations

- BUN = blood urea nitrogen
- DKA = diabetic ketoacidosis.
- DM = diabetes mellitus.
- HHS = hyperosmolar hyperglycemic state.
- USG = urine-specific gravity.

Suggested Reading

Koenig A, Drobatz KJ, Beale AB, King LG. Hyperglycemic, hyperosmolar syndrome in feline diabetics: 17 cases (1995–2001). *J Vet Emerg Crit Care* 2004;14:30–40.

O'Brien MA. Diabetic emergencies in small animals. *Vet Clin North Am Small Anim Pract* 2010;40:317–333.

Rand JS. Diabetic ketoacidosis and hyperosmola hyperglycemia in cats. *Vet Clin North Am Small Anim Pract* 2013;43:367–379.

Trotman, TK, Drobatz KJ, Hess RS. Retrospective evaluation of hyperosmolar hyperglycemia in 66 dogs (1993–2008). *J Vet Emerg Crit Care* 2013;23:557–564.

Author/editor: Heidi Lobprise
Topic adapted from Five Minute Veterinary Consultation, 7th edition, 2021
Original Topic: Diabetes Mellitus with Hypoerosmolar Hyperglycemic State

Author: Thomas Schermerhorn
Consulting Editor: Patty A. Lathan

Chapter 25

Diabetes Mellitus with Ketoacidosis

BASICS

DEFINITION

A medical emergency secondary to absolute or relative insulin deficiency, characterized by hyperglycemia, ketonemia, metabolic acidosis, dehydration, and electrolyte depletion.

PATHOPHYSIOLOGY

- Insulin deficiency causes an increase in lipolysis, resulting in excessive ketone body production and metabolic acidosis; an inability to maintain fluid and electrolyte homeostasis causes dehydration, prerenal azotemia, electrolyte disorders, obtundation, and death.
- Many patients with diabetic ketoacidosis (DKA) have underlying conditions such as infection, inflammation, or heart disease that cause stress hormone (e.g., glucagon, cortisol, growth hormone, epinephrine) secretion; this probably contributes to development of insulin resistance and DKA by promoting lipolysis, ketogenesis, gluconeogenesis, and glycogenolysis.
- Dehydration and electrolyte abnormalities result from osmotic diuresis, promoting the loss of total body water and electrolytes.

SYSTEMS AFFECTED

- Endocrine/metabolic.
- Gastrointestinal.
- Hematologic (cats).

SIGNALMENT

Species

Dog and cat.

Breed Predilections

- Dog—miniature poodle and dachshund.
- Cat—none.

Blackwell's Five-Minute Veterinary Consult Clinical Companion: Small Animal Senior Care, First Edition. Edited by Heidi B. Lobprise.

Companion website: www.wiley.com/go/lobprise/Senior

Mean Age and Range

- Dog—mean age: 8.4 years.
- Cat—median age: 11 years (range: 1–19 years).

Predominant Sex

- Dogs—females 1.5 times more prevalent than males.
- Cats—males 2 times more prevalent than females.

SIGNS

- Shock.
- Dehydration.
- Hypothermia.
- Polyuria.
- Polydipsia or adipsia.
- Anorexia.
- Weakness.
- Vomiting.
- Lethargy.
- Tachypnea.
- Muscle wasting and weight loss.
- Unkempt haircoat.
- Thin body condition.
- Ketone odor on breath.
- Icterus.
- Dandruff.

CAUSES

- Diabetes mellitus.
- Infection (e.g., pyoderma, pneumonia, urinary tract infection, prostatitis, pyelonephritis, pyometra).
- Concurrent disease (e.g., heart failure, pancreatitis, renal insufficiency or failure, asthma, neoplasia, acromegaly).
- Estrus.
- Idiopathic.
- Medication noncompliance.
- Stress.
- Surgery.

RISK FACTORS

- Any condition that leads to absolute or relative insulin deficiency.
- History of corticosteroid or beta blocker administration.

DIAGNOSIS

DIFFERENTIAL DIAGNOSIS

- Hyperosmolar hyperglycemic state.
- Acute hypoglycemic coma/insulin overdose.
- Uremia/azotemia due to renal disease or postrenal obstruction.
- Other cause of metabolic acidosis (e.g., lactic acidosis, ethylene glycol intoxication, renal tubular acidosis).

CBC/BIOCHEMISTRY/URINALYSIS

- Leukocytosis with mature neutrophilia.
- Hyperglycemia—blood glucose concentration usually >250 mg/dL.
- High liver enzyme activity.
- Hypercholesterolemia and lipemia.
- Azotemia.
- Hypochloremia.
- Hypokalemia.
- Hyponatremia.
- Hypophosphatemia.
- Hypomagnesemia.
- High anion gap—anion gap = (sodium + potassium) – (chloride + bicarbonate); normal is 16 ± 4.
- Glucosuria and ketonuria.
- Variable urinary specific gravity with active or inactive sediment.
- Hyperproteinemia.
- Heinz body anemia (cats).

OTHER LABORATORY TESTS

- Metabolic acidosis—HCO_3^- <15 mEq/L (total CO_2 estimates HCO_3^-).
- Hyperosmolarity (>330 mOsm/kg).
- Bacterial culture of urine and blood.

DIAGNOSTIC PROCEDURES

- Abdominal and thoracic radiography and ultrasound may be necessary to identify comorbid diseases.
- ECG and blood pressure monitoring indicated for patients with shock or electrolyte abnormalities.

PATHOLOGIC FINDINGS

Pancreatic islet cell atrophy.

TREATMENT

APPROPRIATE HEALTH CARE

- If the animal is bright, alert, and well hydrated, intensive care and IV fluid administration are not required; start SC administration of insulin (short- or intermediate-acting insulin), offer food, and supply constant access to water; monitor closely for signs of illness (e.g., anorexia, lethargy, vomiting).
- Treatment of animals with DKA that are systemically ill requires intensive inpatient care; goals are to correct depletion of water and electrolytes, reverse ketonemia and acidosis, and increase rate of glucose use by insulin-dependent tissues.

NURSING CARE

- Fluids—necessary to ensure adequate cardiac output and tissue perfusion and to maintain vascular volume; also reduce blood glucose concentration.
- IV administration of isotonic crystalloid supplemented with potassium is initial fluid of choice; volume and rate determined by fluid replacement needs plus maintenance requirements; replace over 24–48 hours.

DIET

Following stabilization, diet should be adjusted to account for patient's diabetes, concurrent disease, and body condition. High-fiber diets are not recommended in underweight pets.

CLIENT EDUCATION

Serious medical condition requiring lifelong insulin administration in most patients.
Confirm that client is prepared to inject twice daily insulin prior to treatment of DKA.

MEDICATIONS

DRUG(S) OF CHOICE

Insulin

- Regular insulin is the insulin of choice until eating; lispro insulin may also be considered.
- Initial dosage—0.2 U/kg IM (or SC if hydration normal).
- Subsequent dosage 0.1–0.2 U/kg IM given 3–6 hours later—may be given hourly if patient is closely monitored; response to previous insulin dosage should be considered when calculating subsequent dosages; ideally, glucose concentration should drop by 50–100 mg/dL/h.
- Regular insulin can also be administered as CRI via designated catheter. Dogs: 2.2 units/kg in 250 mL of 0.9% NaCl; Cats: 1.1 units/kg in 250 mL 0.9% NaCl. Then, allow 50 mL of dilute insulin to flow through IV tubing and discard. If blood glucose >250 mg/dL, administer

at 10 mL/h; if blood glucose 200–250 mg/dL, administer at 7 mL/h; if blood glucose 150–200 mg/dL, administer at 5 mL/h; if blood glucose 100–150 mg/dL, administer at 5 mL/h and add 2.5% dextrose to IV crystalloid fluids; if blood glucose <100 mg/dL, discontinue IV insulin infusion and continue 2.5–5% dextrose in IV crystalloid infusion.

- Check blood glucose q1–3h using automated test strip analyzer (Accu-Chek® III, Alpha Trak® II glucometer), corrected for patient's PCV as indicated.
- Monitor urine or serum ketones daily.
- Administer longer-acting insulin once patient is eating, drinking, and ketosis is resolved; the dosage is based on that of short-acting insulin given in hospital.

Potassium Supplementation

- Total body potassium is depleted and treatment (e.g., fluids and insulin) will further lower serum potassium.
- If possible, check potassium concentration before initiating insulin therapy to guide supplementation; if extremely low, insulin therapy may need to be delayed (hours) until serum potassium concentration increases.
- Refractory hypokalemia may indicate hypomagnesemia, requiring magnesium replacement at 0.75–1 mEq/kg/24 h IV as magnesium chloride or magnesium sulfate.
- Supplementation of potassium should start at 0.2 mEq/kg/h, which can be adjusted to max 0.5 mEq/kg/h. Potassium concentration should be measured q6–8h until stabilized.

Dextrose Supplementation

- Because insulin is required to correct the ketoacidotic state, the supplementation of dextrose allows continuous insulin administration without hypoglycemia.
- Whenever blood glucose <200 mg/dL, 50% dextrose should be added to fluids to produce 2.5% dextrose solution (increase to 5% dextrose if glucose <100 mg/dL). Discontinue dextrose once glucose is maintained above 250 mg/dL.
- Insulin therapy is continued as long as blood glucose >100 mg/dL

Bicarbonate Supplementation

- Controversial; consider if patient's venous blood pH <7.0 or HCO_3^- <11 mEq/L; of little benefit if pH >7.0.
- Dosage—bodyweight (kg) × 0.3 × base deficit (base deficit = normal serum bicarbonate − patient's serum bicarbonate); *slowly* administer ¼ to ½ of dose IV and give remainder in fluids over 3–6 hours.
- Recheck blood gas or serum total carbon dioxide (TCO_2) before further supplementation.

Phosphorus Supplementation

- Pretreatment serum phosphorus is usually normal; however, treatment of ketoacidosis reduces phosphorus, and serum concentrations should be checked q12–24h once supplementation is initiated.
- Dosage—0.01–0.03 mmol/kg/h for 6–12 hours in IV fluids (may need to increase dose to 0.06 mmol/kg/h). Remember to account for additional potassium in potassium phosphate if supplemented.

CONTRAINDICATIONS

If the patient anuric or oliguric or if blood potassium concentration >5 mEq/L, do not supplement potassium until urine flow is established or potassium concentration decreases.

PRECAUTIONS

- Use bicarbonate with caution in patients without normal ventilation (cannot excrete carbon dioxide created during treatment).
- Acidosis results in falsely elevated blood ionized calcium concentrations; calcium should be rechecked as acidosis resolves and supplemented as necessary.

FOLLOW-UP

PATIENT MONITORING

- Attitude, hydration, cardiopulmonary status, urine output, and body weight.
- Blood glucose q1–3h initially; q6h once stable.
- Electrolytes q4–8h initially; q24h once stable.
- Acid–base status q8–12h initially; q24h once stable.

PREVENTION/AVOIDANCE

Appropriate insulin administration.

POSSIBLE COMPLICATIONS

- Hypokalemia.
- Hypoglycemia.
- Hypophosphatemia.
- Cerebral edema.
- Pulmonary edema/heart failure.
- Renal failure.

EXPECTED COURSE AND PROGNOSIS

Guarded

MISCELLANEOUS

Associated Conditions

- Pancreatitis.
- Hyperadrenocorticism.
- Diestrus.
- Bacterial infection.
- Electrolyte depletion.

PREGNANCY/FERTILITY/BREEDING

- Risk of fetal death may be relatively high.
- Glucose regulation is often difficult in pregnant animals.

See Also

- Diabetes Mellitus—Cats and Dogs

Abbreviations

- DKA = diabetic ketoacidosis
- TCO_2 = total carbon dioxide.

Suggested Reading

Behrend E, Holford A, Lathan P, et al. 2018 AAHA diabetes management guidelines for dogs and cats. *J Am Anim Hosp Assoc* 2018;54:1–21.

Difazio J, Fletcher DJ. Retrospective comparison of early- versus late-insulin therapy regarding effect on time to resolution of diabetic ketosis and ketoacidosis in dogs and cats: 60 cases (2003–2013). *J Vet Emerg Crit Care* 2016;26:108–115.

Hume DZ, Drobatz KJ, Hess RS. Outcome of dogs with diabetic ketoacidosis: 127 dogs (1993–2003). *J Vet Intern Med* 2006;20(3):547–555.

Kerl ME. Diabetic ketoacidosis: pathophysiology and clinical and laboratory presentation. *Comp Cont Educ Pract Vet* 2001;23:220–228.

Kerl ME. Diabetic ketoacidosis: treatment recommendations. *Comp Cont Educ Pract Vet* 2001;23:330–339.

Malerba E, Mazzarino M, Del Baldo F, et al. Use of lispro insulin for treatment of diabetic ketoacidosis in cats. *J Fel Med Surg* 2019;21:115–123.

Sieber-Ruckstuhl NS, Klev S, Tschuor F, et al. Remission of diabetes mellitus in cats with diabetic ketoacidosis. *J Vet Intern Med* 2008;22:1326–1332.

Author/editor: Heidi Lobprise
Topic adapted from Five Minute Veterinary Consultation, 7th edition, 2021
Original Topic: Obesity

Author: Katherine Gerken
Consulting Editor: Patty A. Lathan

Chapter 26

Hyperadrenocorticism (Cushing's Syndrome)—Cats

BASICS

OVERVIEW

Feline Cushing's syndrome (FCS) or hyperadrenocorticism is a consequence of abnormally increased functional activity of the adrenal cortex.

Pathophysiology

- Caused by increased glucocorticoid secretion by the adrenal gland(s).
- Approximately 85% of cases due to bilateral adrenocortical hyperplasia from pituitary hyperplasia or tumor—pituitary-dependent hyperadrenocorticism (PDH).
- Remaining 15% caused by adrenal tumor (AT), half of which are benign.
- Regardless of etiology, concurrent unregulated diabetes mellitus (DM) is frequent (90%) and other concurrent diseases (e.g., pancreatitis, chronic kidney, or cardiac disease) are reported.

SIGNALMENT

- Middle-aged-to-old cat.
- No known breed or sex predisposition.

SIGNS

- Dermatologic abnormalities (alopecia; unkempt hair coat; thin, fragile skin that is easily bruised or torn), polyuria, polydipsia, polyphagia, weight loss, muscle wasting, and pot-bellied appearance.
- Weight gain (unless concurrent DM causes weight loss), hepatomegaly and curled pinnae also seen.
- Lethargy (dullness) secondary to muscle weakness or effects of pituitary mass.
- Excess sex hormones can cause signs such as penile barbs and behavioral changes (sexual).

CAUSES AND RISK FACTORS

- Pituitary adenoma with subsequent corticotropic hyperplasia and excess glucocorticoid secretion.
- Autonomously functioning benign adrenal adenoma (50%) or malignant adenocarcinoma (50%).
- Iatrogenic from glucocorticoid administration (rare).

Blackwell's Five-Minute Veterinary Consult Clinical Companion: Small Animal Senior Care, First Edition. Edited by Heidi B. Lobprise.

Companion website: www.wiley.com/go/lobprise/Senior

DIAGNOSIS

DIFFERENTIAL DIAGNOSIS

- Insulin-resistant DM.
- Acromegaly.
- Hepatopathy.
- Renal disease.
- Sex hormone–secreting adrenal tumor.
- Hyperprogesteronism.
- Dermatologic disease.

CBC/BIOCHEMISTRY/URINALYSIS

- Lymphopenia, anemia.
- Hyperglycemia, hypercholesterolemia, hypertriglyceridemia, hypochloremia.
- Elevated urine cortisol : creatinine (UC : Cr) ratio, proteinuria.
- Azotemia, hyperglobulinemia (less common).
- Elevated serum alkaline phosphatase uncommon.

OTHER LABORATORY TESTS

Screening Tests

- UC : Cr—sensitive (good negative predictive value).
- Low-dose dexamethasone-suppression test—good sensitivity. Dose: 0.1 mg/kg IV. Failure to suppress consistent with FCS.
- Adrenocorticotropic hormone (ACTH) stimulation test—specific but poorly sensitive, not recommended as initial diagnostic test.
- Assays for plasma sex hormone and progesterone concentrations may rule out differentials.

Differentiating Tests

- Plasma endogenous ACTH concentration high normal or greater with PDH compared to low plasma ACTH levels with AT (<10 pg/mL). Reference ranges vary with laboratories.
- Imaging.

IMAGING

- Abdominal ultrasound—accurate to differentiate PDH from AT in most cases; operator dependent. Symmetric adrenal glands of normal or enlarged size are suggestive of PDH; unilateral enlargement or asymmetric adrenal glands support AT.
- CT and MRI—visualization and measurement of pituitary tumors or characterization of adrenal tumors.

TREATMENT

- FCS is a debilitating disease. Prognosis is guarded due to severity of complications and concurrent diseases.
- Presurgical medical treatment is beneficial to prevent complications from fragile skin and infections.

- Radiation therapy of macroadenomas allows better control of the disease and insulin resistance.
- Unilateral adrenalectomy for AT and medical therapy for PDH are the most readily available effective treatment options.
- Hypophysectomy (microsurgical transsphenoidal) is effective and available at some institutions.

MEDICATIONS

DRUG(S) OF CHOICE

- Trilostane reversibly blocks steroid synthesis. In most patients with FCS from PDH, trilostane reduces clinical signs and improves endocrine test results. A starting dose of 5–10 mg/cat PO q12h is recommended.
- Mitotane (Lysodren®; *o,p′*-DDD) is not recommended for treatment of FCS.
- Other medications have limited efficacy (ketoconazole, metyrapone, and aminoglutethimide).

FOLLOW-UP

- Clinical improvement and improved diabetic control are indicative of successful drug therapy.
- ACTH stimulation tests are recommended for dose adjustments of trilostane.

MISCELLANEOUS

Abbreviations

- ACTH = adrenocorticotropic hormone
- AT = adrenal tumor.
- DM = diabetes mellitus.
- FCS = feline Cushing's syndrome.
- PDH = pituitary-dependent hyperadrenocorticism.
- UC : Cr = urine cortisol : creatinine.

Suggested Reading

Feldman EC, Nelson RW. Hyperadrenocorticism in cats (Cushing's syndrome). In: Feldman EC, Nelson RW, eds., Canine and Feline Endocrinology and Reproduction, 3rd ed. Philadelphia, PA: Saunders, 2004, pp. 358–393.

Mellet, K, Bruyette, D, Stanley, S. Trilostane therapy for treatment of spontaneous hyperadrenocorticism in cats: 15 cases (2004–2012). J Vet Intern Med 2013, 27:1471–1477.

Valentin SY, Cortright CC, Nelson RH, et al. Clinical findings, diagnostic test results and treatment outcome in cats with spontaneous hyperadrenocorticism: 30 cases. J Vet Intern Med 2014, 28:481–487.

Author/editor: Heidi Lobprise
Topic adapted from Five Minute Veterinary Consultation, 7th edition, 2021
Original Topic: Hyperadrenocorticism (Cushing's Syndrome)—Cats

Author: Suzy Y.M. Valentin
Consulting Editor: Patty A. Lathan

Chapter 27

Hyperadrenocorticism (Cushing's Syndrome)—Dogs

BASICS

DEFINITION

- Spontaneous hyperadrenocorticism (HAC)—disorder due to excessive production of cortisol by adrenal cortex.
- Iatrogenic HAC—from excessive exogenous administration of glucocorticoids by any route.
- Clinical signs due to effects of elevated circulating glucocorticoid concentrations.

PATHOPHYSIOLOGY

- ~80–85% of cases of naturally occurring HAC due to bilateral adrenocortical hyperplasia resulting from pituitary corticotroph adenoma or hyperplasia with oversecretion of adrenocorticotropic hormone (ACTH).
- In remaining 15–20%, cortisol-secreting adrenocortical neoplasia (AN) present; ~50% malignant.
- Rarely caused by ectopic ACTH secretion from nonpituitary tumor.
- Iatrogenic HAC from excessive administration of exogenous glucocorticoids.

SYSTEMS AFFECTED

- Variable.
- Signs referable to urinary tract or skin common.
- Skin—bilaterally symmetric alopecia, comedones, hyperpigmentation, recurrent pyoderma.
- Renal/urologic—polyuria/polydipsia (PU/PD; 85–90% of cases), proteinuria, urinary tract infections (UTIs).
- Endocrine/metabolic—hyperglycemia; diabetes mellitus (DM) in 10%.
- Cardiovascular—hypertension (usually mild).
- Gastrointestinal—polyphagia.
- Hemic/lymphatic/immune—stress leukogram, immunosuppression, mild erythrocytosis and thrombocytosis, occasional nucleated red blood cells.

Blackwell's Five-Minute Veterinary Consult Clinical Companion: Small Animal Senior Care, First Edition. Edited by Heidi B. Lobprise.

Companion website: www.wiley.com/go/lobprise/Senior

- Hepatobiliary—hepatopathy due to glycogen deposition, increased serum alkaline phosphatase (ALP) activity due to corticosteroid-induced isoenzyme; alanine aminotransferase (ALT) activity also increased, but by less.
- Neuromuscular—muscle weakness; CNS signs from macroadenoma may include anorexia, abnormal mentation, blindness, rarely seizures.
- Reproductive—testicular atrophy, anestrus.
- Respiratory—panting, pulmonary thromboembolism possible.

INCIDENCE/PREVALENCE

One of most common endocrine disorders in dogs.

SIGNALMENT

Breed Predilections

Poodle, dachshund, Boston terrier, German shepherd dog, beagle.

Mean Age and Range

Generally, middle-aged-to-older animals; pituitary-dependent HAC (PDH) rarely seen in dogs as young as 1 year.

SIGNS

General Comments

- Severity varies greatly, depending on duration and extent of cortisol excess.
- In some cases physical presence of neoplastic process (pituitary or adrenal) contributes to illness.

Historical and Physical Examination Findings

PU/PD, polyphagia, pendulous abdomen, increased panting, hepatomegaly, hair loss, cutaneous hyperpigmentation, thin skin, muscle weakness, obesity, lethargy, muscle atrophy, comedones, bruising, testicular atrophy, anestrus, calcinosis cutis, facial nerve palsy.

CAUSES

- PDH—adenoma most common; adenocarcinomas rare; anterior pituitary involved in ~80% of cases, intermediate lobe in remainder; exact incidence of pituitary macroadenomas (tumors >1 cm diameter) unknown, may be 10–25%.
- AN—adenoma or carcinoma (50%).
- Ectopic ACTH secretion and food-dependent hypercortisolism—rare.
- Iatrogenic—due to glucocorticoid administration.

RISK FACTORS

Administration of exogenous glucocorticoids (risk for iatrogenic HAC).

DIAGNOSIS

DIFFERENTIAL DIAGNOSIS

- Depends on clinical and laboratory abnormalities.
- Hypothyroidism, sex hormone dermatoses, alopecia X, sex hormone–secreting tumors, acromegaly, DM, hepatopathies, renal disease, other causes of PU/PD.
- Cortisol can decrease concentration of total T_4; important to check for HAC in dogs with weight gain or dermatologic disease that could be misdiagnosed as hypothyroidism.

CBC/BIOCHEMISTRY/URINALYSIS

- Hemogram may show eosinopenia, lymphopenia, leukocytosis, neutrophilia, erythrocytosis, thrombocytosis.
- Serum chemistry may show elevated cholesterol concentration; ALP activity high in ~85–90% and elevations proportionately greater than for ALT.
- Mild hyperglycemia common, but only ~10% of dogs with HAC have concurrent DM.
- Urinalysis may reveal low specific gravity, proteinuria, hematuria, pyuria, and/or bacteriuria.

OTHER LABORATORY TESTS

- Endocrine testing required in dogs with history, clinical signs, and laboratory abnormalities suggestive of HAC; see Appendix II.
- Do not perform HAC testing in sick dogs unless clinical signs consistent with HAC.
- *Screening tests* determine if HAC present or not.
- Once diagnosis of HAC made, perform *differentiation test* to determine if PDH or AN present; differentiation crucial for therapeutic decisions and prognosis.
- To convert cortisol concentration in nmol/L to µg/dL, divide by 27.6.
- All cortisol concentrations below for illustration; normal ranges and cut-off values vary with lab.

Screening Tests

Urine Cortisol : Creatinine Ratio (UC : Cr)

- Urine cortisol excretion increases with augmented adrenal secretion of cortisol, whether due to PDH or AN.
- Should be measured in urine sample collected at home when pet not stressed.
- Elevated UC : Cr is sensitive marker of HAC, present in 90–100% of affected dogs; normal ratio makes diagnosis of HAC very unlikely.
- False-positive results common; only ~20% of dogs with elevated UC : Cr have HAC.
- Due to chance of false-positive, always do ACTH stimulation test or low-dose dexamethasone suppression test to confirm presence of HAC.

Low-Dose Dexamethasone Suppression Test (LDDST)

- Lack of suppression 8h after injection of low dose of dexamethasone consistent with diagnosis of HAC.
- Sensitivity ~95% in dogs.
- In dogs with nonadrenal illness, relatively high chance of false-positive.

- Lack of suppression at 4 hours but full suppression at 8 hours technically not consistent with HAC, but suspicious for its presence; further testing warranted.
- LDDST may also serve as differentiation test; if 8 hours sample >1.4 µg/dL, result consistent with HAC; if also suppression to <1.4 µg/dL at 4 hours post dexamethasone (i.e., "escape" at 8 hours post dexamethasone) or 4 hours and/or 8 hours post-dexamethasone samples <50% of baseline, results consistent with PDH; if criteria for PDH not met, chances still ~⅔ for PDH vs. AN.
- If baseline values close to 1.4 µg/dL or suppression just at 50%, confirm presence of PDH by other means.

ACTH Stimulation Test

- Response > normal consistent with diagnosis of spontaneous HAC, but cannot differentiate between PDH and AN.
- Overall sensitivity of test ~80%; for PDH, sensitivity ~87%; for HAC due to AN sensitivity ~61%.
- More specific in dogs than LDDST (only 15% chance of false-positive with nonadrenal illness).
- Only test that can diagnose iatrogenic HAC; diagnosis made with history of glucocorticoid exposure by any route, consistent clinical signs, and post-ACTH cortisol concentration < reference range.
- Cosyntropin (or tetracosactrin) recommended form; if using compounded ACTH, collect samples before and at 1 and 2 hours post ACTH administration so peak response not missed.

Differentiating Tests

High-Dose Dexamethasone Suppression Test (HDDST)

- Two responses consistent with PDH—suppression to <1.4 µg/dL at 4 and/or 8 hours post dexamethasone; or 4 and/or 8 hours post-dexamethasone samples <50% of baseline.
- If baseline values close to 1.4 µg/dL or suppression just at 50%, confirm presence of PDH by other means.
- Can *never* confirm presence of AN; if criteria for diagnosis of PDH not met, 50/50 chance patient has PDH or AN; since HDDST does not significantly increase ability to differentiate PDH from AN, endogenous ACTH (eACTH) and/or abdominal US used instead.

eACTH Concentration

- Requires only single blood sample, but inappropriate handling can lead to decreased eACTH concentrations due to degradation.
- In patients with PDH, eACTH concentration usually normal to increased; with AN, eACTH concentration < normal.
- If concentration increased, consistent with PDH, but due to episodic secretion of ACTH even in patients with PDH, low value does not always confirm AN.
- If eACTH concentration falls in gray zone, results not diagnostic.

IMAGING

- Abdominal radiographs—~40–50% of canine ANs seen; adrenal mineralization suspicious for AN.
- Thoracic radiographs indicated in patients with AN to check for metastases.
- US—useful for staging AN, but poor screening test (adrenal enlargement occurs with chronic nonadrenal illness, AN may be difficult to see with US); adrenal atrophy can be difficult to

determine with US, but bilaterally enlarged adrenal glands consistent with PDH; vena caval invasion and metastasis may be present with AN.

- CT and MRI—can show pituitary macroadenomas and assess AN invasion into adjacent structures; follow-up and treatment recommendations (e.g., radiation therapy) may vary with tumor size.

DIAGNOSTIC PROCEDURES

Adrenal histopathology following adrenalectomy for AN often needed to differentiate benign vs. malignant tumor; biopsy prior to removal may result in complications.

PATHOLOGIC FINDINGS

- PDH—normal-to-enlarged pituitary and bilateral adrenocortical enlargement.
- Microscopically, pituitary adenoma, adenocarcinoma, or corticotroph hyperplasia of pars distalis or pars intermedia and adrenocortical hyperplasia.
- AN—variable-sized adrenal mass, atrophy of contralateral gland (rarely bilateral tumors), metastasis and invasion into vena cava with thrombosis possible.
- Microscopically, adrenocortical adenoma or carcinoma.

TREATMENT

APPROPRIATE HEALTH CARE

Dictated by severity of clinical signs, patient's overall condition, any complicating factors (e.g., DM, pulmonary thromboembolism).

CLIENT EDUCATION

- For medical therapy, lifelong therapy required.
- If adverse reaction to mitotane or trilostane occurs—discontinue drug, give dexamethasone, have veterinarian re-evaluate next day; if no response noted in few hours, veterinarian should evaluate immediately.

SURGICAL CONSIDERATIONS

- Hypophysectomy—described, but limited availability.
- Bilateral adrenalectomy not used for treatment of PDH.
- Surgery treatment of choice in dogs with adrenocortical adenomas and carcinomas unless patient poor surgical candidate.
- Appropriate personnel and facilities required as adrenalectomy (especially with vena caval thrombi) is technically demanding and intensive postoperative management required.
- Surgery not curative, but long-term survival possible
- Medical control of HAC may be desirable prior to surgery.

MEDICATIONS

DRUG(S) OF CHOICE

Trilostane

- Trilostane (Vetoryl®) inhibits adrenocortical enzyme 3-β-hydroxysteroid dehydrogenase and maybe others, thereby suppressing production of progesterone and its end-products, including cortisol and aldosterone (less than cortisol); efficacy and survival time for treatment of PDH excellent.
- Initial dose 2–3 mg/kg PO q24h (in morning) or divided q12h with food; twice-daily dosing more expensive, but quicker resolution of clinical signs, fewer dose changes and monitoring tests; if q24h dosing elected and patient controlled during day but has more clinical signs at night, splitting daily dose ½ morning and ½ evening may improve clinical signs.
- Side effects: lethargy, decreased appetite, vomiting, diarrhea; within first few days of therapy with gastrointestinal upset due oral medication; hypocortisolemia can also occur due to oversuppression of cortisol production and cause same clinical signs; rarely, idiosyncratic adrenal necrosis with hypocortisolemia and hypoaldosteronism, but less common with lower doses (as recommended above).
- Monitoring—control clinical signs and avoid complications (especially hypocortisolemia); assessment of clinical signs (PU/PD, polyphagia, panting) and cortisol testing (see below) to ensure cortisol not suppressed excessively.
- ACTH stimulation test used to monitor trilostane therapy, 4–6 hours post trilostane administration; 1 μg/kg cosyntropin IV effective for monitoring, but *not* for diagnosis (must use 5 μg/kg); ideal post-ACTH cortisol concentration 2–6 μg/dL, but must consider clinical signs.
- Post-ACTH stimulation cortisol values do not always correlate well with clinical signs, measuring cortisol concentration before morning dose of trilostane may correlate better; assessing clinical signs imperative when using pre-pill cortisol concentration for monitoring; if signs of hypocortisolemia (vomiting, diarrhea, decreased appetite), must use ACTH stimulation test; using pre-pill cortisol concentration: patient not cortisol deficient 2–6 μg/dL clinical signs used to determine whether dose adequate; if <2 μg/dL, perform ACTH stimulation test or decrease dose; if patient still clinical (PU/PD, polyphagic, panting) and pre-pill cortisol >6 μg/dL, safe to increase dose; in clinically uncontrolled patient, and cortisol concentration 2–6 μg/dL: probably safe to increase dose if pre-pill cortisol 5 μg/dL, but probably not at 2.5 μg/dL; perform ACTH stimulation test in this situation.
- Perform either ACTH stimulation test or pre-pill cortisol at 10–14, 30, and 90 days after each dose change; if at 10- to14-day recheck any improvement seen, do not increase dose even if cortisol concentration above ideal; wait until 30-day recheck and change dose then if necessary, as effect of trilostane often increases between 2 and 4 weeks; assess renal profile, including electrolytes, at 14- or 30-day exam; once clinical condition and dose stabilized, perform pre-pill cortisol or ACTH stimulation test, and electrolyte panel, q3–6 months.
- If lethargy, decreased appetite, vomiting, or diarrhea occurs, ACTH stimulation test to confirm dog not hypocortisolemic (<2 μg/dL); if hypocortisolemia confirmed, assess electrolyte panel to ensure hyponatremia and hyperkalemia not present; discontinue trilostane until clinical signs of HAC recur and baseline and/or post-ACTH cortisol concentrations >5–6 μg/dL.

- If signs of hypocortisolemia more severe than mild lethargy, vomiting, decreased appetite, give dexamethasone 0.1 mg/kg/day PO/IV, then taper to lowest effective dose to control signs; if signs of HAC recur, taper dexamethasone and discontinue, then perform baseline cortisol and/or ACTH stimulation test interpreted as above; if dexamethasone unavailable and prednisone used instead, delay cortisol testing until at least 24 hours after last prednisone dose, as prednisone can cross-react with cortisol assay.
- If more severe signs occur, hospitalization with IV fluids, dexamethasone, and other supportive therapy necessary.
- Hypocortisolemia secondary to trilostane administration usually resolves within 48–72 hours of drug discontinuation, but temporary cortisol suppression of weeks to months and even permanent suppression can occur.
- Trilostane can be used to treat hypercortisolemia from AN and usually controls clinical signs; although mitotane theoretically preferred due to chemotherapeutic properties, no difference shown between survival of patients with AN treated with mitotane or trilostane.

Mitotane

- Mitotane (*o,p′*-DDD, Lysodren®) selectively destroys glucocorticoid-secreting cells of adrenal cortex; in patients with AN may destroy tumor cells as well as controlling cortisol secretion, but no difference in survival between dogs with AN receiving mitotane vs. trilostane.
- PDH—initial loading dose 40–50 mg/kg PO divided twice daily; evaluate efficacy with ACTH stimulation test after 8 days, or sooner if decreased appetite, vomiting, diarrhea, listlessness, decreased water intake (<60 mL/kg/day); target for both basal and post-ACTH cortisol concentration 1–5 µg/dL; continue induction with repeat testing as necessary until adequate response, then initiate maintenance therapy at 50 mg/kg/week PO divided in 2–3 doses; adjust dosage based on ACTH stimulation testing (to maintain basal and post-ACTH cortisol levels in ideal range); if serum cortisol concentration pre- or post-ACTH <1 µg/dL, measure electrolyte concentrations, stop administering mitotane, and give physiologic doses of prednisone (0.1 mg/kg PO q12h; do not give within 24 hours before ACTH stimulation test); cortisol secretion usually recovers in weeks to months but can take longer; once cortisol concentration in ideal range, discontinue prednisone and begin maintenance therapy; if dog was on maintenance therapy when became cortisol deficient, restart maintenance at 25% lower dose; if relapse occurs at any time on maintenance therapy (as indicated by cortisol levels above ideal range), dose adjustment required; if post-ACTH serum cortisol concentration 5–10 µg/dL, increase maintenance mitotane dose by 25% and reevaluate in 4 weeks; if post-ACTH serum cortisol concentration >10 µg/dL, repeat loading sequence for 5–7 days and repeat ACTH stimulation test; continue loading until cortisol concentration in ideal range, then reinitiate weekly maintenance dose at ~50% higher dose.
- AN—goal of mitotane to achieve low-to-nondetectable (<1 µg/dL) basal and post-ACTH cortisol concentrations; starting dose 50–75 mg/kg PO divided daily; perform ACTH stimulation test after 10–14 days of therapy to evaluate efficacy, sooner if decreased appetite, vomiting, diarrhea, lethargy, decreased water intake (<60 mL/kg/day); induction typically requires higher doses and longer duration than for treatment of PDH and dose should be increased by 50 mg/kg/day q10–14 days if control not achieved (based on ACTH stimulation test); if adverse effects develop, continue administration at highest tolerable dose; once control achieved, begin maintenance therapy at 75–100 mg/kg/week PO divided into 2–3 doses; if cortisol levels pre- and post-ACTH rise into normal resting range (1–5 µg/dL), increase maintenance dose by 50%; if cortisol levels

rise above normal resting range pre- and post-ACTH, reload until control achieved and increase weekly maintenance dose ~50%; because goal of induction and maintenance is to create glucocorticoid insufficiency, prednisone should be administered at 0.2 mg/kg/day PO.

- Aldosterone deficiency possible from mitotane therapy; if it occurs, patient will likely have permanent complete adrenocortical insufficiency and treatment for hypoadrenocorticism should be initiated.

L-Deprenyl

- L-Deprenyl (selegiline hydrochloride); FDA approved for treatment of PDH; decreases pituitary ACTH secretion, thus decreasing serum cortisol concentration.
- Questionable efficacy; not currently recommended.

Ketoconazole

Ketoconazole (10 mg/kg PO q12 h initially; up to 20 mg/kg PO q12 h in some dogs) inhibits cortisol synthesis; no longer recommended (trilostane causes fewer side effects).

CONTRAINDICATIONS

- Do not use ketoconazole with trilostane therapy (increased potential for hypocortisolism)
- Monitor for hyperkalemia if concurrent angiotensin-converting enzyme inhibitor therapy.

PRECAUTIONS

- Side effects of trilostane include anorexia, lethargy, vomiting, diarrhea; usually mild and resolve with discontinuation and dose adjustment; Addisonian crisis and adrenocortical necrosis reported.
- Use trilostane and mitotane with caution in patients with renal insufficiency and hepatic disease; trilostane contraindicated in pregnancy.
- Side effects of mitotane mild in most dogs; include lethargy, anorexia, vomiting, diarrhea, ataxia, iatrogenic hypoadrenocorticism.
- Side effects more common in dogs with AN given high-dose mitotane.
- In diabetic patients, insulin requirement can decrease with control of HAC.

ALTERNATIVE DRUG(S)

Radiation therapy possible to treat pituitary macroadenomas. Treatment with trilostane or mitotane still usually required afterwards. ACTH levels may take several months to decrease and HAC controlled with drugs in interim.

FOLLOW-UP

PATIENT MONITORING

- Response to therapy—use periodic ACTH stimulation and/or cortisol testing to assess trilostane and mitotane efficacy (see above); once on maintenance mitotane therapy, test at 1, 3, and 6 months and q3–6 months thereafter or if clinical signs of HAC recur

- Adequacy of any mitotane reloading period checked with ACTH stimulation test before higher maintenance dose initiated.
- Adequacy of trilostane dose alterations checked with ACTH stimulation test performed 4–6 hours after dosing.

PREVENTION/AVOIDANCE

For prevention of recurrence and hypocortisolemia, regular administration of medications with appropriate follow-up required.

POSSIBLE COMPLICATIONS

- Hypertension.
- Proteinuria.
- Recurrent infections.
- Urinary calculi (calcium oxalate).
- DM.
- Pulmonary thromboembolism.
- Neurologic signs secondary to pituitary macroadenoma.
- Hypoadrenocorticism secondary to treatment.

EXPECTED COURSE AND PROGNOSIS

- Untreated HAC—progressive disorder with survival of 6–18 months.
- Treated PDH—usually good prognosis; median survival time with mitotane or trilostane treatment ~2 years; at least 10% survive 4 years; dogs living >6 months tend to die of causes unrelated to HAC.
- Macroadenomas in animals with no or mild neurologic abnormalities have fair-to-good prognosis with radiation and medical therapy; in patients with significant neurologic abnormalities, prognosis poor to grave.
- Adrenal adenomas—usually good-to-excellent prognosis; small carcinomas (not metastasized) fair-to-good prognosis overall, good-to-excellent with surgical resection.
- Large carcinomas and AN with widespread metastasis—generally poor-to-fair prognosis, but impressive responses to high doses of mitotane occasionally seen.

MISCELLANEOUS

Associated Conditions

Neurologic signs in dogs with pituitary tumors; glucose intolerance or concurrent DM; pulmonary thromboembolism; increased incidence of infections, especially UTI and skin; hypertension; proteinuria/glomerulopathy.

Abbreviations

- ACTH = adrenocorticotropic hormone
- ALP = alkaline phosphatase.
- ALT = alanine aminotransferase.
- AN = adrenal neoplasia.

- DM = diabetes mellitus.
- eACTH = endogenous ACTH.
- HAC = hyperadrenocorticism.
- HDDST = high-dose dexamethasone-suppression test.
- LDDST = low-dose dexamethasone-suppression test.
- PDH = pituitary-dependent HAC.
- PU/PD = polyuria/polydipsia.
- UC : Cr = urine cortisol : creatinine.
- UTI = urinary tract infection.

Suggested Reading

Behrend EN, Kooistra HS, Nelson R, et al. Diagnosis of spontaneous canine hyperadrenocorticism: 2012 ACVIM consensus statement (small animal). *J Vet Intern Med* 2013;27:1292–1304.

Braddock JA, Church DB, Robertson ID, et al. Trilostane treatment in dogs with pituitary-dependent hyperadrenocorticism. *Aust Vet J* 2003;81:600–607.

Kintzer PP, Peterson ME. Mitotane (o,p′-DDD) treatment of 200 dogs with pituitary-dependent hyperadenocorticism. *J Vet Intern Med* 1991;5:182–190.

Nagata N, Kokima K, Yuki M. Comparison of survival times for dogs with pituitary-dependent hyperadrenocorticism in a primary-care hospital: treated with trilostane versus untreated. *J Vet Intern Med* 2017;31:22–28.

Vaughn MA, Feldman EC, Hoar BR, Nelson RW. Evaluation of twice-daily, low-dose trilostane treatment administered orally in dogs with naturally occurring hyperadrenocorticism. *J Am Vet Med Assoc* 2008;232:1321–1328.

Author/editor: Heidi Lobprise
Topic adapted from Five Minute Veterinary Consultation, 7th edition, 202_
Original Topic: Hyperadrenocorticism (Cushing's Disease)—Dogs

Author: Patty A. Lathan
Consulting Editor: Patty A. Lathan

Chapter 28

Hyperparathyroidism

BASICS

DEFINITION

A pathologic, sustained, high, circulating concentration of parathyroid hormone (PTH).

PATHOPHYSIOLOGY

- PTH is secreted by the parathyroid glands in response to changes in the concentration of ionized calcium in the serum and causes an increase in serum calcium concentration through direct effects on bone and renal tubular calcium resorption and indirectly by vitamin D–dependent intestinal calcium absorption.
- Primary hyperparathyroidism is usually associated with benign adenoma of the parathyroid gland(s), although adenocarcinoma and hyperplasia are possible.
  - Secondary to chronic kidney disease (CKD); impaired renal excretion of phosphorus leading to hyperphosphatemia and ionized hypocalcemia, elevation of FGF-23, and suppression of renal calcitriol synthesis; increased PTH production; PTH as a uremic toxin can promote nephrocalcinosis and CKD progression.
  - secondary hyperparathyroidism can be caused by a deficiency of calcium and vitamin D associated with malnutrition or chronic renal disease.

SYSTEMS AFFECTED

- Cardiovascular.
- Gastrointestinal.
- Neuromuscular.
- Renal/urologic.

GENETICS

- Autosomal dominant with possible age-dependent penetrance in the keeshond; genetic test available from Cornell.
- Secondary hyperparathyroidism can develop in association with hereditary nephropathy.

Blackwell's Five-Minute Veterinary Consult Clinical Companion: Small Animal Senior Care, First Edition. Edited by Heidi B. Lobprise.

Companion website: www.wiley.com/go/lobprise/Senior

INCIDENCE/PREVALENCE

- Prevalence of primary form is unknown.
- More common in dogs than in cats.
- Common among causes of hypercalcemia, but less common than hypercalcemia of malignancy in dogs; more common in middle-aged-to-geriatric dogs.
- Chronic renal failure with secondary hyperparathyroidism is extremely common, more so in cats than in dogs.
- Renal secondary hyperparathyroidism can develop prior to azotemia in cats, without hyperphosphatemia and hypocalcemia.
- Nutritional secondary hyperparathyroidism is decreasing in prevalence as the public becomes more educated in pet nutrition.

SIGNALMENT

Species

Cat and dog.

Breed Predilections

- Keeshond, but seen in almost any breed.
- Siamese and domestic shorthair cats.

Mean Age and Range

- Cats—mean age: 13 years; range: 8–20 years.
- Dogs—mean age: 10 years; range: 4–17 years.

SIGNS

General Comments

- Primary HPT
    - Most dogs and cats do not appear ill.
    - Signs are usually mild and due to the effects of hypercalcemia, or lower urinary tract signs if urolithiasis is present.
    - Signs become apparent when hypercalcemia is severe and chronic.
- Renal Secondary HPT
    - Uremia due to underlying CKD.
    - Renal osteodystrophy or "rubber jaw" most commonly occurs in young dogs with severe renal secondary hyperparathyroidism (RSHPT).
    - Pain around the head or long bones.

Historical Findings

- Polyuria/Polydipsia.
- Anorexia; vomiting
- Lethargy; weakness
- Urolithiasis.
- Stupor and coma.

Physical Examination Findings

- Often unremarkable.
- Parathyroid adenoma is not palpable in dogs but often is in cats.
- Nutritional secondary disease is sometimes associated with pathologic bone fractures and general poor body condition.

CAUSES

- Primary hyperparathyroidism—PTH-secreting adenoma of the parathyroid gland; in most cases only one gland is adenomatous; malignant tumors of the parathyroid glands are uncommon and usually noninvasive.
- Renal secondary hyperparathyroidism (RSHPT)—renal calcium loss and reduced gut absorption of calcium due to deficiency in calcitriol production by the renal tubular cells.
- Nutritional secondary hyperparathyroidism—a nutritional deficiency of calcium and vitamin D.

RISK FACTORS

- Primary hyperparathyroidism—unknown.
- Secondary hyperparathyroidism—renal tubular disease or calcium/vitamin D malnutrition.

DIAGNOSIS

DIFFERENTIAL DIAGNOSIS

Primary HPT

- The differential list includes causes of hypercalcemia (lymphoma, anal sac apocrine gland adenocarcinoma, miscellaneous carcinoma, myeloproliferative disease - cats)
- Chronic kidney disease.
- Hypoadrenocorticism.
- Vitamin D intoxication—cholecalciferol-containing rodenticides, plant sources, human anti-psoriasis topical creams, and vitamin supplements.
- Granulomatous diseases.
- Idiopathic hypercalcemia in cats.

Renal Secondary HPT

- Hypercalcemic nephropathy—kidney disease caused by ionized hypercalcemia; can be difficult to differentiate from longstanding RSHPT, in which hyperplasia of the parathyroid glands disrupts the normal feedback arc between PTH release and ionized calcium (tertiary hyperparathyroidism).
- Ionized serum calcium concentration is usually low or normal with RSHPT, but high with hypercalcemic nephropathy.
- Low serum PTH and PTH-related protein (PTHrP) high in animals with hypercalcemia of malignancy.

CBC/BIOCHEMISTRY/URINALYSIS

Primary HPT

- High serum total and ionized calcium concentrations.
- Low or low–normal serum phosphorus concentration in primary hyperparathyroidism.
- Hyperphosphatemia in renal secondary hyperparathyroidism or hypervitaminosis D.
- Serum blood urea nitrogen (BUN) and creatinine concentrations are usually normal in patients with primary hyperparathyroidism, except those with hypercalcemia-induced renal failure.

Renal Secondary HPT

- Azotemia.
- Hyperphosphatemia.
- Dilute urine.
- Total serum calcium does not reliably predict ionized calcium.

OTHER LABORATORY TESTS

Primary HPT

- Serum ionized calcium high in PHT or hypercalcemia associated with malignancy.
- High serum intact PTH diagnostic for primary hyperparathyroidism in the absence of azotemia; a normal serum PTH with ionized hypercalcemia is *abnormal;* can signal parathyroid-dependent hypercalcemia.
- Measurement of PTH-related peptide (PTH-rp) may detect hyperparathyroidism related to neoplasia.

RSHPT

- Serum ionized calcium often normal (or low) in patients with chronic renal failure
- Definitive diagnosis and monitoring of RSHPT require validated assay of serum PTH.

IMAGING

- Radiography for identifying urolithiasis and occult neoplasia; to assess renal morphology and bone density—(RSHPT) low bone density, loss of the lamina dura around teeth, soft tissue mineralization of gastric mucosa and other tissues.
- Ultrasonography (ventral cervical area) sometimes reveals a parathyroid gland adenoma.
- Ultrasound of the abdomen can reveal lymphadenomegaly, urolithiasis, or renal morphologic abnormalities.

DIAGNOSTIC PROCEDURES

Primary HPT: Surgical exploration of the ventral cervical area.

PATHOLOGIC FINDINGS

Primary HPT

- Parathyroid adenoma is usually a solitary, small (=1 cm), round, light brown or reddish mass located in the proximity of the thyroid gland.
- Occasionally multiple adenomas are found.

- The histologic distinctions between adenomas, hyperplasia, and carcinomas of the parathyroid gland are often unclear.

TREATMENT

APPROPRIATE HEALTH CARE

- Primary hyperparathyroidism generally requires inpatient care and surgery.
- Nutritional or renal secondary hyperparathyroidism in noncritical patients can be managed on an outpatient basis.

DIET

Calcium supplementation for secondary forms.

CLIENT EDUCATION

Explain signs referable to changes in calcium status, because hypocalcemia is a potential complication of parathyroidectomy if Primary HPT

SURGICAL CONSIDERATIONS

Primary HPT

- Surgery is the treatment of choice for primary hyperparathyroidism and is often important in establishing the diagnosis.
- Percutaneous ultrasound-guided heat ablation has been used successfully for treatment of parathyroid adenomas and may be recommended if available.
- Percutaneous ultrasound-guided ethanol ablation has been reported to be less successful than surgery or heat ablation.

MEDICATIONS

DRUG(S) OF CHOICE

Primary HPT

- Normal saline is the fluid of choice for treatment of hypercalcemia.
- Diuretics (furosemide) and corticosteroids can be useful in treating hypercalcemia.
- No medical treatment exists for primary hyperparathyroidism per se.
  RSHPT

Intestinal Phosphate Binders

- Phosphorous binders used to further reduce serum phosphorous if dietary management insufficient. Serum phosphorous targets based on the IRIS stages are stages 1 and 2: >2.7 to <4.6 mg/dL; Stage 3: >2.7 to <5.1 mg/dL; and Stage 4: >2.7 to <6.0 mg/dL.
- Aluminum hydroxide (60–90 mg/kg/day), calcium carbonate (90–150 mg/kg/day), calcium acetate (60–90 mg/kg/day), or lanthanum carbonate (60–90 mg/kg/day)—dose to achieve target serum phosphorus concentration, but do not exceed max dosage. All must be given

with meals. Combine different phosphate binders to reduce the dosage of each and minimize the risk of hypercalcemia or aluminum toxicity.

- Avoid calcium-containing phosphate binders with calcitriol therapy as hypercalcemia may occur.

Calcitriol

- Low-dose calcitriol (2.0–3.5 ng/kg PO q24h)—may use after serum phosphorus is controlled; administered on an empty stomach and before bedtime (no food for 6–8 hours after administration).
- Calcitriol therapy may result in hypercalcemia, especially if combined with a calcium-containing phosphate binder. Increased total calcium concentration may develop in patients with long-standing CKD but is unrelated to calcitriol treatment. Ionized calcium concentration is normal or low in these patients.
- Calcitriol use has not gained uniform acceptance.
- A new class of calcimimetic drugs is being used in humans to treat renal secondary hyperparathyroidism; studies of these drugs in dogs and cats have not been reported and expense limits their use.

CONTRAINDICATIONS

Do not use glucocorticoids until the diagnosis of lymphoma has been excluded; they can obfuscate the diagnosis of a parathyroid adenoma.

PRECAUTIONS

Use furosemide only in patients with adequate hydration.

ALTERNATIVE DRUG(S)

Pamidronate and other bisphosphonate drugs have been used to treat hypercalcemia of various causes in dogs and cats.

FOLLOW-UP

PATIENT MONITORING

Primary HPT

- Postoperative hypocalcemia is relatively common; preoperative ionized calcium and PTH concentrations are poor predictors of postsurgical hypocalcemia, so monitoring is essential in all cases.
- Requires treatment with vitamin D (calcitriol is recommended) and calcium supplements (see treatment of hypoparathyroidism); ionized calcium should be monitored to guide dosage adjustments; contradictory evidence exists with respect to preoperative administration of calcitriol.
- In patients with renal impairment, check serum concentrations of BUN and creatinine.

RSHPT

- Initially and in unstable patients, serum concentrations of calcium, phosphorus, creatinine, and urea nitrogen—monitor weekly to monthly depending on therapy and the severity of CKD.

- Patients receiving calcitriol should be monitored for hypercalcemia and hyperphosphatemia weekly for 4 weeks, then every 3–4 months.
- Serial evaluations of PTH concentration—most treated with low-dose calcitriol achieve near-normal levels of PTH within 3 months; it may be necessary to increase the dose in those with severe parathyroid gland hyperplasia.
- If hypercalcemia develops discontinue calcitriol; calcium should normalize within 5 days of discontinuation. Measurement of ionized calcium is recommended—animals with CKD may develop nonionized hypercalcemia that is unrelated to calcitriol treatment.

PREVENTION/AVOIDANCE

Primary HPT

- Avoid breeding affected keeshonden.
- Nutritional secondary hyperparathyroidism is prevented by proper nutrition.

RSHPT

- Dietary phosphorus restriction may delay the onset of RSHPT.

POSSIBLE COMPLICATIONS

- Irreversible renal failure secondary to hypercalcemia.
- Fractures due to decreased bone density with chronic hyperparathyroidism.

EXPECTED COURSE AND PROGNOSIS

Primary HPT

- Untreated PHT may progress to end-stage kidney or neuromuscular disease depending on severity; many dogs clinically seem to do well even with no treatment, provided urolithiasis does not develop.
- Prognosis for surgical treatment of parathyroid adenoma is excellent.
- Recurrence is seen in a small percentage of cases.
- In animals that develop postoperative hypoparathyroidism, the return of normal parathyroid function is unpredictable and can take weeks to months.

RSHPT

- Progression of the underlying CKD may be slowed by minimizing phosphorus retention and RSHPT.
- Long-term prognosis is guarded to poor for patients with CKD and RSHPT.

MISCELLANEOUS

See Also

- Chronic Kidney Disease
- Nutrition
- Urolithiasis.

Abbreviations

- BUN = blood urea nitrogen
- CKD = chronic kidney disease.
- PTH = parathyroid hormone.
- PTH-rp = PTH-related peptide.
- RSHPT = renal secondary hyperparathyroidism.

Suggested Reading—Hyperparathyroidism

Dear JD, Kass PH, Della Maggiore AM, Feldman EC. Association of hypercalcemia before treatment with hypocalcemia after treatment in dogs with primary hyperparathyroidism. *J Vet Intern Med* 2017;31(2):349–354.

Feldman EC, Hoar B, Pollard R, Nelson RW. Pretreatment clinical and laboratory findings in dogs with primary hyperparathyroidism: 210 cases (1987–2004). *J Am Vet Med Assoc* 2005;227(5):756–761.

Milovancev M, Schmiedt CW. Preoperative factors associated with postoperative hypocalcemia in dogs with primary hyperparathyroidism that underwent parathyroidectomy: 62 cases (2004–2009). *J Am Vet Med Assoc* 2013;242(4):507–515.

Richter KP, Kallet AJ, Feldman EC, Brum DE. Primary hyperparathyroidism in cats: seven cases (1984–1989). *J Am Vet Med Assoc* 1991;199(12):1767–1771.

Schaefer C, Goldstein RE. Canine primary hyperparathyroidism. *Compend Contin Educ Vet* 2009;31(8):382–389.

Suggested Reading—Renal Secondary Hyperparathyroidism

Finch NC, Syme HM, Elliott J. Parathyroid hormone concentration in geriatric cats with various degrees of renal function. *J Am Vet Med Assoc* 2012;241(10):1326–1335.

Foster J. Update on mineral and bone disorders in chronic kidney disease. *Vet Clin North Am Small Anim Pract* 2016;46(6):1131–1149.

Polzin D. Chronic kidney disease. In: Ettinger SJ, Feldman EC (eds) *Textbook of Veterinary Internal Medicine*, 7th edn. St. Louis, MO: Elsevier, 2009; pp. 2036–2067.

Polzin DJ, Ross SJ, Osborne CA. Calcitriol therapy in chronic kidney disease. In Bonagura J (ed.) *Current Veterinary Therapy XIV*. Philadelphia, PA: Saunders, 2008; pp. 892–895.

Author/editor: Heidi Lobprise
Topic adapted from Five Minute Veterinary Consultation, 7th edition, 2021
Original Topic: Hyperparathyroidism

Author: Brett A. Wasik
Consulting Editor: Patty A. Lathan
Topic adapted from Five Minute Veterinary Consultation, 7th edition, 2021
Original Topic: Renal Secondary Hyperparathyroidism

Author: David J. Polzin
Consulting Editor: J.D. Foster

Chapter 29

Hypersomatotropism/ Acromegaly in Cats

BASICS

OVERVIEW

- Caused by excessive growth hormone (GH) secretion from the anterior pituitary by an adenoma or somatotroph hyperplasia.
- GH induces hepatic insulin-like growth factor-1 (IGF-1) secretion. The combination of increased GH and IGF-1 causes lipolysis, protein synthesis, impaired carbohydrate metabolism, and insulin resistance (IR).
- Prevalence in Europe ranges from 1 : 3 to 1 : 5.5 diabetic cats.

SIGNALMENT

- Median age—11 years (range: 9.5–13 years).
- Male : female ratio is 2 : 1.
- No breed predisposition.

SIGNS

- Clinical signs of diabetes mellitus (DM; e.g., polyuria, polydipsia, and polyphagia) occur from GH-induced IR. IR can be variable or persistent, which makes the DM difficult to control.
- Many (~40%) diabetics with hypersomatotropism (HST) lose weight due to poorly controlled DM; a small proportion (~17%) gain weight.
- Anabolic state—patients may present with polyphagia (without DM), or soft-tissue growth resulting in upper airway obstruction, broad facial features, or clubbed feet.
- A small proportion (~2%) develop neurologic signs due to pituitary adenoma.

CAUSES AND RISK FACTORS

- GH-secreting pituitary adenoma or somatotroph hyperplasia.
- In dogs, but not cats, progestins can result in increased GH concentration.

Blackwell's Five-Minute Veterinary Consult Clinical Companion: Small Animal Senior Care, First Edition. Edited by Heidi B. Lobprise.

Companion website: www.wiley.com/go/lobprise/Senior

DIAGNOSIS

DIFFERENTIAL DIAGNOSIS

- Uncomplicated DM.
- Pituitary-dependent hyperadrenocorticism.
- Causes of polyphagia such as exocrine pancreatic insufficiency, gastrointestinal inflammatory diseases, hyperthyroidism, and inflammatory liver diseases. Cats with HST and polyphagia but without DM typically gain weight, unlike other differentials.

CBC/BIOCHEMISTRY/URINALYSIS

- Consistent with DM.
- Diabetic ketoacidosis uncommon.

OTHER LABORATORY TESTS

- Serum IGF-1 concentration using validated assays is test of choice.
    - Positive predictive value of IGF-1 >1000 ng/mL (131 nmol/L) of 95%.
    - Roughly one-third of cats with HST have a low IGF-1 at diagnosis, which increases to >1000 ng/mL after insulin therapy.
    - IGF-1 concentrations between 700 and 1000 ng/mL (92–131 nmol/L) is a "gray" zone—many non-HST diabetic cats are in this range.
- There is no commercially available GH assay.

IMAGING

- Abdominal ultrasound might identify organomegaly.
- Contrast-enhanced CT can assess pituitary size.
- Echocardiographic findings—increased left ventricular wall thickness, left atrial enlargement, aortic insufficiency.

TREATMENT

Surgery

Hypophysectomy most consistently normalizes IGF-1 concentration (80% of cases) and results in highest diabetic remission rates (50% achieve long-term remission).

Medical Management

- Somatostatins (SSTs) are primary negative regulatory hormones of GH secretion.
- Pasireotide is an SST analogue. Short-acting pasireotide (0.03 mg/kg SC q12h) decreased IGF-1 in 12 cats after 3 days of treatment, while long-acting pasireotide (8 mg/kg SC monthly) resulted in normalization of IGF-1 in 2/8 cats; all cats experienced increased insulin sensitivity and 3/8 cats achieved diabetic remission.
- Octreotide is an SST analogue with a different binding profile that temporarily decreases GH without improvement in clinical control of HST or DM.
- Dopamine receptor 2 inhibits GH secretion. Cabergoline, a dopamine receptor 2 agonist, decreases IGF-1 and increases insulin sensitivity in some cats with HST.

Radiotherapy

Fractionated radiotherapy improves neurologic signs and may improve diabetic control. Stereotactic radiotherapy might be more favorable as improved diabetic control and diabetic remission is more likely.

Palliative Treatment

- Maximizing diabetic control (e.g., with insulin and diet) is recommended but may be challenging.
- Comorbidities (e.g., osteoarthritis, cardiac disease) should be managed.
- Controlling polyphagia in some cats with HST is challenging. Despite lack of endocrine improvement after cabergoline, many owners reported normalization of appetite.

MEDICATIONS

See Medical Management.

FOLLOW-UP

- Depends on treatment modality.
- Survival varies from months to years; most euthanized due to poor quality of life or causes unrelated to HST.
- Diabetic control should be monitored as for an uncomplicated diabetic. A small proportion of cats gain weight despite poor diabetic control and have persistent polyphagia despite good diabetic control.

MISCELLANEOUS

Abbreviations

- DM = diabetes mellitus
- GH = growth hormone.
- HST = hypersomatotropism.
- IGF-1 = insulin like growth factor-1.
- IR = insulin resistance.
- SST = somatostatin.

Suggested Reading

Berg RI, Nelson RW, Feldman EC, et al. Serum insulin-like growth factor-I concentration in cats with diabetes mellitus and acromegaly. *J Vet Intern Med* 2007;21(5):892–898.

Gostelow R, Scudder C, Keyte S, et al. Pasireotide long-acting release treatment for diabetic cats with underlying hypersomatotropism. *J Vet Int Med* 2017;31(2):355–364.

Wormhoudt TL, Boss M-K, Lunn K, et al. Stereotactic radiation therapy for the treatment of functional pituitary adenomas associated with feline acromegaly. *J Vet Int Med* 2018;32(4):1383–1389.

Author/editor: Heidi Lobprise
Topic adapted from Five Minute Veterinary Consultation, 7th edition, 2021
Original Topic: Hypersomatotropism-Acromegaly in Cats

Author: Christopher J. Scudder
Consulting Editor: Patty A. Lathan

Chapter 30

Hyperthyroidism

BASICS

DEFINITION

A state of increased metabolism caused by increased circulating concentrations of thyroid hormone.

PATHOPHYSIOLOGY

- Feline hyperthyroidism most often caused by benign adenomatous hyperplasia or follicular cell adenoma, causing increased secretion of thyroxine (T_4) and triiodothyronine (T_3).
- Naturally occurring hyperthyroidism rare in dogs; most often malignant carcinoma (<2% of cats have malignant thyroid carcinoma).
- Oversupplementation with exogenous thyroid hormone may cause hyperthyroidism in dogs.

SYSTEMS AFFECTED

- Cardiovascular—systemic hypertension, thyrotoxic cardiomyopathy.
- Gastrointestinal (GI)—malabsorption, hypermotility.
- Nervous/behavioral—restlessness, irritability, aggression, vocalization, pacing.
- Urologic—increased glomerular filtration rate (GFR).
- Musculoskeletal—catabolism, cachexia.

GENETICS

None known.

INCIDENCE/PREVALENCE

- Most common feline endocrinopathy; affects 3–8% of cats >10 years old.
- Rare in dogs.

SIGNALMENT

- Cats 4–22 years old; mean age of onset is 13 years.
- <5% of affected cats <8 years old.
- Most common in dogs >10 years old.

Blackwell's Five-Minute Veterinary Consult Clinical Companion: Small Animal Senior Care,
First Edition. Edited by Heidi B. Lobprise.

Companion website: www.wiley.com/go/lobprise/Senior

SIGNS

General Comments

- Signs related to increased metabolism.
- Small number of cats show atypical signs; the human term "apathetic hyperthyroidism" is characterized by lethargy, decreased appetite, and muscle weakness; signs may be more common with advanced hyperthyroidism.

Historical Findings

- Weight loss.
- Polyphagia.
- Hyperactivity/irritability/restlessness.
- Polyuria/polydipsia.
- Vomiting.
- Diarrhea.
- Increased vocalization.
- Tachypnea.
- Muscle weakness.

Physical Examination Findings

- Cachexia/muscle loss.
- Palpable thyroid gland (unilateral or bilateral).
- Tachycardia/heart murmur/gallop rhythm.
- Systemic hypertension/retinopathy.
- Unkempt hair/hair loss.
- Thickened nails.
- Ventroflexion of neck (advanced disease).

CAUSES

- In cats, benign adenomatous hyperplasia and follicular cell adenoma lead to oversecretion of T_4 and T_3; thyroid carcinoma is rare.
- In dogs, thyroid carcinoma is more likely; hyperthyroidism in dogs may be secondary to oversupplementation of T_4.

RISK FACTORS

- Increased risk with aging.
- Decreased risk in Burmese, Tonkinese, Persian, Siamese, Abyssinian, and British shorthair cats; possible increased risk in domestic longhair cats.
- Multifactorial environmental contributors are possible, including bisphenol A (BPA) associated with canned food diets, and polybrominated diphenyl ether (PBDE) flame retardants, but further study is needed.

DIAGNOSIS

DIFFERENTIAL DIAGNOSIS

- Any of the differentials for hyperthyroidism can reflect concurrent disease.
- Neoplasia.
- Inflammatory bowel conditions.
- Diabetes mellitus.
- Chronic kidney disease.
- Cardiomyopathy.

CBC/BIOCHEMISTRY/URINALYSIS

- CBC—mild packed cell volume (PCV) elevation or stress leukogram.
- Elevated alanine aminotransferase (ALT) activity is common.
- Elevated alkaline phosphatase (ALP), aspartate aminotransferase (AST) activities, and blood urea nitrogen, creatinine, phosphorus, bilirubin, and glucose concentrations may be seen.
- Urinalysis (UA) shows variable urine specific gravity; pre-treatment specific gravity does not predict post-treatment renal function.
- Glucosuria and evidence of urinary tract infection possible.

OTHER LABORATORY TESTS

- Elevated serum total T_4 (TT_4) concentration is diagnostic for hyperthyroidism in cats with clinical signs.
  - T_4 concentrations naturally decrease with age; early hyperthyroid cats may have T_4 levels in high-normal range.
  - T_4 concentration may be decreased by concurrent disease.
- Free T_4 concentration measured by equilibrium dialysis may be helpful in cats with concurrent disease or early hyperthyroidism, but is not a screening test.
- T_3 concentration is not useful for diagnosis in cats.
- Thyroid-stimulating hormone (TSH) concentration should not be used for diagnosis in cats.
- T_3 suppression test or thyrotropin-releasing hormone (TRH) stimulation test can help to confirm diagnosis in mild cases.
- Fructosamine concentration may be decreased by concurrent hyperthyroidism.
- Cardiac biomarker concentrations (N-terminal pro brain natriuretic peptide, cardiac toponin I) may be elevated; myocardial disease and biomarkers may return to normal after control of hyperthyroidism.

IMAGING

- Thoracic and abdominal radiography helpful to evaluate for neoplasia and cardiac disease.
- Abdominal ultrasound helpful in determining concurrent disease.
- Echocardiography to evaluate cardiac function.
- Thyroid scintigraphy can determine location of abnormal and ectopic thyroid tissues.

DIAGNOSTIC PROCEDURES

- BP measurement is part of baseline database.
- GFR measurement is possible but not always practical.

PATHOLOGIC FINDINGS

- Multinodular adenomatous hyperplasia can be unilateral or bilateral (98% of cats).
- Thyroid carcinoma in dogs and <2% of hyperthyroid cats.

TREATMENT

APPROPRIATE HEALTH CARE

- Advanced hyperthyroidism with concurrent congestive heart failure requires hospitalization for stabilization.
- Most cases managed on an outpatient basis.
- Radioactive iodine and surgical treatments require hospitalization.

ACTIVITY

No activity restrictions.

DIET

- Because of increased metabolism and hypermotility of intestinal tract, highly digestible diets preferred.
- Malabsorption improves with resolution of hyperthyroid state.
- Vitamin B_{12} supplementation may be helpful.
- An iodine-deficient therapeutic diet is available and effective in appropriate situations.

CLIENT EDUCATION

- Hyperthyroidism in cats is common and treatable.
- Treatment with medication or diet restriction is lifelong.
- Medication dosing needs to be monitored regularly and adjusted accordingly.
- Comorbidities are possible.
- Hyperthyroidism in dogs is usually a malignancy and carries a poor long-term prognosis.
- Possible side effects of medication.
- Surgical thyroidectomy—anesthetic risks, risk of damage to parathyroid glands.
- In some cases, radioactive iodine (I-131) treatment may need to be repeated.
- Resolution of thyrotoxicosis may reveal other, previously masked conditions (e.g., renal disease).

SURGICAL CONSIDERATIONS

- Surgical thyroidectomy is an accepted treatment option.

- Thyroidectomy for carcinoma is not curative but may be helpful with or without subsequent radioactive iodine treatment.

MEDICATIONS

DRUG(S) OF CHOICE

- I-131 is treatment of choice for hyperthyroidism.
- Methimazole (2.5–5 mg/cat PO q12–24h) is the most common medication.
  - Methimazole should be dosed below expected therapeutic dose and titrated upward to minimize side effects.
  - Transdermal methimazole is available and effective; ideally, initial management with oral methimazole will stabilize patient, then transition to transdermal; resolution may be prolonged if treatment initiated with transdermal medication.
  - Methimazole may cause anorexia, vomiting, skin excoriations, thrombocytopenia, hepatopathy, and hypothyroidism; side effects occur within first weeks to months of treatment.
  - Anorexia, vomiting, and skin excoriations can be mitigated by starting at very low doses of methimazole and increasing to therapeutic levels; cessation of drug can resolve these issues, and restarting with transdermal methimazole may avoid recurrence of GI side effects.
  - Bleeding disorders, bone marrow dyscrasias, and hepatic issues require discontinuation of methimazole and choosing an alternative therapy.
  - Severe blood dyscrasias may require hospitalization and supportive care, but should resolve with appropriate treatment.
- Atenolol may be used for severe tachycardia.

POSSIBLE INTERACTIONS

Concurrent use of phenobarbital may reduce effectiveness of methimazole.

ALTERNATIVE DRUG(S)

- Carbimazole—converted to methimazole after absorption; effective, may have fewer side effects than methimazole; not available in United States.
- Propylthiouracil—not recommended.
- Ipodate—for short-term treatment only, not effective for most hyperthyroid cats; not recommended in most cases.

FOLLOW-UP

PATIENT MONITORING

- Regardless of treatment option, GFR and renal function may decline after treatment, but will stabilize within 1 month of thyroid control.
- I-131—physical exam (PE), BP, T_4, serum chemistry, and UA at 1-, 3-, 6-, and 12-months post treatment.

- Methimazole—PE, CBC, serum chemistry, T_4, and UA every 2–4 weeks after starting treatment and after every dose change until T_4 is stabilized between 1 and 2.5 µg/L.
- In cats with renal insufficiency, serum T_4 should be maintained in upper half of reference interval.
- Thyroidectomy—hypocalcemia can occur within several days post-surgery (see below with hypoparathyroidism); monitor for postoperative laryngeal paralysis; PE, T_4, serum chemistry, and UA 2–4 weeks post-surgery, then every 3–6 months; supplementation should not be started postsurgically unless T_4 levels remain low after 3 months; hypothyroidism may be transient with subtotal thyroidectomy.
- Therapeutic diet—PE, BP, serum chemistry, CBC, T_4, and UA every 4–6 months; may take as long as 6 months for cats with severe T_4 elevations to become euthyroid, if at all.

POSSIBLE COMPLICATIONS

- Fatal, if untreated.
- Complications of thyroidectomy include hypothyroidism, hypoparathyroidism, laryngeal paralysis.
- I-131, antithyroid drugs, and thyroidectomy can all lead to hypothyroidism; proper dosing of I-131 and methimazole is imperative.
- Iatrogenic hypothyroidism associated with worsening renal function and decreased survival.

EXPECTED COURSE AND PROGNOSIS

- Prognosis is excellent in cats without concurrent disease.
- Cats on methimazole are likely to relapse if medication is not administered correctly.
- Cats eating a therapeutic diet who do not strictly follow diet will not be successful.
- Post I-131 treatment—mean survival time is 4 years.
- Treatment with methimazole—mean survival time is 2 years.
- Overall mean survival time can be up to 5.3 years.
- Cats with preexisting renal disease have a poorer prognosis.
- Cats and dogs with carcinoma have a poor prognosis—best option for treatment may be surgical debulking of tumor followed by high dose I-131; recurrence is common.

MISCELLANEOUS

ASSOCIATED CONDITIONS

- Because hyperthyroidism is life-threatening, treatment of all hyperthyroid cats is recommended, with concurrent management of any comorbidities.
- Less aggressive treatment options should be considered for cats with advanced (IRIS stages 3–4) renal disease.
- Hypoparathyroidism—parathyroid glands damaged or removed during thyroidectomy (10–82% of cats)
  - Lethargy, anorexia, depression (100%); seizures (50%); muscle trembling (83%); panting (33%); bradycardia (17%); posterior lenticular cataracts (33%)
  - Serum PTH—undetectable or very low
- Hypocalcemia (<6.5 mg/dL), normal-to-moderate hyperphosphatemia
  - Evaluate albumin and rule out renal failure (azotemia is not typically due to hypoparathyroidism)

- Hospitalize for medical management until signs are controlled and serum calcium is >7 mg/dL

Emergency Treatment Hypocalcemia

- Calcium gluconate 10% solution—5–15 mg/kg (0.5–1.5 mL/kg); give IV slowly to effect over 10 minutes; monitor heart rate and stop temporarily if bradycardia occurs; if ECG monitoring is possible, QT interval shortening is an indication to temporarily stop administration. Vomiting can indicate excessive calcium administration.
- Calcium chloride 10% solution—also effective but not recommended in small animals because it is extremely caustic if administered extravascularly. Three times more potent than calcium gluconate; mg/kg dosage is the same, but only one-third the volume is needed (0.15–0.5 mL/kg).

Short-Term Treatment Immediately after Correction of Tetany for Hypoparathyroidism

- Relapse of clinical signs can be prevented by use of IV CRI of calcium gluconate 10% solution (60–90 mg/kg/day [6.5–9.75 mL/kg/day]) added to fluids that do not contain bicarbonate.
- Subcutaneous calcium gluconate 10% diluted 2–4 times with saline can be administered 3 or 4 times daily for initial control of tetany (reported to be safe in most patients, but there have been reports of marked and disabling inflammatory calcinosis cutis associated with subcutaneous use).

Long-Term Therapy

- Vitamin D administration is needed indefinitely for primary hypoparathyroidism and total parathyroidectomy; dosage should be adjusted based on serum calcium concentration.
- Shorter-acting preparations of vitamin D are preferred so that overdosage (causing hypercalcemia) can be quickly corrected.
- A more economical approach to treatment is to maximize oral administration of calcium and reduce oral administration of vitamin D; calcium is usually less expensive than vitamin D; dosage is influenced by each product's available elemental calcium content.

PRECAUTIONS

- All calcium preparations given orally can cause nausea and constipation; calcium carbonate may be less irritating because of its high calcium availability and lower dosage requirement.
- Incompatible with many drugs (tetracyclins, cephalothin, dobutamine, methylpred, metoclopramide, amphotericin B).

Synonyms

- Thyrotoxicosis.
- Plummer's disease.

See Also

- Cardiomyopathy, Hypertrophic
- Chronic Kidney Disease.
- Congestive Heart Failure
- Hypertension, Systemic Arterial.

Abbreviations

- ALT = alanine aminotransferase
- ALP = alkaline phosphatase.
- AST = aspartate aminotransferase.
- BPA = bisphenol A.
- GFR = glomerular filtration rate.
- GI = gastrointestinal.
- I-121 = radioactive iodine.
- PBDE = polybrominated diphenyl ether.
- PCV = packed cell volume.
- PE = physical exam.
- T_3 = triiodothyronine.
- T_4 = thyroxine.
- TRH = thyrotropin-releasing hormone.
- TSH = thyroid-stimulating hormone.
- TT_4 = total thyroxine.
- UA = urinalysis.

Internet Resources

Accessed 29 June 2024
https://www.catvets.com/public/PDFs/ClientBrochures/Hyperthyroidism-WebView.pdf

Suggested Reading

Carney HC, Ward CR, Bailey SJ, et al. 2016 AAFP guidelines for the management of feline hyperthyroidism. *J Fel Med Surg* 2016;18:400–416.

Scott-Moncrief JC. Feline hyperthyroidism. In: Feldman EC, Nelson RW, Reusch CE, et al. (eds) *Canine and Feline Endocrinology and Reproduction*, 4th edn. St. Louis, MO: Elsevier, 2015; pp. 136–195.

Stock E, Daminet S, Paepe D, et al. Evaluation of renal perfusion in hyperthyroid cats before and after radioiodine treatment. *J Vet Intern Med* 2017;31:1658–1663.

Walter KM, Lin YP, Kass PH, Puschner B. Association of polybrominated diphenyl ethers (PBDEs) and polychlorinated biphenyls (PCBs) with hyperthyroidism in domestic felines: sentinels for thyroid hormone disruption. *BMC Vet Res* 2017;13:120.

Author/editor: Heidi Lobprise
Topic adapted from Five Minute Veterinary Consultation, 7th edition, 2021
Original Topic: Hyperthyroidism

Author: Renee Rucinsky
Consulting Editor: Patty A. Lathan

Chapter 31

Hypothyroidism

BASICS

DEFINITION

Clinical manifestations that result from inadequate production of thyroxine (T_4) and 3,5,3′-triiodothyronine (T_3) by the thyroid gland. Characterized by a generalized decrease in cellular metabolic activity.

PATHOPHYSIOLOGY

Acquired Hypothyroidism

- In dogs, acquired hypothyroidism can be primary, secondary, or tertiary.
- Primary hypothyroidism is associated with a defect localized to the thyroid gland. The thyroid tissue has been destroyed or replaced, and thus becomes less responsive to thyroid-stimulating hormone (TSH). T_3 and T_4 levels gradually decline, with a compensatory increase in TSH.
  - Lymphocytic thyroiditis is an immune-mediated process characterized by chronic and progressive lymphocytic infiltration and destruction of the thyroid gland. This process is gradual and accounts for the slow onset of clinical signs associated with hypothyroidism. The immune-mediated process is associated with production of autoantibodies, predominantly against thyroglobulin; however, autoantibodies against T_3 and T_4 have been reported.
  - Idiopathic thyroid atrophy does not demonstrate an inflammatory component and is caused by the replacement of normal thyroid tissue with adipose tissue.
  - Together, these processes account for 95% of the clinical cases of hypothyroidism in dogs; each accounts for 50% of reported cases.
  - Rare causes of primary hypothyroidism include neoplastic destruction of thyroid tissue, iodine deficiency, infection, and iatrogenic destruction secondary to drugs, surgery, or radioiodine treatment.
- Secondary acquired hypothyroidism is rare. The defect is localized to the pituitary, where the ability to synthesize and secrete TSH is impaired. Secondary hypothyroidism may be caused by pituitary tumors, congenital malformation of the pituitary, infection, or TSH suppression. Drugs, hormones, or concurrent illness can cause TSH suppression.
- Tertiary hypothyroidism (not reported in the veterinary literature) is hypothalamic in origin, and production of thyrotropin-releasing hormone (TRH) is either decreased or nonexistent.
- Hypothyroidism may occur following radioactive iodine (I-131) therapy for hyperthyroidism in cats.

Blackwell's Five-Minute Veterinary Consult Clinical Companion: Small Animal Senior Care,
First Edition. Edited by Heidi B. Lobprise.

Companion website: www.wiley.com/go/lobprise/Senior

SYSTEMS AFFECTED

- Behavioral.
- Cardiovascular.
- Endocrine/metabolic.
- Gastrointestinal (GI).
- Nervous.
- Neuromuscular.
- Ophthalmic.
- Reproductive.
- Skin/exocrine.

INCIDENCE/PREVALENCE

- Primary hypothyroidism is the most common endocrinopathy in dogs. Prevalence appears to average about 1 : 250.
- Hypothyroidism is rare in cats.

GEOGRAPHIC DISTRIBUTION

Worldwide

SIGNALMENT

Species

Dog, rarely cat.

Breed Predilections

Larger-breed dogs are more likely to develop hypothyroidism (golden retriever, Doberman pinscher, Great Dane, Irish setter), though several smaller-breed dogs do appear to also be predisposed (miniature schnauzer, cocker spaniel, poodle, dachshund).

Mean Age and Range

Most commonly seen in middle-aged dogs, with the average age of onset being 7 years (in larger dogs, this would be considered senior for most).

Predominant Sex

None

SIGNS

General Comments

Clinical signs associated with hypothyroidism are vague and involve many different systems.

Historical Findings

- Lethargy, weight gain, and hair loss are the most common signs (40–50% of all cases).

- Pyoderma (often recurrent), hyperpigmentation of the skin, and a dry, brittle hair coat (10% of cases).
- Rarely (<5% of cases), facial paralysis, weakness, or conjunctivitis.

Physical Examination Findings

- Most changes appear to be secondary to decreased metabolism due to a lack of circulating thyroid hormones.
- The most common findings include dermatologic abnormalities (88% of hypothyroid dogs):
    - Bilateral symmetric nonpruritic truncal alopecia; hair loss is noted in areas of increased wear and usually includes the ventral thorax and neck, ventral abdomen, elbows, and tail. Loss of primary hair is most common, with retention of guard hairs, resulting in a short, fine hair coat.
    - Dry, lackluster hair coat.
    - Seborrhea is common - localized or more generalized distribution pattern.
    - Pyoderma in 14% of hypothyroid dogs; may be recurrent. Generalized demodicosis and *Malassezia* spp. infections are common. Pruritis may accompany secondary parasitic, yeast, or bacterial infections. Chronic changes to the skin can result in thickening and hyperpigmentation.
- Otitis externa.
- Weight gain.
- Decreased activity/lethargy.
- Most neurologic signs are associated with polyneuropathy and include weakness, facial nerve paralysis, vestibular signs (usually peripheral), and hyporeflexia. No data support a direct association between megaesophagus or laryngeal paralysis and hypothyroidism.
- CNS signs, including seizures, ataxia, and coma (myxedema coma), are rare.
- In females, increased periparturient mortality and lower birth rate in pups. In males, decreased fertility has been reported, but not confirmed.
- Cardiovascular abnormalities are rare. Bradycardia, arrhythmias, decreased conduction, decreased contractility, and diastolic dysfunction have been reported.
- Ocular changes including corneal cholesterol deposits, keratoconjunctivitis sicca (KCS), and conjunctivitis are seen in less than 1% of hypothyroid dogs.

CAUSES

- Lymphocytic thyroiditis.
- Idiopathic thyroid atrophy.
- Neoplasia.
- Pituitary disease.
- Congenital abnormalities.
- Iodine deficiency (dietary).
- Iatrogenic (secondary to surgery or radiation).

RISK FACTORS

- Surgical removal (bilateral) of the thyroid gland.
- I-131 therapy for hyperthyroidism in cats.

DIAGNOSIS

DIFFERENTIAL DIAGNOSIS

- Primary dermatologic disease.
- Other endocrinopathies (hyperadrenocorticism, diabetes mellitus, growth hormone deficiency).
- Pancreatitis.
- Nephrotic syndrome.
- Hepatobiliary disease.

CBC/BIOCHEMISTRY/URINALYSIS

- Useful to rule out nonthyroidal illness.
- Normochromic, normocytic, and nonregenerative anemia is a common finding (28–32% of hypothyroid dogs).
- Hyponatremia.
- Hypercholesterolemia (present in over 75% of hypothyroid dogs).
- Hypertriglyceridemia.
- Elevated levels of cholesterol and triglycerides have been associated with atherosclerosis in dogs, although this is rare.
- No specific changes are noted on urinalysis.

OTHER LABORATORY TESTS

- Diagnosing hypothyroidism is complex. The TSH stimulation test is a reliable single test considered the gold standard. However, there is limited access to test reagents and the cost is often prohibitive.
- Tests to assess thyroid function, thyroid hormone levels, and antithyroglobulin antibody levels including total T_4, free T_4, endogenous TSH, antithyroglobulin antibodies, anti-T_3 antibodies, anti-T_4 antibodies, total T_3, reverse T_3, and free T_3.
- Combination testing will yield a reliable result.

Total T_4

- Initial screening (high sensitivity) test of thyroid function.
- This test measures both protein-bound and free T_4 levels, a direct assessment of the ability of the thyroid gland to produce hormone.
- Decreased total T_4 level is common in hypothyroid animals but is not diagnostic of hypothyroidism as concurrent illness can cause an artificial decrease in total T_4 level.

Free T_4

- Measures metabolically active portion of total T_4 level.
- Hypothyroid animals would be expected to have a low free T_4 level.
- Concurrent illness has less effect on the free T_4 level compared with the total T_4 level.
- Measurement by equilibrium dialysis (fT_4ED)—more reliable than radioimmunoassay, as it mitigates the influence of antithyroglobulin antibodies.
- Newer methods utilize chemiluminescent technology with comparable sensitivity and specificity to fT_4ED, but the effect of antibodies on this assay is unclear, and the fT_4ED is still the gold standard.

Endogenous TSH Level

- Available for canine endogenous TSH
- Cross-reactivity allows this assay to be used in cats; accurate only 50% of the time.
- High specificity and low sensitivity; best as a confirmatory test (not screening).
- Due to loss of negative feedback, TSH level should be elevated in primary hypothyroid animals but 20–40% of hypothyroid dogs have TSH values in the reference range.
- Interpretation of the TSH level requires knowledge of the total or free T_4 level.
- Methods of assessing TSH levels are less sensitive at low levels and evaluation of endogenous TSH cannot be used to diagnose secondary hypothyroidism.

Antithyroglobulin Antibodies

- Antithyroglobulin antibodies include antithyroglobulin, anti-T_3, and anti-T_4 antibodies.
- A positive titer is predictive of immune-mediated thyroiditis, and suggestive of hypothyroidism, but only 20% of euthyroid dogs with antibodies develop hypothyroidism within 1 year.
- Anti-T_3 and -T_4 antibodies are similar to T_3 and T_4 and can cross-react to falsely elevate these assay levels. In animals who are slightly hypothyroid (as measured by total T_4), the presence of anti-T_4 antibodies may make it appear as if these animals are euthyroid, leading to a delay in the diagnosis and treatment of hypothyroidism.

TSH Stimulation Test

- Historically considered the gold standard for diagnosing hypothyroidism.
- Pharmaceutical-grade bovine TSH was used to conduct this test; however, this is no longer available.
- Recombinant human TSH can be used safely in both dogs and cats to effectively conduct the test, but is expensive. Therefore, this test is unlikely to become routine.

Total T_3, Reverse T_3, and Free T_3

- Total T_3 measurement is an unreliable indicator of thyroid function.
- The total T_3 level has been demonstrated to be normal in up to 90% of hypothyroid dogs.
- The reverse T_3 level has not been validated in companion animals.
- Evaluation of total T_3, reverse T_3, and free T_3 levels is not recommended to assess thyroid function.

Nonthyroid Factors That Alter Thyroid Function Tests

- Sick euthyroid syndrome and other factors can alter the results of thyroid function tests, which may result in a misdiagnosis.
- Most nonthyroid factors cause an artificial *decrease* in thyroid hormone levels.
- Some drugs can decrease thyroid hormone levels, but do not usually result in developing clinical signs.
    - Glucocorticoids inhibit the entire hypothalamic–pituitary–thyroid axis and have a direct effect against thyroid hormone.
    - Phenobarbital causes a decrease in thyroid levels only in animals receiving long-term treatment. Phenobarbital should not be administered for 4 weeks prior to thyroid function testing.
    - The influence of NSAIDs is variable and evaluation of thyroid function should be made with caution, and preferably after stopping NSAIDs well in advance of testing.
- Sulfonamides can decrease thyroid hormone levels and lead to clinical disease. This effect is noted to occur within weeks of initiation of therapy and disappears 2 weeks after therapy has been discontinued.

- Well-conditioned and athletic dogs consistently have lower total and free T_4 levels. Certain breeds have total T_4 concentrations that are well below the mean concentrations for other dogs (greyhound, Scottish deerhound, saluki, and whippet). Alaskan sled dogs have serum T_4, T_3, and free T_4 concentrations below the normal reference range.
- Vaccination causes a transient increase in circulating autoantibody levels, so thyroid function testing should not be conducted if a patient has been vaccinated within the previous 2 weeks.

IMAGING

Radiographic Findings

Developmental bone problems (delayed epiphyseal ossification or dysgenesis) are usually noted with congenital hypothyroidism.

Ultrasonographic Findings

- Significant differences in thyroid gland volume and echogenicity exist between hypothyroid and euthyroid patients, but interpretation is highly user dependent.
- No significant difference is noted between euthyroid and sick euthyroid subjects.

PATHOLOGIC FINDINGS

- Lymphocytic thyroiditis—chronic and progressive lymphocytic infiltration and destruction of the thyroid gland. Cytotoxic T cells initiate inflammation, leading to thyrocyte destruction and parenchymal fibrosis.
- Idiopathic thyroid atrophy has replacement of normal thyroid parenchyma with adipose and connective tissue.
- Many cutaneous changes are nonspecific. However, certain findings, including dermal thickening, myxedema, and vacuolation of arrector pili muscles, are most characteristic.

TREATMENT

APPROPRIATE HEALTH CARE

Outpatient medical management.

CLIENT EDUCATION

- Lifelong therapy required.
- Easily managed with oral thyroid hormone supplementation.
- Dose adjustments are common in the early stages of treatment.
- Most clinical signs will resolve over time with appropriate thyroid hormone supplementation.

MEDICATIONS

DRUG(S) OF CHOICE

- Synthetic thyroid hormone supplementation easily treats hypothyroidism.
- Levothyroxine sodium is available as both human and veterinary products.

- Generic forms should be avoided, as human studies have demonstrated wide variability in the bioavailability of generic forms. If a generic form is used, always prescribe the same formulation.
- Hormone supplementation is initiated at 0.02 mg/kg PO q12h.
- Supplementation can often eventually be decreased to once daily after proper control is achieved.
- Levothyroxine doses for dogs exceed those for humans and may confuse pharmacists or human endocrinologists.
- Humans are instructed to take the medication on an empty stomach and proton pump inhibitors can impede absorption. This should be considered if a dog is difficult to regulate.

PRECAUTIONS

Patients with concurrent metabolic conditions (hepatic disease, endocrinopathies, renal disease, cardiac disease) should have supplementation started slowly (about 25% of recommended dose) and slowly increased over time (3 months) to the recommended maintenance level.

POSSIBLE INTERACTIONS

- Glucocorticoids, NSAIDs, furosemide may increase metabolism of levothyroxine.
- GI protectants can decrease absorption and administration should be separated from thyroid hormone supplementation by 2 hours.

ALTERNATIVE DRUG(S)

- If T_4 levels do not normalize after attempting monitoring and treatment, treatment can be attempted with liothyronine (4–6 mg/kg PO q8–12h).
- Monitoring is based on T_3 levels. However, there is no reliable method by which to measure T_3.

FOLLOW-UP

PATIENT MONITORING

- Assessment of clinical signs, weight, and thyroid function testing is recommended 6–8 weeks after therapy has begun, 2–4 weeks after each dose change, and then once to twice yearly. Patients should also be monitored if signs of thyroid toxicosis (e.g., polyuria/polydipsia [PU/PD], polyphagia) occur.
- The total T_4 level with blood taken 4–6 hours after pill administration.
- Once stable and well controlled, the total treatment dose may be given once daily in some dogs.
- For animals receiving supplementation once daily, blood should be taken immediately before the medication is given and then again 4–6 hours later, to measure trough and peak concentrations.
- The total post dose T_4 level should be in the upper half of the reference range, or slightly above it. If significantly increased above normal, the medication dose should be decreased or the frequency of administration reduced.

- If the total T_4 level is low, an increase in the dose may be necessary.
- Before increasing dose, assess client compliance, evaluate GI status to ensure there is no impact on absorption, and confirm there has been no change in the levothyroxine formulation.

PREVENTION/AVOIDANCE

Adequate hormone supplementation with routine monitoring should avoid recurrence of this condition.

POSSIBLE COMPLICATIONS

- If untreated hypothyroid animals are at increased risk of developing myxedema, myxedema coma, and atherosclerosis.
- Oversupplementation of thyroid hormone can result in iatrogenic hyperthyroidism.

EXPECTED COURSE AND PROGNOSIS

- Primary hypothyroidism can be successfully controlled; with an excellent prognosis. Resolution of clinical signs is an important predictor of adequate supplementation therapy.
- Significant improvement in attitude, activity level, and alertness should occur within 1 week of starting therapy.
- Dermatologic abnormalities improve slowly, with complete resolution taking up to 3 months.
- Polyneuropathies usually begin improving quickly; complete resolution may take several months.
- Anemia and serum cholesterol levels gradually resolve in the first weeks of therapy.
- Life expectancy usually normal.
- Myxedema and Myxedema Coma—severe hypothyroidism with a precipitating event (often infection) that overwhelms normal homeostatic mechanisms; edema—pitting and brain (mental dullness)

MISCELLANEOUS

Abbreviations

- fT_4ED = Free T_4 measured by equilibrium dialysis
- GI = gastrointestinal.
- I-131 = radioactive iodine.
- KCS = keratoconjunctivitis sicca.
- NSAID = nonsteroidal anti-inflammatory drug.
- PU/PD = polyuria/polydipsia.
- TRH = thyrotropin-releasing hormone.
- TSH = thyroid-stimulating hormone.

Suggested Reading

Bellumori TP, Farnula TR, Bannasch DL, et al. Prevalence of inherited disorders among mixed-breed and purebred dogs; 27,254 cases (1995–2010). *J Am Vet Assoc* 2013;242(11):1549–1555.

Scott-Moncrieff JCR. Hypothyroidism. In: Ettinger SJ, Feldman EC (eds) *Textbook of Veterinary Internal Medicine*, 7th edn. St. Louis, MO: Elsevier, 2010; pp. 1751–1761.

Author/editor: Heidi Lobprise
Topic adapted from Five Minute Veterinary Consultation, 7th edition, 2021
Original Topic: Hypothyroidism

Author: Patty A. Lathan
Consulting Editor: Patty A. Lathan

Gastrointestinal

Chapter 32

Anorexia

BASICS

DEFINITION

Anorexia is the lack or loss of appetite for food. Hyporexia is a reduction in appetite, while dysrexia is a change in appetite or lack of consistent appetite. Anorexia results in decreased food intake, which then leads to weight loss, dehydration, nutritional deficiencies, and/or sarcopenia.

PATHOPHYSIOLOGY

- A complex interaction between the central nervous system, the environment, and the gastrointestinal (GI) tract.
- Sensory signals include the odor, taste, texture, and temperature of food as well as gastric and duodenal distention.
- Environmental factors including the location and timing of meals, as well as learned behaviors and circadian rhythms, modulate appetite.
- Fear, pain, and stress may decrease appetite.
- In patients with neoplastic and advanced cardiac diseases, the expected upregulation of dietary intake in response to increased energy expenditure is frequently absent.
- Inflammatory and neoplastic diseases can cause hyporexia by the release of proinflammatory cytokines.
- Exogenous and endogenous toxins (e.g., renal and liver failure), neoplasia, metabolic disorders, pancreatitis, and primary GI diseases can cause hyporexia.

SIGNS

Historical Findings

- Refusal to eat is a common presenting complaint and causes owners' significant distress.
- Weight loss may be reported.

Physical Examination Findings

- Findings vary depending on the underlying cause.
- Low body condition score and muscle wasting may be evident depending upon the duration of decreased food intake.

Blackwell's Five-Minute Veterinary Consult Clinical Companion: Small Animal Senior Care,
First Edition. Edited by Heidi B. Lobprise.

Companion website: www.wiley.com/go/lobprise/Senior

- Pseudoanorectic patients commonly display halitosis, excessive drooling, difficulty with prehension or mastication, and odynophagia (painful swallowing).

CAUSES

Anorexia/Hyporexia/Dysrexia

- Possible manifestations of a myriad of systemic disorders (see above)
- Psychological—food aversion, stress, alterations in routine or environment.
- Pain.
- Animals lacking a sense of smell (anosmia) often show a lack of interest in food.
- Miscellaneous (e.g., motion sickness, high environmental temperature).

Pseudoanorexia

Any disease causing painful or dysfunctional prehension, mastication, or swallowing. These patients are hungry but unable to eat due to disorders causing dysfunction or pain of the face, neck, oropharynx, and esophagus.

DIAGNOSIS

CBC/BIOCHEMISTRY/URINALYSIS

- Abnormalities vary with different underlying diseases.
- May be normal.

OTHER LABORATORY TESTS

- Additional diagnostic tests may be necessary to investigate specific diseases suggested by history, physical examination, and preliminary tests.
- A baseline cortisol or an adrenocorticotropic hormone (ACTH) stimulation test to rule out hypoadrenocorticism is warranted even when there are no significant laboratory changes.

IMAGING

- Thoracic and abdominal imaging (radiographs and ultrasound) studies are often included in the minimum database to detect anatomic or functional abnormalities.
- Videofluoroscopy and endoscopy may be indicated to specifically evaluate pharyngeal, esophageal, and GI function and appearance.

DIAGNOSTIC PROCEDURES

- Nutritional assessment with a thorough dietary history, evaluate food intake, and obtain body and muscle condition scores.
- History regarding the patient's environment, changes in routine, people, or other pets, to help identify potential sources of psychologic stress.
- Observe the patient's interest in food and ability to prehend, masticate, and swallow food.
- Complete a thorough physical examination to determine the presence of disease.

TREATMENT

APPROPRIATE HEALTH CARE

- Assisted feeding (enteral and/or parenteral feeding) should be considered immediately for significantly malnourished patients (≥10% body weight loss, hypoalbuminemia, poor body condition score, evidence of muscle wasting, and/or chronic disease processes).
- In well-conditioned patients with decreased appetite, assisted feeding should be considered if food consumption is less than the resting energy requirement [RER = $70 \times (\text{body weight}_{kg}{}^{0.75})$] for 3–5 days without trends toward improvement.
- Force feeding should be avoided, particularly in cats, considering the association with conditioned food aversions.
- Appetite Stimulants—see below

NURSING CARE

- Medications the patient is receiving should be reviewed for possible side effects leading to reduced appetite.
- Provide comfort and nutrition to the patient while efforts are directed at identifying and correcting the underlying disease so that more specific treatment can be provided.
- Symptomatic therapy includes correcting fluid deficits and electrolyte derangements, control of pain and/or nausea, reduction in environmental stressors, and modification of the diet to improve palatability.

DIET

- Palatability can be improved by adding flavored toppings such as low-sodium broth, increasing the moisture, fat, or protein content of the food, and warming the food to body temperature.
- For senior pets—small meals served on a more frequent basis can be helpful for appetite and digestion.

MEDICATIONS

DRUG(S) OF CHOICE

- Appetite stimulants should not replace diagnostic efforts to identify the specific cause(s) of decreased appetite.
- Mirtazapine: Canine dosing is 0.5 mg/kg q24h orally, or 1.88 mg/cat PO q24–48h (for cats with chronic kidney disease).
    - Mirataz® is FDA approved for use in cats, with a recommended dose of a 1.5 in. strip applied to the inner pinna once daily for 14 days.
- Capromorelin is a ghrelin receptor agonist that stimulates appetite centrally in the hypothalamus.
    - Entyce® is approved by the FDA for dogs as an appetite stimulant. Dosing at 3 mg/kg PO q24h is safe for long-term administration.

    - Elura® specifically is FDA approved for use in cats with chronic kidney disease (CKD) to help them gain weight.
- Diazepam (0.1 mg/kg IV q24h) is a short-acting appetite stimulant with sedative properties.
- Cyproheptadine (0.2–0.4 mg/kg PO, 10–20 minutes prior to feeding), an antihistamine with antiserotonergic properties, has been used as an appetite stimulant with mixed success.
- Antiemetics are useful in decreasing nausea or vomiting, but are not appetite stimulants.
    - Ondansetron (0.5–1.0 mg/kg SC/IV/PO q12h) and dolasetron (0.6–1.0 mg/kg SC/IV/PO q24h) are potent antiemetics as 5-HT3 antagonists.
    - Maropitant is a substance P analogue, inhibiting vomiting.
        - Cerenia® approved by the FDA for dogs and cats as an antiemetic (dogs: 1 mg/kg SC/IV or 2 mg/kg PO q24h; cats: 1 mg/kg SC/IV/PO q24h).
- Prokinetics such as metoclopramide (0.2–0.4 mg/kg SC/PO q8–12h), ranitidine (2 mg/kg SC/IV/PO q12h), or erythromycin (0.5–1 mg/kg PO q8–12h) are useful if anorexia is associated with ileus (NOT with obstruction)
- Omega-3 fatty acids can reduce inflammatory cytokines and have modest benefit for appetite.

CONTRAINDICATIONS

Avoid antiemetics and prokinetics if GI obstruction is present or suspected.

POSSIBLE INTERACTIONS

Mirtazapine should not be combined with drugs that interact with or affect serotoninergic systems including monoamine oxidase inhibitors (MAOIs), tricyclic antidepressants (TCAs), and selective serotonin reuptake inhibitors (SSRIs). Ondansetron and dolasetron, as well as metoclopramide, are 5-HT3 antagonists, and care should be used with combining these drugs with mirtazapine.

FOLLOW-UP

PATIENT MONITORING

- Body weight, body and muscle condition score, and hydration assessment.
- Monitor caloric intake to ensure return of appetite is sufficient to meet nutritional needs.

POSSIBLE COMPLICATIONS

- Dehydration, malnutrition, cachexia, and sarcopenia are sequelae of prolonged anorexia/hyporexia/dysrexia; these exacerbate the underlying disease.
- A loss of more than 25–30% of body protein compromises the immune system and muscle strength, and death results from infection and/or cardiopulmonary failure.
- Hepatic lipidosis is a possible complication of anorexia, particularly in cats.
- Breakdown of the intestinal mucosal barrier further compromises debilitated patients.

EXPECTED COURSE AND PROGNOSIS

Depends on the underlying cause(s).

MISCELLANEOUS

See Also

- Weight loss, sarcopenia, and cachexia
- Nutrition

Abbreviations

- ACTH = adrenocorticotropic hormone
- CKD = chronic kidney disease
- FDA = Food and Drug Administration
- MAOI = monoamine oxidase inhibitors
- SSRI = selective serotonin uptake inhibitors
- TCA = tricyclic antidepressants

Suggested Reading

Forman MA. Anorexia. In: Ettinger SJ, Feldman EC, Côté E (eds) *Textbook of Veterinary Internal Medicine*, 8th edn. St. Louis, MO: Elsevier Saunders, 2017; pp. 97–100.

Quimby JM, Lunn KF. Mirtazapine as an appetite stimulant and anti-emetic in cats with chronic kidney disease: a masked placebo-controlled crossover clinical trial. *Vet J* 2013;197(3):651–655.

Schermerhorn T. Gastrointestinal endocrinology. In: Ettinger SJ, Feldman EC, Côté E (eds) *Textbook of Veterinary Internal Medicine*, 8th edn. St. Louis, MO: Elsevier Saunders, 2017; pp. 1833–1838.

Wofford JA, Zollers B, Rhodes L, et al. Evaluation of the safety of daily administration of capromorelin in cats. *J Vet Pharmacol Ther* 2018;41(2):324–333.

Author/editor: Heidi Lobprise
Topic adapted from Five Minute Veterinary Consultation, 7th edition, 2021
Original Topic: Anorexia

Author: Andrea Wang Munk
Consulting Editor: Mark P. Rondeau

Chapter 33

Constipation

BASICS

DEFINITION

- *Constipation* is defined as infrequent, incomplete, or difficult defecation with passage of hard or dry feces; not abnormal motility or loss of function.
- *Obstipation* denotes intractable constipation that has failed several consecutive treatments; defecation is impossible in the obstipated patient.

PATHOPHYSIOLOGY

- Constipation can develop with any disease that impairs the passage of feces through the colon (vertebral malformation, spinal cord disease, pelvic canal narrowing (trauma), rectal mass lesions and painful perianal disease).
- Often in cats no underlying etiology can be identified.
- Delayed fecal transit allows removal of additional salt and water, producing drier feces. Clinical signs are attributable to dehydration and potential toxemia resulting from fecal retention.
- Peristaltic contractions may increase during constipation, but eventually motility diminishes because of smooth muscle degeneration secondary to chronic overdistension.

Species

- Dog and cat.
- More common in cat, especially older cats

SIGNS

Historical Findings

- Reduced, absent, or painful defecation.
- Hard, dry feces.
- Small amount of liquid, mucoid stool, sometimes with blood present produced after prolonged tenesmus.
- Occasional vomiting, inappetence, and/or lethargy.

Physical Examination Findings

- Colon filled with hard feces; Severe impaction may cause abdominal distention.
- Other findings depend on underlying cause.

Blackwell's Five-Minute Veterinary Consult Clinical Companion: Small Animal Senior Care, First Edition. Edited by Heidi B. Lobprise.

Companion website: www.wiley.com/go/lobprise/Senior

- Rectal examination may reveal mass, stricture, perineal hernia, anal sac disease, foreign body or material, prostatic enlargement, or narrowed pelvic canal

CAUSES

Dietary

- Ingesting bones, hair, foreign material, excessive fiber.
- Inadequate water intake.

Environmental

- Lack of exercise.
- Change of environment—hospitalization, dirty litter box.
- Inability to ambulate.

Drugs

- Anticholinergics, antihistamines, opioids.
- Barium sulfate.
- Sucralfate, antacids, kaopectolin.
- Iron supplements.
- Diuretics.

Painful Defecation (Dyschezia)

- Anorectal disease—anal sacculitis, anal sac abscess, perianal fistula, anal stricture, anal spasm, rectal foreign body, rectal prolapse, proctitis.
- Trauma—fractured pelvis, fractured limb, dislocated hip, perianal bite wound or laceration, perineal abscess.

Mechanical Obstruction

- Extraluminal—healed pelvic fracture with narrowed pelvic canal, prostatic hypertrophy, prostatitis, prostatic neoplasia, intrapelvic neoplasia, sublumbar lymphadenopathy.
- Intraluminal and intramural—colonic or rectal neoplasia or polyp, rectal stricture, rectal foreign body, rectal diverticulum, perineal hernia, rectal prolapse, congenital defect (atresia ani).

Neuromuscular Disease

- Central nervous system—paraplegia, spinal cord disease, intervertebral disc disease, cerebral disease (lead toxicity, rabies).
- Peripheral nervous system—dysautonomia, sacral nerve disease, sacral nerve trauma (e.g., tail fracture/pull injury).
- Colonic smooth muscle dysfunction—idiopathic megacolon in cats.

Metabolic and Endocrine Disease

- Impaired colonic smooth muscle function—hyperparathyroidism, hypothyroidism, hypokalemia (chronic renal failure), hypercalcemia.
- Debility—general muscle weakness, dehydration, neoplasia.

RISK FACTORS

- Manx cats may be predisposed due to vertebral (sacral) abnormalities.
- Drug therapy—anticholinergics, narcotics, barium sulfate.

- Metabolic disease causing dehydration.
- Feline dysautonomia.
- Intact male—perineal hernia, benign or infectious prostatic disease.
- Castrated male—prostatic neoplasia.
- Perianal fistula.

DIAGNOSIS

DIFFERENTIAL DIAGNOSIS

- Dyschezia and tenesmus (e.g., caused by colitis or proctitis)—unlike constipation, associated with increased frequency of attempts to defecate and frequent production of small amounts of liquid feces containing blood and/or mucus; rectal examination reveals diarrhea and lack of hard stool.
- Stranguria (e.g., caused by cystitis/urethritis)—unlike constipation, can be associated with hematuria and abnormal findings on urinalysis (pyuria, crystalluria, bacteriuria).

CBC/BIOCHEMISTRY/URINALYSIS

- Usually unremarkable.
- May detect hypokalemia, hypercalcemia.
- High packed cell volume (PCV) and total protein in dehydrated patients.
- High white blood cell (WBC) count in patients with severe obstipation secondary to bacterial or endotoxin translocation, abscess, perianal fistula, prostatic disease.
- Pyuria and hematuria with prostatitis.

OTHER LABORATORY TESTS

- If hypercholesterolemic, rule out hypothyroidism.
- If hypercalcemic, consider parathyroid hormone assay.

IMAGING

- Abdominal radiography documents severity of colonic impaction. Other findings may include colonic or rectal foreign body, colonic or rectal mass, prostatic enlargement, fractured pelvis, dislocated hip, or perineal hernias.
- Pneumocolon (after enemas to clean colon) may better define intraluminal mass or stricture.
- Ultrasonography may help define extraluminal mass and prostatic disease.

DIAGNOSTIC PROCEDURES

Colonoscopy may be needed to identify a mass, stricture, or other colonic or rectal lesion; rectal/colonic mucosal biopsy specimens should always be obtained.

PATHOLOGIC FINDINGS

Dependent on underlying disease process.

TREATMENT

APPROPRIATE HEALTH CARE

- Remove or ameliorate any underlying cause if possible.
- Discontinue any medications that may cause constipation.
- May need to treat as inpatient if obstipation and/or dehydration present.

NURSING CARE

Dehydrated patients should receive IV (preferably) or SC balanced electrolyte solutions (with potassium supplementation if indicated).

ACTIVITY

Encourage activity.

DIET

Dietary supplementation with a bulk-forming agent (bran, methylcellulose, canned pumpkin, psyllium) is often helpful, though they can sometimes worsen colonic fecal distension; in this instance, feed a low-residue diet.

CLIENT EDUCATION

- Feed appropriate diet and encourage activity.
- Survey cat boxes daily to ensure level of defecation activity.

SURGICAL CONSIDERATIONS

- Manual removal of feces through the anus with the animal under general anesthesia (after rehydration) may be required if enemas and medications are unsuccessful.
- Subtotal colectomy may be required with recurring obstipation that responds poorly to assertive medical therapy.

MEDICATIONS

DRUG(S) OF CHOICE

- Laxatives
  - Emollient—docusate sodium or docusate calcium (dogs: 50–100 mg PO q12–24h; cats: 50 mg PO q12–24h).
  - Stimulant—bisacodyl (5 mg/animal PO q8–24h); if not obstructed
  - Saline—isosmotic mixture of polyethylene glycol and poorly absorbed salts; usually administered as a trickle amount via nasoesophageal tube over 6–12 hours.
  - Disaccharide—lactulose (1 mL/4.5 kg PO q8–12h to effect).

- Enemas
- Warm water enemas; a small amount of mild soap or docusate sodium can be added but is usually not needed;
  - Sodium phosphate retention enemas (e.g., Fleet®) are contraindicated because of their association with severe hypocalcemia.
  - Suppositories can be used as a replacement for enemas; use glycerol, bisocodyl, or docusate sodium products.
- Motility modifiers—cisapride (dogs: 0.3–0.5 mg/kg PO q8–12h; cats: 2.5–10 mg/cat PO q8–12h) may stimulate colonic motility; indicated with early megacolon.

CONTRAINDICATIONS

- Avoid mineral oil and white petrolatum lubricants (danger of fatal lipid aspiration pneumonia due to their lack of taste).
- Fleet (sodium phosphate) enemas.
- Anticholinergics.
- Diuretics.

PRECAUTIONS

Cisapride and cholinergics—can be used with caution; contraindicated in obstructive processes. Avoid the use of metoclopramide because it does not affect the colon.

POSSIBLE INTERACTIONS

N/A

ALTERNATIVE DRUG(S)

- Ranitidine causes contraction of colonic smooth muscle in vitro.
- Misoprostol causes contraction of colonic smooth muscle in vitro.
- Newer-generation cisapride-like drugs may be available soon.
- One recent pilot study using multistrain probiotic SLAB51® showed clinical improvement in a feline cohort having chronic constipation and idiopathic megacolon.

FOLLOW-UP

PATIENT MONITORING

Monitor frequency of defecation and stool consistency at least twice a week initially, then weekly or biweekly in response to dietary and/or drug therapy.

PREVENTION/AVOIDANCE

Keep pet active and feed appropriate diet. Subcutaneous fluids to ensure hydration can help reduce frequency of constipation, particularly in cats.

POSSIBLE COMPLICATIONS

- Chronic constipation or recurrent obstipation can lead to acquired megacolon.
- Overuse of laxatives and enemas can cause diarrhea.
- Colonic mucosal damage - improper enema technique, repeated rough mechanical breakdown of feces, or ischemic necrosis secondary to pressure of hard feces.
- Perineal irritation and ulceration can lead to fecal incontinence.

EXPECTED COURSE AND PROGNOSIS

- Fair-to-good prognosis with early diagnosis and intervention.
- Recurring bouts of constipation/obstipation may occur dependent on underlying cause.

MISCELLANEOUS

Associated Conditions

Vomiting—with severe/prolonged obstipation.
Constipation—reduction in removal of toxins that are cleared out during sleep.

Synonyms

- Colonic impaction.
- Fecal impaction.

Suggested Reading

Chandler M. Focus on nutrition: dietary management of gastrointestinal disease. *Compend Contin Educ Vet* 2013;35(6):E1–E3.

Rossi G, Jergens A, Cerquetella M, et al. Effects of a probiotic (SLAB51™) on clinical and histologic variables and microbiota of cats with chronic constipation/megacolon: a pilot study. *Benef Microbes* 2018;9:101–110.

Tam FM, Carr AP, Myers SL. Safety and palatability of polyethylene glycol 3350 as an oral laxative in cats. *J Feline Med Surg* 2011;13(10):694–697.

Author/editor: Heidi Lobprise
Topic adapted from Five Minute Veterinary Consultation, 7th edition, 20[illegible]
Original Topic: Constipation and Obstipation

Author: Albert E. Jergens
Consulting Editor: Mark P. Rondeau

Chapter 34

Inflammatory Bowel Disease

BASICS

DEFINITION

A group of chronic enteropathies characterized by persistent or intermittent gastrointestinal (GI) signs with histopathologic evidence of intestinal inflammation. Inflammatory bowel disease (IBD) is generally categorized by the predominant mucosal cellular infiltrate, such as lymphocytic-plasmacytic, eosinophilic, or granulomatous enteritis.

PATHOPHYSIOLOGY

- Poorly understood but likely due to complex interplay between mucosal immunity and environmental factors (i.e., dietary and bacterial antigens) in genetically susceptible dogs; aberrant host immune responses are likely triggered by antigens derived from resident microbiota.
- Damage results from elaboration of cytokines, release of proteolytic and lysosomal enzymes, complement activation secondary to immune complex deposition, and generation of oxygen free radicals.
- Host genetic susceptibility involving defects in innate immunity is suspected in dogs and possibly cats.

SYSTEMS AFFECTED

- GI.
- Hepatobiliary.
- Hemic/lymphatic/immune—rarely.
- Musculoskeletal—rarely.
- Ophthalmic—rarely.
- Respiratory—rarely.
- Skin/exocrine—rarely.

GENETICS

Defects in host susceptibility genes have been identified in German shepherd dog, boxer, and soft-coated wheaten terrier.

Blackwell's Five-Minute Veterinary Consult Clinical Companion: Small Animal Senior Care, First Edition. Edited by Heidi B. Lobprise.

Companion website: www.wiley.com/go/lobprise/Senior

INCIDENCE/PREVALENCE

IBD is most common histopathologic diagnosis in dogs and cats with chronic GI signs in which other causes have been eliminated through clinical trials and diagnostic testing.

SIGNALMENT

Species

Dog and cat.

Breed Predilections

- Increased risk in German shepherd, boxer, and soft-coated wheaten terrier, in addition to breed-specific forms described elsewhere.
- Siamese cats may be predisposed.

Mean Age and Range

- Most common in middle-aged animals, but younger animals may be affected.
- While the mean age of onset may not be in the senior life stage parameters, this condition requires life-long management and can be a critical factor in senior health.

SIGNS

Historical Findings

- Intermittent or persistent chronic GI signs (>3 weeks' duration).
- May include vomiting, small/large bowel diarrhea, decreased appetite, and/or weight loss.
- Severe IBD may cause protein-losing enteropathy (PLE) in dogs.

Physical Examination Findings

- Vary from apparently healthy to a thin, lethargic animal.
- Poor hair coat with chronic disease and nutritional deficiencies.
- Abdominal palpation may reveal pain, thickened bowel loops, and mesenteric lymphadenopathy (especially in cats).
- Ascites may occur in dogs with PLE.
- Hematochezia, fecal mucus, and tenesmus seen with colonic involvement.

CAUSES

Pathogenesis unknown but most likely multifactorial, involving complex interactions between host genetics, mucosal immunity, and environmental (diet, intestinal bacteria) factors.

Infectious Agents

- Adherent and invasive *Escherichia coli* has been associated with granulomatous colitis in dogs.
- *Giardia*, *Salmonella*, *Campylobacter*, and resident microbiota have been implicated.

Dietary Agents

Meat proteins, milk proteins, gluten (wheat), and additives are all proposed causative agents, likely playing an important role.

Genetic Factors

- Some forms of IBD more common in certain breeds.
- Defects in innate immunity (e.g., mutations in *TLR2*, *TLR5*, and *nod2* as seen in German shepherd dogs) that perturb mucosal homeostasis may predispose individual to IBD.

RISK FACTORS

Current hypotheses suggest that IBD is multifactorial disorder conditioned by genetic, immunologic, and environmental factors.

DIAGNOSIS

DIFFERENTIAL DIAGNOSIS

- Cats—hyperthyroidism, intestinal neoplasia (especially small cell lymphoma), adverse food reactions, feline infectious peritonitis and other viral infections (e.g., feline leukemia virus [FeLV] and feline immunodeficiency virus [FIV]), renal and hepatic insufficiency, exocrine pancreatic insufficiency, intestinal parasitism, and antibiotic-responsive diarrhea (ARD) are primary differentials.
- Dogs—intestinal neoplasia, motility disorders, adverse food reactions, lymphangiectasia, exocrine pancreatic insufficiency, intestinal parasitism, and ARD are primary differentials.

CBC/BIOCHEMISTRY/URINALYSIS

- Often unremarkable; these tests more often serve to eliminate other differential diagnoses.
- Anemia of chronic disease; mild leukocytosis ± left shift sometimes seen with mucosal disruption (e.g., erosions); mild eosinophilia may be seen with eosinophilic enteritis, food allergy, and intestinal parasites among other causes.
- Cats may show alterations in serum total protein (i.e., hyperproteinemia) and albumin concentrations, with increased liver enzyme activities.
- Hypoproteinemia more common in dogs than cats.
- Cobalamin deficiency in both dogs and cats with involvement of ileum.

OTHER LABORATORY TESTS

- Useful to eliminate other differentials.
- Dogs—evaluation of exocrine pancreatic function: canine trypsin-like immunoreactivity (cTLI); serology for pancreatitis: canine pancreatic lipase activity (Spec cPL), and serum cobalamin and folate assays to localize small intestinal disease.
- Cats—T_4 and FeLV/FIV serology; fasting serum TLI (if exocrine pancreatic insufficiency suspected); serology for pancreatitis (Spec fPL), and serum cobalamin and folate assays to localize small intestinal disease.

IMAGING

- Survey abdominal radiographs—usually unremarkable.
- Barium contrast studies—may reveal mucosal abnormalities and thickened bowel loops; normal findings do not eliminate possibility of IBD.

- Ultrasonography—may indicate increased intestinal wall thickness (particularly muscularis propria and submucosal layers) and mesenteric lymphadenopathy; however, these abnormalities not specific for IBD.

DIAGNOSTIC PROCEDURES

- Perform elimination dietary trial to rule out adverse food reactions; if GI signs resolve within 2 weeks, then diagnosis of adverse food reaction is made.
- Perform fecal testing for nematode and protozoal parasites; treat for *Giardia* spp. and endoparasitic infection with fenbendazole (50 mg/kg for 5 days).
- Definitive diagnosis of IBD requires intestinal biopsy and histopathology usually obtained via GI endoscopy; WSAVA guidelines should be used to define severity of mucosal inflammation.
- Laparotomy indicated if GI endoscopy unavailable or to collect full-thickness mucosal specimens; *always be sure to collect ileal biopsies*.
- Use scoring indices (canine inflammatory bowel disease activity index—CIBDAI) to define clinical severity and assess response to therapy.
    - Six Categories: (1) attitude/activity; (2) appetite; (3) vomiting; (4) stool consistency; (5) stool frequency; (6) weight loss
    - Scored 0–3
        - 0 = normal
        - 1 = mild change
        - 2 = moderate change
        - 3 = severe change
    - Summation of variables—total composite score
        - 0–3—clinically insignificant disease
        - 4–5—mild IBD
        - 6–8—moderate IBD
        - 9 or greater—severe IBD

PATHOLOGIC FINDINGS

Morphologic evidence of mucosal inflammation including epithelial changes, architectural distortion (e.g., erosion/ulceration, crypt hyperplasia, fibrosis, loss of colonic goblet cells), and increased lamina propria cellularity. Histopathologic guidelines for defining severity of GI inflammation have been described.

TREATMENT

APPROPRIATE HEALTH CARE

Outpatient, unless patient is debilitated from dehydration, hypoproteinemia, or cachexia.

NURSING CARE

- If patient is dehydrated or must have food restricted because of intractable vomiting, any balanced crystalloid fluid is adequate (for a patient without concurrent disease); otherwise, select fluids on basis of secondary diseases.
- If severe hypoalbuminemia from PLE, consider use of colloids.

ACTIVITY

No restrictions.

DIET

- Feed novel intact protein or hydrolysate elimination diet to help reduce intestinal inflammation.
- Fiber supplementation (e.g., fermentable fiber such as pumpkin, Metamucil®) suggested in dogs and cats with colitis.
- Fish oil (n-3 fatty acids) as free radical scavenger to reduce inflammation.
- Probiotics may be of benefit in some animals but clinically unproven at this time; must be given continuously over several weeks for potential benefit to be realized.

CLIENT EDUCATION

- Emphasize that IBD is not cured but is controllable in most instances.
- Relapses are common; clients should be patient during the various food and medication trials that are often necessary to control the disease.

SURGICAL CONSIDERATIONS

Surgery only indicated for collection of intestinal biopsies in dogs and intestinal and/or liver, pancreatic and/or mesenteric biopsies in cats.

MEDICATIONS

DRUG(S) OF CHOICE

- Evidence-based data indicate glucocorticoids are effective drugs for inducing remission in majority of dogs and cats; use prednisone or prednisolone in dogs at 1–2 mg/kg PO daily for 21 days to induce remission, then taper dose by 25% every 2 weeks.
- Dogs weighing >30 kg will require lower steroid dosage to provide comparable clinical efficacy; this will also reduce adverse effects; *dose large dogs by body surface area.*
- Treat cats with oral prednisolone at 1–2 mg/kg for 14–21 days, then taper as above; avoid glucocorticoids in cats with diabetes mellitus and those with history of adverse effects.
- Budesonide may be used to minimize adverse steroid effects and maintain remission in some dogs and cats; dosage ranges dogs: 1–3 mg/m^2 daily; cats: 1 mg/day.
- Correct hypocobalaminemia by weekly parenteral cobalamin injections for first 6 weeks and thereafter every 2–3 weeks or as needed based on repeat testing of cobalamin concentrations; oral cobalamin therapy requires daily administration; antibiotics (metronidazole, tylosin) generally *not* indicated for treatment of IBD; these drugs may cause significant disruption to gut microbiota even after administration discontinued.
- Some evidence that oral cyclosporine is of value in dogs with steroid-refractory disease and PLE; dose at 5 mg/kg PO daily for 4–6 weeks or as needed to induce remission.
- Use of other immunosuppressive drugs, including azathioprine, chlorambucil, leflunomide, or mycophenolate, has been reported.

- Empirical deworming with fenbendazole (50 mg/kg PO q24h for 5 days).
- Fecal microbiota transplant anecdotally effective in cases of refractory IBD; however, clinical trial data yet to be reported.

FOLLOW-UP

PATIENT MONITORING

- Periodic (q2–4 weeks) physical and laboratory evaluations may be necessary until the patient's condition stabilizes; serum albumin provides important prognostic information in dogs; serum cobalamin deficiency will delay complete clinical recovery in both dogs and cats.
- Monitor serum cobalamin concentrations in hypocobalaminemic dogs and cats.
- No other follow-up may be required except yearly physical examination and assessment during relapse.

POSSIBLE COMPLICATIONS

Dehydration, malnutrition, adverse drug reactions, hypoproteinemia, hypocobalaminemia, anemia, and diseases secondary to therapy.

EXPECTED COURSE AND PROGNOSIS

- Generally good-to-excellent short-term prognosis.
- Poor long-term prognosis in dogs with IBD has been associated with severe clinical disease, marked endoscopic (duodenal) abnormalities, ascites, and hypoalbuminemia; long-term prognosis worse compared to food-responsive diarrhea and ARD, other forms of canine chronic enteropathy.

MISCELLANEOUS

Associated Conditions

- See discussion under specific diseases.
- Cats may demonstrate concurrent inflammatory lesions in the liver and/or pancreas ("triaditis").

Abbreviations

- ARD = antibiotic-responsive diarrhea
- cPL = canine pancreatic lipase.
- FeLV = feline leukemia virus.
- FIV = feline immunodeficiency virus.
- fPL = feline pancreatic lipase.
- GI = gastrointestinal.
- IBD = inflammatory bowel disease.
- PLE = protein-losing enteropathy.
- TLI = trypsin-like immunoreactivity.

Internet Resources

Accessed 29 June 2024
Gastrointestinal Guidelines—WSAVA

Suggested Reading

Allenspach K, Culverwell C, Chan D. Long-term outcome in dogs with chronic enteropathies: 203 cases. *Vet Rec* 2016;178:368.

Day MJ, Bilzer T, Mansell J, et al. International standards for the histopathological diagnosis of gastrointestinal inflammation in the dog and cat: a report from the World Small Animal Veterinary Association Gastrointestinal Standardization Group. *J Comp Pathol* 2008;138(Suppl 1):S1–S43.

Jergens AE, Schreiner CA, Frank DE, Niyo Y, Ahrens FE, Eckersall PD, Benson TJ, Evans R. A scoring index for disease activity in canine inflammatory bowel disease. *J Vet Intern Med* 2003;17:291–297. https://doi.org/10.1111/j.1939-1676.2003.tb02450.x (accessed 4-12-2024).

Makielski K, Cullen J, O'Connor A, Jergens AE. Narrative review of therapies for chronic enteropathies in dogs and cats. *J Vet Intern Med* 2019;33(1):11–22.

Simpson KW, Jergens AE. Pitfalls and progress in the diagnosis and management of canine inflammatory bowel disease. *Vet Clin North Am Small Anim Pract* 2011;41(2):381–398.

Author/editor: Heidi Lobprise
Topic adapted from Five Minute Veterinary Consultation, 7th edition, 2021
Original Topic: Inflammatory Bowel Disease

Author: Albert E. Jergens
Consulting Editor: Mark P. Rondeau

Chapter 35

Pancreatitis—Dogs

BASICS

DEFINITION

Inflammation of the pancreas, acute (no pathologic changes) or chronic (continuously or intermittently) with fibrosis and atrophy (chronic pancreatitis).

PATHOPHYSIOLOGY

- Premature intrapancreatic activation of pancreatic enzymes and inflammatory cytokines results in local inflammation, edema, and necrosis of the pancreas and peripancreatic fat.
- Local effects (abdominal pain, vomiting) and possible systemic effects (pyrexia, systemic inflammatory response syndrome [SIRS], multiple organ dysfunction syndrome [MODS], and acute kidney injury [AKI]).
- An autoimmune mechanism is suspected in English cocker spaniels but remains unproven.

SYSTEMS AFFECTED

- Altered GI motility (ileus) due to regional chemical peritonitis; local or generalized peritonitis due to enhanced vascular permeability.
- Cardiac arrhythmias may result from release of myocardial depressant factor.
- Circulating proinflammatory cytokines and altered endothelial cell function can result in complications such as SIRS and/or disseminated intravascular coagulation (DIC).
- Hepatocellular damage secondary to regional inflammation and extrahepatic bile duct obstruction.
- Acute kidney injury can occur as a consequence of MODS.
- Regional respiratory vasculitis - pulmonary edema and/or pleural effusion, even life-threatening acute respiratory distress syndrome.

GENETICS

Miniature schnauzers - possible genetic basis where mutations in the *SPINK1* gene may confer increased susceptibility.

Blackwell's Five-Minute Veterinary Consult Clinical Companion: Small Animal Senior Care,
First Edition. Edited by Heidi B. Lobprise.

Companion website: www.wiley.com/go/lobprise/Senior

SIGNALMENT

Breed Predilections

- Acute—miniature schnauzer, Yorkshire terrier, other terriers.
- Chronic—cocker spaniel and cavalier King Charles spaniel.

Mean Age and Range

Acute pancreatitis is most common in middle-aged and older (>7 years) dogs.

Predominant Sex

Females overrepresented in some reports.

SIGNS

Historical Findings

- Variable duration and severity, depending on the form of disease (acute vs. chronic).
- Lethargy/anorexia.
- Vomiting.
- Weakness.
- Abdominal pain (may be absent in chronic disease).
- Diarrhea—small or large bowel type.

Physical Examination Findings

- Lethargy.
- Dehydration—common; due to GI losses.
- Abdominal pain—may adopt a "prayer position."
- Mass lesions may be palpable.
- Fever—common with more severe acute pancreatitis.
- Less common—respiratory distress, bleeding, and cardiac arrhythmias.

RISK FACTORS AND CAUSES

- Breed—miniature schnauzers, terriers.
- Obesity.
- Prior GI or endocrine disease. (duodenal reflux, pancreatic trauma/ischemia)
- Dietary indiscretion—access to garbage or fatty foods.
- Hypertriglyceridemia—while an association exists between hypertriglyceridemia and pancreatitis, a causative link remains unclear.
- Pancreatic duct obstruction.
- Hypercalcemia (shown in other species)
- Infectious agents—vectorborne diseases (babesiosis, ehrlichiosis, and leishmaniasis) have been identified in some cases of acute pancreatitis.
- Drugs/toxins—idiosyncratic reactions to certain drugs (L-asparaginase, azathioprine, chlorpromazine, clomipramine, potassium bromide) zinc toxicosis, mainly from ingestion of pennies minted after 1982, may cause pancreatitis.
- Surgery—possible; secondary to hypoperfusion or traumatic manipulation of the pancreas.

DIAGNOSIS

DIFFERENTIAL DIAGNOSIS

- Other GI or hepatobiliary diseases can often be differentiated with abdominal imaging.
- Genitourinary (AKI) or hypoadrenocorticism—appropriate diagnostics to differentiate.

CBC/BIOCHEMISTRY/URINALYSIS

- CBC—hemoconcentration; inflammatory leukogram; thrombocytopenia.
- Biochemistry—azotemia; increased liver enzyme activities; hyperbilirubinemia; electrolyte abnormalities associated with vomiting; hyperglycemia; hypoalbuminemia; hypercholesterolemia; and hypertriglyceridemia.
- Urinalysis—may show evidence of proteinuria or may be unremarkable.

OTHER LABORATORY TESTS

- Serum amylase and lipase activities are unreliable serologic markers.
- Serum pancreatic lipase immunoreactivity (cPL) is a sensitive and specific marker of acute pancreatic inflammation (less for chronic cases), In house cPL assay (SNAP cPL) is a useful screening tool and should be followed up by serum Spec cPL for quantitation.

IMAGING

- Abdominal radiographs—increased soft-tissue opacity in the right cranial abdomen; loss of visceral detail ("ground glass appearance") due to abdominal effusion; static gas pattern in the proximal duodenum; widened pyloroduodenal angle.
- Abdominal radiographs are insensitive for pancreatitis and are of greater value for ruling out other causes of vomiting such as gastric or intestinal foreign bodies.
- Thoracic radiographs—may be normal, reveal pleural effusion or pulmonary edema.
- Abdominal ultrasound—imaging modality of choice; nonhomogeneous mass lesions suggest pancreatic abscess; pancreas is usually enlarged and irregular; may be a pancreatic mass or hypoechogenicity in the area of the pancreas due to edema; surrounding mesentery is typically hyperechoic due to peritonitis; may see peritoneal effusion and extrahepatic biliary obstruction.
- cPL assay and ultrasound in combination have the highest sensitivity for an antemortem diagnosis of acute pancreatitis.

DIAGNOSTIC PROCEDURES

- Ultrasound-guided needle-aspiration cytology may confirm inflammation, abscess, or cyst.
- Laparoscopy with pancreatic biopsy for histologic diagnosis.
- Histopathologic evaluation may miss focal or segmental pancreatic inflammation and must be interpreted with caution.

TREATMENT

APPROPRIATE HEALTH CARE

- Inpatient management typically required.
- Identify and remove any predisposing causes.

NURSING CARE

- Care to maintain lethargic patients in sternal recumbency with elevated head, and management of vomiting should be done to avoid risk of aspiration pneumonia.
- Aggressive IV fluid resuscitation with isotonic crystalloids should be administered to correct dehydration and encourage perfusion of the pancreas.
- If hypoalbuminemic, synthetic colloids may be needed (10–20 mL/kg/day).
- If hypokalemia, IV potassium supplementation (not to exceed 0.5 mEq/kg/h) is often required.

ACTIVITY

Clinical status will determine.

DIET

- Food withheld if vomiting uncontrolled.
- Enteral feeding should be encouraged as it supports enterocyte health, decreases bacterial translocation, and decreases incidence of vomiting episodes.
- Feeding cranial to the duodenum (prepyloric) is safe. If not eating voluntarily, nasoesophageal, nasogastric, or esophageal feeding tubes should be used to deliver low-fat diets.

CLIENT EDUCATION

Discuss possible complications, variable clinical severity, and risk of recurrence associated with pancreatitis.

SURGICAL CONSIDERATIONS

- Surgery should be avoided if possible; minimally invasive techniques (laparoscopy) or alternatives to surgery (ultrasound-guided percutaneous drainage) should be used.
- Surgical intervention may be indicated if there is suspicion of an infected necrotic area of the pancreas, pancreatic abscess, or pancreatic enlargement causing extrahepatic biliary obstruction.

MEDICATIONS

DRUG(S) OF CHOICE (EMPHASIS ON ACUTE PANCREATITIS)

- Analgesic—fentanyl 2–5 µg/kg/h IV CRI; buprenorphine 0.01–0.02 mg/kg q6–8h IV or IM.
- Antiemetics—maropitant 1 mg/kg SQ q24h; ondansetron 0.5–1.0 mg/kg IV or SQ q8h; metoclopramide 2 mg/kg/day IV CRI.

- Antibiotics—usually not indicated. If bacterial translocation from the GI tract is suspected, broad-spectrum antibiotic therapy is recommended (e.g., ampicillin/sulbactam 30 mg/kg IV q8h).
- Fresh frozen plasma—no clinical benefit has been shown.
- Glucocorticoids—limited evidence to support benefit. Dogs with chronic autoimmune pancreatitis (English cocker spaniels are predisposed) may be treated with prednisone 2 mg/kg PO as induction therapy and then tapered as based on cPL levels and clinical signs.

CONTRAINDICATIONS

- Anticholinergics.
- Azathioprine.
- Chlorothiazide.
- L-Asparaginase.
- Meglumine antimonite.
- Potassium bromide.

FOLLOW-UP

PATIENT MONITORING

- Monitor hydration status and electrolyte levels frequently. Special attention should be paid to development of systemic signs suggestive of SIRS or MODS (increased respiratory rate, decreased urine production, bleeding).
- Reassess need for more or less aggressive pain control frequently.
- Ultrasound findings and cPL levels can lag behind clinical improvement; decide on discharge from veterinary care based on the overall clinical disease activity.

PREVENTION/AVOIDANCE

Feed a low-fat diet and avoid medications known to be triggers for pancreatitis.

POSSIBLE COMPLICATIONS

- Acute complications—extrahepatic biliary tract obstruction, aspiration pneumonia, SIRS, MODS.
- Chronic complications—exocrine pancreatic insufficiency, diabetes mellitus.

EXPECTED COURSE AND PROGNOSIS

Prognosis is generally good for mild cases. Severe cases with development of SIRS/MODS have a more guarded prognosis. Negative prognostic factors—increases in blood urea/creatinine, thrombocytopenia, and marked increases in Spec cPL have been associated with increased mortality. Increased alanine aminotransferase has been associated with extended hospitalization in dogs with acute pancreatitis.

MISCELLANEOUS

FELINE PANCREATITIS EXCERPTS

- A separate topic was not included in this text due to major similarities to pancreatitis in dogs, and that the mean age for acute pancreatitis in cats at 7.3 years of age (any age can be affected, not just seniors)
- Some unique attributes in cats include:
  - No sex predilection; Siamese cats are over-represented.
  - Necropsy surveys suggest an increased prevalence in cats with cholangitis and IBD. The unique feline pancreaticobiliary anatomy and intestinal microbiota likely contribute to multiorgan inflammatory disease in this species.
  - Excessively lean body mass is associated with ANP (acute necrotizing pancreatitis).
  - Diarrhea—small bowel and large bowel diarrhea and fever are less common in cats than in dogs.
  - CBC—often reveals nonregenerative anemia (40%).
  - Potassium chloride (KCl) supplementation usually needed.
  - While most nutritionists agree that excessive dietary fat restriction is not necessary in cats with pancreatitis, neither should a diet with excessive amounts of fat should be used.
  - Patient monitoring
    - First 24 hours—evaluate hydration closely (physical examination, body weight, hematocrit, total plasma protein, BUN and urine output); adjust flow rates as needed.
    - Watch closely for systemic complications, including IBD, diabetes mellitus, exocrine pancreatic insufficiency (EPI), and/or hepatic lipidosis in cats with ANP.
    - Gradually taper fluids down.
    - Maintain oral alimentation.
  - Prognosis
    - Cats with multiorgan inflammation may be less responsive to treatment.
    - More guarded to poor for patients with severe necrotizing pancreatitis, decreased ionized calcium fraction, hyperkalemia, fPL >20 µg/L, and systemic conditions.

Abbreviations

- AKI = acute kidney injury.
- cPL = canine pancreatic lipase immunoreactivity
- DIC = disseminated intravascular coagulation.
- GI = gastrointestinal.
- MODS = multiple organ dysfunction syndrome.
- PLI = pancreatic lipase immunoreactivity.
- SIRS = systemic inflammatory response syndrome.

Internet Resources

Veterinary Information Network: https://www.vin.com/VIN.plx

Suggested Reading

Mansfield C. Pathophysiology of acute pancreatitis: potential applications from experimental models and human medicine to dogs. *J Vet Intern Med* 2012;26:875–887.

Watson P. Chronic pancreatitis in dogs. *Top Companion Anim Med* 2012;27:133–139.

Xenoulis PG, Steiner JM. Pancreas: necrosis and inflammation: canine. In: Washabau RJ, Day MJ (eds) *Canine and Feline Gastroenterology*. St. Louis, MO: Elsevier, 2013; pp. 812–821.

Author/editor: Heidi Lobprise
Topic adapted from Five Minute Veterinary Consultation, 7th edition, 2021
Original Topics: Pancreatitis—Dogs, and Pancreatitis—Cats

Author: Albert E. Jergens
Consulting Editor: Mark P. Rondeau

Hematologic

Chapter 36

Myelodysplastic Syndromes

BASICS

OVERVIEW

- Category of diseases characterized by nonregenerative anemias or cytopenias and dysplastic features in the blood or bone marrow.
- Primary myelodysplastic syndromes (MDS) result from a clonal expansion of a genetically altered pluripotent stem cell resulting in a hypercellular bone marrow with maturation arrest as a consequence of apoptosis.
- Subcategorized as MDS with excessive blasts, which may progress to acute myeloid leukemia, MDS with refractory cytopenia, and MDS with erythroid predominance.
- Secondary MDS in dogs is associated with neoplasia (lymphoma, multiple myeloma), drug or toxin exposure, immune-mediated disease, infections, or ionizing radiation exposure.
- Secondary MDS in cats is typically associated with feline leukemia virus (FeLV) infection.

SIGNALMENT

- Dog and less commonly cat.
- Primary MDS typically older dogs.

SIGNS

- Lethargy.
- Exercise intolerance.
- Depression.
- Anorexia.
- Fever.
- Pale mucous membranes.
- Petechiation.
- Heart murmur due to anemia.

CAUSES AND RISK FACTORS

- Viral—FeLV, feline immunodeficiency virus (FIV), parvovirus.
- Neoplasia—lymphoma, multiple myeloma.

Blackwell's Five-Minute Veterinary Consult Clinical Companion: Small Animal Senior Care, First Edition. Edited by Heidi B. Lobprise.

Companion website: www.wiley.com/go/lobprise/Senior

- Autoimmune—immune-mediated hemolytic anemia, immune-mediated thrombocytopenia.
- Drugs—chemotherapeutics, estrogen, chloramphenicol, cephalosporins, phenylbutazone, trimethoprim-sulfadiazine, quinidine, thiacetarsamide, griseofulvin, albendazole.
- Iron deficiency, folic acid deficiency.
- Lead toxicity.
- Infectious—ehrlichiosis, bacterial septicemia, and endotoxemia.

DIAGNOSIS

DIFFERENTIAL DIAGNOSIS

- Need to differentiate between primary and secondary MDS.
- Other causes of nonregenerative anemias—anemia of chronic disease, chronic renal failure, myeloproliferative diseases, lymphoproliferative diseases, myelofibrosis.

CBC/BIOCHEMISTRY/URINALYSIS

Nonregenerative anemia, cytopenias.

OTHER LABORATORY TESTS

To diagnose underlying causes of secondary MDS—viral antigen/antibody titers, iron levels, tick titers, Coombs' test.

IMAGING

- As needed to rule out secondary causes of MDS.
- Abdominal radiography—evaluate for lead foreign bodies.
- Abdominal ultrasonography—evaluate for abdominal masses consistent with retained testes and Sertoli cell tumors associated with estrogen secretion.

DIAGNOSTIC PROCEDURES

Bone marrow aspirate or biopsy.

TREATMENT

- Inpatient or outpatient.
- If secondary MDS—treat underlying disease (e.g., discontinue drug, treat underlying infection).
- If neutropenic—limit exposure to other sick animals.
- Blood transfusions for anemic patients.

MEDICATIONS

DRUG(S) OF CHOICE

- For neutropenia—broad-spectrum antibiotics and filgrastim 3–5 µg/kg SC q24h in dogs and cats.
- For anemia—erythropoietin 35–50 U/kg SC 3 times a week or darbepoetin 0.45 µg/kg once a week.
- Chemotherapy for primary MDS has been reported—hydroxyurea, cytosine arabinoside, prednisone, cyclosporine A, vincristine.
- Interferon α (cats with FeLV).

FOLLOW-UP

- Serial monitoring of CBC for resolution of cytopenias.
- Prognosis dependent on primary vs. secondary.
- Increasing blast percentage, multiple cytopenias, marked cellular atypia are poor prognostic factors for patients with primary MDS.

MISCELLANEOUS

Abbreviations

- FeLV = feline leukemia virus
- FIV = feline immunodeficiency virus.
- MDS = myelodysplastic syndromes.

Suggested Reading

Juopperi TA, Bienzle D, Bernreuter DC, et al. Prognostic markers for myeloid neoplasms: a comparative review of the literature and goals for future investigation. *Vet Pathol* 2011;48(1):182–197.

Author/editor: Heidi Lobprise
Topic adapted from Five Minute Veterinary Consultation, 7th edition, 2021
Original Topic: Myelodysplastic Syndromes

Author: Rebecca G. Newman
Consulting Editor: Timothy M. Fan

Chapter 37

Pulmonary Thromboembolism

BASICS

DEFINITION

Develops when a thrombus lodges in the pulmonary arterial (PA) tree, occluding blood flow to the portion of lung supplied by that artery.

PATHOPHYSIOLOGY

- Pulmonary thromboembolism (PTE) associated with heartworm disease (HWD) occurs *in situ* in the pulmonary vessels; in most other instances, thrombus origin is unclear.
- Potential sites of origin include right atrium, venae cavae, and jugular, femoral or mesenteric veins; thrombi are carried in the venous circulation to the lungs, and lodge in the pulmonary arteries.
- Abnormal blood flow (stasis), vascular endothelial damage, and hypercoagulability are believed to predispose to thrombus formation.
- Often a complication of another primary disease process.

SYSTEMS AFFECTED

- Cardiovascular—pulmonary hypertension (PH) may result, leading to right ventricular enlargement, right ventricular failure (cor pulmonale), and reduced cardiac output.
- Respiratory—diminished pulmonary blood flow leads to arterial hypoxemia and dyspnea.

INCIDENCE/PREVALENCE

- Unknown—likelihood of PTE increases with abnormal coagulation or severe systemic disease.
- Uncommon in the dog and cat; likely underdiagnosed due to nonspecific clinical signs, lack of clinical suspicion, and paucity of noninvasive, definitive diagnostic tests.

SIGNALMENT

Mean Age and Range

- More frequently seen in middle-aged-to-older dogs.
- Bimodal age distribution reported in cats; peak occurrence <4 years and >10 years of age.

Blackwell's Five-Minute Veterinary Consult Clinical Companion: Small Animal Senior Care, First Edition. Edited by Heidi B. Lobprise.

Companion website: www.wiley.com/go/lobprise/Senior

SIGNS

Historical Findings

- Often reflect the primary disease process.
- May include peracute dyspnea, anorexia, syncope, collapse, cough, hemoptysis, weakness, exercise intolerance, and inability to sleep or get comfortable.

Physical Examination Findings

- Tachypnea and dyspnea in most animals; adventitious lung sounds in some animals.
- Tachycardia, weak pulses, jugular vein distension, pale or cyanotic mucous membranes, delayed capillary refill time, right-sided heart murmur, and split or loud S2 in severe cases.

CAUSES

- HWD.
- Neoplasia.
- Hyperadrenocorticism (Cushing's disease) or corticosteroid administration.
- Protein-losing nephropathy or enteropathy.
- Immune-mediated hemolytic anemia (IMHA).
- Pancreatitis.
- Pulmonary hypertension (PH).
- Orthopedic trauma or surgery.
- Sepsis.
- Disseminated intra-vascular coagulation.
- Liver disease.

RISK FACTORS

- Coagulopathy, especially any hypercoagulable state.
- Diseases listed under Causes are associated.
- Estrogen administration, immobility, and air travel may be causative in humans.

DIAGNOSIS

DIFFERENTIAL DIAGNOSIS

- Other diseases that cause clinically important dyspnea and hypoxemia without profound radiographic findings include upper airway obstruction, laryngeal paralysis, and diffuse airway disease processes (e.g., toxin inhalation and interstitial lung disease).
- Upper airway obstruction often manifests as inspiratory dyspnea; breath sounds often loudest over trachea or larynx.
- PTE should be a leading diagnostic consideration in a patient with acute onset of dyspnea or collapse and a known associated disease.

CBC/BIOCHEMISTRY/URINALYSIS

CBC—may be normal; thrombocytopenia may be seen in up to 50% of dogs with PTE; leukocytosis may develop. Biochemistry—results often reflect underlying disease.

Urinalysis—results often reflect underlying disease; evaluate for proteinuria.

OTHER LABORATORY TESTS

- Arterial blood gases often show arterial hypoxemia (PaO_2 often <65 mmHg) and low $Paco_2$ with respiratory alkalosis.
- Metabolic and respiratory acidosis may develop in severely affected patients.
- D-dimers result from the breakdown of crosslinked fibrin, indicate physiologic or pathologic thrombosis, and testing plays a pivotal role in diagnostic algorithms for PTE in humans; however, utility for PTE diagnosis in veterinary patients is uncertain.
- Thromboelastography provides a global assessment of coagulation and thrombolysis; may be useful in diagnosing systemic hypercoagulability but not widely available.
- Coagulation profile may show high fibrin degradation products, abnormal fibrinogen, or alterations in one-stage prothrombin time (PT), and activated partial thromboplastin time (PTT).
- Heartworm serology (antigen testing in dogs; antigen and antibody testing in cats) should be performed in any animal with suspected PTE.
- Cardiac biomarkers—cardiac troponin I and B-type natriuretic peptide (NT-proBNP) levels may be elevated.

IMAGING

Thoracic Radiography

- May be normal.
- PA enlargement or pruning.
- Cardiomegaly.
- Interstitial and alveolar lung patterns.
- Small-volume pleural effusion.
- Areas of regional hyperlucency (Westermark sign).

Echocardiography

- Right ventricular enlargement.
- Enlarged PA segment.
- Flattening of the interventricular septum.
- Reduced left ventricular cavity size.
- High-velocity tricuspid or pulmonic regurgitation jets provide evidence of PH in some patients.
- Infrequently a thrombus is imaged in the right heart or the main PA segments.

CT, Angiography, and Radionuclide Studies

- One or more of these tests usually required for definitive diagnosis.
- CT angiography is gold standard for the diagnosis of PTE.
- Spiral CT nonselective angiography may show intraluminal filling defects created by emboli, peripheral wedge-shaped pulmonary infiltrates, or pleural effusion.

- Right-sided cardiac catheterization with pulmonary angiography may permit identification of intraluminal filling defects or regions of reduced pulmonary blood flow.
- Nonselective angiography using conventional radiographic techniques has a low level of diagnostic success.
- Combined ventilation and perfusion scans with radioisotopes permit identification of well-ventilated lung regions that are not receiving normal blood flow.

DIAGNOSTIC PROCEDURES

ECG

- Acute cor pulmonale—right-axis deviation, P pulmonale, ST segment deviation, large T waves.
- Arrhythmias.

PATHOLOGIC FINDINGS

- Thrombi in major PA branches.
- Some patients exhibit multiple smaller thrombi in small PA vessels, eventually leading to marked respiratory dysfunction and death.
- Concurrent lung pathology (e.g., pneumonia, pulmonary edema, neoplasia, interstitial fibrosis) is common.

TREATMENT

APPROPRIATE HEALTH CARE

Hospitalize patients documented with PTE until hypoxemia is resolved.

NURSING CARE

- Administer IV fluids cautiously unless preexisting volume depletion; they may precipitate right-sided congestive heart failure.
- Administer oxygen if dyspneic and/or PaO_2 <65 mmHg; response to oxygen therapy is variable.

CLIENT EDUCATION

- Alert that condition is often fatal; further episodes likely unless an underlying cause is identified and corrected; sudden death is not unusual.
- Traditional anticoagulants can lead to bleeding complications requiring frequent clotting time reevaluation (e.g., PT and PTT) for successful management; low-molecular-weight heparins (LMWHs) are safer and require less monitoring but are more expensive; anticoagulants may be required for several months, even after resolution of the causative disease

MEDICATIONS

DRUG(S) OF CHOICE

- Always identify and treat underlying disease; if this is unlikely to be successful, aggressive efforts to treat PTE will probably be in vain.
- Unfractionated heparin may help to prevent further thrombi from developing; low dosages are probably inadequate for initial management; a dosage of 200–300 units/kg SC q8h or alternatively a bolus of 200 units/kg IV followed by a CRI at 15–30 units/kg/h adjusted to maintain the PTT at 1.5–2 times the baseline value.
- Thrombolytics (e.g., urokinase, streptokinase, or tissue plasminogen activator) may also be useful in hemodynamically unstable cases; these are expensive and carry a higher risk of bleeding complications.
- Warfarin—may occasionally be considered for long-term treatment (0.1 mg/kg q24h), with dosage adjustments to maintain a PT 1.5–2 times the baseline value; animals must be heparinized prior to warfarin therapy to avoid initial hypercoagulable phase.
- LMWHs are likely associated with fewer bleeding complications than unfractionated heparin or warfarin, require less intensive monitoring, and are more suitable for long-term management; however, their cost may be a limiting factor.
- Thromboprophylactic effects have been demonstrated for dalteparin 150 units/kg SC q12h in the absence of prolonged bleeding times or adverse effects; enoxaparin has been used at 1 mg/kg SC q12h.
- Sildenafil 1–2 mg/kg PO q8h may help in some animals with PTE and concomitant PH.

PRECAUTIONS

Warfarin—interacts with many other drugs; degree of anticoagulation may change after giving these drugs, or with diet alterations.

Dose titration may be difficult in patients with diseases that result in coagulopathy. Review mechanism of action and pharmacology of antithrombotic drugs before use.

POSSIBLE INTERACTIONS

See Precautions for warfarin.

FOLLOW-UP

PATIENT MONITORING

Serial arterial blood gases and/or pulse oximetry—may help determine improvement in respiratory function.

PREVENTION/AVOIDANCE

- Activity or physical therapy may improve venous blood flow and prevent development of venous thrombi in immobile patients with severe systemic disease.

- Aspirin (0.5–5 mg/kg PO q12–24h) may have some preventive role but is inadequate as treatment.
- Clopidogrel (1–2 mg/kg PO q24h) is an alternative antiplatelet drug that may have some role in prevention. A single loading dose, up to 10 mg/kg, can be administered for rapid platelet inactivation in cases with active thrombosis.
- Heparin may be administered to hospitalized animals predisposed to the development of PTE (200 units/kg IV initially and 75–200 units/kg SC q8h).
- Alternatively, dalteparin (150 units/kg SC q12h) or enoxaparin (1 mg/kg SC q12h) may be used for thromboprophylaxis.
- Rivaroxaban, an oral factor Xa inhibitor, has been used in small animals (1 mg/kg PO q24h). Rivaroxaban and other newer oral antithrombotics, such as fondaparinux, apixaban, or dabigatran, may be as effective as warfarin for prevention of recurrent thrombosis in people and require less monitoring; these drugs may play a future role in longer-term anticoagulation of veterinary patients, but further study on dosing and safety in animals is needed.

POSSIBLE COMPLICATIONS

Bleeding complications may arise with anticoagulants. Bleeding may occur from any organ system. Anticipate active bleeding or anemia necessitating blood or plasma transfusion and have blood products readily available.

EXPECTED COURSE AND PROGNOSIS

Generally guarded to poor; depends on resolution of the precipitating cause. For irreversible diseases (e.g., some neoplasias and advanced protein-losing nephropathy), prognosis is poor; it is somewhat better for patients with PTE due to trauma or sepsis.

MISCELLANEOUS

Age-Related Factors

Predisposing conditions more likely in middle-aged and older animals.

See Also

- Anemia, Immune-Mediated.
- Hyperadrenocorticism (Cushing's Syndrome)—Cats.
- Hyperadrenocorticism (Cushing's Syndrome)—Dogs.

Abbreviations

- HWD = heartworm disease
- IMHA = immune-mediated hemolytic anemia.
- LMWH = low-molecular-weight heparin.
- NT-ProBNP = B-type natriuretic peptide.
- PA = pulmonary artery/arterial.
- PH = pulmonary hypertension.
- PT = prothrombin time.
- PTE = pulmonary thromboembolism.
- PTT = partial thromboplastin time.

Suggested Reading

Goggs R, Blais MC, Brainard BM, et al. American College of Veterinary Emergency and Critical Care (ACVECC) Consensus on the Rational Use of Antithrombotics in Veterinary Critical Care (CURATIVE) guidelines: small animal. *J Vet Emerg Crit Care* 2019;29:12–36.

Hackner SG. Pulmonary thromboembolism. In: Bonagura JD, Twedt DC (eds) *Kirk's Current Veterinary Therapy XV*. St. Louis, MO: Saunders Elsevier, 2014; pp. 705–710.

Marschner CB, Kristensen AT, Rozanski EA. Diagnosis of canine pulmonary thromboembolism by computed tomography and mathematical modelling using haemostatic and inflammatory variables. *Vet J* 2017;229:6–12.

Schermerhorn T, Pembleton-Corbett JR, Kornreich B. Pulmonary thromboembolism in cats. *J Vet Intern Med* 2004;18:533–535.

Author/editor: Heidi Lobprise
Topic adapted from Five Minute Veterinary Consultation, 7th edition, 2021
Original Topic: Pulmonary Thromboembolism

Authors: Suzanne M. Cunningham and John E. Rush
Consulting Editor: Michael Aherne

Hepatic

Chapter 38

Cholecystitis and Cholelithiasis

BASICS

OVERVIEW

- Cholecystitis = gallbladder (GB) inflammation.
- Choledochitis = large bile duct inflammation.
- Associated with cholelithiasis; secondary to GB mucocele (GBM); extrahepatic bile duct obstruction (EHBDO); inflammation of intrahepatic biliary structures (common in ductal plate malformation [DPM]).
- Severe GB inflammation can lead to rupture and subsequent bile peritonitis, necessitating combined surgical and medical interventions.
- Bile duct obstruction increases risk for biliary infection: enteric bacteria transmigrate bowel wall, pass into portal circulation, disseminate within liver, bile, and the GB, dispersing endotoxins and bacteria that may cause systemic sepsis or septic peritonitis.

SIGNALMENT

- Dog and cat.
- No breed or sex predilection.
- Necrotizing cholecystitis (dogs)—usually middle-aged or older animals.
- GBM—predisposition for elderly dogs, dogs with certain conditions (see Gallbladder Mucocele).

SIGNS

- Choledochitis—vague signs, variable icterus.
- Sudden onset—inappetence, lethargy, vomiting, vague abdominal pain
- Chronic postprandial discomfort/distress (cholecystitis or GBM)—position of comfort, stretching, pacing, panting.
- Mild to moderate—jaundice and fever common.
- Severe disease—shock due to endotoxemia, bacteremia, hypovolemia.
- Soft-tissue mass in right cranial abdomen palpable in small dogs and cats reflecting inflammation or adhesions between GB and pericholecystic tissues.

CAUSES AND RISK FACTORS

- Impaired bile flow at cystic duct or GB (cholelithiasis, mass lesions), GB dysmotility or ischemic insult to GB wall (from GB distention)—may precede cholecystitis ± necrotizing lesions.

Blackwell's Five-Minute Veterinary Consult Clinical Companion: Small Animal Senior Care, First Edition. Edited by Heidi B. Lobprise.

Companion website: www.wiley.com/go/lobprise/Senior

- Irritants in sludged bile (e.g., lysolecithin, prostaglandins, choleliths, flukes) or retrograde flow of pancreatic enzyme into bile duct in cats may initiate/augment GB or duct inflammation.
- Previous enteric disorders, trauma, abdominal surgery—may be contributing factors.
- Bacterial infection—common; retrograde duct bacterial invasion from intestines or hematogenous dispersal from splanchnic circulation.
- Toxoplasmosis and biliary coccidiosis—rare causes.
- Necrotizing cholecystitis (dogs)—ruptured GB (common, often secondary to cholelithiasis or hypermature GBM); *Escherichia coli* and *Enterococcus* spp.: common isolates.

DIAGNOSIS

DIFFERENTIAL DIAGNOSIS

- EHBDO.
- GBM.
- Cholelithiasis.
- Cholangitis/cholangiohepatitis.
- Pancreatitis.
- Focal or diffuse peritonitis.
- Bile peritonitis.
- Gastroenteritis with biliary involvement.
- Hepatic necrosis or abscessation.
- Septicemia.

CBC/BIOCHEMISTRY/URINALYSIS

- Variable leukocytosis, toxic neutrophils, and inconsistent left shift if necrosis or sepsis.
- High bilirubin and bilirubinuria common.
- High alanine aminotransferase (ALT), aspartate aminotransferase (AST), alkaline phosphatase (ALP), and γ-glutamyl transferase (GGT) activity.
- Low albumin with peritonitis.
- High cholesterol and bilirubin if EHBDO.
- Hypercholesterolemia and/or hypertriglyceridemia—breed related, endocrine related, pancreatitis, nephrotic syndrome, EHBDO, GBM.

OTHER LABORATORY TESTS

- Abdominocentesis—inflammatory effusion
- Bile culture (dogs and cats)
- Coagulation tests

IMAGING

- Abdominal radiography—may reveal loss of cranial abdominal detail with focal or diffuse peritonitis or effusion; ileus; radiodense choleliths; gas in biliary structures; radiodense GB (dystrophic mineralization due to chronic inflammation; porcelain GB is rare).

- Ultrasonography—
  - Diffusely thick GB wall, segmental hyperechogenicity and/or laminated wall or double-rimmed GB wall observed with necrotizing cholecystitis;
  - Double-rimmed GB wall also observed with acute cholecystitis, hepatitis, cholangiohepatitis; GB lumen filled with amorphous echogenic stellate or finely striated pattern, resembling sliced kiwi fruit (“kiwi sign”) in mature GBM;
  - GB rupture implicated by discontinuous GB wall (or failure to image), pericholecystic fluid, or generalized effusion, and hyperechogenicity of pericholecystic tissue;
  - Mineralized GB (dystrophic mineralization—limey or porcelain GB); chronic cholecystis (sacculated GB or bile ducts in DPM: Caroli’s phenotype;
  - Intrahepatic bile ducts may be difficult to visualize or be thick and prominent;
  - Ascending cholangitis or EHBDO (dilated ducts, “too many tubes sign” defined with color-flow Doppler);
  - Pericholecystic fluid: necrotizing cholecystitis and surgical emergency.
- Choledochitis involving common bile duct (CBD)—thick wall, intraluminal debris, extends into hepatic ducts.

TREATMENT

- Inpatient—provision of critical care during diagnostic/presurgical evaluation or if septic.
- IV polyionic fluids and blood component therapy as needed.
- Restore fluid and electrolyte balance; monitor electrolytes frequently.
- Vitamin K—if jaundiced; give parenterally (see Medications) before surgical interventions, cystocentesis, jugular venipuncture, other iatrogenic trauma.
- Plasma—preferred colloid; indicated if hypoalbuminemia *and* coagulopathy or anticipated surgical interventions and complicating coagulopathy uncorrected.
- Whole blood or fresh frozen plasma—for surgical cases with bleeding tendencies; if septic, artificial colloids may delay recovery; if bleeding, some artificial colloids impair platelet aggregation.
- Monitor urine output.
- Remain vigilant for vasovagal reflex (abrupt bradycardia, hypotension, cardiac arrest) during biliary tree manipulation or cholecystocentesis; be prepared with anticholinergics (atropine) and pressor drugs.
- Remain vigilant for cholangiovenous reflux—systemic dispersal of endotoxin or bacteria while handling septic biliary tree: give IV antibiotics promptly (but after culture collection).
- GB resection advised for cholecystis, best based on surgical evaluations, ultrasound images, bedside cytology of bile—bacterial infection mandates cholecystectomy.

MEDICATIONS

DRUG(S) OF CHOICE

- Antibiotics—*before surgery*; broad spectrum; surgical manipulations may cause bacteremia; select antibiotics for *Enterococcus* spp., enteric Gram-negative and anaerobic flora; refine treatment using culture and sensitivity results; good initial choice is triad combination of metronidazole, ticarcillin (or clavamox), and a fluorinated quinolone; reduce standard dose for metronidazole by 50% if cholestatic jaundice.

- Ursodeoxycholic acid—10–15 mg/kg PO daily divided BID with food; requires decompression of EHBDO *prior to treatment*.
- Antioxidants—vitamin E (α-tocopherol acetate): 10 IU/kg (water-soluble form if EHBDO); S-adenosylmethionine (SAMe): use enteric-coated bioavailable product; on empty stomach: used as glutathione (GSH) donor (20 mg/kg PO q24h), 2 hours before feeding; nonbile acid-dependent (GSH) choleresis (40 mg/kg PO q24h); n-acetylcysteine (NAC) IV if oral administration of antioxidants not possible; loading dose 140 mg/kg IV over 20 minutes, follow by 70 mg/kg over 20 minutes q6–8h.
- Vitamin K_1—0.5–1.5 mg/kg SC/IM q12h for three doses; *caution*: never administer IV (anaphylactoid reaction); treat early to allow response before surgical manipulations.

CONTRAINDICATIONS/POSSIBLE INTERACTIONS

Ursodeoxycholic acid—contraindicated in uncorrected EHBDO or bile peritonitis.

FOLLOW-UP

PATIENT MONITORING

- After critical crisis resolution and surgery—physical examination and pertinent diagnostic testing: repeat every 1–2 weeks until abnormalities resolve.
- If septic—continue antibiotics until enzymes, hyperbilirubinemia, leukocytosis, left shift, and fever resolve.

POSSIBLE COMPLICATIONS

Anticipate protracted clinical course with ruptured biliary tract or peritonitis; postoperative pancreatitis.

MISCELLANEOUS

Associated conditions

- Cholelithiasis.
  - Most are clinically silent; radiopaque (50% in cats) or radiolucent
  - Hyperlipidemic and hypercholesterolemic dogs—predisposed to GBM; may relate to endocrine disorders, idiopathic condition, or other disorders
  - Bile sludge accumulation and mineralization
  - When accompanied by infection or causing intermittent or complete EHBDO (with or without peritonitis)—vomiting; meal-related discomfort, vague abdominal pain; fever; ± jaundice.
  - Fused feline pancreatic and bile duct predisposes to concurrent biliary/pancreatic cholelithiasis, choledochitis, and bile stasis
  - If surgical removal done, biopsy for histopathology of contributing liver disease(s)
  - Choleresis with UDCA may help move sludged biliary debris, but not in asymptomatic patients
  - If chronic and recurrent, strong indication for cholecystectomy.
  - Fat-restricted diets

- Ursodeoxycholic acid—10–15 mg/kg/day PO, divided BID, given with food to increase bioavailability; provides choleretic, hepatoprotectant, anti-endotoxic, antifibrotic effects, and may facilitate cholesterol stone dissolution; therapy often continued lifelong if no cause for cholelithiasis.
- Antioxidant - Vitamin E, SAMe (S-adenosylmethionine)

See also

Gallbladder Mucocele.

Abbreviations

- ALP = alkaline phosphatase
- ALT = alanine aminotransferase.
- AST = aspartate aminotransferase.
- CBD = common bile duct.
- DIC = disseminated intravascular coagulation.
- DPM = ductal plate malformation.
- EHBDO = extrahepatic bile duct obstruction.
- GB = gallbladder.
- GBM = gallbladder mucocele.
- GGT = γ-glutamyltransferase.
- GSH = glutathione.
- NAC = n-acetylcysteine.
- SAMe = S-adenosylmethionine.

Suggested Reading

Center SA. Diseases of the gallbladder and biliary tree. *Vet Clin North Am Small Anim Pract* 2009;39(3): 543–598.

Lawrence YA, Ruaux CG, Nemanic S, et al. Characterization, treatment, and outcome of bacterial cholecystitis and bactibilia in dogs. *J Am Vet Med Assoc* 2015;246:982–989.

Tamborini A, Jahns H, McAllister H, et al. Bacterial cholangitis, cholecystitis, or both in dogs. *J Vet Intern Med* 2016;30:1046–1055.

Author/editor: Heidi Lobprise
Topic adapted from Five Minute Veterinary Consultation, 7th edition, 2021
Original Topic: Cholecystitis with Choledochitis; Cholelithiasis

Author: Sharon A. Center
Consulting Editor: Kate Holan

Chapter 39

Cirrhosis and Fibrosis of the Liver

BASICS

DEFINITION

- Hepatic fibrosis—replacement of hepatic parenchyma, intrasinusoidal, variable zonal, reflecting injury-associated release of cytokines/mediators stimulating accumulation of extracellular matrix (ECM).
- Cirrhosis— due to chronic hepatic injury, fibrogenesis, and hepatic regeneration; regenerative nodules with dissecting fibrotic partitions and regions of parenchymal extinction, deranging hepatic architecture; usually reflects chronic necroinflammatory liver injury.

PATHOPHYSIOLOGY

- Cirrhosis—typified by regenerative nodules, reduced functional hepatic mass, collagen deposition in sinusoids (space of Disse) or portal tracts, compromising parenchymal perfusion.
- Cirrhosis/fibrosis—leads to hepatic dysfunction, capillarization and collagenization of hepatic sinusoids, sinusoidal hypertension, intrahepatic shunting through sinusoids, recanalized vascular pathways in fibrotic partitions between regenerative nodules; these microcirculatory disturbances impair exchanges between blood and hepatocytes.
- Sinusoidal hypertension—leads to hepatofugal portal flow (away from liver); splanchnic hypertension; acquired portosystemic shunt (APSS) formation; episodic hepatic encephalopathy (HE); splanchnic pooling of blood, decreased effective systemic blood volume, stimulation of renal sodium and water retention, with ascites formation; hypertensive splanchnic vasculopathy predisposing to enteric bleeding.

SYSTEMS AFFECTED

- Gastrointestinal (GI)—splanchnic portal hypertension leads to ascites ± enteric bleeding.
- Neurologic—HE.
- Hemic—red blood cell (RBC) microcytosis reflects APSS; bleeding tendencies: failed factor synthesis or activation, thrombocytopenia; reduced anticoagulants increase risk for thrombosis.

Blackwell's Five-Minute Veterinary Consult Clinical Companion: Small Animal Senior Care, First Edition. Edited by Heidi B. Lobprise.

Companion website: www.wiley.com/go/lobprise/Senior

- Renal/urologic—ammonium biurate crystalluria; isosthenuria: polyuria/polydipsia (PU/PD); hepatorenal syndrome (rare) may follow therapeutic paracentesis of large-volume ascites (postcentesis hypotension syndrome [PHS]).
- Endocrine/metabolic—hypoglycemia if end-stage liver failure.
- Respiratory—tachypnea if tense ascites or pleural effusion.
- Skin—superficial necrolytic dermatitis, unkempt coat.

GENETICS

Familial predisposition for chronic hepatitis—Doberman pinscher, cocker spaniel, Labrador retriever, Maltese, Bedlington terrier (copper related), West Highland white terrier, others.

INCIDENCE/PREVALENCE

High in dogs with chronic necroinflammatory liver disease, animals with chronic extrahepatic bile duct occlusion (EHBDO), dogs with severe hepatic copper accumulation.

SIGNALMENT

Species

- Cirrhosis—dogs with chronic hepatitis; cats with chronic cholangitis/cholangiohepatitis; dogs and cats with chronic EHBDO.
- Severe fibrosis—dogs and cats with severe DPM-CHF phenotype.

Breed Predilection

- Many breeds and mixed-breed dogs.
- • Copper-associated hepatopathy (CuAH)
- DPM-CHF phenotype—boxers may be predisposed. many breeds of dogs and cats; cats with polycystic malformations at risk.

Mean Age and Range

- Cirrhosis (dogs)—any age; more common in middle-aged to older; CuAH any age.
- Biliary cirrhosis (cats)—with chronic cholangiohepatitis often >7 years old.
- Fibrosis—ECM accumulates with aging (suspected).

Predominant Gender

- Cocker spaniels—may be higher in males.
- Doberman pinschers and Labrador retrievers—no sex predilection.

SIGNS

General Comments

- Initially—vague and nonspecific.
- Later—relate to complications of portal hypertension (e.g., HE, ascites, gastroduodenal bleeding) and impaired hepatic function.

Historical Findings

- Chronic intermittent lethargy, anorexia, reduced body condition.
- GI signs—vomiting, diarrhea or constipation. Melena—late stage or as APSS develop.
- PU/PD.
- Late onset—ascites, bleeding, HE.
- Jaundice—with necroinflammatory disease;
- Cats—ascites uncommon with acquired necroinflammatory disease, ptyalism, aggression, seizures with HE.

Physical Examination Findings

- Lethargy.
- Poor body condition/coat.
- ±Variable jaundice.
- ±Ascites.
- ±HE.
- Obstructive uropathy—ammonium biurates.
- Anasarca—rare; may develop with overzealous fluid therapy.
- Liver size—dogs: microhepatia; cats: variable.
- Coagulopathy—variable
- Cutaneous lesions—superficial necrolytic dermatitis (see Hepatocutaneous Syndrome).

CAUSES

- Chronic necroinflammatory, oxidant, or immune-mediated liver injury has many causes; may develop subsequent to chronic inflammatory bowel disease (IBD) or pancreatitis.
- CuAH.
- Drug- or toxin-induced liver injury—anticonvulsants; azole antifungals; nonsteroidal anti-inflammatory drug (NSAID) oxibendazole; trimethoprimsulfamethoxazole; chronic food-borne toxins (aflatoxins), others.
- Infections—leptospirosis, canine adenovirus I, leishmanial, histoplasmosis, protozoal (toxoplasmosis).
- Chronic cholangiohepatitis (cats).
- Chronic EHBDO (>6 weeks, dogs and cats).
- Single episode of massive hepatic necrosis; sago palm (cycad toxicity), xylitol, NSAIDs in dogs with substantial Cu accumulation.

RISK FACTORS

- Breed predisposition.
- Dietary Cu intake >patient tolerance.
- Hepatic iron accumulation—supplementation.
- Chronic hepatobiliary inflammation.
- Chronic EHBDO.
- Chronic phenobarbital administration (dogs).
- NSAIDS—dogs, especially carprofen.

DIAGNOSIS

DIFFERENTIAL DIAGNOSIS

- Various hepatic diseases.
- Chronic IBD or pancreatitis.
- Metastatic neoplasia or carcinomatosis.
- Right-sided heart failure, pericardial disease.
- Cats—hepatic lipidosis, feline infectious peritonitis, toxoplasmosis.
- Hemolytic anemia (jaundice differential).

CBC/BIOCHEMISTRY/URINALYSIS

CBC

- Microcytic RBCs: APSS; mild anemia: small RBCs with normal cell count; anemia of chronic disease; microangiopathic shearing: sinusoidal fibrosis, APSS.
- Mild thrombocytopenia variable.
- Leukogram variable.

Biochemistry

- Bilirubin variable.
- Liver enzyme activities—high (alanine transaminase [ALT] > alkaline phosphatase [ALP]) noted before clinical signs or liver dysfunction; at end-stage enzymes may decline.
- Normal to hypoalbuminemia.
- Normal to hyperglobulinemia.
- Hypocholesterolemia—reflects APSS.
- Low blood urea nitrogen (BUN)—reduced urea cycle activity, APSS, protein restricted diet, PU/PD.
- Hypoglycemia—rare.
- Hypokalemia—may predispose to HE.
- Hyponatremia—fluid imbalance with ascites.

Urinalysis

- Isosthenuria—with PU/PD.
- Ammonium biurate crystalluria.
- Bilirubinuria, bilirubin crystalluria.

OTHER LABORATORY TESTS

- Ascitic fluid—pure or modified transudate.
- Coagulation tests—inconsistently prolonged prothrombin time (PT), activated partial thromboplastin time, buccal mucosal bleeding time (BMBT).
- Low protein C and antithrombin activity—reflects APSS, synthetic failure, or disseminated intravascular coagulation (DIC).
- Serum bile acids—high; reflects APSS or cholestasis in cirrhosis.
- Hyperammonemia—inferred from ammonium biurate crystalluria.

IMAGING

Radiography

Abdominal—small-to-normal-sized liver; ascites may obscure details; urate calculi radiolucent unless calcium complexed.

Ultrasonography

- Abdominal—hyperechoic or mixed echogenic liver parenchyma; ± nodularity; often small with cirrhosis; abdominal effusion (ascites); APSS (color-flow Doppler); enlarged portal lymph nodes; no parenchymal change in some cases.
- Doppler interrogation of portal vasculature—may confirm hepatofugal flow or nests of APSS, esp. near left kidney or splenic vessels.

DIAGNOSTIC PROCEDURES

- Fine-needle aspiration cytology—helps rule out neoplasia; rule in bacterial infection; *cannot define fibrosis* or *nonsuppurative inflammation*.
- Liver biopsy—for definitive diagnosis; accuracy increased by multiple biopsy samples.
- Ultrasound guided—14–16G.
- Laparoscopy/laparotomy—best methods, permits gross visualization, documents APSS, biopsy access to multiple liver lobes and focal lesions.

PATHOLOGIC FINDINGS

Gross

- Fibrosis—small, firm irregular-to-finely nodular liver; DPM-CHF may not be small; fibrotic liver may display APSS, ±ascites.
- Cirrhosis—firm irregular liver; prominent micro- or macronodules, APSS, ±ascites.

Histopathology

- Immune-mediated hepatitis—periportal, lobular, or centrilobular lymphoplasmacytic infiltrates, hepatic cord disorganization, sinusoidal fibrosis, biliary hyperplasia.
- Postnecrotic fibrosis—fibrosis marks regenerative repair, disorganized wide hepatic cords; engorged lymphatics reflect sinusoidal hypertension.
- Cirrhosis—diffuse lesion; fibrosis, nodular regeneration distorting lobular architecture, periportal or sinusoidal fibrosis depending on zone of chronic injury, engorged lymphatics; single hepatocyte necrosis if active disease.

TREATMENT

APPROPRIATE HEALTH CARE

- Outpatient—minimally symptomatic patients.
- Inpatient—diagnostic tests; treatment for dehydration, severe HE, enteric bleeding, tense ascites.

NURSING CARE

- Fluids—avoid lactate if hepatic failure; avoid sodium loading if ascites.
- B complex vitamins (esp. cats)—2 mL/L fluid advised.
- Vitamin K_1—0.5–1.5 mg/kg SC q12h for three doses initially; titrate with proteins invoked by vitamin K absence or antagonism (PIVKA; if available) or PT.
- Glucose—if hypoglycemia; 2.5–5% dextrose in polyionic solution; titrate to response.
- Potassium chloride—in fluids, as needed.
- Avoid alkalosis—worsens HE.
- Therapeutic large-volume abdominocentesis if tense ascites nonresponsive to medical treatment; *caution*: PHS—hypotensive crisis and acute renal failure.

ACTIVITY

Limit

DIET

- Withhold oral food in acute severe HE if stupor, coma, or vomiting associated with enteric bleeding or pancreatitis.
- Consider partial parenteral nutrition or total parenteral nutrition.
- If HE—restrict protein intake, use soy or dairy protein sources (dogs) with medical interventions to increase nitrogen tolerance (see Hepatic Encephalopathy).
- Supplement water-soluble vitamins.

CLIENT EDUCATION

- Treatment palliative and symptomatic.
- Fibrosis diminished by control of inflammation and provocative diseases.
- Attenuate factors provoking HE—azotemia, dehydration; infection; catabolism; high-protein meals hypokalemia; alkalemia; constipation, endoparasitism; enteric bleeding; certain drugs.

SURGICAL CONSIDERATIONS

- Cirrhosis—high anesthetic risk; gas anesthesia preferred: isoflurane or sevoflurane.
- Coagulopathy—predisposes to bleeding; BMBT may better assess risk for bleeding.
- Postoperative intensive care—avoid HE, maintain hydration, euglycemia, electrolytes, acid–base balance (avoid alkalemia).
- Predisposed to enteric bacterial translocation—judiciously administer antibiotics, esp. if surgical procedures involve alimentary canal or biliary structures.

MEDICATIONS

DRUG(S) OF CHOICE

- Treatments for specific etiologies—withdraw potentially hepatotoxic drugs, herbal or natural remedies.
- No clinical trials prove efficacy of specific regimens in animals.

Immune Modulation

- Prednisolone/prednisone—1–2 mg/kg q24h PO; taper to 0.5 mg/kg q48h; do not exceed 40 mg/day/dog.
- Azathioprine—2 mg/kg (or 50 mg/m^2) q24h for 14 days, then q48h; contraindicated in cats (toxic); dogs: with prednisone, antioxidants, antifibrotics, and polyenylphosphatidylcholine (PPC).
- Cyclosporine—5 mg/kg BID tapered to q24h; has been successful as single agent or with corticosteroids.
- Mycophenolate—10–15 mg/kg BID; has been successful as first- or second-line treatment with corticosteroids.

Antifibrotics

- Immunomodulation, S-adenosylmethionine (SAMe), silybin, vitamin E—considered antifibrotics as well as hepatoprotectants.
- Ursodiol—7.5 mg/kg/day PO q12h with food; use indefinitely.
- Polyunsaturated phosphatidylcholine with dilinolylphosphatidylcholine (PhosChol®)—25 mg/kg/q24h, mix with food.
- Colchicine—0.025–0.03 mg/kg q24–48h; no evidence of chronic benefit; side effects complicate use; no longer recommended.
- Losartan and telmisartan—losartan: 0.5 mg/kg/q24h; telmisartan: 0.5–1 mg/kg q24h initial dose; closely monitor blood pressure, renal function, and potassium, reducing dose if hypotension or hyperkalemia; angiotensin receptor blockers used in humans as antihypertensives and have been shown to be nephroprotective, to protect against some forms of drug-induced hepatotoxicity, and to inconsistently limit hepatic fibrosis.

Antioxidants

- Necroinflammatory disorders.
- SAMe—20 mg/kg q24h PO, *empty stomach*.
- Vitamin E mixed tocopherols—10 U/kg q24h PO with food.

Hepatoprotectants

- Necroinflammatory disorders.
- Ursodeoxycholate, vitamin E, SAMe.
- Silibinin—efficacy unclear, use PPC complexed form (bioavailable), 2–5 mg/kg q24h PO.
- Elemental zinc—1.5–3 mg PO q24h (if low liver zinc confirmed); adjust dose with plasma zinc measurements; avoid ≥800 µg/dL; contraindicated with concurrent D-penicillamine administration.

Gastroprotectants

- Gastric acid inhibitors—if enteric bleeding (see Hepatitis, Chronic).
- Eliminate endoparasitism.

Ascites

- Restrict activity
- Dietary sodium restriction (0.2% dry matter basis or <0.05 g/100 kcal).
- Diuretics (see Hypertension, Portal; Hepatitis, Chronic); slowly mobilize effusion: furosemide (0.5–1 mg/kg IV/SC/PO q12h) with spironolactone (0.5–2 mg/kg PO q12h); adjust dose to response (7–10 day recheck; if no response titrate up q3–5 days to max dose 4 mg/kg/day).

- Therapeutic large-volume abdominocentesis if nonresponsive ascites mobilization after 7–14 days of diuretics and sodium restriction.
- Consider vasopressin V_2 antagonists with low-dose diuretics for treatment-resistant ascites (no published data for dogs or cats).

CONTRAINDICATIONS

NSAIDs—avoid; potentiate enteric bleeding; may worsen ascites; potentiate centrilobular hepatic necrosis-hepatotoxic metabolites and CuAH.

PRECAUTIONS

- Diuretics—dehydration, hypokalemia, alkalemia worsen HE.
- Glucocorticoids—increase susceptibility to infection, enteric bleeding, sodium and water retention, ascites, protein catabolism, HE.
- Avoid drugs or reduce dose if first-pass hepatic extraction, if require hepatic conjugation or biotransformation (e.g., metronidazole—reduce conventional dose to 7.5 mg/kg PO q12h, as used for HE).

ALTERNATIVE DRUG(S)

- Dexamethasone—if ascites, replace prednisone/prednisolone to avoid mineralocorticoid effect); divide dose by 7–10, administer q3–4 days; taper dose to efficacy.

FOLLOW-UP

PATIENT MONITORING

- Liver enzymes, albumin, BUN, cholesterol, bilirubin—monthly to quarterly.
- Serial monitoring of total serum bile acids—adds no prognostic or diagnostic information.
- Body condition score, weight, muscle mass—reflects nutritional adequacy/nitrogen balance.
- Abdominal girth—reflects ascites volume.
- Azathioprine, mycophenolate, colchicine—monitor for bone marrow toxicity (serial CBCs) and other side effects.

POSSIBLE COMPLICATIONS

HE, septicemia, bleeding—may be life-threatening; DIC—may be terminal event.

EXPECTED COURSE AND PROGNOSIS

- Flare-ups of HE and ascites may require hospitalization to adjust nutritional and medical interventions.
- Sodium restriction and diuretics may require titration to achieve optimal control of ascites.
- Presence of ascites indicates severe disease.

- Cirrhosis—variable: poor long-term prognosis in limited studies, <6 months; however, some can survive years (>5) with careful interventional management depending on whether histologic changes truly "end-stage" or not.

MISCELLANEOUS

Zoonotic Potential

Dogs with leptospirosis-associated chronic liver disease (rare) may shed organisms.

Abbreviations

- ALP = alkaline phosphatase
- ALR = alanine transaminase.
- APSS = acquired portosystemic shunt.
- BMBT = buccal mucosal bleeding time.
- BUN = blood urea nitrogen.
- CHF = congenital hepatic fibrosis.
- CuAH = copper associated hepatopathy.
- DIC = disseminated intravascular coagulation.
- DPM = ductal plate malformation.
- ECM = extracellular matrix.
- EHBDO = extrahepatic bile duct occlusion.
- GI = gastrointestinal.
- HE = hepatic encephalopathy.
- IBD = inflammatory bowel disease.
- NSAID = nonsteroidal anti-inflammatory drug.
- PHS = postcentesis hypotension syndrome.
- PIVKA = proteins invoked by vitamin K absence or antagonism.
- PPC = polyenylphosphatidylcholine.
- PT = prothrombin time.
- PU/PD = polyuria/polydipsia.
- RBC = red blood cell.
- SAMe = S-adenosylmethionine.

Suggested Reading

Center SA. Metabolic, antioxidant, nutraceutical, probiotic, and herbal therapies relating to the management of hepatobiliary disorders. *Vet Clin North Am Small Anim Pract* 2004;34:67–172.

Eulenberg VM, Lidbury JA. Hepatic fibrosis in dogs. *J Vet Intern Med* 2018;32:26–41.

Strickland JM, Buchweitz JP, Smedley RC, et al. Hepatic copper concentrations in 546 dogs (1982–2015). *J Vet Intern Med* 2018;32:1943–1950.

Webster CRL, Center SA, Cullen JM, et al. ACVIM consensus statement on the diagnosis and treatment of chronic hepatitis in dogs. *J Vet Intern Med* 2019;33(3):1173–1200.

Author/editor: Heidi Lobprise
Topic adapted from Five Minute Veterinary Consultation, 7th edition, 2021
Original Topic: Cirrhosis and Fibrosis of the Liver

Authors: Alysha Vincent and Kate Holan
Consulting Editor: Kate Holan

Chapter 40

Gallbladder Mucocele

BASICS

OVERVIEW

- Gallbladder (GB) accumulation of tenacious, thick, mucin-rich, inspissated bile sludge, impairing GB reservoir capacity and GB contraction and expulsion (post-prandial); often associated with episodic abdominal pain.
- Sludge expands GB lumen, flattens/thins GB wall; when severe, provokes necrotizing cholecystitis and occasional GB rupture.
- Initiated by GB dysmotility.

SIGNALMENT

- Dog.
- Shetland sheepdogs, miniature schnauzers, cocker spaniels, bichon frisé, shih tzu overrepresented in one study of 219 dogs.
- Middle-aged-to-older adults.
- No sex predilection.
- Associated with endocrinopathies—adrenal hyperplasia (typical or sex hormone atypical form) hypothyroidism, diabetes mellitus, and administration of glucocorticoids; these likely associated with GB dysmotility, hypertriglyceridemia, or hypercholesterolemia that may impart negative influence on GB contraction.
- Notably associated with hypertriglyceridemic syndromes.

SIGNS

General Comments

- Symptomatic or asymptomatic—depending on stage at diagnosis: mature vs immature gall bladder mucocele (GBM).
- Asymptomatic GBM—often serendipitously discovered on abdominal US

Historical Findings: Symptomatic

- Episodic periprandial abdominal discomfort, anorexia and vomiting.
- Lethargy.
- ±Polyuria/polydipsia—reflects underlying endocrinopathy.
- Collapse—vasovagal episode or bile peritonitis.

Blackwell's Five-Minute Veterinary Consult Clinical Companion: Small Animal Senior Care,
First Edition. Edited by Heidi B. Lobprise.

Companion website: www.wiley.com/go/lobprise/Senior

Physical Examination Findings

- May demonstrate no physical signs if immature GBM.
- ±Lethargy.
- ±Cranial abdominal discomfort—GB dysmotility and maturing GBM.
- Jaundice late in syndrome.
- ±Dehydration.
- ±Fever—secondary infection.

CAUSES AND RISK FACTORS

- Inborn errors of lipid metabolism (hypertriglyceridemia)—miniature schnauzer, Shetland sheepdogs, beagles, others.
- Medical/dietary conditions provoking hypercholesterolemia or dyslipidemia—endocrinopathies, recurrent pancreatitis, feeding high-fat diet to dog with predisposing disorder or dyslipidemia.
- GB dysmotility.
- Cystic mucosal hyperplasia—common in older dogs; may be aggravated by sex hormones (e.g., progestins).

DIAGNOSIS

DIFFERENTIAL DIAGNOSIS

Conditions causing GB bile stasis—GB dysmotility; or other causes of incomplete GB emptying such as cystic duct or GB wall neoplasia, pedunculated adenomatous mucosal lesions, ball-valve cholelith obstructions.

CBC/BIOCHEMISTRY/URINALYSIS

CBC

- Inflammatory leukogram—variable, depends on GB wall viability and hepatic impact of GBM.
- Stress leukogram—if underlying hyperadrenocorticism.
- Nonregenerative anemia—if chronic inflammation or hypothyroidism.

Biochemistry

- High liver enzymes—may be noted on acute presentation for GBM or discovered on routine health assessments; alkaline phosphatase (ALP), γ-glutamyltransferase (GGT), alanine aminotransferase (ALT), ±aspartate aminotransferase (AST) variably affected; ALP activity predominant.
- High ALP—often associates with glycogen-type vacuolar hepatopathy (VH), may reflect adrenal endocrinopathy or glucocorticoid therapy.
- Variable hyperbilirubinemia; depends on GBM maturation and common bile duct patency.
- Low albumin—if ruptured biliary tree and bile peritonitis.
- Prerenal azotemia—if ruptured GB, sepsis, or dehydration from vomiting.
- Electrolyte abnormalities with fluid and acid–base disturbances—due to bile peritonitis or persistent vomiting.

Urinalysis

No specific features.

OTHER LABORATORY TESTS

- Triglyceride concentrations.
- Coagulation tests—normal unless chronic extrahepatic bile duct obstruction (EHBDO), GB rupture, bile peritonitis, sepsis, or disseminated intravascular coagulation (DIC).

IMAGING

- Abdominal radiography—normal or large liver; loss of detail in cranial abdomen if focal peritonitis with GB rupture or concurrent pancreatitis; rarely intrahepatic gas.
- Abdominal US—liver may be normal, or large with rounded margins; diffuse-to-multifocal hyperechoic hepatic parenchyma (associated with glycogen-type VH); may have hypoechoic nodular appearance if severe VH;
    - Typical GBM US image: lumen filled with amorphous echogenic "organizing" non-gravitational debris with stellate or finely striated pattern resembling sliced kiwi fruit ("kiwi sign");
    - Distended GB (>1.2 mL/kg bodyweight) and sometimes distended common bile duct ± cystic duct if EHBDO; pericholecystic edema may enhance GB wall imaging; pericholecystic or generalized effusion with hyperechogenicity of surrounding tissues may indicate focal peritonitis and bile leakage (even if GB wall not ruptured);
    - Diffusely thick GB wall with segmental hyperechogenicity and double-rimmed or laminated appearance associates with necrotizing cholecystitis;
    - GB rupture associated with discontinuous GB wall or difficult-to-image GB;
    - Ruptured GBM may have inspissated congealed biliary material released into abdominal cavity where discrete free-floating "mass" may be discovered; intrahepatic bile ducts may be difficult to visualize or appear prominent or distended.
- GB motility study—indicated if suspected developing GBM serendipitously recognized if GB volume ≥1.2 mL/kg bodyweight.
    - Sequential GB volume measurements determined after meal ingestion (100 g food; may include 0.5 mg/kg erythromycin as motilin agonist provoking GB contraction if no response with food alone).
    - Normal GB contraction results in ≥25% decline of initial or baseline GB volume on one or more recorded postprandial images.
    - Procedure: image GB at 0, 15, 30, 45, 60, 90, 120 minutes relative to feeding.
    - GB volume in mL = [length (cm) × width (cm) × height (cm)] × 0.52.

DIAGNOSTIC PROCEDURES

- Aspiration sampling—fluid *adjacent* to biliary structures or free in abdominal cavity; clarifies GB rupture and/or infection.
- *CAUTION*: do *not* perform cholecystocentesis on suspected GBM as this may cause bile peritonitis.
- Laparotomy—for diagnosis, cholecystectomy, perhaps cholecystenterostomy.
- Laparoscopy—*not* advised as CBD should be flushed to patency.
- Liver biopsy—collect biopsy distant to GB; biopsy from GB area often interpreted as severely fibrotic or as cholangitis.

- Bacterial culture/sensitivity—any effusion; GB wall, mucinous debris clinging to GB wall (scrape GB wall for best sample), liver (single inoculum); request aerobic and anaerobic bacterial culture. Positive ranging from 17 to 33% in different studies; histologic identification of bacteria unreliable.
- Cytology—impression smears of GB wall mucinous debris and liver assist prompt recognition of suppurative septic inflammation or rarely neoplasia.

TREATMENT

Outpatient management—

- Ursodeoxycholic acid and *S*-adenosylmethionine (SAMe) induce bile acid and non-bile-acid-mediated choleresis and provide hepatoprotection—*but* medical therapy is *not* advised to resolve GBM.
- While medical management has occasionally resolved immature GBM in some dogs, these patients remain at risk for GBM recurrence. Naïve unmonitored treatment with choleretics may eventuate in ruptured GB.

Inpatient management

- Inpatient—depends on whether patient presents with severe acute necrotizing cholecystitis, suppurative cholecystitis, intact nonurgent mature GBM, or incidentally discovered immature GBM.
    - If patient hyperlipidemic, investigate cause, restrict dietary fat, avoid glucocorticoids.
    - Symptomatic patients require exploratory surgery for cholecystectomy and evaluation/treatment for potential bile peritonitis.
    - Cholecystotomy and mucocele removal with GB retention *not* advised; high risk for recurrent GBM and potential bile peritonitis.
    - Fluid therapy—balanced polyionic solutions to correct hydration and electrolyte status.
    - Be prepared for blood component therapy.
    - Abdominal lavage—at surgery if bile peritonitis encountered.

MEDICATIONS

DRUG(S) OF CHOICE

Antimicrobials

Initiate combined broad-spectrum antimicrobials *before* surgery; continue treatment 4–8 weeks if septic complications; adjust drugs based on culture and sensitivity test reports and biochemical appraisals. If no histologic or culture evidence of infection and postoperative recovery unremarkable, discontinue antimicrobials 7–10 days after surgery.

Vitamin K1

0.5–1.5 mg/kg IM/SC q12h for three doses—*if jaundiced*; oral route ineffective if EHBDO.

Antiemetics/Antacids/Gastroprotectants

- Antiemetics—may be needed during preoperative interval.
    - Maropitant citrate (Cerenia®), NK-1 antagonist—2 mg/kg PO or 1 mg SC q24h up to 5 days.
    - Ondansetron—0.1–0.3 mg/kg PO 30 minutes before feeding, maximum q8h, or 0.1–0.2 mg/kg slow IV push q6–12h if vomiting.

- Antacids—preoperative interval, proton pump inhibitors preferred: omeprazole 0.7–1.0 mg/kg PO/IV q24h or pantoprazole 0.7–1.0 mg/kg IV q24h.
- Gastric prokinetics—if postoperative gastric atony: metoclopramide 0.2–0.5 mg/kg PO/IV/SC q6–8h or 1–2 mg/kg/day CRI.

- Gastroprotectant—if suspected gastritis, esophagitis, or upper gastrointestinal bleeding: sucralfate—0.5–1.0 g PO q8–12h.

Choleretics

- Maintain hydration status to optimize choleresis.
- Ursodeoxycholic acid—choleretic, hepatoprotectant, anti-inflammatory, anti-endotoxic effects: 10–15 mg/kg PO divided BID daily with food for best bioavailability; treat until complete biochemical recovery or chronically if suspect persistent cholangitis.
- SAMe—choleretic, antioxidant, and metabolic benefits; choleretic dose (40 mg/kg PO q24h on empty stomach) higher than antioxidant dose.

Antioxidants

- Vitamin E—α-tocopherol 10 IU/kg/day PO with food: antioxidant, anti-inflammatory, antifibrotic influence.
- SAMe—20 mg/kg PO daily 2 hours before feeding: give until liver enzymes normalize or indefinitely if chronic hepatitis or cholangitis.

CONTRAINDICATIONS/POSSIBLE INTERACTIONS

N/A

FOLLOW-UP

PATIENT MONITORING

- Repeat sequential hematology, biochemistry, and imaging to monitor surgical recovery; if GBM caused clinicopathologic abnormalities, all changes should resolve within weeks.
- Persistent clinicopathologic abnormalities implicate underlying endocrinopathy, intrahepatic cholangiopathy, or other liver disease.
- At-risk dogs should have US assessment of GB as part of routine health appraisal when middle-aged to geriatric.

POSSIBLE COMPLICATIONS

- Suppurative cholangitis or cholangiohepatitis.
- Bile peritonitis.
- EHBDO.

EXPECTED COURSE AND PROGNOSIS

- Good with successful surgery, chronic choleretic therapy, correction/management of comorbid conditions, dietary and/or medical management of hypertriglyceridemia.
- Anticipate protracted clinical course if ruptured biliary tract or peritonitis—dogs with ruptured GBM 2–3 times more likely to succumb to GBM-related illness.

- Recrudescence may occur if mucocele contents removed and GB retained, with or without chronic medical therapy.
- Chronic postoperative jaundice may reflect iatrogenic stricture at site of cholecystectomy.

MISCELLANEOUS

See Also

- Cholecystitis and Choledochitis.
- Cholelithiasis.
- Glycogen-Type Vacuolar Hepatopathy.
- Hepatitis, Chronic.

Abbreviations

- ALP = alkaline phosphatase
- ALT = alanine aminotransferase.
- AST = aspartate aminotransferase.
- DIC = disseminated intravascular coagulation.
- EHBDO = extrahepatic bile duct obstruction.
- GB = gallbladder.
- GBM = gallbladder mucocele.
- GGT = γ–glutamyltransferase.
- SAMe = S-adenosylmethionine.
- VH = vacuolar hepatopathy.

Suggested Reading

Aguirre AL, Center SA, Randolph JF. Gallbladder disease in Shetland Sheepdogs: 38 cases (1995–2005). *J Am Vet Med Assoc* 2007;231:79–88.

Jaffey JA, Graham A, VanEerde E, et al. Gallbladder mucocele: variables associated with outcome and the utility of ultrasonography to identify gallbladder rupture in 219 dogs (2007–2016). *J Vet Intern Med* 2018;32:195–200.

Author/editor: Heidi Lobprise
Topic adapted from Five Minute Veterinary Consultation, 7th edition, 2021
Original Topic: Gallbladder Mucocele

Author: Sharon A. Center
Consulting Editor: Kate Holan

Chapter 41

Glycogen-Type Vacuolar Hepatopathy

BASICS

DEFINITION

- Glycogen-type vacuolar hepatopathy (VH)—reversible hepatocellular cytosolic vacuolation.
- Reflects many primary disorders including glucocorticoid treatment, hyperadrenocorticism, atypical adrenal hyperplasia (sex hormone hyperplasia), chronic systemic illnesses (inflammatory, neoplastic), and rarely congenital glycogen storage disorders.
- Typified by high alkaline phosphatase (ALP) activity—usually without hyperbilirubinemia or hepatic insufficiency.
- Similar but remarkably severe VH in hepatocutaneous disease; may reflect chronic phenobarbital administration.
- Glycogen VH may coexist with cytosolic lipid vacuolation—comparatively rare in dogs, but may associate with idiopathic hyperlipidemia, diabetes mellitus, hypothyroidism, and rare inborn errors of glycogen/lipid metabolism.

PATHOPHYSIOLOGY

- Glucocorticoids—induce reversible increase in hepatocyte glycogen within 2–3 days; injectable or reposital drug induces most severe VH compared to PO or topical routes.
- Variable response relates to drug type; route; dose; treatment duration; individual sensitivity
- Cell expansion—causes hepatomegaly, ballooning degeneration leads to parenchymal collapse; when severe, nodularity grossly mistaken for cirrhosis.
- May reflect stress response, cytokines, or acute-phase response proteins initiated by nonhepatic systemic disorders or neoplasia (especially lymphoma)
- VH common in dogs with gallbladder mucocele.

SYSTEMS AFFECTED

- Hepatobiliary—normal hepatic function usually; severe degenerative VH can lead to hepatic dysfunction, jaundice, ascites, liver failure.
- All systems affected by steroid hormones or primary systemic disease.

Blackwell's Five-Minute Veterinary Consult Clinical Companion: Small Animal Senior Care, First Edition. Edited by Heidi B. Lobprise.

Companion website: www.wiley.com/go/lobprise/Senior

INCIDENCE/PREVALENCE

- Dogs—common, often accompanies primary necroinflammatory liver disorders.
- Cats—rare; liver vacuolation with triglyceride accumulation more common (see Hepatic Lipidosis).

SIGNALMENT

Species

Dog; rarely cat.

Breed Predilections

Breeds predisposed to hyperadrenocorticism, Scottish terriers (sex hormone adrenal hyperplasia, hyperlipidemia), and others with hyperlipidemia (miniature schnauzers, Shetland sheepdogs) may develop mixed glycogen/lipid VH.

Mean Age and Range

- Middle-aged-to-old dogs—spontaneous hyperadrenocorticism (>75% older than 9 years); chronic systemic inflammation or neoplasia.
- Dogs of any age—iatrogenic VH subsequent to glucocorticoid administration.
- Young dogs or cats—genetic glycogen storage disease.

SIGNS

General Comments

- Reflect glucocorticoids or underlying systemic illness.
- Rarely, signs of hepatic disease or failure; hepatic failure can develop with severe chronic VH.
- Hepatic encephalopathy observed in some dogs with hepatocutaneous syndrome.

Historical Findings

- Glucocorticoid excess—polyuria and polydipsia; polyphagia; endocrine alopecia; abdominal distention: weak muscles, loss of elasticity; skeletal muscle weakness; excessive panting; lethargy; friable skin; bruising tendencies; urinary tract infections, may be asymptomatic; corneal ulcer.
- Adrenal sex hormone hyperplasia—may display some signs of glucocorticoid excess but often fewer and less severe; endocrine alopecia may be only sign; some dogs remain asymptomatic except for chronic progressive marked ALP activity and degenerative VH.
- Other causes—depend on system affected; chronic phenobarbital may cause severe VH.
- Sex hormone hyperplasia causing VH may increase risk for dysplastic hepatic foci and hepatocellular carcinoma (e.g., Scottish terriers).

Physical Examination Findings

- Hepatomegaly.
- Relate to steroid hormone excess or underlying disease; depend on severity and duration.

CAUSES

- Glucocorticoid administration.
- Typical hyperadrenocorticism (spontaneous).
- Atypical adrenal hyperplasia—overproduction of cortisol precursor sex hormones (spontaneous).
- Systemic disease provoking acute-phase response or stress—e.g., severe dental disease, inflammatory bowel disease, chronic pancreatitis, systemic neoplasia (especially lymphoma), chronic infections (urinary tract, skin), hypothyroidism, many others.
- Dogs receiving chronic phenobarbital.

DIAGNOSIS

DIFFERENTIAL DIAGNOSES

- Other diffuse hepatopathies

CBC/BIOCHEMISTRY/URINALYSIS

CBC

- Depends on underlying disease.
- Nonregenerative anemia—anemia of chronic disease or hypothyroidism.
- Relative polycythemia—steroid excess.
- Stress leukogram—hyperadrenocorticism; glucocorticoid exposure; stress of illness.
- Thrombocytosis—neoplasia; hyperadrenocorticism; splenic disease.

Biochemistry

- ALP markedly increased (> ALT or AST); ALP glucocorticoid isoenzyme cannot differentiate cause of VH as other liver disorders also induce this isoenzyme; variable γ-glutamyltransferase (GGT), ALT, AST activity.
- Normal/mild increase in total serum bile acids (TSBA).
- Serum albumin and total bilirubin—usually normal; high bilirubin typically implicates another hepatobiliary or hemolytic process.
- Hypercholesterolemia—hyperadrenocorticism, sex hormone adrenal hyperplasia; breed-related hyperlipidemias; hypothyroidism; pancreatitis; nephrotic syndrome.

OTHER LABORATORY TESTS

- ALP glucocorticoid isoenzyme—see above, lacks specificity and thus clinical utility.
- TSBA—may be modestly increased; ammonia tolerance test: usually normal.
- Pituitary adrenal axis—adrenocorticotropic hormone (ACTH) response test or low-dose ± high-dose dexamethasone suppression test (LDDST ± HDDST) and endogenous ACTH may help differentiate nonadrenal illness, adrenal or pituitary disorders.
- Urine cortisol : creatinine ratio—at-home urine collection helps rule out hyperadrenocorticism; high ratio may reflect stress or nonadrenal illness.

- Thyroid testing—rules out hypothyroidism.
- Triglycerides (fasting)—hyperlipidemia.
- Canine pancreatic lipase immunoreactivity (cPLI)—may indicate "subclinical" pancreatic inflammation or inflammatory bowel disease.

IMAGING

- Abdominal radiography—reveals hepatomegaly or other underlying conditions.
- Thoracic radiography—may reveal lymphadenopathy, metastatic disease, cardiac or pulmonary disorders.
- Abdominal ultrasonography—discloses hepatomegaly, diffuse hyperechoic hepatic parenchyma or multifocal nodular "mottling"; multifocal lesions suggest nodules ("Swiss cheese pattern") formed by progressive hepatocellular ballooning degeneration; may disclose underlying primary visceral abnormalities (e.g., mesenteric lymphadenopathy, neoplasia) or adrenal disorders (size/shape): adrenals may be large with hyperadrenocorticism, sex hormone adrenal hyperplasia, chronic stress, or neoplasia.

DIAGNOSTIC PROCEDURES

- Fine-needle aspiration cytology—22 gauge, 2.5–3.75 cm (1–1.5 in) US-guided needle aspiration; target nodules and normal parenchyma.
- Cytology—glycogen vacuolation common in many primary liver disorders; used to rule out vacuolar change; cannot definitively confirm illness caused only by VH.
- Hepatic biopsy—verifies VH; excludes other primary hepatic disease;
  - Needle biopsy to confirm VH, but may miss primary hepatic disease,
  - Laparoscopy or laparotomy if biopsy needed.
- Cytologic features—hepatocellular cytosolic distention: "rarefication" or granular appearance with increased cell fragility; canalicular bile casts may be observed;
  - Primary VH not associated with inflammatory infiltrates; common association with extramedullary hematopoiesis (EMH) may be misinterpreted as suppurative inflammation.
- Tissue culture and sensitivity—if suppurative inflammation suspected, submit aerobic and anaerobic bacterial cultures.
- Coagulation assessments—prothrombin time (PT), activated partial thromboplastin time (APTT), fibrinogen, and mucosal bleeding time: usually normal; bench assessments have low predictive value in predicting iatrogenic hemorrhage; buccal mucosal bleeding time may be more relevant.

TREATMENT

DIET

- Hyperlipidemia or pancreatitis—restrict dietary fat and fatty supplements.
- Obesity—gradual energy restriction; treat predisposing disorders.

SURGICAL CONSIDERATIONS

- Depend on underlying conditions.
- Adrenal masses may be resected.
- Hypophyseal masses—resection only by experienced surgeons; pituitary mass lesions may respond to radiation therapy.

MEDICATIONS

DRUG(S) OF CHOICE

- Depend on underlying disease.
- Pituitary-dependent hyperadrenocorticism or adrenal hyperplasia syndrome (sex hormone)—usually treated medically: op′-DDD (mitotane or Lysodren®), trilostane, or ketoconazole; op′-DDD preferred for sex hormone adrenal hyperplasia, as trilostane augments sex hormone accumulation; L-deprenyl and melatonin ineffective.
- Primary inflammatory disorders necessitating immunosuppressive or anti-inflammatory medications—use polypharmacy to minimize glucocorticoid exposure if symptomatic or progressive VH; see Alternative Drug(s).
- Neoplasia—tumor resection, chemotherapy, or radiation, as appropriate.
- Dental disease—antibiotics and dentistry.
- Inflammatory bowel disease—hypoallergenic/hydrolyzed protein diets and immunomodulation (avoid glucocorticoids).
- Pyelonephritis, chronic dermatitis, or other infectious disorders—long-term antimicrobial treatment based on microbial culture and sensitivity tests; other appropriate medications.
- Hypothyroidism—supplemental thyroxine.

CONTRAINDICATIONS

- Avoid hepatotoxic drugs if severe VH.
- Beware of drug interactions if using ketoconazole for adrenal disease.
- Avoid drugs with hepatic ALP induction effects.

PRECAUTIONS

Glucocorticoids—caution in VH patients; use lowest effective dose regimen (e.g., alternate-day protocol if prednisone or prednisolone); special caution in hyperlipidemia: may worsen clinical signs of abdominal pain, vomiting, pancreatitis; increase insulin requirements in diabetes mellitus; may augment gallbladder mucocele formation; may provoke hepatic lipidosis in cats.

ALTERNATIVE DRUG(S)

Polypharmacy protocol—may reduce glucocorticoid usage in management of immune-mediated or inflammatory disorders; e.g., metronidazole, azathioprine, chlorambucil, cyclophosphamide, mycophenolate, or cyclosporine.

FOLLOW-UP

PATIENT MONITORING

- Hepatomegaly—abdominal palpation; imaging.
- Normalizing enzymes—biochemistry.
- Adrenal function—ACTH stimulation tests.
- Neoplasia—physical exams and imaging.
- Control of infection—repeat cultures.
- Hyperlipidemia—assess gross plasma lipemia; measure triglycerides and cholesterol.

PREVENTION/AVOIDANCE

- Limit glucocorticoid exposure.
- Use alternate-day therapy with prednisone/prednisolone; titrate to lowest effective dose; use alternative medications to control primary illness.

POSSIBLE COMPLICATIONS

Numerous—related to multisystemic effects of glucocorticoids and associated conditions.

EXPECTED COURSE AND PROGNOSIS

- Most patients are asymptomatic for VH despite high ALP; however, progressive degenerative hepatopathy leading to diffuse nodule formation and hepatic insufficiency may develop in chronic VH in dogs with high ALP activity.
- Laboratory and pathologic features reversible before degenerative parenchymal collapse.
- Dogs with sex hormone hyperplasia, VH, and dysplastic hepatocellular foci appear at risk for development of hepatocellular carcinoma.

MISCELLANEOUS

Associated Conditions

- Pulmonary thromboembolism and myopathy due to hyperadrenocorticism.
- Pancreatitis associated with hyperlipidemia.
- Gallbladder mucocele.

Synonyms

- Glucocorticoid hepatopathy.
- Steroid hepatopathy.
- Corticosteroid hepatopathy.
- Vacuolar change.

See Also

- Gallbladder Mucocele.
- Hyperadrenocorticism (Cushing's Disease)—Cats.
- Hyperadrenocorticism (Cushing's Disease)—Dogs.

Abbreviations

- ACTH = adrenocorticotropic hormone
- ALP = alkaline phosphatase.
- ALT = alanine aminotransferase.
- APTT = activated partial thromboplastin time.
- AST = aspartate aminotransferase.
- cPLI = canine pancreatic lipase immunoreactivity.
- EMH = extramedullary hematopoiesis.
- GGT = γ-glutamyltransferase.
- HDDST = high-dose dexamethasone suppression test.
- LDDST = low-dose dexamethasone suppression test.
- PT = prothrombin time.
- TSBA = total serum bile acids.
- VH = vacuolar hepatopathy.

Suggested Reading

Cortright CC, Center SA, Randolph JF, et al. Clinical features of progressive vacuolar hepatopathy in Scottish Terriers with and without hepatocellular carcinoma: 114 cases (1980–2013). *J Am Vet Med Assoc* 2014;245:797–808.

Sepesy LM, Center SA, Randolph JF, et al. Vacuolar hepatopathy in dogs: 336 cases (1993–2005). *J Am Vet Med Assoc* 2006;229:246–252.

Author/Editor: Heidi Lobprise
Topic adapted from Five Minute Veterinary Consultation, 7th edition, 2021
Original Topic: Glycogen-Type Vacuolar Hepatopathy

Author: Sharon A. Center
Consulting Editor: Kate Holan

Chapter 42

Hepatic Nodular Hyperplasia

BASICS

OVERVIEW

Hepatic Nodular Hyperplasia (HNH)

- Benign parenchymal feature; nonencapsulated, ≤2 cm (rarely up to 5 cm), expansile nodule of hepatocellular hyperplasia, maintaining a modified lobular architecture with recognizable central and portal elements that are irregularly spaced, organized hepatic cord structure 1 cell wide, without marginal parenchymal collapse or fibrosis (is not a regenerative nodule), smooth margins; hepatocyte phenotype may be similar to surrounding parenchyma but may contain glycogen of lipid vacuoles.
- May associate with increased liver enzymes in elderly dogs, especially alkaline phosphatase (ALP).
- Clinical concern derives from association with increased liver enzyme activity and US detection of hepatic nodules or hepatic nodularity during exploratory surgery.
- HNH etiology—unknown; metabolic factors, prior injurious events. In humans associated with infarcts, but no evidence of this in dogs.

SIGNALMENT

HNH

- Age-related lesion.
- Nodules develop by 6–8 years of age; one study documented lesions in all geriatric dogs >14 years of age.

SIGNS

Physical Examination Findings

- HNH does not cause clinical illness.
- Large nodules that rupture and bleed or nodules impairing hepatic sinusoidal perfusion likely represent misdiagnosed hepatic adenomas or well-differentiated hepatocellular carcinoma.

Blackwell's Five-Minute Veterinary Consult Clinical Companion: Small Animal Senior Care, First Edition. Edited by Heidi B. Lobprise.

Companion website: www.wiley.com/go/lobprise/Senior

DIAGNOSIS

DIFFERENTIAL DIAGNOSIS

- Necroinflammatory liver disease—regenerative nodular hyperplasia of entire liver with areas of parenchymal collapse, fibrous connective tissue, and loss of lobular architecture.
- Neoplasia—hepatic adenoma or adenocarcinoma

CBC/BIOCHEMISTRY/URINALYSIS

- CBC—no association with HNH.
- Biochemistry profile—increased serum ALP activity may be encountered; usually normal total protein, albumin, bilirubin, and cholesterol.
- Urinalysis—no consistent findings.

OTHER LABORATORY TESTS

Total serum bile acids (TSBA)—usually normal, unless lesions are diffuse and severe.

IMAGING

- Abdominal radiography—no abnormalities except hepatomegaly with HDH due to VH.
- Abdominal US—variable echogenicity relating to histologic features, nodule number and size, and associated VH. HNH often not noted until liver grossly inspected at surgery or laparoscopy.

DIAGNOSTIC PROCEDURES

- Aspiration cytology—may yield normal hepatocytes, hepatocytes with cytosolic rarefication and fragility consistent with VH (glycogen retention), or cells with discrete lipid (triglyceride) vacuoles (HNH); occasional binucleate hepatocytes may reflect cell proliferation or other concurrent disease (common in portosystemic vascular anomalies/microvascular dysplasia); hepatocytes may be small with size variation in HDH.
- Liver biopsy—collection of a needle biopsy specimen may not clearly differentiate HNH lesion because of small specimen size; definitive diagnosis requires targeted sampling of a large enough tissue specimen to include lesion and adjacent normal hepatic tissue.
- Special stains may be needed to differentiate from regenerative nodules secondary to chronic liver injury; periodic acid-Schiff staining with and without amylase predigestion confirms excess glycogen in vacuolated hepatocytes (see Glycogen-Type Vacuolar Hepatopathy).

PATHOLOGIC FINDINGS

- HNH gross—single or multiple mass lesions, rarely >2 cm in diameter; color similar to adjacent normal hepatic tissue or paler if vacuolated with glycogen or lipid.

TREATMENT

Usually none required; rupture of large nodules indicates hepatocellular carcinoma misdiagnosis; may necessitate blood transfusion and emergency mass excision. Palliate or alleviate underlying cause of VH.

FOLLOW-UP

PATIENT MONITORING

- Quarterly biochemical profiles.
- Sequential abdominal US to evaluate progression of hepatic nodules.

POSSIBLE COMPLICATIONS

Distinction of HNH from neoplastic foci is not possible based only on clinical, laboratory, or imaging data, although lesions >2 cm are unlikely to be this diagnosis.

EXPECTED COURSE AND PROGNOSIS

More extensive numbers of nodules may develop in some dogs with HNH and HDH; HDH predicts risk for primary hepatocellular neoplasia, which requires surveillance and surgical treatment.

MISCELLANEOUS

Hepatocellular Dysplastic Hyperplasia (HDH)

- Potentially preneoplastic (hepatocellular carcinoma HCA) proliferative hepatocellular foci in dogs with glycogen-type vacuolar hepatopathy (VH); nonencapsulated, variably sized, reduced reticulin substructure, expansile nodules of nonvacuolated hepatocytes forming wide (2 cells wide, normal = 1 cell width) disorganized hepatic cords, an irregular (serrated) margin interfacing with adjacent "normal VH" affected hepatocytes, and lacking remodeled marginal lesions (fibrosis, parenchymal collapse).
- Associated with VH-related increased liver enzymes, dominated by increased ALP activity (2 5 to 15 times normal), CBC changes,
- Seemingly associated with increased sex hormone concentrations (androgens, progestins); reflect adrenal hyperplasia syndromes
- Variable US appearance depending on size, number, distribution.
    - Hepatocytes may be small with size variation on aspiration; adequate biopsies of normal and abnormal tissue needed; may be mistaken for nodular regeneration without special stains to detail reticulin substructure and collagen fibril deposition.
    - Sequential assessment of biochemistry and US for indication of transformation of mass to a neoplastic phenotype
    - If increased sex hormones with hyperadrenocorticism, consider modulation with a drug that does not increase sex hormones (Lysodren or mitotane); trilostane increases sex hormones.
- Scottish terrier syndrome does not respond to adrenal modulation; instead use surveillance to detect emerging hepatocellular carcinoma.

See Also

- Cirrhosis and Fibrosis of the Liver.
- Glycogen-Type Vacuolar Hepatopathy.
- Hepatitis, Chronic.

Abbreviations

- ALP = alkaline phosphatase
- ALT = alanine aminotransferase.
- HDH = hepatic dysplastic hyperplasia.
- HNH = hepatic nodular hyperplasia.
- TSBA = total serum bile acids.
- VH = vacuolar hepatopathy.

Suggested Reading

Cortright CC, Center SA, Randolph JF, et al. Clinical features of progressive vacuolar hepatopathy in Scottish Terriers with and without hepatocellular carcinoma: 114 cases (1980–2013). *J Am Vet Med Assoc* 2014;245:797–808.

Sepesy LM, Center SA, Randolph JF, et al. Vacuolar hepatopathy in dogs: 336 cases (1993–2005). *J Am Vet Med Assoc* 2006;229:246–252.

Stowater JL, Lamb CR, Schelling SH. Ultrasonographic features of canine hepatic nodular hyperplasia. *Vet Radiol* 1990;31:268–272.

Author/editor: Heidi Lobprise
Topic adapted from Five Minute Veterinary Consultation, 7th edition, 2021
Original Topic: Hepatic Nodular Hyperplasia

Author: Sharon A. Center
Consulting Editor: Kate Holan

Chapter 43

Hepatitis—Chronic, Copper-Associated, and Suppurative

BASICS

DEFINITION

- Hepatic injury (active chronic necroinflammatory; not "chronic active hepatitis"), nonsuppurative inflammation.
- Chronicity—progressive remodeling, regenerative nodule formation, sinusoidal fibrosis to cirrhosis.

PATHOPHYSIOLOGY

- A variety of causes (see below) with oxidative injury to hepatic cells and/or organelle membranes; activated cytokines and cell-mediated immune responses widen and perpetuate inflammation.
- Lesion progression is variable; chronic inflammation leads to progressive fibrosis with bridging of involved zones and regenerative nodules that distort tissues; then fibrosis (injury from sustained inflammation) and portal hypertension, impaired function that evolve into cirrhosis and hepatic failure at a late stage.
- Progressive cholestasis due to mechanical compression/distortion of bile ducts may occur.

SYSTEMS AFFECTED

- Hepatobiliary—inflammation; necrosis; cholestasis; fibrosis.
- Gastrointestinal (GI)—emesis; diarrhea; anorexia, portal hypertension, ascites, enteric bleeding.
- Neurologic—HE (advanced stage, associated with APSS—acquired portosystemic shunt).
- Hemic—red blood cell (RBC) microcytosis (APSS); coagulopathies typically observed with advanced injury or severe diffuse hepatic necrosis.
- Renal/urologic—polyuria/polydipsia (PU/PD); isosthenuria; ammonium biurate crystalluria (advanced stage with APSS and HE).
- Endocrine/metabolic—hypoglycemia (end-stage failure)
- Respiratory—tachypnea if tense ascites; bicavitary effusion or pulmonary edema.

Blackwell's Five-Minute Veterinary Consult Clinical Companion: Small Animal Senior Care, First Edition. Edited by Heidi B. Lobprise.

Companion website: www.wiley.com/go/lobprise/Senior

GENETICS

- Breed or familial predisposition for chronic hepatitis—Doberman pinscher, Labrador retriever, West Highland white terrier, and Dalmatian—secondary to pathologic Cu accumulation; cocker spaniel hepatopathy, anecdotal in other breeds or breeding lines.
- Inherited Cu-associated hepatopathy only proven in Bedlington terrier—autosomal recessive, genetic test available.

SIGNALMENT

Species

Dog

Mean Age and Range

Average age 6–8 years (range: 2–14 years).

Predominant Gender

Inconsistent

SIGNS

General Comments

- Initially—vague and nonspecific, often includes lethargy and inappetence
- Later—relate to complications of portal hypertension; impaired hepatic function including cholestasis.

Historical and Physical Examination Findings

- May be no signs in early disease or mild lethargy.
- Anorexia, vomiting, weight loss, reduced body condition, poor coat
- PU/PD.
- Jaundice—variable; later stage unless portal hepatitis involves bile duct injury.
- Ascites—late stage.
- HE—late stage, infers APSS with cirrhosis.
- Liver size—normal to small, depends on chronicity.

Late-Stage Physical Findings

- Ascites.
- HE.
- Obstructive uropathy—ammonium biurates.
- Bleeding or thrombotic tendencies.

CAUSES

- Chronic necroinflammatory, oxidant, and immune-mediated liver injury has many causes.

- Infectious—canine hepatitis virus; leptospirosis, enteric-portal bacteremia, or endotoxemia affiliated with inflammatory bowel disease; accidental parenteral administration of intranasal *Bordetella* vaccine.
    - Infectious etiologies are an uncommon cause of CH, however, should be ruled out if there are pertinent clinical history or findings or where there is pyogranulomatous hepatitis (ACVIM).
- Immune-mediated—autoimmune with positive antinuclear antibody (ANA); acquired immune sensitization, nonsuppurative inflammation. ACVIM.
    - Immune-mediated CH is presumed to occur in dogs; however, a careful search for a primary underlying etiology should be undertaken before instituting immunosuppressive therapy for suspected immune-mediated CH.
- Toxic—Cu-associated hepatopathy (see below); acute or chronic exposure to drugs—predictable or idiosyncratic toxicity: e.g., azole antifungals, trimethoprim-sulfa, zonisamide, phenobarbital, primidone, phenytoin, CCNU, NSAIDs (esp. carprofen); repeat exposure to environmental or food-borne toxins, e.g., dimethylnitrosamine, aflatoxin, cycad, cyanobacteria.
    - Every biopsy should be evaluated for abnormal hepatic Cu as this is a common cause of liver injury and is treatable.

RISK FACTORS

- Immunostimulants (vaccinations?) and molecular mimicry of cell epitopes by infectious agents or infection of sinusoidal endothelium.
- Cu-associated hepatopathy.
- Hepatic iron accumulation—from inappropriate supplementation.
- Xenobiotics (drugs, herbal, holistic, or Chinese remedies), inducers or inhibitors of microsomal enzymes, impaired hepatic antioxidant status; xenobiotic metabolites foster inflammation or augment direct initial liver injury.

DIAGNOSIS

DIFFERENTIAL DIAGNOSIS

- Acute hepatitis, other hepatic conditions
- Chronic pancreatitis.
- Other causes of abdominal effusion—hypoalbuminemia; passive congestion; carcinomatosis; chemical peritonitis (bile, urine, pancreatitis), hepatic or nonhepatic causes of portal hypertension: see Hypertension, Portal.
- Jaundice—extrahepatic bile duct occlusion (EHBDO); bile peritonitis, cholangitis/cholangiohepatitis syndrome, ductopenia, hemolysis.

CBC/BIOCHEMISTRY/URINALYSIS

Hemogram

CBC—nonregenerative anemia; RBC microcytosis if APSS; variable leukogram, occasional thrombocytopenia; low total protein if chronic disease with synthetic failure and portal hypertension causing enteric protein loss.

Biochemistry

High liver enzymes; variable bilirubin, albumin, blood urea nitrogen (BUN), glucose, cholesterol; hepatic failure—suggested by low albumin, BUN, glucose, and cholesterol in absence of alternative causes.

- Hyperbilirubinemia in approximately 50%; is a negative prognostic indicator (ACVIM).
- Hypoalbuminemia—late marker of synthetic failure; occurs in most dogs with LCH.

Urinalysis

Variable urine concentration; escalated bilirubinuria; ammonium biurate crystalluria if APSS.

OTHER LABORATORY TESTS

- Total serum bile acids (TSBA)—variable; depends on extent of hepatic remodeling, sinusoidal hypertension, and cholestasis; *superfluous test if hepatic hyperbilirubinemic.*
- Ammonia intolerance—reflects APSS; insensitive to cholestasis, lability impairs accuracy.
- Coagulation tests—reflect panlobular injury, chronicity, vascular injury, impaired synthetic capacity or vitamin K adequacy; early disease: few abnormalities except possible high fibrinogen; advanced stage or severe panlobular injury: single or multiple abnormalities including prolonged prothrombin, activated partial thromboplastin time, low fibrinogen, increased D-dimers.
- Low protein C or antithrombin activity—may reflect PSVA, APSS, hepatic failure, or consumptive coagulopathy.
- Abdominal effusion—chronic liver disease portal hypertension: pure or modified transudate.
- Liver tissue zinc—low with chronic disease and APSS.
- Serologic or PCR tests—possible infectious agents, e.g., leptospirosis, rickettsial diseases, *Borrelia*, *Bartonella*, endemic fungal agents.
- ANA titer—if potential for autoimmune disease; *note*: low-level positive titers nonspecific and more common with advanced age.
- Immunohistochemical staining of liver biopsy—can confirm infectious agents or phenotype of infiltrating cells (inflammatory or neoplastic).

IMAGING

Abdominal Radiography

- Microhepatia—suggests late-stage disease or APSS causing lobular atrophy.
- Abdominal effusion—obscures image.
- Ammonium biurate calculi—radiolucent unless combined with radiodense minerals.

US

- Liver size depends on disease stage.
- Normal-to-variable parenchymal and biliary tract echogenicity; may note nodularity and irregular liver margins with chronicity due to regenerative nodules.
- APSS—tortuous vessels most commonly identified caudal to left kidney or near splenic vein.
- Abdominal effusion—US facilitates fluid sampling.
- Uroliths—renal pelvis or urinary bladder; may signify ammonium biurate urolithiasis (need stone analysis).
- Enables fine-needle aspiration—cytology and cholecystocentesis for bile collection.

DIAGNOSTIC PROCEDURES

Aspiration Cytology

- Fine-needle aspiration cytology—*cannot define* fibrosis or nonsuppurative inflammation; *cannot* recommend therapy.
- Cannot definitively diagnose chronic hepatitis, hepatic fibrosis, or Cu-associated hepatopathy.

Liver Biopsy

- Liver biopsy—needed for definitive diagnosis; acquire biopsies from multiple liver lobes.
- Tru-Cut® needle biopsy—use 14–16G.
- Laparoscopy—best biopsy method; lower morbidity and faster recovery vs. exploratory laparotomy.

Bacterial Culture

Aerobic and anaerobic bacterial culture and sensitivity of liver and bile; use particulate biliary debris if possible.

Metal Analyses

- Measure Cu, iron, and zinc concentrations in liver (dry matter basis).
- Low hepatic zinc associated with portosystemic shunting requires supplementation.
- Iron commonly accumulates in necroinflammatory disorders.
- Cu quantification and rhodanine staining—ascertains relevance to parenchymal injury.

PATHOLOGIC FINDINGS

Histopathology

- Immune-mediated hepatitis—periportal, lobular, centrilobular, or panlobular with lymphoplasmacytic infiltrates, hepatic cord injury causing disorganization, sinusoidal fibrosis, biliary hyperplasia.
- Cu-associated hepatopathy—initially centrilobular, may evolve panlobular immune-mediated hepatitis.
- Cirrhosis—diffuse, unresolvable; fibrosis, nodular regeneration distorting lobular architecture.

TREATMENT

APPROPRIATE HEALTH CARE

- Inpatient—for diagnostic testing, supportive care, treatment initiation in severe illness.
- Outpatient—if condition stable at diagnosis; slowly titrated onto medical therapy.

NURSING CARE

- Depends on underlying condition.
- Fluid therapy—balanced polyionic fluids supplemented to correct hydration, electrolyte aberrations, or hypoglycemia; restricted sodium if ascites, may require fresh frozen plasma, avoid synthetic colloids.

- Water-soluble vitamins—2 mL/L fluids.
- Ascites (see Cirrhosis and Fibrosis of the Liver).

ACTIVITY

Keep patient warm and hydrated; restricted activity may improve hepatic regeneration, euglycemia, and ascites mobilization.

DIET

- Conserve body condition and muscle mass.
- Adequate calories and protein—to avoid negative nitrogen balance and catabolism.
- Dietary protein—restrict protein quantity *only* if signs of HE or observe ammonium biurate crystalluria; feed balanced species-specific diet; if HE, avoid fish and red meat source protein (dogs).
- Fat restriction rarely needed.
- Meal frequency—feed several small meals per day.
- Sodium restriction—with ascites or severe hypoalbuminemia: <100 mg/100 kcal or <0.2% dry matter basis formula.
- Balanced vitamin supplements (water soluble, fat soluble)
- Thiamin—ensure repletion to avoid metabolic complications and neurologic signs; 50–100 mg PO q24h; *caution*: anaphylactoid reactions may occur with injectable thiamin.
- Parenteral nutrition: partial to meet energy requirements or total if inappetence >7 days; branched-chain amino acids remain controversial in dogs with liver dysfunction.

CLIENT EDUCATION

- Control, not cure, is the goal; medications usually required for life; chronic hepatitis is cyclic and will minimally require re-evaluations q4–6 months after initial control.
- CU—ACVIM
- Antifibrotics—best control of fibrosis through control of inflammation and underlying primary process.
- Attenuate factors provoking HE—dehydration; azotemia, infection; catabolism; constipation; hypokalemia; alkalemia; high-protein meals; endoparasitism; enteric bleeding; certain drugs.

SURGICAL CONSIDERATIONS

- APSS—do not ligate APSS or band vena cava.
- Cirrhosis—high anesthetic risk; gas anesthesia preferred: isoflurane or sevoflurane.

MEDICATIONS

DRUG(S) OF CHOICE

- Treatments for specific etiologies.
- Withdraw plausible hepatotoxic drugs.
- No clinical trials prove efficacy of specific therapeutic regimens at this time (ACVIM).

Immunomodulation

- ACVIM—in dogs with histologically identified inflammatory infiltrates, short courses of an anti-inflammatory dosage of corticosteroids may be beneficial
- At present, however, not enough evidence is available to recommend an optimal immunosuppressive protocol.
    - Corticosteroids effective as first-line treatment, but adverse effects should be considered; combine with other immunosuppressive drugs to enable more rapid tapering to every other day anti-inflammatory doses, with maintenance on the second drug alone.
        - Prednisolone/prednisone—1–2 mg/kg daily PO; taper to lowest effective dose (0.25–0.5 mg/kg PO q48h)
        - If ascites, replace prednisone or prednisolone with dexamethaxone to avoid mineralocorticoid effect; divide dose by 7–10, administer q3 days.
        - Use microemulsified cyclosporine (2.5–5 mg/kg PO) with glucocorticoids to increase drug efficacy and permit lower dose
    - Cyclosporine can be considered as first-line treatment, twice daily tapered to once daily.
    - Mycophenolate as first- or second-line treatment and in combination with corticosteroids. 10–15 mg/kg PO q12h; doses ≥10 mg/kg PO BID
        - If diarrhea, lower initial dose and/or divide total daily dose into 3–4 doses.
        - More GI issues than azathioprine; avoid dosing with food or proton pump inhibitors.
    - Azathioprine 2 mg/kg (50 mg/m^2) PO q24h × 14 days then titrate to q48h
        - Bone marrow side effect, but not GI
        - If failure to respond, go to cyclosporine
        - If toxicity—go to mycophenolate
    - Azathioprine and mycophenolate
        - Monitor q7–14 days for hematopoietic, hepatic, or pancreatic toxicity
        - Adjust dose (25–50% dose reduction) in 2–6 months with biochemical improvement (normalized total bilirubin and marked decline in liver enzyme activity).
        - If acute toxicity—stop therapy, allow recovery then reintroduce with 25% reduction in dose; if insidious chronic toxicity, discontinue and change to alternate drug

Hepatoprotectants

- There is no large body of veterinary evidence-based information to substantiate efficacy of the hepatoprotective agents ursodeoxycholate, S-adenosylmethionine (SAMe), and vitamin E in chronic hepatitis (CH) in dogs. However, based on their safety profile and extensive preclinical study and investigated utility in human liver diseases, these agents are routinely used as adjunctive treatment (ACIVM).
- Ursodeoxycholate (UDSA); also immunomodulatory, antifibrotic, choleretic, anti-endotoxic, and antioxidant effects; 10–15 mg/kg PO SID or divided q12h; administer with food for best bioavailability; may use as aqueous solution; no deleterious side effects; maintain indefinitely.
    - Vitamin E—α-tocopherol, 10 IU/kg PO q24h with food; anti-oxidant.
    - SAMe—S-adenosylmethionine with thionine; 20 mg/kg/day enteric-coated tablet PO, give on empty stomach for best bioavailability, 1–2 hours before feeding; anti-oxidant,

- Antifibrotic: PPC (Polyunsaturated phosphatidylcholine) dilinolylphosphatidylcholine (DLPC—PPC containing DLPC): primarily antifibrotic, also immunomodulatory, antioxidant, and improves membrane fluidity; 25–50 mg/kg/day PO with food;
    - PhosChol® with preformed DLPC (52%) has benefit in some forms of liver disease (humans, animal models); may have corticosteroid-sparing effect (allows reduced glucocorticoid dosing);
    - Safely prescribed without liver biopsy.

- Silybin with PPC (milk thistle)—studies suggest potential hepatoprotectant, antifibrotic, antioxidant effects, and possibly promoting hepatocyte regeneration.
    - Low bioavailability of oral forms significantly limits biologic effect at traditional oral dosing: 2–5 mg/kg/day PO (PPC complexed form);
    - Only bioavailable form IV formulation (Legalon® SIL) used for *Amanita* death cap mushroom toxicity with high dose protocol; orphan drug.

Antioxidants (In Addition to Above)

- Avoid vitamin C (ascorbate).
- Zinc (zinc acetate)—antioxidant and antifibrotic benefits,
    - If low liver zinc (<120 µg/g dry weight liver); may improve control of HE 1.5–3 mg/kg PO daily.
    - Avoid plasma concentrations ≥800 µg/dL to prevent hemolysis; plasma zinc levels do not correlate with tissue levels.
    - Unreliable for limiting enteric Cu uptake.

CONTRAINDICATIONS

- NSAIDs—avoid; may provoke enteric ulceration and bleeding; may worsen ascites; metabolites cause centrilobular hepatocyte injury.
- Avoid drugs requiring extensive hepatic metabolism or judiciously adjust dose if APSS, HE, jaundice, or hepatic failure evident.

PRECAUTIONS

- Avoid drugs or reduce dose for those dependent on first-pass hepatic extraction if APSS or those requiring hepatic conjugation or biotransformation for detoxification, e.g., metronidazole—reduce conventional dose to 7.5 mg/kg PO q12h (often used for HE).
- Zinc overdose may cause hemolysis.
    - Cyclosporine side effects: gingival hyperplasia (managed with azithromycin), rare cholestatic liver injury, hyperlipidemia, hypercholesterolemia, worsening preexisting hypertension, risk for GB disease, risk for opportunistic infections high dose can lead to nephrotoxicity; risk for neoplasia with chronic use; avoid concurrent use of p450 inhibitors unless cyclosporin dose substantially reduced.

POSSIBLE INTERACTIONS

- Avoid medications altering hepatic p450 cytochrome biotransformation/elimination pathways (cimetidine, quinidine, ketoconazole).
- Avoid concurrent treatment with metoclopramide if spironolactone used for diuresis (causes aldosterone release).

FOLLOW-UP

PATIENT MONITORING

- At-home behavior/cognitive function, bodyweight, body condition, and muscle mass scores monitored.
- CBC, biochemistry, urinalysis—depending on immunosuppressive medications (see above), initially q2 weeks for 2 months, then monthly or quarterly; depends on patient status and drugs administered; monitor for opportunistic infections.
- Serial monitoring of TSBA—usually does not add prognostic or diagnostic information.
    - Azathioprine—monitor for bone marrow toxicity; GI or pancreatic toxicity
    - Mycophenolate—monitor for GI toxicity; rare bone marrow toxicity
- Cyclosporine—renal function, infectious complications, avoid cytochrome p450 inhibitor drugs; remain aware of possible drug-provoked hyperlipidemia, hypercholesterolemia, related GB disease (dysmotility, GBM, cholelithiasis).

POSSIBLE COMPLICATIONS

HE, septicemia, bleeding—may be life-threatening; disseminated intravascular coagulation—may be terminal event.

EXPECTED COURSE AND PROGNOSIS

- Chronic hepatitis often cyclic; occasional flare-ups inconsistently associated with clinical illness, more consistently associated with vacillating liver enzymes or hyperbilirubinemia.
- Some dogs achieve solid long-term remission.
- Development of ascites—severe liver injury, APSS, potential for HE, shorter survival.
- Severe disease—with APSS, HE, and ascites may require occasional hospitalizations to adjust nutritional and medical interventions.

MISCELLANEOUS

Copper-Associated Hepatopathy (CuAH)

While CuAH can be diagnosed first in an older pet, breed disposition often means this is found in young-to-middle-aged dogs. Some distinctions are below:

- Initial injury with pathologic or toxic Cu accumulation
- Injury zone 3 (centrilobular) may progress to panlobular inflammation
- Inherited Cu-associated hepatopathy only proven in Bedlington terrier—autosomal recessive, genetic test available.
- Breed or familial predisposition for chronic hepatitis secondary to pathologic Cu accumulation - Doberman pinscher, Labrador retriever, West Highland white terrier, and Dalmatian.
- Metal analysis of Cu, iron, and zinc concentrations in liver (dry matter basis): Normal hepatic Cu ≤400 µg/g.
  Cu quantification and rhodamine staining—ascertains relevance to parenchymal injury.
- Diet—Cu-restricted diets for their lifetime with reduction in dietary protein only when exhibiting signs of HE
- Chelation (see Supplemental reading)

- D-Penicillamine—10–15 mg/kg PO q12h on empty stomach (1 hour before feeding).
  - Supplement vitamin B6 (pyridoxine) and water-soluble vitamins other than Vit.C
  - Monitoring with subsequent biopsies optimal; but ALT can be used as a surrogate marker.
  - Can cause anorexia and vomiting; additional side effects.
- Trientine hydrochloride—as effective as d-penicillamine but expensive: 5–7 mg/kg PO q12h given 1 hour before meals.
- Ammonium tetrathiomolybdate—alternative method; limited use in dogs.
- Zinc—unreliable for limiting enteric Cu uptake; effects too slow; may help in early CuAH

Prognosis

- If mild-to-moderate hepatic injury (detected before liver remodeling or hepatitis), good prognosis with treatment.
- Poor in young dogs with acute hepatic failure or older dogs with cirrhosis

Suppurative Hepatitis

- Suppurative septic cholangitis/cholangiohepatitis—most common in young-to-middle-aged male cats.
- Hepatic abscesses—most common in old dogs with HCA (hepatic carcinoma), or secondary to immunosuppression or diabetes mellitus.
- Ultrasonography—best noninvasive method of abscess detection (>0.5 cm lesions); solitary, variably echogenic, cavitated, hyperechoic rim.
- In middle-aged/older dogs—lobectomy for abscess removal and possible wide-margin resection of an HCA.
- Abscess—drain via lobectomy during laparotomy or under ultrasound guidance before surgery; judiciously repeat drainage (may require insertion of an indwelling catheter for short-term continuous drainage); consider alcoholization of abscess after drainage with ultrasound monitoring at 24 and 48 hours post procedure and 15, 30, 60, and 120 days.

Zoonotic Potential

- Dogs with leptospirosis-associated chronic liver disease (rare) may shed organisms.
- *Bartonella* and rickettsial infections are sentinels for endemic vectors.

See Also

- Cirrhosis and Fibrosis of the Liver.
- Glycogen-Type Vacuolar Hepatopathy.

Abbreviations

- ANA = antinuclear antibody
- APSS = acquired portosystemic shunt.
- BUN = blood urea nitrogen.
- CRS = colorectal scintigraphy.
- DLPC = dilinolylphosphatidylcholine.
- EHBDO = extrahepatic bile duct occlusion.
- GBM = gallbladder mucocele.
- GI = gastrointestinal.
- HE = hepatic encephalopathy.
- NSAID = nonsteroidal anti-inflammatory drug.
- PPC = polyunsaturated phosphatidylcholine.

- PSVA = portosystemic vascular anomaly.
- PU/PD = polyuria/polydipsia.
- RBC = red blood cell.
- SAMe = S-adenosylmethionine.
- SPS = splenoportal scintigraphy.
- TSBA = total serum bile acids.

Suggested Reading

Webster CRL, Center SA, Cullen JM, et al. ACVIM consensus statement on the diagnosis and treatment of chronic hepatitis in dogs. *J Vet Intern Med* 2019;33(3):1173–1200.

Author/editor: Heidi Lobprise
Topic adapted from Five Minute Veterinary Consultation, 7th edition, 2021
Original Topic: Hepatitis, Chronic; Copper-Associated Hepatopathy and Hepatitis, Suppurative and Hepatic Abscess

Author: Sharon A. Center—Hepatitis, Chronic and Copper-Associated Hepatopathy

Author: Ashleigh Seigneur—Hepatitis, Suppurative and Hepatic Abscess
Consulting Editor: Kate Holan

Chapter 44

Hepatocutaneous Syndrome

BASICS

OVERVIEW

- Liver lesion—severe degenerative vacuolar hepatopathy, hepatocyte degeneration leads to parenchymal collapse associated with marked proliferative hepatocyte response; this process leads to severe hepatic nodularity; hepatocutaneous syndrome (HCS) hepatopathy often associated with syndromic pressure point crusting, painful dermatosis, and diabetes mellitus (DM)
- Liver lesions—may precede cutaneous lesions and DM.
- Hepatopathy—recognized on abdominal US, pursued because of marked alkaline phosphatase (ALP) increase.
- Occasionally HCS hepatopathy develops in dogs treated chronically with phenobarbital.

SIGNALMENT

- Middle-aged-to-older dogs.
- Males may have a greater predilection.
- Familial syndrome in shih tzu dogs described.

SIGNS

Historical Findings

- Acute-to-subacute onset; may be few initial signs.
- Common signs—anorexia, weight loss, lethargy, polyuria/polydipsia, diarrhea, vomiting, ± jaundice, often with prominent cutaneous pressure point and painful foot pad lesions characterized as fissured crusted oozing wounds.

Physical Examination Findings

- Lethargy, poor body condition, with foot pad and elbow lesions causing pain in standing and recumbent postures, may be jaundiced.
- Cutaneous lesions
- Normal, small-to-large hepatic size.
- Rare abdominal effusion—signifies late-stage HCS hepatopathy.

Blackwell's Five-Minute Veterinary Consult Clinical Companion: Small Animal Senior Care,
First Edition. Edited by Heidi B. Lobprise.

Companion website: www.wiley.com/go/lobprise/Senior

CAUSES AND RISK FACTORS

- Etiology—associated with pathologic hypoaminoacidemia and aminoaciduria; low amino acid (AA) concentrations seemingly have causal association with cutaneous and liver lesions. Most significantly low AA affiliated with urea cycle and synthesis of glutathione and collagen.
- Hyperglucagonemia associated with glucagonoma—originally proposed as causal mechanism but that remains unproven; ~30–40% of tested dogs have increased plasma glucagon concentrations; glucagonoma confirmed in <15% of reported cases.
- Insulin-resistant DM—commonly associated with HCS; may reflect increased glucagon.
- Contributing role hypothesized for ill-defined deficiencies of zinc, fatty acids, or niacin.
- Similar cutaneous lesions described with primary hepatopathies caused by phenobarbital or rarely chronic mycotoxicosis.

DIAGNOSIS

DIFFERENTIAL DIAGNOSIS

- Cirrhosis—unresolvable architectural remodeling with fibrosis, sinusoidal hypertension, and regenerative nodules.
- Chronic hepatitis—inflammatory infiltrates and individual hepatocyte necrosis.
- Copper-associated hepatopathy—pathologic copper accumulation initially with zone 3 associated with oxidative necroinflammatory hepatocyte injury.
- Diffuse nodular hyperplasia—rare cause of hepatic nodularity of similar magnitude.
- Degenerative glycogen-type vacuolar hepatopathy (VH)—may evolve similar nodular hepatic US pattern.

CBC/BIOCHEMISTRY/URINALYSIS

- CBC—mild-to-moderate nonregenerative to mild regenerative anemia; red blood cell microcytosis; neutrophilic leukocytosis reflecting cutaneous lesion inflammation or infection.
- Biochemistry—high liver enzymes (especially ALP); variable hypoproteinemia with hypoalbuminemia, low cholesterol, and blood urea nitrogen; euglycemic to fasting hyperglycemia.
- Urinalysis—ammonium biurate crystalluria reflects hepatic insufficiency in end-stage hepatopathy; occasionally develop acquired portosystemic shunts, with shunting contributing to hyperammonemia.

OTHER LABORATORY TESTS

- Total serum bile acids—normal or increased.
- Insulin—inappropriately increased before development of diabetes mellitus.
- Plasma glucagon—inconsistently increased.
- Plasma AA profile—30–50% reduction in AA concentrations of healthy dogs; dogs with cutaneous lesions have more severe AA deficiencies than dogs with only HCS hepatopathy.
- Urine AA profile—prodigious renal wasting of lysine and proline; profile of urine AA concentrations must be normalized with urine creatinine concentration for interpretation.

IMAGING

- Abdominal radiography—variable liver size (small, normal, to large); rare effusion.
- Abdominal US—may disclose irregular liver margin; characteristic nodular pattern: hypoechoic foci (proliferative nodules) with background hyperechoic parenchyma (glycogen-type VH and lipid-type VH) typified as "Swiss cheese pattern"; although suggested as pathognomonic, other causes of severe degenerative VH also may demonstrate this pattern; occasional diffuse nodularity cannot be imaged in HCS; pancreatic mass <15% of dogs.

DIAGNOSTIC PROCEDURES

- Aspiration sampling—hepatocytes display glycogen- and lipid-type vacuolation.
- Liver biopsy—needle biopsy may compromise definitive diagnosis due to limited sampling of distinctive proliferative hepatocyte foci between regions with massive degenerative VH; needle biopsy may be best option for dogs with extensive skin lesions, larger laparoscopic samples preferred; avoid laparotomy as dogs with cutaneous lesions may not promptly heal.
- Skin biopsy; usually diagnostic for HCS.
- AA profiles in plasma and urine with urine AA normalized using urine creatinine disclose profound reduction of plasma AA and severe aminoaciduria with prominent losses of lysine and proline.
- Glucagonomas often express somatostatin receptors; these might be identified using radioisotope somatostatin label; however, prohibitively expensive for most clients
- If pancreatic mass discovered, should be resected, submitted for routine and special stains (request immunohistochemical stains for neuroendocrine neoplasia); like other islet cell tumors, glucagonomas may produce other hormones (see Suggested Reading).

Note: Positive immunohistochemical staining does not confirm pathologic hormone secretion.

TREATMENT

- Diet—use high-quality/high-quantity protein, energy-dense diets; enteral or parenteral feeding may be required for some dogs at initial diagnosis.
- If hepatic encephalopathy (HE) observed—improve nitrogen tolerance with lactulose and metronidazole (see Hepatic Encephalopathy) and use liver-specific diet as baseline formula.
- Supplemental AA therapy is cornerstone of treatment—IV route superior to oral route.
- Oral AA supplementation—historically done with egg yolk (3–6 yolks/day) but *not* very effective; dietary supplementation with anabolic whey protein powder increases protein intake, but alone *not* very effective; oral treatment may lack efficacy due to reduced enteral AA uptake.
- IV AA infusion with IV lipid infusion—*most* effective therapy (lesion resolution and survival).
- IV AA infusion—8.5–10% solution of crystalline AA (Aminosyn®); using 10% solution (100 mL delivers 10 g AA) dose: 25 mL/kg bodyweight over 6–8 hours through peripheral vein.
- IV 20% Intralipid® (or generic 20% IV fat emulsion)—dose: 7 mL/kg bodyweight over 6–8 hours; given concurrently with IV AA using Y-adaptor for combined infusions through one line; combined therapy achieves best response to date.
- IV infusion treatment interval—initially q7–10 days until evidence of improvement: skin easiest to appraise with photo documentation and evidence of foot pad pain resolution; hepatic lesions require US imaging for assessment: these take months to improve; liver enzymes may be used to infer improvement but do not normalize (remain vacillating). RBC

microcytosis resolves with significant recovery. After initial strong response, frequency of IV AA and IV Intralipid determined based on dog's physical and lesional status and trends in hematologic and biochemical profiles. Chronically managed patients typically receive IV infusions at 6-week intervals, titrated frequency achieved by gradually lengthening intervals between infusions while monitoring for relapse.

- Essential fatty acid supplementation—omega-3 fatty acids; double normal dose.
- Metastatic pancreatic tumors secreting glucagon may be controlled with long-acting somatostatin analogue (octreotide: 2–3.7 µg/kg q6–12h); prohibitively expensive.
- Manage DM with insulin and judicious dose titration to response.
- Other supplements—see Medications.

MEDICATIONS

DRUG(S) OF CHOICE

- Insulin for DM management; may demonstrate insulin resistance.
- AA infusion and lipid infusions and diet—see above.
- Cutaneous or nail bed infections—systemic antimicrobials or antifungals; germicidal baths.
- Ketoconazole—for secondary yeast infection; anti-inflammatory and antipruritic effects: monitor liver enzymes for drug-induced liver injury warranting drug discontinuation.
- Zinc supplementation—2–4 mg/kg elemental zinc q24h; avoid zinc methionine if HE.
- Niacinamide—250–300 mg/dog q12h (500 mg for dogs >10 kg); watch for toxic effects; avoid extended-release form.
- Topical glucocorticoids—if unresponsive inflammatory skin lesions, after infection managed (*caution*: systemic glucocorticoids may promote HE, enteric ulceration, infection, may complicate DM management).
- Ursodeoxycholic acid—10–15 mg/kg PO daily, divided dose given with food; hepatoprotectant against bile-acid-mediated membrane injury.
- Antioxidants—vitamin E (10 IU/kg daily PO with food); S-adenosylmethionine (20 mg/kg PO daily, empty stomach) provides additional metabolic and hepatoprotective influences.
- If associated with phenobarbital, discontinue this drug.

CONTRAINDICATIONS/POSSIBLE INTERACTIONS

- HE induction—high-protein diet supplements and AA infusions.
- Toxic effects of ketoconazole and its interference with p450 drug metabolism.
- Toxic effects of niacinamide and zinc.

FOLLOW-UP

PATIENT MONITORING

- Weekly-to-monthly physical exam, CBC, biochemistry, and urinalysis to assess need for IV AA and lipid infusions and treatments for secondary infections.
- As needed for management of DM.

POSSIBLE COMPLICATIONS

- With HCS, IV infusions may cause thrombophlebitis and risk for thromboembolism.
- Ketoacidosis—uncommon.
- Hepatic encephalopathy.
- Sepsis—due to diabetes and skin lesions or IV catheter-related infections.
- Pain—from skin lesions may require analgesics.

EXPECTED COURSE AND PROGNOSIS

- Liver and skin lesions often improve with IV infusions.
- Some dogs achieve cutaneous remission ≥3 years with described therapies.
- Some dogs have unremitting HCS progression, necessitating euthanasia.

MISCELLANEOUS

Synonyms

- Superficial necrolytic dermatitis.
- Necrolytic migratory erythema.
- Metabolic epidermal necrosis.
- Glucagonoma syndrome.

Abbreviations

- AA = amino acids
- ALP = alkaline phosphatase.
- DM = diabetes mellitus
- HE = hepatic encephalopathy
- HCS = hepatocutaneous syndrome
- VH = vacuolar hepatopathy

Suggested Reading

Bach JF, Glasser SA. A case of necrolytic migratory erythema managed for 24 months with intravenous amino acid and lipid infusions. *Can Vet J* 2013;54:873–875.

Hall-Fonte DL, Center SA, McDonough SP, et al. Hepatocutaneous syndrome in Shih Tzus: 31 cases (1996–2014). *J Am Vet Med Assoc* 2016;248(7):802–813.

Oberkirchner U, Linder KE, Zadronzny L, et al. Successful treatment of canine necrolytic migratory erythema (superficial necrolytic dermatitis) due to metastatic glucagonoma with octreotide. *Vet Dermatol* 2010;21:510–516.

Author/editor: Heidi Lobprise
Topic adapted from Five Minute Veterinary Consultation, 7th edition, 2021
Original Topic: Hepatocutaneous Syndrome

Authors: Sharon A. Center and John P. Loftus
Consulting Editor: Kate Holan

Immune System

Chapter 45

Anemia, Immune-Mediated

BASICS

DEFINITION

Accelerated removal or hemolysis of red blood cells (RBCs) due to a type II hypersensitivity reaction.

PATHOPHYSIOLOGY

- Antibodies form against endogenous RBC antigens (primary/nonassociative immune-mediated hemolytic anemia [IMHA]), or RBC membrane antigens, or antigens altered by infectious organisms, drugs, or neoplasia (secondary/associative IMHA).
- Immunoglobulin deposited on RBC membrane, causing either direct intravascular hemolysis or accelerated extravascular removal by monocyte/macrophage system.
- Intravascular hemolysis occurs when adsorbed antibodies (especially immunoglobulin [Ig] M) activate complement.
- Extravascular removal of RBCs occurs when RBCs coated with antibodies (especially IgG) are engulfed by splenic macrophages.
- RBC agglutination occurs when IgM or high titers of IgG cause RBC bridging.
- Nonregenerative IMHA caused by immune-mediated destruction of RBC precursors in bone marrow.

SYSTEMS AFFECTED

- Hemic/lymphatic/immune—destruction of RBCs, release of proinflammatory mediators, disseminated intravascular coagulation (DIC).
- Cardiovascular—signs of anemia, thromboembolism.
- Hepatobiliary—hyperbilirubinemia, icterus, bilirubinuria; centrilobular necrosis.
- Respiratory—tachypnea (secondary to anemia or inflammation), hypoxemia (pulmonary thromboembolism [PTE]).
- Integument—rare: cold-type IMHA causes necrosis of extremities and ear tips.

GENETICS

Cocker spaniels are at increased risk.

Blackwell's Five-Minute Veterinary Consult Clinical Companion: Small Animal Senior Care, First Edition. Edited by Heidi B. Lobprise.

Companion website: www.wiley.com/go/lobprise/Senior

INCIDENCE/PREVALENCE

Most common hemolytic anemia of dogs, relatively rare in cats.

GEOGRAPHIC DISTRIBUTION

Secondary IMHA may have higher prevalence where associated infectious diseases endemic; incidence may vary seasonally.

SIGNALMENT

Species

Dog and cat.

Breed Predilections

- Cocker spaniel, English springer spaniel, Old English sheepdog, Doberman pinscher, collie, bichon frise, miniature pinscher, Finnish spitz.
- Domestic shorthair cats.

Mean Age and Range

- Dogs—mean age: 5–6 years (range: 1–13 years).
  While the mean age of onset may not be in the senior life stage parameters, this condition requires life-long management and can be a critical factor in senior health.
- Cats—mean age: 2 years (range: 0.5–9 years).

Predominant Sex

- Female dogs at higher risk.
- Male cats overrepresented.

SIGNS

Historical Findings

- Lethargy/weakness/collapse.
- Anorexia.
- Dyspnea, tachypnea.
- Vomiting and/or diarrhea.
- Pigmenturia.
- Pica (cats).

Physical Examination Findings

- Pale mucous membranes, tachycardia, tachypnea.
- Splenomegaly/hepatomegaly.
- Icterus and pigmenturia (hemoglobin or bilirubin).
- Fever/lymphadenopathy.
- Systolic heart murmur.
- Petechiae, ecchymoses, or melena (if concurrent thrombocytopenia or DIC).

- Other findings possible (e.g., joint pain) when IMHA is component of systemic lupus erythematosus (SLE).
- Necrosis of extremities and ear tips in cold-type IMHA (rare).

CAUSES AND RISK FACTORS

Primary IMHA

Poorly characterized immune dysregulation.

Secondary IMHA

- Infectious causes—hemotrophic *Mycoplasma* spp., *Ehrlichia* spp., *Anaplasma phagocytophilum*, *Anaplasma platys*, *Babesia* spp., *Leishmaniasis*, *Dirofilaria immitis*, feline leukemia virus (FeLV), feline immunodeficiency virus (FIV), chronic bacterial infection.
- Neoplasia—lymphoma, lymphoid leukemia, hemangiosarcoma, hemophagocytic histiocytic sarcoma.
- Drugs—penicillins, cephalosporins, propylthiouracil, methimazole, sulfonamides.
- SLE.
- Neonatal isoerythrolysis.
- Dog erythrocyte antigen (DEA) incompatible blood transfusion.
- Vaccination, surgery, hormonal changes, or other stressful events hypothesized as potential triggers.

DIAGNOSIS

DIFFERENTIAL DIAGNOSIS

Dogs

- Toxicity (zinc, onions, garlic, naphthalene, skunk musk).
- Snake/spider envenomation (coral snakes, recluse spiders).
- Severe hypophosphatemia.
- Anemia due to hemorrhage, hemoperitoneum.
- Microangiopathic anemia due to splenic neoplasia or torsion.
- Pyruvate kinase or phosphofructokinase deficiency.

Cats

- Toxicity (acetaminophen, zinc, onions, garlic).
- Severe hypophosphatemia.
- Congenital feline porphyria.
- Increased osmotic fragility (Abyssinian, Somali).

CBC/BIOCHEMISTRY/URINALYSIS

- CBC—anemia, normal-to-high mean cell volume (MCV), spherocytosis, polychromasia, ghost cells, leukocytosis with neutrophilia and left shift, monocytosis; anemia nonregenerative in 30% of dogs and 50% of cats.
- Serum biochemistry—hyperbilirubinemia, high alanine aminotransferase (ALT).
- Urinalysis—hemoglobinuria, bilirubinuria.

OTHER LABORATORY TESTS

- Positive saline agglutination test.
- Direct antiglobulin (Coombs) test—positive in up to 75% of animals with IMHA.
- Reticulocytosis if regenerative.
- Thrombocytopenia—60% of dogs.
- Prolonged activated partial thromboplastin time (APTT), ±prolonged prothrombin time (PT), increased fibrin degradation products (FDP) and d-dimer, decreased antithrombin in animals with DIC.
- Blood smear—evidence of hematologic parasites.
- Infectious disease testing—especially *Babesia* spp. (serology, PCR), *Mycoplasma hemofelis* (PCR), other vector-borne pathogens.

IMAGING

Abdominal radiography, ultrasonography—hepatomegaly/splenomegaly, neoplasia.

DIAGNOSTIC PROCEDURES

Bone marrow aspirate to identify nonregenerative (RBC precursor-directed) IMHA or myelofibrosis in chronic cases.

PATHOLOGIC FINDINGS

- Hepatosplenomegaly, centrilobular hepatic necrosis.
- Splenic and hepatic extramedullary hematopoiesis.
- PTE and DIC.

TREATMENT

APPROPRIATE HEALTH CARE

- Inpatient intensive care during acute hemolytic crisis and if complications such as DIC, PTE, thrombocytopenia, gastrointestinal (GI) bleeding, or need for multiple transfusions occur.
- Outpatient when PCV stable, hemolysis controlled, and clinical signs of anemia resolved.

NURSING CARE

- Fluid therapy as needed.
- Packed RBCs (or whole blood), fresh frozen plasma (FFP) if coagulopathic.
- Oxygen therapy as needed.
- Monitor for complications.

CLIENT EDUCATION

- IMHA can be fatal and difficult to treat, with guarded prognosis.
- Lifelong maintenance therapy may be needed; side effects may be severe.
- Disease may recur.

SURGICAL CONSIDERATIONS

Splenectomy can be considered if medical management fails.

MEDICATIONS

DRUG(S) OF CHOICE

- Corticosteroids—prednisone 2–3 mg/kg/day PO; dexamethasone sodium phosphate (0.2–0.4 mg/kg IV q24h) can be used in patients unable to take oral medication.
- Adjunctive immunosuppressants (if poor response to corticosteroids or to avoid side effects of prednisone)—cyclosporine 5 mg/kg PO q12h, cats: 0.5–3 mg/kg PO q12h; mycophenolate mofetil 8–12 mg/kg PO/IV q12h; azathioprine 2 mg/kg PO q24h, can decrease to 0.5–1.0 mg/kg PO q48h after 3 weeks or if bone marrow suppression occurs, monitor for side effects; *do not use in cats.*
- Once PCV above 30%, decrease prednisone dosage to 1 mg/kg PO q12h; then taper by maximum rate of 25–50% per month over 3–6-month period, depending upon PCV and severity of side effects; additional immunosuppressant drugs may be tapered as well.
- For prevention of thromboembolism consider unfractionated heparin 150–300 U/kg SC q6–8h (dose adjusted based on APTT prolongation or measurement of anti-Xa activity) and/or clopidogrel 1–2 mg/kg PO q24h; low-molecular-weight heparins (enoxaparin 0.8 mg/kg SC q6–8h or dalteparin 150 U/kg SC q8h) or rivaroxaban (0.5–1.0 mg/kg PO q24h) may be considered in lieu of unfractionated heparin.
- Address underlying cause (secondary IMHA).
- Therapeutic plasma exchange/plasmapheresis may be useful adjunctive therapy.

CONTRAINDICATIONS

Anticoagulant medications should be used cautiously in patients with thrombocytopenia (<40,000 platelets/µL).

PRECAUTIONS

- Prednisone/prednisolone can cause signs of hyperadrenocorticism and may increase risk of PTE, pancreatitis, diabetes mellitus, secondary infection, gastric ulcers (consider gastric protectants).
- Immunosuppressive drugs can cause bone marrow suppression, secondary infection, pancreatitis (azathioprine), GI upset (cyclosporine, azathioprine, mycophenolate mofetil), gingival hyperplasia, papillomatosis (cyclosporine), infertility.

ALTERNATIVE DRUG(S)

- Chlorambucil—for cats, 0.1–0.2 mg/kg PO q24h initially, then q48h.
- Human IV immunoglobulin (hIVIG; 0.5–1 g/kg IV) in dogs not responding to other therapies.

FOLLOW-UP

PATIENT MONITORING

- Monitor heart rate, respiratory rate, body temperature frequently.
- Monitor for adverse reactions to treatment.
- If PTE suspected, CT angiography indicated for diagnosis; oxygenation can be assessed with pulse oximetry or arterial blood gas analysis.
- Initially, check packed cell volume (PCV) daily until stable, then every 1–2 weeks for 2 months; if still stable, recheck monthly for 6 months, then 2–4 times/year.
- CBC and reticulocyte count at least monthly; if neutrophil count falls <3000 cells/μL, discontinue cytotoxic drugs until count recovers; reinstitute at lower dosage.

PREVENTION/AVOIDANCE

Consider need for vaccination on case-by-case basis in dogs with IMHA; measurement of titers prior to elective vaccinations may be indicated.

POSSIBLE COMPLICATIONS

- Pulmonary/multiorgan thromboembolism.
- DIC.
- Centrilobular hepatic necrosis and renal tubular necrosis secondary to hypoxia.
- Infection secondary to immunosuppressive therapy.
- GI ulceration due to high-dose glucocorticoids.
- Iatrogenic hyperadrenocorticism.

EXPECTED COURSE AND PROGNOSIS

- Mortality—30–70% (dog), 24% (cat).
- Hyperbilirubinemia >5 mg/dL, autoagglutination, intravascular hemolysis, severe thrombocytopenia, hypoalbuminemia associated with poorer prognosis.
- Response to treatment may take weeks to months; nonregenerative IMHA may have more gradual onset than typical IMHA and be slower to respond to treatment. Most patients receive immunosuppressive therapy for 4–8 months.

MISCELLANEOUS

Abbreviations

- ALT = alanine aminotransferase
- APTT = activated partial thromboplastin time.
- DEA = dog erythrocyte antigen.
- DIC = disseminated intravascular coagulation.
- FDP = fibrin degradation products.
- FeLV = feline leukemia virus.
- FFP = fresh frozen plasma.
- FIV = feline immunodeficiency virus.
- GI = gastrointestinal.
- hIVIG = human IV immunoglobulin.
- Ig = immunoglobulin.
- IMHA = immune-mediated hemolytic anemia.
- MCV = mean cell volume.
- PCV = packed cell volume.
- PT = prothrombin time.
- PTE = pulmonary thromboembolism.
- RBC = red blood cell.
- SLE = systemic lupus erythematosus.

Suggested Reading

Garden OA, Kidd L, Mexas AM, et al. ACVIM consensus statement on the diagnosis of immune-mediated hemolytic anemia in dogs and cats. *J Vet Intern Med* 2019;33(2):313–334.

Kohn B, Weingart C, Eckmann V, et al. Primary immune-mediated hemolytic anemia in 19 cats: diagnosis, therapy, and outcome (1998–2004). *J Vet Intern Med* 2006;20:159–166.

Swann JW, Garden OA, Fellman CL, et al. ACVIM consensus statement on the treatment of immune-mediated hemolytic anemia in dogs. *J Vet Intern Med* 2019;33(3):1141–1172.

Author/editor: Heidi Lobprise
Topic adapted from Five Minute Veterinary Consultation, 7th edition, 2021
Original Topic: Anemia—Immune Mediated

Author: Bridget C. Garner
Consulting Editor: Melinda S. Camus

Chapter 46

Pemphigus

BASICS

DEFINITION

- A group of autoimmune dermatoses characterized by varying degrees of erosion, ulceration, crusting, pustule, and vesicle formation.
- Affects the skin and sometimes mucous membranes.
- Forms identified in animals—pemphigus foliaceus (PF), pemphigus erythematosus (PE), pemphigus vulgaris (PV), paraneoplastic pemphigus (PP), and panepidermal pustular pemphigus (PEP)/pemphigus vegetans (PVeg).

PATHOPHYSIOLOGY

- Tissue-bound autoantibody directed at intraepidermal cell antigens (desmoglein and desmocollin) and acetylcholine receptors is deposited within the intercellular spaces, causing epidermal cell separation and cell rounding (acantholysis).
- Severity of ulceration and disease—related to depth of autoantibody deposition within the skin.
- PF—autoantibody deposition in the superficial layers of the epidermis.
- PV—lesions more severe; auto-antibody deposition just above the basement membrane zone; rapidly leads to ulcer formation.
- The disease is typically considered to be idiopathic. Possible drug association has been proposed in dogs and cats with PF. Sunlight exposure is suspected to induce flares of PF and PE. Thymoma has been associated with pemphigus variants in dogs and cats.

SYSTEMS AFFECTED

Skin/exocrine

INCIDENCE/PREVALENCE

- PF—most common autoimmune skin disease in dogs and cats.
- PE—relatively common.
- PV/PP—more severe forms, much rarer than PF/PE.
- PEP/PVeg—rarest form; may represent a more severe variant of PF.

Blackwell's Five-Minute Veterinary Consult Clinical Companion: Small Animal Senior Care, First Edition. Edited by Heidi B. Lobprise.

Companion website: www.wiley.com/go/lobprise/Senior

SIGNALMENT

Species

Dogs and cats.

Breed Predilections

PF—Dogs: Akita, chow chow, dachshund, cocker spaniel, Labrador retriever, and English bulldog. Cats: possibly short-haired and Siamese.

Mean Age and Range

Usually middle-aged-to-old animals.

Predominant Sex

None reported.

SIGNS

PF

- Scales, crust, pustules, epidermal collarettes, erosions, erythema, alopecia, and footpad hyperkeratosis with fissuring.
- Common involvement—head, face, ears, and footpads.
- Most cases develop extensive disease within one month.
- Nasal depigmentation may develop, but this is a late event.
- Head and facial distribution is an important distinction from a staphylococcal pyoderma.
- Cats—nipple and ungual fold involvement common.
- Lymphadenopathy, edema, depression, fever, and lameness (if footpads involved) when severe or generalized.
- Variable pain and pruritus.
- Secondary bacterial infection possible.

PE

- May be a variant of PF or a crossover between PF and discoid lupus erythematosus (DLE).
- Dogs and cats—pustules, erosions, and crusts on face and pinnae. Along with depigmentation, erythema and erosion/ulceration of the nasal planum and dorsal muzzle. Rare patients exhibit nonfacial lesions.
- Depigmentation more common than with other pemphigus forms, often precedes crusting.

PV/PP

- Oral cavity lesions frequent and may precede skin lesions.
- Initially vesiculobullous lesions rapidly progressing to ulcerations and erosions.
- More severe than PF and PE.
- Affects mucous membranes, mucocutaneous junctions, and skin; may become generalized.
- Footpads and ungual folds may be involved, with resultant onychomadesis.
- Positive Nikolsky sign (new or extended erosive lesion created when lateral pressure is applied to the skin near an existing lesion).
- Variable pruritus and pain.

- Anorexia, depression, and fever.
- Secondary bacterial infections common.

PEP/PVeg

- Pustule groups become eruptive papillomatous lesions with exudation.
- No oral involvement.
- No systemic illness.

DIAGNOSIS

DIFFERENTIAL DIAGNOSIS

PF

- Superficial pyoderma.
- Dermatophytosis.
- Demodicosis.
- Candidiasis.
- Keratinization disorders.
- Cutaneous lupus erythematosus or DLE.
- PE.
- Subcorneal pustular dermatosis.
- Drug eruption.
- Zinc-responsive dermatitis.
- Dermatomyositis.
- Tyrosinemia.
- Mycosis fungoides.
- Metabolic epidermal necrosis.
- Linear IgA dermatosis.

PE

- PF
- DLE.
- Mucocutaneous pyoderma.
- Demodicosis.
- Dermatophytosis.
- Epidermolysis bullosa simplex.
- Uveodermatologic syndrome.

PV/PP

- Subepidermal blistering diseases.
- Systemic lupus erythematosus.
- Toxic epidermal necrolysis.
- Drug eruption.
- Mycosis fungoides.
- Ulcerative stomatitis causes.
- Erythema multiforme.

PEP/PVeg

- PF.
- PV.
- Superficial pyoderma.
- Lichenoid dermatoses.

CBC/BIOCHEMISTRY/URINALYSIS

- Abnormalities uncommon.
- Leukocytosis and hyperglobulinemia with chronicity and/or secondary infection.

OTHER LABORATORY TESTS

Antinuclear antibody—may be weakly positive in PE only.

DIAGNOSTIC PROCEDURES

- Cytology of pustules—aspirates or impression smears from pustules or under crusts: acantholytic keratinocytes (rounded and deeply staining isolated keratinocytes) and neutrophils; occasionally with eosinophils.
- Biopsy of pustules or crusted lesions (submit crusts with the biopsy samples of the skin).

PATHOLOGIC FINDINGS

- Histopathology:
  - PF—subcorneal pustules with acantholytic cells and neutrophils; eosinophils often present; follicles may be involved.
  - PE—intragranular and subcorneal pustules, eosinophils, neutrophils, lichenoid interface dermatitis.
  - PV—suprabasilar intraepidermal cleft with the remaining basal cells exhibiting a tombstone appearance.
  - PP—suprabasilar clefting with interface dermatitis and apoptotic keratinocytes.
  - PEP/PVeg—pustules present throughout the epidermal layers and includes follicular epithelium.
- Immunopathology of biopsied skin via immunofluorescent antibody assays or immunohistochemical testing—may demonstrate positive staining in the intercellular spaces in 50–90% of cases; results can be affected by concurrent or previous corticosteroid (or other immunosuppressive drug) administration; indirect immunofluorescence usually negative; PE may demonstrate staining of basement membranes and intercellular spaces.

TREATMENT

APPROPRIATE HEALTH CARE

- Initial inpatient supportive therapy for severely affected patients.
- Outpatient treatment with initial frequent hospital visits (every 1–3 weeks); taper to every 1–3 months when remission is achieved and the patient is on a maintenance medical regimen.

NURSING CARE

Severely affected patients may require antibiotics and hydrotherapy/soaks.

CLIENT EDUCATION

Sun avoidance/use of sunblock—ultraviolet light may exacerbate lesions (PF and PE).

MEDICATIONS

DRUG(S) OF CHOICE

PF

Corticosteroids—Dogs

- Prednisone or prednisolone 2 mg/kg/day PO divided q12h to initiate control. An attempt to reduce this dose should be made when the disease undergoes remission.
- Minimum maintenance—0.5 mg/kg PO q48h to twice weekly.
- High pulse therapy—10 mg/kg once daily for three consecutive days, followed by standard dosage (<2 mg/kg/day). Pulses can be repeated if new lesions continue to appear in spite of the lower doses. Pulse should not be repeated more than once weekly.

Corticosteroids—Cats

- Prednisolone—2 mg/kg/day until clinical resolution. Majority of cats achieve disease control with corticosteroids monotherapy.

Cytotoxic Agents

- Most patients require additional immuno-modulating drugs.
- Work synergistically with corticosteroids to allow reduction in dose and side effects.
- Azathioprine 1.5–2.5 mg/kg PO q24h, then q48h. Recommended for canine cases that fail to achieve adequate control with glucocorticoids alone (dogs only; potential for marked bone marrow suppression in cats).
- Chlorambucil 0.1–0.2 mg/kg every other day; best option for cats with disease control that is not achieved with corticosteroid monotherapy.
- Cyclosporine 5–10 mg/kg PO q24h; variable efficacy in dogs and cats.
- Mycophenolate mofetil 10–20 mg/kg twice daily.

PE

- Oral prednisone or prednisolone 1.1 mg/kg PO q24h; then q48h; then to the lowest maintenance dose possible; may be stopped when in remission.
- Topical steroids may be sufficient in mild cases.
- Topical tacrolimus.

PV

- Aggressive therapy with corticosteroids and azathioprine or chlorambucil + systemic antibiotic therapy.

PP

- Aggressive therapy with corticosteroids and azathioprine or chlorambucil ± systemic antibiotic therapy.
- Identification and treatment or removal of underlying neoplasia.

PEP/PVeg

- Treatment similar to PF.
- Response more variable; some patients may achieve remission with conservative treatment.

PRECAUTIONS

- Corticosteroids—polyuria, polydipsia, polyphagia, temperament changes, diabetes mellitus, pancreatitis, and hepatotoxicity.
- Azathioprine—pancreatitis, bone marrow suppression.
- Cytotoxic drugs—leukopenia, thrombocytopenia, nephrotoxicity, hepatotoxicity, and gastrointestinal upset.
- Immunosuppression—can predispose animal to demodicosis, cutaneous and systemic bacterial and fungal infection.

ALTERNATIVE DRUG(S)

Alternative Corticosteroids

- Use instead of prednisone if undesirable side effects or poor response noted.
- Methylprednisolone 0.8–1.5 mg/kg PO q12h; for patients that tolerate prednisone poorly.
- Triamcinolone or dexamethasone 0.2–0.3 mg/kg PO q12h; then 0.05–0.1 mg/kg q48–72h.

Topical Steroids

- Hydrocortisone cream.
- Potent topical corticosteroids—0.1% betamethasone valerate, fluocinolone acetonide, or 0.1% triamcinolone; q12h; then q24–48h.

Miscellaneous

- PF cases—doxycycline 5 mg/kg twice daily and niacinamide 500 mg twice daily for dogs >10 kg; 250 mg for dogs <10 kg.

FOLLOW-UP

PATIENT MONITORING

- Monitor response to therapy.
- Monitor for medication side effects—routine hematology and serum biochemistry, especially patients on high doses of corticosteroids and cytotoxic drugs; check every 1–3 weeks, then every 1–3 months when in remission.

EXPECTED COURSE AND PROGNOSIS

PV and PF

- Dogs—poor (PV/PP) to fair (PF/PEP): life-long or long-term therapy with corticosteroids and cytotoxic drugs usually needed; good (PE): relatively benign and self-limiting.
- Cats—good (PF), but long-term treatment required, tendency to relapse spontaneously or with treatment changes.
- Regular monitoring necessary.
- Side effects of medications may affect quality of life.
- May be fatal if untreated (especially PV).
- Secondary infections cause morbidity and possible mortality (especially PV).

MISCELLANEOUS

Abbreviations

- DLE = discoid lupus erythematosus
- PE = pemphigus erythematosus.
- PEP/PVeg = panepidermal pustular pemphigus/pemphigus vegetans.
- PF = pemphigus foliaceus.
- PP = paraneoplastic pemphigus.
- PV = pemphigus vulgaris.

Suggested Reading

Ackermann AL, May ER, Frank LA. Use of mycophenolate mofetil to treat immune-mediated skin disease in 14 dogs: a retrospective evaluation. *Vet Dermatol* 2017;28:195–e44.

Bizikova P, Burrows A. Feline pemphigus foliaceus: original case series and a comprehensive literature review. *BMC Vet* 2019;15:22.

Bizikova P, Olivry T. Oral glucocorticoid pulse therapy for induction of treatment of canine pemphigus foliaceus—a comparative study. *Vet Dermatol* 2015;26:354, e77.

Helton Rhodes KA, Werner A. *Blackwell's Five-Minute Veterinary Consult: Clinical Companion: Small Animal Dermatology*, 3rd edn. Hoboken, NJ: Wiley-Blackwell, 2018.

Author/editor: Heidi Lobprise
Topic adapted from Five Minute Veterinary Consultation, 7th edition, 2021
Original Topic: Pemphigus

Author: Clarissa P. Souza
Consulting Editor: Alexander H. Werner Resnick

Chapter 47

Perianal Fistula

BASICS

OVERVIEW

Chronic inflammatory condition characterized by multiple, painful, progressive, ulcerating sinuses or, less frequently, true fistulous tracts involving the perianal region.

SIGNALMENT

- Dog.
- German shepherd dogs primarily; Irish setters.
- Mean age: 5–7 years; range: 7 months–14 years.
  While the mean age of onset may not be in the senior life stage parameters, this condition requires life-long management and can be a critical factor in senior health.
- Males more commonly affected.

SIGNS

- Dyschezia.
- Tenesmus.
- Hematochezia.
- Constipation.
- Diarrhea.
- Malodorous mucopurulent anal discharge.
- Ulceration of the perianal skin with sinus tract formation.
- Licking and self-mutilation.
- Reluctance to sit; posturing difficulties; personality changes.
- Pain on manipulation of tail and examination of perianal area.
- Fecal incontinence.
- Anorexia.
- Weight loss.

CAUSES AND RISK FACTORS

- Multifactorial immune-mediated mechanism is suspected.
- Appears to be an inappropriate T-cell mediated response.

Blackwell's Five-Minute Veterinary Consult Clinical Companion: Small Animal Senior Care,
First Edition. Edited by Heidi B. Lobprise.

Companion website: www.wiley.com/go/lobprise/Senior

- An association with colitis has also been proposed, particularly in German shepherd dogs.
- A genetic predisposition has been proposed but not proven.
- Low tail carriage and a broad-based tail may contribute in German shepherd dogs.
- High density of apocrine sweat glands in the cutaneous zone of the anal canal of German shepherd dogs.

DIAGNOSIS

DIFFERENTIAL DIAGNOSIS

- Other inflammatory processes—e.g., anusitis, hydradenitis suppurativa.
- Chronic anal sac abscess.
- Perianal adenoma or adenocarcinoma with ulceration and drainage.
- Squamous cell carcinoma.
- Atypical bacterial infection.
- Oomycosis.
- Rectal fistula.

CBC/BIOCHEMISTRY/URINALYSIS

- Usually unremarkable.
- May have an inflammatory leukogram.

DIAGNOSTIC PROCEDURES

- Presumptive diagnosis—clinical signs and physical examination.
- Definitive diagnosis—biopsy of the affected area.
- Colonoscopy with biopsy—may reveal associated colitis.

TREATMENT

- Outpatient medical therapy recommended initially in all cases.
- Clipping and cleaning the perianal area facilitates local therapy.
- Bathing with an antimicrobial shampoo may be helpful.
- Dietary modification—strictly enforced hydrolyzed or novel protein elimination diet.
- Stool softeners—with pain or tenesmus.
- Surgery is considered for patients with incomplete resolution following appropriate medical therapy.
- Anal sacculectomy—if anal sac involvement.
- Surgical options—resection of inflammatory tissue and/or ablation of remaining sinuses with carbon dioxide laser is preferred.
- Surgical debridement (deroofing) with fulguration by chemical cautery or electrocautery; surgical resection followed by primary closure or second intention healing are other options.
- Radical excision of the rectal ring with modified rectal pull-through is rarely necessary and is associated with a higher risk of fecal incontinence.

MEDICATIONS

DRUG(S) OF CHOICE

- Cyclosporine (CsA) ± ketoconazole is treatment of choice but is expensive
  - Ketaconazole reduces dose of cyclosporine required by inhibiting CsA-metabolizing enzymes:
  - Give CsA orally at 1–5 mg/kg/day PO and ketoconazole at 5–10 mg/kg/day PO and then taper CsA as clinical signs resolve.
  - Continue treatment at least 4 weeks after complete resolution of fistula(e). Many patients require chronic treatment at reduced frequency to prevent recurrence.
- Tacrolimus (0.1% ointment) topically as maintenance therapy may be sufficient to control lesions; begin application as dose of oral medications is reduced:
  - Apply q12h with gloved hand, then taper to q24–72h.
- Oral prednisone and topical tacrolimus appear to be efficacious and economical in less severe cases:
  - Prednisone 2 mg/kg PO q24h for 2 weeks, decrease to 1 mg/kg q24h for 4 weeks and then 1 mg/kg q48h for 10 weeks.
  - Tacrolimus 0.1% ointment as above.
  - Chronic maintenance therapy with tacrolimus and possibly prednisone likely necessary for long-term control.
- Azathioprine alone or combined with prednisone is another treatment option.

ALTERNATIVE DRUG(S)

- Analgesics may be necessary.
- Metronidazole 10 mg/kg q12h for 2 weeks at initiation of therapy to control secondary infection.

FOLLOW-UP

PATIENT MONITORING

- Assess CsA trough levels if improvement is not seen or if toxicity is suspected.
- Reexamine to assess healing, signs of recurrence, and associated complications.

POSSIBLE COMPLICATIONS

- Reversible alopecia.
- Vomiting, diarrhea, anorexia.
- Weight loss.
- Recurrence.
- Failure to heal.
- Surgical dehiscence.
- Tenesmus.
- Fecal incontinence.
- Anal stricture.

- Flatulence.
- Iatrogenic Cushing's disease from corticosteroids.
- Gingival hyperplasia from CsA.

EXPECTED COURSE AND PROGNOSIS

- Guarded for complete resolution except in mildly affected patients.
- Chronic treatment may be necessary.

MISCELLANEOUS

Associated Conditions

- Colitis.
- Constipation and/or obstipation may develop.

Abbreviations

- CsA = cyclosporine

Suggested Reading

Fallipowicz D. Nonsurgical management of perianal fistulae. In: Bojrab MJ, Waldron D, Tombs JR (eds) *Currrent Techniques in Small Animal Surgery*, 5th edn. Jackson, KY: Teton Newmedia, 2014; pp. 309–315.

Pieper J, McKay L. Perianal fistulas. *Compend Contin Educ Vet* 2011;33(9):E4.

Author/editor: Heidi Lobprise
Topic adapted from Five Minute Veterinary Consultation, 7th edition, 2021
Original Topic: Perianal Fistula

Author: Eric R. Pope
Consulting Editor: Mark P. Rondeau

Chapter 48

Polyarthritis, Erosive, Immune-Mediated

BASICS

DEFINITION

- An autoimmune disease of the joint that results in destruction of articular cartilage, subchondral bone, and surrounding ligaments. This damage can result in joint instability, laxity, and deformation with chronicity.
- Canine syndromes:
  - Rheumatoid arthritis—antibody response against rheumatoid factors or autoantibodies that results in severe damage to the articular cartilage, periarticular bone, and ligaments.
  - Felty's syndrome—constellation of arthritis, neutropenia, and splenomegaly.
  - Erosive polyarthritis of greyhounds—minimal subchondral changes despite necrosis of the articular cartilage and proliferative synovitis; peripheral lymphadenopathy.
- Feline erosive polyarthritis:
  - Periosteal proliferative polyarthritis—acute onset of pain and systemic manifestations (fever, lymphadenopathy) related to arthropathy with prolific periarticular periosteal bone formation.
  - Feline rheumatoid arthritis—insidious development of joint deformity accompanied by less systemic illness and periosteal bone formation.

PATHOPHYSIOLOGY

- Immune-complex deposition within the synovial membrane results in an inflammatory response (involving complement and cytokines) leading to cartilage erosion.
  - Release of matrix-degrading enzymes (metalloproteases) responsible for cartilage destruction. Chronic synovitis results in a pannus, or granulation tissue, across the articular cartilage that extends into subchondral bone, replacing areas of destruction.
  - Destruction of joint ligaments leads to joint instability and luxation.

SYSTEMS AFFECTED

Musculoskeletal

Blackwell's Five-Minute Veterinary Consult Clinical Companion: Small Animal Senior Care,
First Edition. Edited by Heidi B. Lobprise.

Companion website: www.wiley.com/go/lobprise/Senior

GENETICS

No genetic predisposition known.

INCIDENCE/PREVALENCE

- Uncommon to rare.
- Nonerosive disease more common.

SIGNALMENT

Species

Dog and cat.

Breed Predilections

- More common in small-breed dogs; Shetland sheepdogs, cocker spaniels, collies appear more affected.
- Siamese cats.

Mean Age and Range

- Canine—middle age (3–9.5 years).
- Feline—bimodal distribution of young adults and middle-aged to older cats.

While this primarily affects middle-aged dogs, in larger dogs, once identified, it needs life-long management.

Predominant Sex

- Feline—predominantly male.
- Dogs—none.

SIGNS

General Comments

- Typically affects more distal joints (carpus, elbow, stifle, and tarsal joints more frequently, digital joints and vertebral column may be affected).
- Clinically, it can appear as though only one joint is affected.
- Evaluate cats for causes of reactive polyarthritis (septic arthritis, systemic infection, and neoplasia).

Historical Findings

- Progressive, intermittent, or shifting-leg lameness.
- Reluctance to walk or stand, inappetence, and weight loss.

Physical Examination Findings

- Pain and/or effusion detected on palpation of one or more joints.
- Deformation, instability, and luxation of the joint is unique to erosive (as compared to non-erosive) arthritis; occurs with chronicity. May be associated with cranial cruciate ligament rupture (CCLR).

- Stiffness on gait evaluation, decreased range of motion, and muscle atrophy
- Pyrexia and/or peripheral lymphadenopathy.
- Cats may resent handling. May present with acute signs or may be more insidious over weeks to months.

CAUSES

- Underlying etiology has yet to be identified.
- Canine distemper virus within synovial fluid can result in sustained inflammation within the joint possibly predisposing a dog to erosive arthritis.
- Feline leukemia virus (FeLV) and feline syncytium-forming virus are associated with feline periosteal proliferative polyarthritis (FPPP), but causation has not been shown.

RISK FACTORS

None currently known.

DIAGNOSIS

DIFFERENTIAL DIAGNOSIS

- Other causes of arthropathy—infectious arthritis, degenerative joint disease, neoplasia (e.g., synovial cell sarcoma), hemarthrosis, congenital arthropathies (elbow dysplasia, osteochondrosis dissecans), tick-borne disease.
- Hypertrophic osteodystrophy.
- Panosteitis.
- Polymyositis.
- Steroid-responsive meningitis-arteritis.
- Systemic lupus erythematosus (SLE).
- Reactive polyarthritis due to antigenic stimulation from systemic disease.
- Drug-induced polyarthritis (sulfa drugs, phenobarbital, erythropoietin, penicillins, cephalosporins, vaccines).
- Trauma.

CBC/BIOCHEMISTRY/URINALYSIS

- Hemogram—a mild, non-regenerative anemia and mild leukocytosis may be present although hemogram can be unremarkable.
- Chemistry—hyperglobulinemia may be present.
- Urinalysis and urine culture—generally unremarkable. Proteinuria should be quantified with a UPC.

OTHER LABORATORY TESTS

- Synovial fluid analysis—aseptic, neutrophilic, or mixed inflammation with greater than 10% non-degenerate neutrophils:
  - Protein concentration often >3.0 g/dL and total nucleated cell count (TNCC) usually >3000 cells/μL (not associated with severity).
  - Make a direct smear prior to lab submission.

- Synovial fluid culture (bacteria and mycoplasma)—negative results do not entirely rule out septic arthritis.
- Antinuclear antibody titers—usually negative, unlikely to be clinically useful unless SLE suspected.
- Rheumatoid factor testing—positive test is supportive only when erosive disease is present; other causes of joint disease can elevate rheumatoid factor levels:
  Positive results seen in cats with rheumatoid arthritis, not in FPPP.
- Testing for infectious diseases (tick-borne disease (*Borrelia*, *Ehrlichia*, *Rickettsia*), FeLV/feline immunodeficiency virus (FIV) testing, systemic mycoses, *Leishmania* if endemic, blood and urine culture, ±echocardiogram for bacterial endocarditis.
- CSF collection, serum creatine kinase, and direct Coombs' testing can be considered on an individual basis to evaluate for systemic diseases.

IMAGING

- Joints:
  - Imaging of multiple joints is recommended; initial radiographs may be unremarkable without obvious change for 6 or more months.
  - Progressive disease results in subchondral bone lysis, irregular joint surface, and narrowing or widening of the joint space, calcification of soft tissues around the joint, and extensive bone destruction.
  - Cats can have periosteal new bone formation and enthesophytes.
- Thoracic and vertebral radiographs with abdominal ultrasound can help rule out reactive polyarthritis.

DIAGNOSTIC PROCEDURES

Arthrocentesis (joint tap): four joints should be sampled.

PATHOLOGIC FINDINGS

- Grossly, the synovium can be discolored, thickened, and ulcerated with extension of granulation tissue into the subchondral bone.
- Histopathology of synovial membrane is rarely necessary, but may reveal synovial hypertrophy and hyperplasia, necrosis, and mononuclear inflammation (often lymphoplasmacytic).

TREATMENT

APPROPRIATE HEALTH CARE

Outpatient

NURSING CARE

Larger dogs may require more assistance and support during treatment.

ACTIVITY

Strict rest is recommended while symptomatic and painful.

DIET

No dietary restrictions.

CLIENT EDUCATION

- Management is lifelong.
- Erosive disease is often progressive and less responsive to treatment.
- Importance of weight management.

SURGICAL CONSIDERATIONS

- Arthrodesis (primarily carpal) has been used for joint luxation to improve quality of life.
- Surgical repair of CCLR if necessary.
- Synovectomy, arthroplasty, or joint replacement can be considered.
- Splenectomy as last resort in Felty's syndrome.

MEDICATIONS

DRUG(S) OF CHOICE

Antibiotics

- Doxycycline or minocycline recommended in cats and dogs while infectious disease testing is pending.
- Tylosin trial in greyhounds for mycoplasma.

Dogs

Initial Therapy

- Prednisone or prednisolone 1–2 mg/kg/day or 50 mg/m^2, until remission encountered (often 4 weeks), then taper.
- Cyclosporine 5 mg/kg PO q12—suitable alternative to corticosteroids.

Combination Therapy

Can be helpful to achieve remission, allow for tapering of corticosteroids and aid in refractory cases; each can be combined with corticosteroids:

- Mycophenolate mofetil 10 mg/kg PO q12h; taper by 50% after 2–3 weeks or if hemorrhagic gastrointestinal signs noted.
- Leflunomide 3–4 mg/kg PO q24h; allow 4–6 weeks before decreasing dose to every 48 hours then every 72 hours.
- Azathioprine 1.6–2 mg/kg PO q24h for 2 weeks or until remission, then taper to every 48 hours.
- Other immunosuppressives to consider include chlorambucil, cyclophosphamide, levamisole, methotrexate.

Cats

- Prednisolone 2 mg/kg PO q12h followed by a taper; ~50% of cats with FPPP show improvement in signs and slowing of progression when used with analgesia.
- 58% of cats improved using a protocol of methotrexate + leflunomide: methotrexate 2.5 mg/cat PO q12h for three consecutive doses (7.5 mg/24 hours) repeated weekly until improvement then 2.5 mg/cat PO weekly; leflunomide 10 mg/cat PO q24h until improvement then 10 mg/cat PO twice weekly.
- Other immunosuppressive agents that can be considered include cyclosporine or chlorambucil.

Other

Omega-3 fatty acid supplementation.

Analgesia

Gabapentin 5–15 mg/kg PO q8–12h; amantadine 3–5 mg/kg PO q24h; nonsteroidal anti-inflammatory drug (NSAIDs) as appropriate if not using corticosteroids.

CONTRAINDICATIONS

Glucocorticoids should not be given with NSAIDs.

PRECAUTIONS

- Tapering immunosuppressive therapy too soon can lead to relapses.
- Confirm aseptic inflammation prior to initiating immunosuppressive therapy.
- Consider secondary immunosuppressive agent if unable to attain remission or if symptoms relapse while still on glucocorticoids.
- Monitor for infectious diseases and opportunistic infections.

POSSIBLE INTERACTIONS

Concurrent use of multiple immunosuppressives with the same mechanism of action.

FOLLOW-UP

PATIENT MONITORING

- Monitor for potential side effects of treatments (liver enzymes, hyperglycemia, etc.) and concurrent disorders (e.g., hematologic abnormalities and proteinuria) as necessary.
- Tapering of medications often possible after 4 weeks of therapy. A 50% taper every month or dose reduction of 25–30% every 2–3 weeks with a minimum of 4 months of therapy can be considered.
- If relapse occurs during taper, increase corticosteroid to the most recent effective dose and/or consider a second agent, if not already utilized.
- If relapse occurs after the taper, a short course of corticosteroid and the dose of the second agent that maintained clinical control can be utilized long term.

- Serial or repeated arthrocentesis can be performed to rule out poor control of immune-mediated disease in cases of ongoing or recurrent lameness. In some dogs, this may identify degenerative joint disease as the cause of lameness rather than relapse of polyarthritis.

EXPECTED COURSE AND PROGNOSIS

- Erosive disease is typically progressive; ~50% of cats will improve with good quality of life.
- Monitoring recommended if initially nonerosive.
- Tick-borne disease usually responds to appropriate antibiotic therapy within 7 days.

MISCELLANEOUS

See Also

- Osteoarthritis—Degenerative Joint Disease

Abbreviations

- CCLR = cranial cruciate ligament rupture
- FeLV = feline leukemia virus.
- FIV = feline immunodeficiency virus.
- FPPP = feline periosteal proliferative polyarthritis.
- SLE = systemic lupus erythematosus.
- TNCC = total nucleated cell count.

Suggested Reading

Lemetayer J, Taylor S. Inflammatory joint disease in cats: diagnostic approach and treatment. *J Feline Med Surg* 2014;16(7):547–562.

Shaughnessy M, Sample S, Abicht C, et al. Clinical features and pathological joint changes in dogs with erosive immune-mediated polyarthritis: 13 cases (2004–2012). *J Am Vet Med Assoc* 2016;249(10):1156–1164.

Author/Editor: Heidi Lobprise
Topic adapted from Five Minute Veterinary Consultation, 7th edition, 2021
Original Topic: Obesity

Author: J.D. Foster
Consulting Editor: Mathieu M. Glassman

Chapter 49

Polyarthritis, Non-Erosive, Immune-Mediated, Dogs

BASICS

DEFINITION

- Nonerosive polyarthritis—a non-infectious inflammatory disease of multiple (>2) joints without radiographic evidence of bone or cartilage involvement.
- Most common polyarthropathy in dogs, idiopathic or type I immune-mediated polyarthritis (IMPA).
- Reactive polyarthropathy, where inflammation in the joints is secondary to distant disease, includes types II, III, and IV—disease is secondary to chronic inflammatory or infectious disease, chronic gastrointestinal disease, and neoplasia, respectively.
- Systemic lupus erythematosus (SLE), familial shar-pei fever (FSF), and familial juvenile-onset polyarthritis of Akitas are less common nonerosive polyarthritides.

PATHOPHYSIOLOGY

- All causes of nonerosive polyarthritis are immune-mediated.
- Immune complex deposition is the underlying mechanism in idiopathic IMPA (type I) and reactive polyarthropathy (types II, III, and IV).
- Reactive polyarthropathy involves immune stimulus distant to the joints due to underlying infectious, inflammatory, or neoplastic disease, as well as adverse drug reactions, with subsequent immune complex deposition in the synovium.
- SLE is the result of immune complex deposition secondary to autoantibodies (antinuclear antibodies [ANA]) formed against tissue proteins and DNA.
- FSF is the result of amyloid deposition in the synovium.

SYSTEMS AFFECTED

- Musculoskeletal:
    - Appendicular joints are more commonly affected than axial joints. Intervertebral joints are not usually affected.
    - Distal joints (carpus, tarsus) are more commonly affected than proximal joints (stifle, shoulder, coxofemoral) in IMPA.
    - The hock joints are typically affected in FSF.

Blackwell's Five-Minute Veterinary Consult Clinical Companion: Small Animal Senior Care, First Edition. Edited by Heidi B. Lobprise.

Companion website: www.wiley.com/go/lobprise/Senior

- Hemic/lymphatic/immune:
  - Immune stimulus may result in fever, lethargy, and poor appetite.
  - Hemolytic anemia and thrombocytopenia may be present in SLE.
- Skin/exocrine:
  - Immune-mediated skin disease targeting the mucocutaneous junctions is common in SLE.
- Renal/urologic:
  - Immune-complex deposition in the kidneys and protein-losing nephropathy may be present in SLE.
  - Glomerulonephropathy and proteinuria secondary to amyloidosis may occur in FSF.

GENETICS

MTBP gene missense mutation is believed to be responsible for FSF.

INCIDENCE/PREVALENCE

- Idiopathic IMPA is common in dogs.
- Reactive polyarthritis accounts for only 25% of nonerosive polyarthritis cases in dogs.
- IMPA is rare in cats.

SIGNALMENT

Species

Dog and cat.

Breed Predilections

- Large-breed dogs, such as Labrador retrievers, golden retrievers, Rottweilers, Irish setters, Shetland sheepdogs, cocker spaniels, and American Eskimo dogs are over-represented for idiopathic IMPA.
- Doberman pinschers are overreported in cases of polyarthropathy secondary to sulfonamide administration.

Mean Age and Range

Mean age: 4–6 years old, range: 6 months to 12 years.

While the mean age is 4–6 years old, in larger dogs, this is near the senior life stage; once identified, it needs life-long management.

Predominant Sex

None reported.

SIGNS

Historical Findings

- Shifting limb lameness, stiff gait, reluctance to walk, exercise intolerance
- Fever.
- Lethargy.
- Inappetence.
- Lymphadenopathy.

Physical Examination Findings

- Joint pain and effusion.
- Fever.
- Lameness.

CAUSES

- Type I IMPA—idiopathic.
- Immune-mediated dermatopathy and hepatopathy are among the most common noninfectious causes of type II IMPA.
    - Infectious sources to consider include endocarditis, discospondylitis, prostatitis, deep pyoderma, and systemic infections (fungal, protozoal).
    - Drugs implicated in adverse drug reaction-related polyarthropathy (type II) include human albumin, erythropoeitin, phenobarbital, and antibiotics such as sulfonamides, cephalosporins, penicillins, lincosamides, and macrolides. This should be considered a potential cause when administered 5–20 days prior to the onset of signs.
    - Reports of postvaccinal polyarthropathy have included canine distemper and Lyme vaccines, typically within 30 days of vaccine administration.
- Type III IMPA occurs secondary to chronic gastrointestinal disease such as inflammatory bowel disease, but is rare.
- Type IV IMPA has been reported secondary to renal carcinoma, mammary carcinoma, leiomyoma, Sertoli cell tumor, and seminoma.

DIAGNOSIS

DIFFERENTIAL DIAGNOSIS

- Infectious polyarthritis, including rickettsial disease, *Mycoplasma*, bacterial, and fungal etiologies:
    - *Borrelia burgdorferi*, *Anaplasma phagocytophilum*, *Rickettsia rickettsii*, *Ehrlichia canis*, *Ehrlichia ewingii*, and *Ehrlichia chaffeensis* are among the rickettsial diseases that should be considered for polyarthropathy.
- Leishmaniasis should be considered, particularly in instances of significant systemic involvement, presence of skin lesions, and/or history of travel to the Mediterranean/southern Europe, Africa, India, or South America within the past 7 years.
- Panosteitis and hypertrophic osteodystrophy should be considered, particularly in young dogs with lameness and fever.
- Degenerative joint disease (DJD) should be considered in middle-age-to-older animals.
- Viral etiologies have been implicated as a cause of polyarthritis in cats, including feline calicivirus and feline coronavirus associated with feline infectious peritonitis.

CBC/BIOCHEMISTRY/URINALYSIS

- CBC—mild non-regenerative anemia and mild leukocytosis; leukopenia is also possible. Presence of thrombocytopenia may be suggestive of tick-borne disease or when severe, SLE.

- Chemistry—often normal, except when distant (reactive polyarthropathy) or polysystemic disease (SLE) is present.
- Urinalysis—proteinuria may be present and should prompt obtaining a UPC.

OTHER LABORATORY TESTS

- Definitive diagnosis can be obtained by arthrocentesis and cytology of multiple joints.
- Aerobic and anerobic joint culture to definitively exclude septic arthritis in all cases; sensitivity is ~50% and can be improved with broth-enrichment media and incubation prior to culture.
- Fungal cultures of joint fluid may be considered, though direct joint involvement is rare.
- Mycoplasmal PCR or culture of synovial fluid may be considered, with PCR being more sensitive.
- Tick PCR panels to exclude rickettsial disease should be performed in all cases. Quantitative serology may be considered, but positive results may lag behind onset of clinical signs, and false-negative results are common. Qualitative tests for antibody production, including SNAP ELISA tests, may be indicated in cases with high index of clinical suspicion for rickettsial diseases such as Lyme disease.
- Serologic fungal titers may be considered where fungal disease is endemic or there has been travel history to rule it out as a cause of reactive polyarthropathy.
- Blood and urine cultures should be considered to exclude bacterial causes of reactive polyarthropathy in cases where no obvious infectious or inflammatory focus is identified. Positive blood cultures may be indicative of primary septic polyarthritis of hematogenous origin given relatively low sensitivity of bacterial culture of synovial fluid.
- C-reactive protein (CRP) can be measured as a nonspecific indicator of inflammation and reassessed for response to therapy.
- ANA titer may be submitted in cases where there is multisystemic immune-mediated involvement.

IMAGING

- Appendicular radiographs including affected joints are necessary to exclude erosive causes of polyarthropathy, though these diseases are uncommon in dogs and may not be radiographically visible initially. Absence of palpable joint effusion should not preclude recommendation to obtain radiographs in cases where clinical suspicion is otherwise suggestive of polyarthritis and screening radiographs of multiple joints should be obtained.
- Joint effusion is the main radiographic finding. Radiographic signs of osteoarthritis may be concurrently present and do not exclude nonerosive polyarthritis as a diagnosis.
- Thoracic radiography, abdominal ultrasonography, and echocardiography should ideally be performed to assess for causes of reactive polyarthropathy.

DIAGNOSTIC PROCEDURES

- Arthrocentesis should be performed aseptically on 3–5 joints for synovial fluid collection, under sedation or general anesthesia.
- Synovial biopsy can be used for confirmation in challenging cases.

PATHOLOGIC FINDINGS

- Turbid ± reduced viscosity of synovial fluid, ±voluminous fluid.
- Synovial fluid cytology characterized by predominantly neutrophilic (>10%) inflammation without evidence of infectious agents in the synovial fluid.

TREATMENT

APPROPRIATE HEALTH CARE

- Typically outpatient therapy.
- Systemic signs (i.e., fever, inappetence) may necessitate hospitalized supportive care.

ACTIVITY

Activity restriction to avoid exacerbation of pain and lameness.

DIET

Weight reduction as applicable to avoid undue stress on joints.

CLIENT EDUCATION

Discuss failure to control clinical signs, particularly in cases where underlying disease cannot be eliminated, and possibility or recurrence and/or need for lifelong medication and monitoring.

MEDICATIONS

DRUG(S) OF CHOICE

- Immunosuppressive dose of steroids, i.e., prednisone (dog) or prednisolone (cat): 2 mg/kg/day PO for 4 weeks, then gradually tapered over at least 4 months unless combination immunosuppressive protocols are used.
- Nonsteroidal anti-inflammatory drugs (NSAIDs) for FSF, i.e., carprofen 2.2 mg/kg PO twice daily.

PRECAUTIONS

Consider risks and complications of prolonged steroid courses, including immunosuppression, diabetes mellitus, risk for congestive heart failure, and muscle-wasting.

POSSIBLE INTERACTIONS

NSAIDs and steroids should not be given together due to increased risk of gastrointestinal ulceration; a 7-day washout period is indicated between medications.

ALTERNATIVE DRUG(S)

- Cyclosporine—dog: 5 mg/kg PO twice daily; cat: 4 mg/kg PO twice daily.
- Mycophenolate mofetil—dog: 10 mg/kg PO or IV twice daily.
- Leflunomide—dog: 2–4 mg/kg PO once daily; cat: 10 mg/cat PO once daily.
- Azathioprine—dog: 2 mg/kg PO once daily, tapered to 0.5–2 mg/kg PO every other day.
- Chlorambucil—dog: 1–2 mg/m² PO once daily; cat: 15 mg/m² PO once daily for 4 days once every 3 weeks or 2 mg/cat every other day.
- Cyclophosphamide—dog: 1.5 mg/kg PO when patient >25 kg, 2 mg/kg PO when patient 5–25 kg, 2.5 mg/kg PO when patient <5 kg every other day or 4 consecutive days of the week; cat: 2.5 mg/kg once daily.
- Analgesics may be considered for additional pain control (e.g., gabapentin (dog), 5–10 mg/kg PO twice daily).
- Given the disease is rare in cats, consider doxycycline 5 mg/kg PO twice daily for 14 days to treat infectious etiologies prior to initiating immunosuppression.

FOLLOW-UP

PATIENT MONITORING

- Repeat arthrocentesis may be considered for evaluation of response to treatment, especially prior to medication changes (i.e., at 4 weeks, prior to beginning steroid taper).
- CRP has a modest correlation to synovial fluid cytology and may be performed as a noninvasive means of patient monitoring.
- CRP and IL-6 may be used to distinguish recurrence of IMPA from osteoarthritis.

PREVENTION/AVOIDANCE

Avoid nonessential vaccination for prevention of recurrence. Canine distemper vaccine should not be given if seroprotective antibody titer levels are present.

POSSIBLE COMPLICATIONS

- Immunosuppression and risk of secondary infection, particularly when multiple immunosuppressive drugs are used.
- Subsequent DJD may occur following IMPA. Patients may show lameness when steroid therapy is tapered; however, most are afebrile.

EXPECTED COURSE AND PROGNOSIS

- Good prognosis for idiopathic IMPA with expected improvement in clinical signs within 7 days.
- Recurrence is possible and reported in almost 30% of cases.
- 10% of cases fail to respond to immunosuppressive therapy.
- Variable prognosis for reactive polyarthropathy, depending on the ability to eliminate or control the underlying disease process.
- Guarded prognosis for SLE.

MISCELLANEOUS

Abbreviations

- ANA = antinuclear antibody
- CRP = C-reactive protein.
- DJD = degenerative joint disease.
- FSF = familial shar-pei fever.
- IL-6 = interleukin-6.
- IMPA = immune-mediated polyarthritis.
- NSAID = nonsteroidal anti-inflammatory drug.
- SLE = systemic lupus erythematosus.

Suggested Reading

Clements DN, Gear RNA, Tattersall J, et al. Type I immune-mediated polyarthritis in dogs: 39 cases (1997–2002). *J Am Vet Med Assoc* 2004;224:1323–1327.

Hillstrom A, Bylin J, Hagman R, et al. Measurement of serum C-reactive protein concentration for discriminating between suppurative arthritis and osteoarthritis in dogs. *BMC Vet Res* 2016;12:240–249.

Lemetayer J, Taylor S. Inflammatory joint disease in cats: diagnostic approach and treatment. *J Feline Med Surg* 2014;16:547–562.

Stone M. Immune-mediated polyarthritis and other polyarthritides. In: Ettinger SJ (ed.) *Textbook of Veterinary Internal Medicine*, 8th edn. St. Louis, MO: Elsevier, 2017; pp. 3055–3070.

Author/editor: Heidi Lobprise
Topic adapted from Five Minute Veterinary Consultation, 7th edition, 2021
Original Topic: Polyarthritis, Non-Erosive, Immune-Mediated

Authors: Ashley E. Bava and J.D. Foster
Consulting Editor: Mathieu M. Glassman

Chapter 50

Thrombocytopenia, Primary Immune-Mediated

BASICS

DEFINITION

- Immune-mediated destruction of platelets with no identifiable cause.
- In secondary immune-mediated thrombocytopenia (ITP), infectious diseases, neoplasia, vaccination, or drugs (e.g., sulfonamides, cephalosporins, phenobarbital, nonsteroidal anti-inflammatory drugs [NSAIDs]) trigger the production of antibodies.

PATHOPHYSIOLOGY

- Antiplatelet autoantibodies result in premature platelet destruction by splenic macrophages.
- In secondary ITP, platelet-bound antibodies can be antibodies bound to platelet antigens altered during course of disease or antibodies bound to foreign antigens or immune complexes.
- Autoantibodies can be directed against megakaryocytes.
- Antibody-mediated impairment of platelet function possible.

SYSTEMS AFFECTED

- Nervous.
- Gastrointestinal.
- Ophthalmic.
- Respiratory.
- Skin/exocrine.
- Renal/urologic.

GENETICS

Autoimmunity is frequently recognized in particular dog breeds and is often familial, suggesting a genetic influence.

PREVALENCE

Approximately 6% of dogs and 3% of cats with thrombocytopenia

Blackwell's Five-Minute Veterinary Consult Clinical Companion: Small Animal Senior Care, First Edition. Edited by Heidi B. Lobprise.

Companion website: www.wiley.com/go/lobprise/Senior

SIGNALMENT

Species

- Dog.
- Rare in cat.

Breed and Familial Predilections

Cocker spaniel, Maltese, bearded collie, poodle, Old English sheepdog, Irish setter.

Mean Age and Range

- Middle-aged dogs.
  - While the mean age of onset may not be in the senior life stage parameters, this condition requires life-long management and can be a critical factor in senior health.
- Reported age range in dogs: 0.3–15 years (mean: 5 years); in cats: 0.7–12 years (mean: 6 years).

Predominant Sex

Female dogs.

SIGNS

Historical Findings

- Acute-onset mucosal hemorrhage.
- Chronic, low-grade blood loss.
- Lethargy, weakness, inappetence.
- Asymptomatic.
- Recent drug administration, vaccines, travel to tick-endemic area.

Physical Examination Findings

- Mucosal and cutaneous petechiae/ecchymoses.
- Melena, hematemesis, hematochezia.
- Epistaxis.
- Ocular hemorrhage, hyphema.
- Hematuria.
- Neurologic signs due to CNS bleeding.
- Dyspnea if bleeding into respiratory tract.
- Prolonged hemorrhage after trauma or venipuncture, hematoma formation.
- Hemorrhagic shock—pale mucous membrane, tachycardia, weak pulses.
- Fever.
- Palpably enlarged spleen.

DIAGNOSIS

- Severe thrombocytopenia (generally <20,000 platelets/μL).
- Careful exclusion of underlying diseases or potential triggers.
- Response to immunosuppressive therapy.

DIFFERENTIAL DIAGNOSIS

- Measurement error due to platelet clumping, especially in cats.
- Pseudomacrothrombocytopenia of cavalier King Charles and English toy spaniels, Cairn and Norfolk terriers.
- Decreased production—infectious diseases, irradiation, primary bone marrow disorders (myelopthisis or myelofibrosis).
- Sequestration in the spleen.
- Increased utilization or consumption:
  - Neoplasia, disseminated intravascular coagulation (DIC), thrombosis, vasculitis/vascular damage, infectious diseases.
  - Severe hemorrhage or thrombosis may result in mild-to-moderate thrombocytopenia.

CBC/BIOCHEMISTRY/URINALYSIS

- Thrombocytopenia often severe (<20,000–30,000/µL), high risk of spontaneous bleeding.
- Blood smear examination—to confirm low platelet count; to identify potential causes for secondary ITP.
- Anemia may be present.
- Leukogram can be normal; mild-to-moderate leukocytosis in 30% of dogs.
- Concurrent neutropenia may indicate primary bone marrow or infectious disease.
- Coagulation testing generally normal; if abnormal consider secondary ITP, DIC.
- Chemistry results unspecific for ITP. Hypoproteinemia and hypoalbuminemia due to blood loss, hyperbilirubinemia due to hematoma resorption (rare), hyperglobulinemia may indicate underlying infectious disease (e.g., ehrlichiosis, leishmaniosis, feline infectious peritonitis [FIP]).
- Hematuria.

OTHER LABORATORY TESTS

- Infectious disease testing—secondary ITP reported in association with anaplasmosis, ehrlichiosis, Rocky Mountain spotted fever, bartonellosis, babesiosis, leishmaniosis, dirofilariasis, *Angiostrongylus* infection, distemper, infectious hepatitis, and bacterial infections in dogs; feline leukemia virus, feline immunodeficiency virus, and FIP in cats.
- Platelet-bound antibody detection—flow cytometric assay in specialized laboratories.
- Adjunct immunodiagnostic testing such as Coombs' test or antinuclear antibody titer if systemic lupus erythematosus is suspected.

IMAGING

- Splenomegaly, rarely hepatomegaly.
- Radiography and ultrasonography to exclude other causes of thrombocytopenia (e.g., neoplasia) or internal bleeding.

DIAGNOSTIC PROCEDURES

- Bone marrow evaluation not indicated with response to therapy; indicated if unexplained cytopenias or poor treatment response.
- Number of megakaryocytes increased unless immune reaction targeted against megakaryocytes.

TREATMENT

APPROPRIATE HEALTH CARE

- Uncomplicated cases with low bleeding risk and good owner compliance may be treated as outpatients.
- Patients with severe thrombocytopenia have very high risk of bleeding and warrant strict confinement.
- Management of hypovolemia with crystalloid solutions (colloids may impair platelet function).
- Packed red blood cells or whole blood to correct anemia.
- Transfusion of platelet products: 10–20 mL/kg fresh whole blood, 1 unit/10 kg body weight of whole blood-derived platelet-rich plasma (containing approximately 8×10^{10} platelets/L) (minimum dose of 1 unit/30 kg) in animals with critical hemorrhage (caution if risk of hypervolemia). Platelet concentrates (lower total volume) if available. Platelets may be destroyed rapidly but may protect against catastrophic hemorrhage. DMSO-stabilized and lyophilized platelet concentrates are commercially available in the United States.

NURSING CARE

- Limit IM or SC injections. Apply extended pressure after IV injections. Avoid cystocentesis and jugular venipuncture. Bone marrow aspiration is safe.
- Intensive nursing care in patients with moderate-to-severe hemorrhage, hypovolemia, CNS abnormalities.
- Avoid hard foods, chew toys.

SURGICAL CONSIDERATIONS

- Splenectomy is a controversial option for refractory cases not responding to medical therapy.
- High risk of bleeding in dogs with severe thrombocytopenia.
- May need extensive peri- and intraoperative transfusions with red blood cells and platelets.

MEDICATIONS

DRUG(S) OF CHOICE

- Immunosuppression:
  - Corticosteroids—methyl prednisolone 10 mg/kg IV once or dexamethasone 0.2–0.3 mg/kg q24h, IV until able to take oral medication; prednisolone or prednisone (dogs 1 mg/kg PO q12h; cats 1.5–2 mg/kg PO q12h initially).

- Additional or long-term therapy, usually in combination with corticosteroid (initial dosages)—cyclosporine 5 mg/kg PO q12h (dogs), mycophenolate mofetil 3–10 mg/kg PO q12h (dogs/cats), can also be given in the acute setting at 7–10 mg/kg IV q12h, azathioprine 2 mg/kg PO q24h (dogs), leflunomide 2–3 mg/kg PO q24h (dogs), chlorambucil 0.1–0.2 mg/kg PO q24h (cats).

- Other acute management—vincristine 0.02 mg/kg IV once (dogs) or human IV immunoglobulin (hIVIG) 0.5–1 g/kg over 6–8 hours once (dogs/cats).
- Antibiotics—consider doxycycline 5 mg/kg PO q12h if tick-borne disease is possible.
- Gastrointestinal protectants—sucralfate 20–50 mg/kg PO q6–8h or proton pump inhibitors (omeprazole 1 mg/kg PO q12h; pantoprazole 1 mg/kg IV/PO q12h).
- Once the platelet count is within the reference interval, the initial prednis(ol)one dose should be tapered by approximately 1/4 to 1/5 every 2 weeks, finally switching to alternate-day therapy. This and other therapies should be tapered slowly over approximately 6 months if no relapse.

PRECAUTIONS

- Discontinue any unnecessary medications.
- Corticosteroids—gastrointestinal ulceration; iatrogenic hyperadrenocorticism.
- Immunosuppression—predisposes to opportunistic infections, mycophenolate associated with gastrointestinal upset.
- Cytotoxic medications (azathioprine, mycophenolate mofetil, chlorambucil, vincristine)—bone marrow suppression.
- Dose tapering too rapidly after remission may predispose to recurrence.

FOLLOW-UP

PATIENT MONITORING

- Hematocrit measurements and physical examination as indicated in cases with severe hemorrhage.
- Measure platelet count daily until >50,000/μL; then every few days until platelet counts normalize. Then every 1–3 weeks during the period of drug dose tapering.
- CBC and biochemistry every 2–4 weeks.
- Urinalysis every 4–6 weeks due to risk of secondary infections.

PREVENTION/AVOIDANCE

Use vaccines judiciously. Role in recurrence is uncertain.

POSSIBLE COMPLICATIONS

- Spontaneous bleeding in specific areas (CNS, lungs) can be fatal.
- Side effects of medications.

EXPECTED COURSE AND PROGNOSIS

- Platelet counts will usually increase >50,000/μL a few days after starting treatment.
- Vincristine or hIVIG in addition to prednisone led to a shorter hospital stay or more rapid increase to 50,000 platelets/μL (median 2.5–4 days), respectively.
- Most dogs achieve normal platelet counts.
- Failure to respond to therapy should prompt diagnostic reconsideration.
- 5 of 19 dogs (26%) relapsed after 19–286, median 66 days; causes for relapse were dose reduction of immunosuppression, lack of owner compliance.
- If relapses occur, add a second immunosuppressive drug.
- Survival to discharge in recent studies—84–97% (dogs); prognosis is more favorable with intensive therapy including blood/platelet products if needed.
- Mortality rate in cats is 15% (2/13).

MISCELLANEOUS

Abbreviations

- DIC = disseminated intravascular coagulation
- FIP = feline infectious peritonitis.
- hIVIG = human intravenous immunoglobulin.
- ITP = immune-mediated thrombocytopenia.
- NSAID = nonsteroidal anti-inflammatory drug.

Suggested Reading

Putsche J, Kohn B. Primary immune-mediated thrombocytopenia in 30 dogs (1997–2003). *J Am Anim Hosp Assoc* 2008;44:250–257.

Wondraschek C, Weingart C, Kohn B. Primary immune-mediated thrombocytopenia in cats. *J Am Anim Hosp Assoc* 2010;46:12–19.

Author/editor: Heidi Lobprise
Topic adapted from Five Minute Veterinary Consultation, 7th edition, 2021
Original Topic: Thrombocytopenia, Immune-Mediated

Author: Barbara Kohn
Consulting Editor: Melinda S. Camus

Musculoskeletal

Chapter 51

Hypertrophic Osteopathy

BASICS

OVERVIEW

- Periosteal proliferation of the distal extremities resulting from peripheral blood flow changes that stimulate an overgrowth of vascular connective tissue.
- Increased blood circulation in the limb due to neural or humoral mechanisms is likely secondary to an underlying disease process: most notably intra-thoracic or intra-abdominal neoplasia.
- Predominantly affects the diaphyseal region of phalanges, metacarpals, and metatarsals.

SIGNALMENT

- More common in dogs than cats.
- Age of highest frequency >8 years; coincides with the peak incidence of neoplasia.

SIGNS

Historical Findings

- Chronic or acute lameness with pain in one or more limbs.
- Reluctance to move or use affected limb(s).
- Large firm swelling of affected limb(s).
- Respiratory clinical signs if intra-thoracic disease present (rare).

Physical Examination Findings

- Long bone or distal extremities—enlarged, firm, taut, thickened; not edematous.
- Single or multiple limbs.
- Firm swelling may extend proximally with progression of disease.
- Lameness and pain noted in affected limb(s).

CAUSES AND RISK FACTORS

- Primary and metastatic neoplasia—lung tumors; esophageal sarcoma; rhabdomyosarcoma; adenocarcinoma of the adrenal gland, liver, or prostate; nephroblastoma; renal cell carcinoma; thoracic and abdominal mesotheliomas.

Blackwell's Five-Minute Veterinary Consult Clinical Companion: Small Animal Senior Care,
First Edition. Edited by Heidi B. Lobprise.

Companion website: www.wiley.com/go/lobprise/Senior

- Non-neoplastic conditions—pneumonia, lung abscess/granulomas, dirofilariasis; congenital or acquired heart disease, bronchial foreign bodies; *Spirocerca lupi* infestation of the esophagus; focal lung atelectasis; obscure toxins; hypertension; hyperestrogenism; congenital idiopathic megaesophagus.

DIAGNOSIS

DIFFERENTIAL DIAGNOSIS

- Osteomyelitis—asymmetric; edematous; lytic bone lesions; history of penetrating trauma or systemic infection.
- Metastatic neoplasia—asymmetric.
- Hypervitaminosis A (feline)—asymmetric; generally involves joint surface.
- Hypertrophic osteodystrophy and multiple cartilaginous exostosis—metaphyseal abnormality, young dogs.
- Degenerative joint disease—involves articular surface changes in multiple joints.

CBC/BIOCHEMISTRY/URINALYSIS

Dependent on underlying cause and concurrent conditions.

OTHER LABORATORY TESTS

Fecal examination—rule out gastrointestinal and respiratory parasitism.

IMAGING

- Radiographs of affected long bones—bilaterally symmetric extensive, aggressive, or nonaggressive periosteal new bone formation on diaphysis; palisading periosteal reaction; joints not affected.
- Thoracic and abdominal imaging (radiographs, ultrasound, and/or CT)—identify and differentiate primary lesions.

DIAGNOSTIC PROCEDURES

Bone biopsy and culture (bacterial and fungal)—in atypical cases to rule out neoplasia and osteomyelitis.

TREATMENT

- Directed at managing, treating, or removing the underlying cause.
- Options in selected cases—unilateral vagotomy on the side of a lung lesion or bilateral cervical vagotomy; incising through parietal pleura; subperiosteal rib resection.

MEDICATIONS

DRUG(S) OF CHOICE

- Dictated by underlying cause.

- Analgesics/anti-inflammatories—as needed.
- No known clinically proven benefit for steroid therapy.

FOLLOW-UP

PATIENT MONITORING

Condition indicates other disease processes—identify the primary cause.

EXPECTED COURSE AND PROGNOSIS

- Clinical signs and bone changes may resolve with treatment of underlying disease.
- Bone changes may take several months to regress.
- Prognosis—guarded to poor due to the common occurrence of neoplastic causes; non-neoplastic lesions may resolve with appropriate treatment of primary cause.
- Tumor recurrence or metastasis may result in recurrence of osteopathy.
- No relationship between size, site, or histologic type of primary lesion, the development of or recurrence of hypertrophic osteopathy postoperatively.

MISCELLANEOUS

SYNONYMS

- Hypertrophic pulmonary osteopathy/osteoarthropathy (HPO/HPOA).
- Hypertrophic osteoarthropathy (HOA).

Suggested Reading

Crumlish PT, Sweeney T, Jones B, Angles JM. Hypertrophic osteodystrophy in the Weimaraner dog: lack of association between DQA1 alleles of the canine MHC and hypertrophic osteodystrophy. *Vet J* 2006;171(2):308–313.

Dunn ME, Blond L, Letard D, Difruscia R. Hypertrophic osteopathy associated with infective endocarditis in an adult boxer dog. *J Small Anim Pract* 2007;48(2):99–103.

Foster SF. Idiopathic hypertrophic osteopathy in a cat. *J Feline Med Surg* 2007;9(2):172–173.

Huang C-H, Jeng C-R, Lin C-T, Yeh L-S. Feline hypertrophic osteopathy: a collection of seven cases in Taiwan. *JAAHA* 2010;46:346–352.

Liptak JM, Monnet E, Dernell WS, Withrow SJ. Pulmonary metastatectomy in the management of four dogs with hypertrophic osteopathy. *Vet Comp Oncol* 2004;2(1):1–12.

Author/editor: Heidi Lobprise
Topic adapted from Five Minute Veterinary Consultation, 7th edition, 2021
Original Topic: Hypertrophic Osteopathy

Author: Marian E. Benitez
Consulting Editor: Mathieu M. Glassman

Chapter 52

Intervertebral Disc Disease

BASICS

DEFINITION

Degeneration of the intervertebral discs that may result in protrusion or extrusion of disc material into the spinal canal. The protruded or extruded disc material causes spinal cord compression (myelopathy) and/or nerve root compression (radiculopathy), as well as concussive spinal cord injury in varying degrees.

PATHOPHYSIOLOGY

- Hansen type I—degeneration of the nucleus pulposus and acute rupture of the annulus fibrosus with extrusion of the nucleus pulposus into the spinal canal.
    - Typically seen in chondrodystrophic breeds at 3–6 years of age.
- Hansen type II—fibrinoid degeneration and protrusion of the dorsal annulus fibrosus into the vertebral canal (can involve a dynamic component).
    - Large-breed dogs (Doberman pinscher, Labrador retriever)—8–10 years of age
    - The most common case presentation is of gradual onset of neurologic dysfunction and slow progression.
    - ANNPE (acute noncompressive nucleus pulposus extrusion) - extrusion of apparently healthy, hydrated nucleus pulposus with or without spinal cord compression,
- Disc extrusion or protrusion into the spinal canal causes focal compression of the spinal cord (myelopathy) and/or focal compression of a nerve root (radiculopathy) in addition to a variable degree of contusion injury.
- Consequences of spinal cord compression are ischemia and demyelination.
- Consequences of spinal cord contusion include axonal and vascular injury as well as secondary cellular injury.
- Disc extrusion may be secondary to trauma, but this rarely occurs aside from those patients with hydrated disc herniations.
- Surgical fusion of cervical vertebrae may alter the biomechanics of adjacent vertebral bodies and therefore predispose discs to protrusion or extrusion; this is termed the domino effect.

SYSTEMS AFFECTED

Cervical—Nervous system—either focal myelopathy or focal radiculopathy.

Thoracolumbar—loss of normal neurologic function to the pelvic limbs, bladder, and anal sphincter.

Blackwell's Five-Minute Veterinary Consult Clinical Companion: Small Animal Senior Care, First Edition. Edited by Heidi B. Lobprise.

Companion website: www.wiley.com/go/lobprise/Senior

- Renal/urologic (loss of voluntary urethral sphincter control).
- Digestive (loss of voluntary anal sphincter control).
- Musculoskeletal (muscle atrophy in chronic disease).
- Thoracolumbar disc disease comprises 85% of all disc herniations; 70% occur from T11 to L3.

SIGNALMENT

Species

Dogs, rarely cats.

- Type II—8–10 years of age in large dogs; cats: mean age of 10 years.

SIGNS

- Severity of clinical signs and spinal cord injury is dependent on several factors, including the rate and volume of disc protrusion or extrusion, spinal cord diameter relative to vertebral canal diameter, and the velocity of disc material that is extruded.
- Herniation in the cervical region can result in fewer neurologic deficits compared to similar lesions in the thoracolumbar region, because the spinal canal area is greater and can accommodate more disc material before spinal cord compression.

Signs also depend on location of effect within the spinal cord (upper motor neuron [UMN] or lower motor neuron [LMN]), and regional spinal canal/spinal cord diameter ratio (cervical vs. thoracolumbar).

Historical Findings

- Cervical
  - Neck pain—most common owner complaint.
  - Stiff, stilted gait, lameness, or reluctance to move the head and neck.
  - Lowered head stance and muscle spasms of the head, neck, and shoulder
  - Inability to rise or falling forward frequently.
- Thoracolumbar
  - Larger dogs or smaller dogs with type II disease have a more insidious onset and tend to worsen with time.

Physical Examination Findings

- Cervical
  - Neck pain—elicited upon slow manipulation of the neck or by deep palpation of the cervical muscles.
  - Apparent forelimb lameness or nerve root signature (e.g., a thoracic limb that knuckles, appears lame, or is held in partial flexion).
  - Paresis with or without general proprioceptive deficits involving one or both thoracic and pelvic limbs may be present.
  - Pelvic limb paresis may be more severe than thoracic limb paresis.
  - Pelvic limb spinal reflexes may be normal to exaggerated.
  - Thoracic limb spinal reflexes may be normal to exaggerated when lesions are located in the C1–C6 spinal cord segment and may be normal to decreased when the C6–T2 spinal cord segment is affected, although this finding is not reliable in some patients.
  - Severity of clinical signs and degree of compression are not always correlated.
  - Bladder function may be upper motor neuron in nature or normal.

- Thoracolumbar
  - Thoracolumbar pain is a common finding in dogs; reluctant to ambulate and hunched posture; careful palpation of spinous processes and epaxial musculature produces distinct localized pain; often some degree of paraparesis with decreased or absent proprioception or decreased motor ability in the pelvic limbs.
  - Myotactic spinal reflexes in the pelvic limbs are exaggerated (hyper-reflexive) when the lesion is between T3 and L3; reflexes are decreased (hyporeflexive) when lesion is caudal to L3.
  - Superficial and deep pain perception may be decreased or absent in the pelvic limbs.
  - Presence of deep pain sensation is the single most reliable prognostic factor for return to acceptable function; pain perception should be conscious in nature and not confused with a withdrawal reflex (local spinal reflex); in animals with diminished conscious deep pain response, observation of mydriasis or tachycardia may be useful in confirming the presence of deep pain.
  - Forelimb function is normal with thoracolumbar disc rupture; occasionally Schiff–Sherrington phenomena may cause increased muscle tone in the forelimbs, but this clinical sign is location related only and does not indicate a poor prognosis.
  - Urinary incontinence or retention is common when the lesion affects motor function.
  - Pain is less obvious in cats; the site of herniation is often lumbar.

CAUSES

- Degeneration of the intervertebral disc material and subsequent herniation or protrusion.
- Trauma may lead to extrusion of healthy material or otherwise degenerative material.

RISK FACTORS

Obesity and repeated traumatic events in those breeds predisposed to intervertebral disc disease.

DIAGNOSIS

DIFFERENTIAL DIAGNOSIS

- Cervical—neoplasia, atlantoaxial instability, spinal fracture/luxation, discospondylitis, meningitis, fibrocartilaginous embolism, cervical vertebral instability, spondylomyelopathy
- Systemic illness—hypoadrenocorticism, hypothyroidism.
- Thoracolumbar, Type II—degenerative myelopathy, spinal neoplasia, discospondylitis, orthopedic disease; differentiated by history, radiographic modalities, and careful orthopedic and neurologic examination.

CBC/BIOCHEMISTRY/URINALYSIS

Often performed in anticipation of medication administration, general anesthesia, and/or surgery.

- Elevation of liver enzymes is common if the patient has received previous corticosteroids for pain or neurologic disease.
- Urine retention/incontinence increases risk of urinary tract infection characterized by leukocytes, protein, and bacteriuria on urinalysis.

OTHER LABORATORY TESTS

- Cerebrospinal fluid (CSF) analysis—performed under general anesthesia (prior to myelography if performed).
- CSF analysis reveals nonspecific changes such as mild-to-moderate elevation in protein levels and mild-to-moderate pleocytosis, which is more pronounced in Hansen type I disc extrusion.
- CSF analysis is an important addition when alternative causes of neuropathy are likely differential diagnoses or when imaging findings are equivocal or nondiagnostic.
- Electromyography may be useful if the underlying cause is associated with denervation.

IMAGING

Cross-Sectional Imaging

- Cervical
  - MRI and CT are most sensitive for diagnosis of cervical intervertebral disc disease and intervertebral disc herniation (IVDH) as well as for surgical planning
  - MRI is the best available method for early recognition of intervertebral disc degeneration (IVDD) in dogs and is capable of the most complete evaluation of the spinal cord parenchyma.
  - CT is also useful in diagnosis of spinal cord compression, especially by degenerative disc material; the spinal cord parenchyma is not as well assessed with this modality compared with MRI.
- Thoracolumbar
  - MRI is now considered the diagnostic mode of choice when available due to the noninvasive nature and superior information regarding location and extent of disease; presence of a hyperintense spinal cord lesion as long as the body of L2 on a T2-weighted image in deep-pain-negative dogs is associated with a poorer prognosis.
  - CT with or without contrast is often diagnostic in chondrodystrophic dogs; dystrophic calcification of extruded material is easily visualized and lateralization can be easily determined; contrast enhancement can different disc disease from neoplastic or granulomatous processes.

Spinal Radiography

- Cervical
  - Well-positioned lateral and ventrodorsal survey radiographs of the cervical spine aid in excluding other differentials (i.e., discospondylitis, fracture/luxation, atlantoaxial instability, or lytic vertebrae suggestive of a bone tumor), but are not reliable for many patients with IVDH.
  - Classic findings include narrowed intervertebral disc space or disc space wedging, collapse of the articular facets, or calcified disc material present in the intervertebral foramen or in the spinal canal, although many of these findings can be seen without clinical signs, especially in over-represented breeds.
  - Hansen type II disc disease may be associated with spondylosis deformans.
- Thoracolumbar
  - Thoracolumbar spinal radiography with the patient anesthetized; unanesthetized radiographs can be used to rule out neoplasia and other processes, but can be misleading for thora-columbar disc disease.

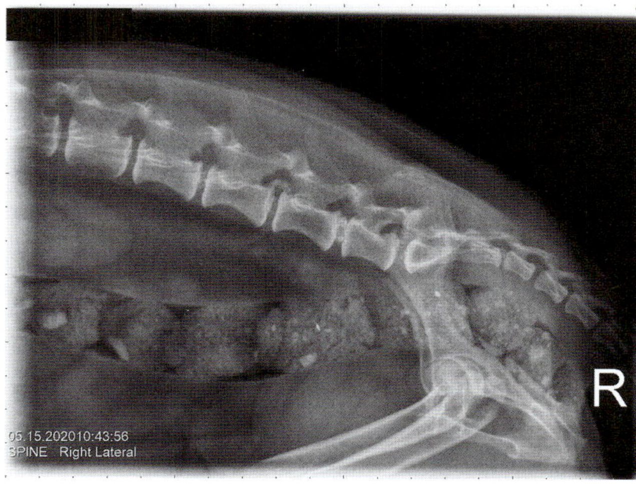

■ **Figure 52.1** Calcified matter L5–L6 beginning to intrude into the spinal canal space.

- Survey radiographs rule out some other disease processes.
- Diagnostic radiographs taken under general anesthesia may reveal a narrowed or wedged disc space, collapsed articular facet space, and small intervertebral foramen with increased or mineralized density within the spinal canal (see Figure 52.1).
- Accuracy and sensitivity of survey radiographs for determining a specific site of disc herniation are low; in conjunction with careful neurologic examination, the exact location can often be narrowed down to a small vertebral area, but the extent of herniation and pressure on the meninges from herniation of disc material may extend over more than one space.

Myelography

- Cervical
  - Survey cervical radiographs may be misleading; therefore, myelography is more sensitive compared to survey radiographs, although cross-sectional imaging has replaced this modality in most practices.
  - Lateral radiographs reveal dorsal deviation of the ventral contrast column over the intervertebral disc space consistent with extradural compression; intraforaminal or dorsolateral disc herniation is best seen on an oblique views.
  - Acute cases with spinal cord swelling can cause blockage of contrast material and prevent it from flowing past the obstruction, limiting the diagnostic capabilities of the image.
- Thoracolumbar
  - Myelography performed with iohexol was previously the method of choice and is still indicated when CT or MRI is not available; the contrast agent is usually introduced at L5–L6; positive diagnosis is an extradural mass lesion causing spinal cord compression adjacent to the affected disc; spinal cord swelling may be evidenced by thinning of contrast columns over several intervertebral spaces.
  - Lateralization is more consistent when determined from both oblique and dorsoventral myelogram views.

TREATMENT

Guidelines for Therapy Based on Classification of Clinical Condition

- Class 1—back pain only, first episode.
- Class 2—recurrent back pain, ataxia, mild paraparesis, motor ability good.
- Class 3—severe paraparesis, proprioceptive deficits, motor ability affected but still present; voluntary control of urination may be diminished; bladder many be easy to manually express or difficult due to detrusor dysfunction.
- Class 4A—complete paralysis (no motor ability) with deep pain perception present; voluntary control of urination and defecation absent, bladder usually easy to express manually.
- Class 4B—complete paralysis, no deep pain perception present.

Treatment Recommendations Based on Classification of Clinical Condition

- Class 1—treated medically unless pain persists.
- Class 2—treated medically initially with serial neurologic exam; surgery is performed if patient remains static or condition declines.
- Classes 3 and 4A—immediate surgical decompression recommended; prognosis good.
- Class 4B—surgical decompression and fair prognosis if within the first 12–48 hours of occurrence or for slower onset of clinical signs (clinical signs progressive over 12 hours); poor prognosis if deep pain perception has been absent for >48 hours or if the clinical signs progressed rapidly (<6 hours) from normal to loss of deep pain.
- Serial neurologic examination important for all affected animals

APPROPRIATE HEALTH CARE

- Cervical
  - Conservative or surgical management dependent on patient's history and presenting neurologic status.
  - In general, conservative management can be considered with a gradual onset of clinical signs or clinical signs that are limited to hyperpathia or mild ataxia.
  - Surgical management is often indicated in patients with repeated episodes of neck pain, severe neck pain and neurologic deficits, or a lack of response to conservative management.
  - Patients with hydrated intervertebral disc herniations may perform similarly with conservative and surgical treatment.
- Thoracolumbar

Guidelines for Therapy Based on Classification of Clinical Condition

- Class 1—back pain only, first episode.
- Class 2—recurrent back pain, ataxia, mild paraparesis, motor ability good.
- Class 3—severe paraparesis, proprioceptive deficits, motor ability affected but still present; voluntary control of urination may be diminished; bladder may be easy to manually express or difficult due to detrusor dysfunction.
- Class 4A—complete paralysis (no motor ability) with deep pain perception present; voluntary control of urination and defecation absent, bladder usually easy to express manually.
- Class 4B—complete paralysis, no deep pain perception present.

Treatment Recommendations Based on Classification of Clinical Condition

- Class 1—treated medically unless pain persists.
- Class 2—treated medically initially with serial neurologic exam; surgery is performed if patient remains static or condition declines.
- Classes 3 and 4A—immediate surgical decompression recommended; prognosis good.
- Class 4B—surgical decompression and fair prognosis if within the first 12–48 hours of occurrence or for slower onset of clinical signs (clinical signs progressive over 12 hours); poor prognosis if deep pain perception has been absent for >48 hours or if the clinical signs progressed rapidly (<6 hours) from normal to loss of deep pain.
- Serial neurologic examination important for all affected animals.

NURSING CARE

- Cervical
  - Level of nursing care needed depends on the severity of the injury; if unable to be cared for at home, patients should be monitored as inpatients.
  - Minimal manipulation of the head and neck to avoid worsening discomfort.
  - Urination—monitor patients for complete emptying of the bladder; patients may need to have bladder manually expressed or intermittent bladder catheterization; in some cases, indwelling urinary catheter may need to be placed.
  - Defecation—patients typically defecate normally, although frequent cleaning and management of any soft stool are important.
  - Recumbent patients—should be kept on a well-padded mat and turned frequently (often every 4 hours); should be checked for pressure sores over bony prominences; should be diligently cleaned and kept dry.
  - Physical therapy—passive range of motion of all joints should be performed as often as possible to prevent severe muscle atrophy, especially in patients with minimal voluntary motor ability; hydrotherapy can be considered in tetraparetic patients as well.
- Thoracolumbar
  - Absolute restricted confinement for 2–4 weeks or until ambulatory.
  - Minimize spinal manipulation and support spine when handling patient.
  - Ensure ability to urinate or consider bladder expression, intermittent catheterization, or indwelling urinary catheter for patients in classes 3–4B.
  - Recumbent patients should be kept clean on padded bedding placed on elevated cage racks and turned frequently to prevent formation of decubital ulcers.
  - Manual evacuation of the bowel or enemas may be necessary to promote defecation.
  - Physical therapy with passive manipulation of pelvic limbs begun early followed by more intense therapy (hydrotherapy) for animals with neurologic deficits but regaining motor function; rehabilitation protocols are not contraindicated, but recent research suggests that they may not be beneficial in improving the speed of return to function.
  - Carts useful in many patients in promoting return to function; patient tolerance is limiting factor.

ACTIVITY

- Cervical
  - Activity should be very limited; no running or jumping, and confined to a crate-sized space; when patients are being walked, a harness should be used instead of a collar.

- With conservative or postoperative management, patients should be strictly confined to cage rest for 4 weeks, followed by a gradual return to normal activity over the course of another 4 weeks.

■ Thoracolumbar
- Restricted movement most important part of medical management.
- Cage rest in hospital or enforced cage rest as an outpatient for 2–4 weeks for class 1 patients or postoperative animals

DIET

For obese patients, a decrease in caloric intake should be instituted.

CLIENT EDUCATION

■ Cervical
- Appropriate expectations for clinical improvement or signs of worsening should be discussed.
- Confinement is very important for recovery.
- Weight loss if the animal is obese.

■ Thoroacolumbar
- Some degree of restricted activity may be important for the remainder of the animal's life since it has disc disease.
- Most animals in classes 1–4A have a good-to-excellent prognosis for return to function, i.e., ambulation with bowel and bladder continence; patients in class 4B have a poorer but not hopeless prognosis; percentages vary, but up to approximately 50% may regain deep pain and some function, especially if appropriate surgical decompression occurs early in the disease process.

SURGICAL CONSIDERATIONS

■ Cervical
- The goal of surgery is to remove disc material from the spinal canal and therefore decompress the spinal cord and/or nerve root.
- Surgery usually provides rapid pain relief and significantly improved motor function.
- A ventral cervical slot is the most common surgical approach for the removal of disc material; disc material that has extruded dorsolaterally into the intervertebral foramen or dorsally is removed via a lateral approach or through a dorsal laminectomy.
- Fenestration alone for dogs with neck pain usually does not resolve clinical signs and is no longer recommended.

■ Thoracolumbar
- Surgery strongly indicated for animals in classes 3 and 4, also within the first 12–48 hours for class 4B dogs; also indicated for static or worsening class 1 and 2 dogs.
- Primary surgical goal is to relieve spinal cord compression by disc mass removal via hemilaminectomy, dorsal laminectomy, or pediculectomy; disc fenestration alone is not effective for treating acute disc extrusions, but is frequently recommended as an adjunct to decompression at the primary site.
- Hemilaminectomy on the side of predominant disc extrusion is the surgical procedure of choice for most thoracolumbar discs; studies indicate improved return to function,

minimized spinal destabilization, and decreased formation of compressive laminectomy scars in the long-term postoperative period.
- Foramenotomy and pediculectomy are similar to hemilaminectomy and may allow a more limited approach and decreased cord manipulation.
- Dorsal laminectomy is the procedure of choice for disc herniation in the region of the lumbosacral plexus or where extensive examination of the spinal cord is necessary.
- Recurrence of clinical signs in animals in the immediate postoperative period may be due to further extrusion of disc from the original site if fenestration is not adjunctively performed at the site of disc disease during hemilaminectomy or dorsal laminectomy; later recurrence of clinical signs after recovery is usually due to protrusion/extrusion at adjacent sites; several studies document approximately 8% long-term recurrence of clinical signs in dogs after initial hemilaminectomy and active site fenestration due to protrusion/extrusion at other sites.
- Controversy remains over the efficacy of multiple site prophylactic disc fenestrations performed during the decompressive surgery, because evidence that fenestration prevents recurrence of clinical signs is not definitive and fenestration causes osteoarthritis to form at the intervertebral space of each site of fenestration, leading to potential chronic patient discomfort and pain.

MEDICATIONS

DRUG(S) OF CHOICE

- Cervical
  - Anti-inflammatory therapy (low-dose glucocorticoid or nonsteroidal anti-inflammatory drugs [NSAIDs]) is often beneficial in order to decrease the pain in animals that are being treated conservatively as well as those recovering from surgery; use of high-dose glucocorticoids is not well supported by the literature and is generally not recommended.
  - Analgesic medications such as gabapentin and muscle relaxants such as methocarbamol can also be used in conjunction with anti-inflammatories to improve pain control in both conservative as well as surgical treatment.
- Thoracolumbar
  - Nonsteroidal anti-inflammatory drugs (NSAIDs) or narcotics may be used as analgesics in class 1 cases to alleviate patient discomfort during recovery; use of analgesics is not a substitute for the cage rest period required of all patients.
  - Narcotic analgesics may be necessary postoperatively; hydromorphone (0.05–0.2 mg/kg IV/IM/SC q4h) or similar narcotic injectable used at appropriate doses are the treatment of choice in the immediate postoperative period; oral narcotics such as codeine (1–2 mg/kg PO q8h) or tramadol (5–8 mg/kg PO q8h) are useful to alleviate patient discomfort within the first week after decompression; transdermal lidocaine or fentanyl may be useful modes of analgesic administration in some animals, particularly those intractable to frequent dosing of injectable or oral agents.
  - Gabapentin (5–10 mg/kg PO q12h), an NMDA receptor antagonist in dogs with chronic pain sensitization, is not an appropriate analgesic used alone in the immediate postoperative period.
  - Methocarbamol (25–45 mg/kg q8h) may be useful in cases where muscle spasm is contributing to pain; more applicable with cervical disease.

- Bethanechol (5–15 mg/dog PO) and phenoxybenzamine (0.25 mg/kg PO q8–12h) or prazosin (1 mg/15 kg PO q8–12h) are variably helpful in managing bladder dysfunction associated with spinal cord lesion.
- Previous indications for methylprednisolone sodium succinate for treatment of acute pain are now controversial for efficacy; the high potential for side effects may outweigh the small gains from the drug.
- Corticosteroids are no longer commonly recommended in the treatment of acute intervertebral disc disease due to lack of demonstrated clinical efficacy.

CONTRAINDICATIONS

Systemic status should be considered when choosing medications.

PRECAUTIONS

- Cervical
  - Anti-inflammatories or analgesic medications given to animals without simultaneous strict cage confinement could exacerbate disc extrusion by encouraging activity.
- Thoracolumbar
  - Glucocorticoid use is discouraged in cases of IVDD where drug side effects such as gastrointestinal hemorrhage and intestinal perforation often far outweigh benefits; potent glucocorticoids such as dexamethasone should never be used.
  - Glucocorticoids are contraindicated within 48 hours of using an NSAID in dogs.
  - Use of glucocorticoids without cage confinement may decrease pain, thereby encouraging excessive activity and leading to further disc herniation and deterioration of clinical condition.

ALTERNATIVE DRUG(S)

Alternative Therapies

- Acupuncture use has been described, but consistent efficacy has not been demonstrated.
- Chiropractic therapy has no proven benefits for IVDD and may potentially be harmful to the animal.
- Percutaneous therapeutic lasers do not reach the site of inflammation and are not efficacious; one recent study did demonstrate slightly more rapid recovery from IVDD if laser therapy regimens occurred as an adjunct to surgical decompression procedures.
- Discolysis by enzymatic injection or laser ablation has been described but is not proven therapy in dogs.
- Targeted pulsed electromagnetic field therapy (PEMF) has been shown to decrease post-surgical pain and enhance healing.

FOLLOW-UP

PATIENT MONITORING

- Cervical
  - Weekly evaluations should be performed until resolution of clinical signs or until clinical progress plateaus.

  - All patients should be fitted with a harness, and neck collars should be avoided.
- Thoracolumbar
  - Patients treated medically should be reevaluated two to three times daily for worsening neurologic signs for the first 48 hours after onset.
  - If stable, reevaluate daily, then weekly, until clinical signs have resolved.
  - Patients treated surgically are evaluated twice daily until improvement is noted; urinary bladder function or awaiting development of an autonomic bladder are the limiting factors for hospitalization.

PREVENTION/AVOIDANCE

- Inherent in particular breeds.
- Keeping patients at an ideal weight may help.

POSSIBLE COMPLICATIONS

- Cervical
  - Complications are uncommon.
  - Conservative management—continued neck pain, deteriorating motor status.
  - Surgical management—hemorrhage, infection, neurologic deterioration, respiratory compromise, subluxation/luxation of vertebral bodies, collapse of intervertebral disc space, and foraminal collapse.
- Thoracolumbar
  - Recurrence of signs associated with disc herniation at original or at new site.
  - Deterioration of clinical signs with or without surgery; continued inflammatory processes initiated by the initial extrusion may result in myelomalacia or diminished function.
  - Rarely, development of ascending or descending myelomalacia; occurs in class 4A or 4B dogs 3–5 days following injury and is characterized by variable and progressive neurologic deterioration, possible fever, possible dyspnea, and extreme pain, with the cranial movement of the inflammation; careful monitoring of the anatomic position of detection of the panniculus reflex is recommended; cranial movement of the reflex can indicate ascending myelomalacia and provide early warning of a grave condition; such animals are often euthanized when diagnosed.

EXPECTED COURSE AND PROGNOSIS

- Cervical
  - Prognosis for patients treated surgically or conservatively depends on neurologic signs at the time of presentation; lack of nociception leads to a poor prognosis for recovery of function long term (<50%) and duration of clinical signs beyond days likely worsens the prognosis.
  - Prognosis is generally favorable for most patients; surgical treatment often leads to rapid improvement in pain control, especially in patients undergoing a ventral slot procedure.
  - Some patients treated conservatively have recurrence of disease or deterioration and may require surgical intervention.
  - Patients who experience IVDH may be predisposed to IVDH at other sites in the future due to the underlying pathology (IVDD).

- Thoracolumbar
    - Overall prognosis for dogs in classes 1–4A good to excellent (85–95%); those treated conservatively may experience recurrence of clinical signs
    - Recurrence rates of dogs without fenestration at the time of laminectomy range from 5–30%.
    - Dogs in class 4B have a variable (10–75%) chance of recovery; overall a guarded but seemingly favorable prognosis if surgery is performed within 48 hours and the animal is allowed sufficient time to recover.

MISCELLANEOUS

Abbreviations

- ANNPE = acute noncompressive nucleus pulposus extrusion
- CSF = cerebrospinal fluid.
- IVDD = intervertebral disc degeneration.
- IVDH = intervertebral disc herniation.
- NSAID = nonsteroidal anti-inflammatory drug.

Suggested Reading—Cervical IVDD

Jeffery ND, Levine JM, Olby NJ, Stein VM. Intervertebral disc degeneration in dogs: consequences, diagnosis, treatment and future directions. *J Vet Intern Med* 2013;27(6):1318–1333.

Lorenz MD, Coates J, Kent M. *Handbook of Veterinary Neurology*, 5th edn. St. Louis, MO: Saunders, 2011.

Suggested Reading—Thoracolumbar IVDD

Dewey CW. Surgery of the thoracolumbar spine. In: Fossum TW (ed.) *Small Animal Surgery*, 4th edn. St. Louis, MO: Elsevier Mosby, 2013; pp. 1508–1528.

Kerwin SC, Levine JM, Mankin JM. Thoracolumbar vertebral column. In: Johnston SA, Tobias KM (eds) *Veterinary Surgery: Small Animal*, 2nd edn. St. Louis, MO: Elsevier, 2018; pp. 485–513.

Zidan N, Sims C, Fenn J, et al. A randomized, blinded, prospective clinical trial of postoperative rehabilitation in dogs after surgical decompression of acute thoracolumbar intervertebral disc herniation. *J Vet Int Med* 2018;32:1133–1144.

Author/editor: Heidi Lobprise
Topic adapted from Five Minute Veterinary Consultation, 7th edition, 2021
Original Topic: Intervertebral Disc Disease—Cervical, and—Thoracolumbar

Author: Lindsay Boozer—IVDD—Cervical

Author: James K. Roush—IVDD—Thoracolumbar
Consulting Editor: Mathieu M. Glassman

Chapter 53

Osteoarthritis

BASICS

DEFINITION

Osteoarthritis (OA) or degenerative joint disease (DJD) is a chronic and progressive disease process that involves the entire joint, leading to loss of articular cartilage and ultimately failure of the joint. It is due to both primary (idiopathic) and secondary causes.

PATHOPHYSIOLOGY

- Secondary OA initiated by mechanical stress—traumatic injury, instability, abnormal conformation, abnormal activity, etc.
- Inflammatory mediators and free radicals are released from damaged chondrocytes and synovium, resulting in breakdown of extracellular matrix of articular cartilage, causing collagen degradation and loss of collagen cross-linking.
    - Collagen synthesis is altered.
    - Extracellular matrix further compromised by increased breakdown of proteoglycans.
    - Nitric oxide released along with other free radicals, which mediates cartilage breakdown and supports chronic inflammation.
- Chondrocyte apoptosis facilitated by cyclooxygenase-2 enzymes and oxidative stress.
- Synovitis—inflammatory cascade in OA with decreased viscosity of synovial fluid, reducing lubrication.
    - Reduces oxygen and nutrient supply to chondrocytes as well as waste removal.
- Subchondral bone becomes sclerotic, worsening loading qualities of bone and overlying cartilage.
- Quiet periods and flare-ups
- Pain
    - Joint capsule distention and stimulation of pain receptors.
    - Synovial inflammation and increased mechanical loading of subchondral bone.
    - Alteration of function of surrounding tendons and ligaments.
    - Development of periarticular fibrosis.
- Progressive cartilage degradation from fibrillation to deep fissuring of cartilage and eventual full-thickness cartilage loss
- Periarticular fibrosis with a reduction of joint motion (and pain); poorer vascularity of synovial membrane and lack of functionality of synovium due to lack of motion in joint.
- Osteophytes and enthesiophytes develop to increase load-bearing surface area.
- These changes reduce functionality and may eventually lead to ankylosis.

Blackwell's Five-Minute Veterinary Consult Clinical Companion: Small Animal Senior Care, First Edition. Edited by Heidi B. Lobprise.

Companion website: www.wiley.com/go/lobprise/Senior

- The chronic inflammation associated with OA can impact accumulative inflammation that effects many body systems, even aging (see Inflammaging in Section 1—Aging Definitions).

GENETICS

- Dogs—secondary OA due to hip and elbow dysplasia, osteochondritis dessicans (OCD), patellar luxations, congenital shoulder luxation, Legg–Perthes, cranial cruciate ligament rupture, intra-articular fractures, obesity, as well as many other causes.
- Cats—primary OA more likely; secondary OA due to patellar luxation, hip dysplasia, obesity, and arthropathy

INCIDENCE/PREVALENCE

- Dog—very common; 20% of dogs older than 1 year have some degree of OA.
- Cat—90% of cats over 12 years of age had evidence of OA on radiographs.
- Clinical problems are more prevalent in larger, overweight, or very active animals.

SIGNALMENT

Species

Dog and cat.

Mean Age and Range

- Secondary OA due to congenital disorders (OCD, hip dysplasia) in immature animals; some present with OA signs when mature (hip and elbow dysplasia)
- Secondary to trauma—any age.
- Common issue in senior dogs and cats -chronic inflammatory process

CAUSES

- Primary—no known cause.
- Secondary-to-abnormal wear on normal cartilage (e.g., joint instability, joint incongruity, trauma to cartilage or supporting soft tissues, obesity) or normal wear on abnormal cartilage (e.g., osteochondral defects).

RISK FACTORS

- Working and athletic dogs, or obese dogs place more stress on their joints.
- Dogs with disorders that affect collagen or cartilage (Cushing's disease, diabetes mellitus, hypothyroidism, hyperlaxity, prolonged steroid use).

SIGNS

Historical Findings

- Dogs—intermittent lameness or stiff gait that slowly progresses, decreased activity levels, behavioral issues (see Figure 53.1).
  - Possible history of joint trauma, OCD, or developmental disorders.

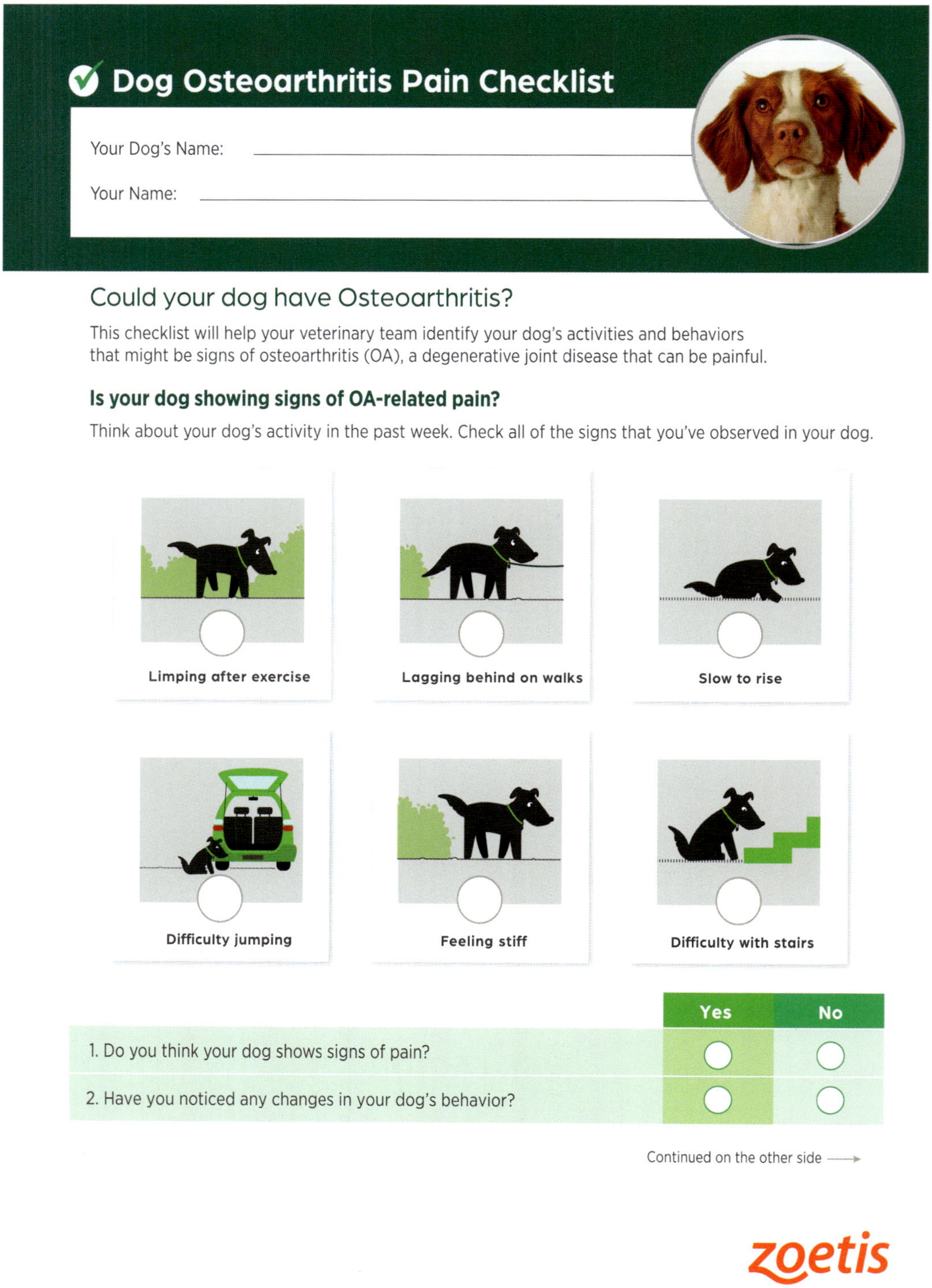

Dog Osteoarthritis Pain Checklist

Your Dog's Name: ____________________

Your Name: ____________________

Could your dog have Osteoarthritis?

This checklist will help your veterinary team identify your dog's activities and behaviors that might be signs of osteoarthritis (OA), a degenerative joint disease that can be painful.

Is your dog showing signs of OA-related pain?

Think about your dog's activity in the past week. Check all of the signs that you've observed in your dog.

- Limping after exercise
- Lagging behind on walks
- Slow to rise
- Difficulty jumping
- Feeling stiff
- Difficulty with stairs

	Yes	No
1. Do you think your dog shows signs of pain?	○	○
2. Have you noticed any changes in your dog's behavior?	○	○

Continued on the other side →

zoetis

■ **Figure 53.1** Dog osteoarthritis pain check list. Source: Zoetis.

OA has both physical and emotional aspects.

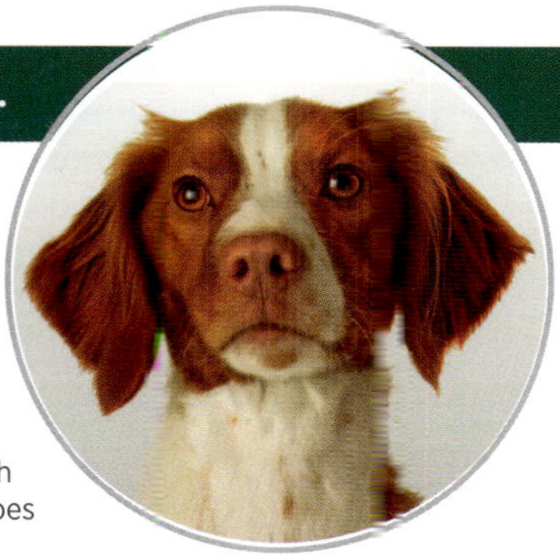

For a dog, OA can be very painful. And, just like in humans, pain can negatively impact dogs not just physically, but also emotionally. The good news is that this pain can be managed. In a recent study, dogs showed significant improvement in both their emotional and physical well-being with the pain under control.[1]

Think about your dog's behavior in the past week. This scale helps measure your dog's pain based on how your dog is feeling. For each statement, circle the number that you think most accurately describes your dog.

Is your dog...	My dog couldn't be less				My dog couldn't be more		
Energetic & enthusiastic?	0	1	2	3	4	5	6
Happy & content?	0	1	2	3	4	5	6
Active & comfortable?	0	1	2	3	4	5	6
Calm & relaxed?	0	1	2	3	4	5	6

1. Reid J, Wright A, Gober M, Nolan AM, Noble C, Scott EM. Measuring chronic pain in osteoarthritic dogs treated long-term with carprofen, through its impact on health-related quality of life (HRQL). *Vet Comp Orthop Traumatol.* 2018; 31(S 01): A1-A6.

Sharing additional history can help your veterinary team help your dog.

	Yes	No
1. Has your dog ever been injured?	○	○
2. Have you ever given your dog medication for pain, such as aspirin?	○	○
3. Has your dog gained weight in the past year?	○	○

Osteoarthritis can affect dogs of all ages, breeds, and sizes. If left untreated, the pain can become worse over time. This checklist is designed to help with the recognition of OA pain to help keep your dog happy and active. Your veterinary team will review the results of this checklist with you to identify if your dog might be suffering from OA, or to monitor how your dog is doing if he or she is already being treated for OA. This checklist is not a medical diagnostic tool and is not intended to replace discussions with an animal healthcare professional. Discuss medical concerns with your veterinarian.

zoetis

■ **Figure 53.1** (Continued)

  - May be exacerbated by exercise, long periods of recumbency, and cold weather.
  - Difficult to perform certain tasks—rising from lying down, climbing up or down stairs or into vehicle, posturing to eliminate.
- Cats—overt lameness may not be seen; unkempt appearance, difficulty accessing litter box, and increased irritability (see Figure 53.2).
  - Difficulties in activities—jumping up and down from surfaces, climbing up and down stairs, running, chasing moving objects[1] (see Table 53.1).

Physical Examination Findings

- Stiff-legged or altered gait or non-use of leg.
- Decreased range of motion.
- Crepitus.
- Joint swelling (effusion and/or thickening of the joint capsule), pain, and instability.
- Early diagnosis—brief orthopedic examination
  - Walk-in, posture, transition (lie–sit–stand)
  - Hands-on:
    - Elbow—medial periarticular fibrosis (PAF), lateral effusion
    - Stifle—effusion, early signs CCL; medial buttress or PAF
    - Tarsus—PAF
- Comprehensive examination
  - Add in neurological examination (proprioception, hopping, reflexes)
  - Assess muscle atrophy: pelvic limb—stifle
  - Range of motion—in lateral
- Pain assessment tools
  - Gait Analysis
  - Feline Grimace Scale
  - Pain biosignal with skin sensor (PainTrace®)
  - Thermography

COAST—Canine OsteoArthritis Staging Tool

- Incorporates pet owner and veterinary team evaluations
- Stages
  - Pre-clinical
    - Stage 0—clinically normal no OA risk factors
    - Stage 1—clinically normal, OA risk factors present
  - Clinical
    - Stage 2—Mild OA
    - Stage 3—Moderate OA
    - Stage 4—Severe OA
- Grade the dog: Clinical Metrology Instrument (CMI), Degree of Dog's discomfort, Static Posture, Motion
- Grade the Joint: pain upon manipulation, passive range of motion, radiography
- Highest "grade" from evaluating the dog or joint determines the final COAST stage.
  - Re-evaluate if there is disparity between the two results.

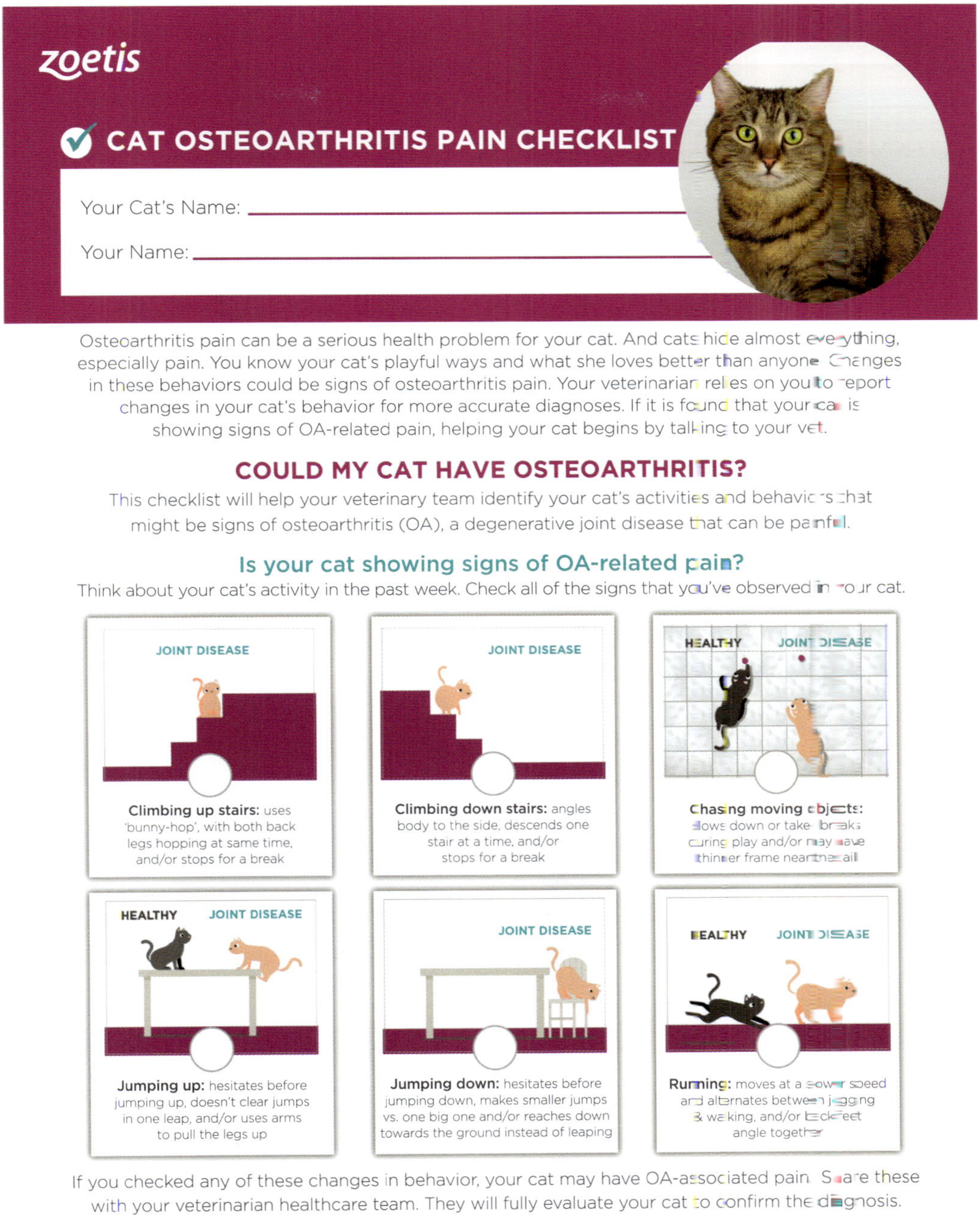

zoetis

CAT OSTEOARTHRITIS PAIN CHECKLIST

Your Cat's Name: ____________

Your Name: ____________

Osteoarthritis pain can be a serious health problem for your cat. And cats hide almost everything, especially pain. You know your cat's playful ways and what she loves better than anyone. Changes in these behaviors could be signs of osteoarthritis pain. Your veterinarian relies on you to report changes in your cat's behavior for more accurate diagnoses. If it is found that your cat is showing signs of OA-related pain, helping your cat begins by talking to your vet.

COULD MY CAT HAVE OSTEOARTHRITIS?

This checklist will help your veterinary team identify your cat's activities and behaviors that might be signs of osteoarthritis (OA), a degenerative joint disease that can be painful.

Is your cat showing signs of OA-related pain?

Think about your cat's activity in the past week. Check all of the signs that you've observed in your cat.

JOINT DISEASE
Climbing up stairs: uses 'bunny-hop', with both back legs hopping at same time, and/or stops for a break

JOINT DISEASE
Climbing down stairs: angles body to the side, descends one stair at a time, and/or stops for a break

HEALTHY / JOINT DISEASE
Chasing moving objects: slows down or takes breaks during play and/or may have thinner frame near the tail

HEALTHY / JOINT DISEASE
Jumping up: hesitates before jumping up, doesn't clear jumps in one leap, and/or uses arms to pull the legs up

JOINT DISEASE
Jumping down: hesitates before jumping down, makes smaller jumps vs. one big one and/or reaches down towards the ground instead of leaping

HEALTHY / JOINT DISEASE
Running: moves at a slower speed and alternates between jogging & walking, and/or back feet angle together

If you checked any of these changes in behavior, your cat may have OA-associated pain. Share these with your veterinarian healthcare team. They will fully evaluate your cat to confirm the diagnosis.

This questionnaire is not a medical diagnostic tool and is not intended to replace discussions with an animal healthcare professional. Discuss medical concerns with your veterinarian.

Figure 53.2 Cat osteoarthritis pain check list. Source: Zoetis.

Osteoarthritis has physical and emotional effects

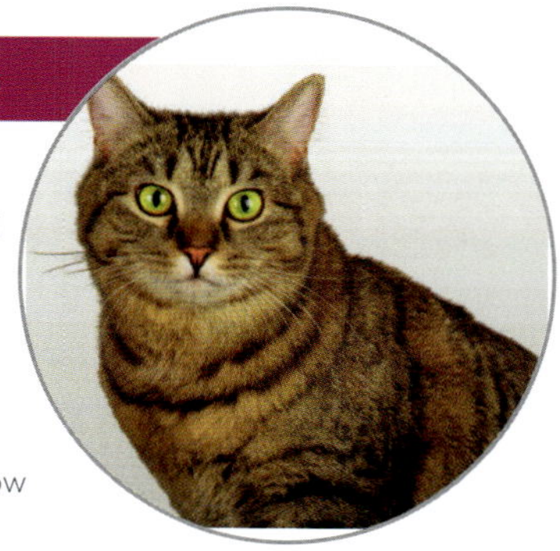

Just as in humans, chronic pain negatively impacts your cat's quality of life, not just physically, but also emotionally. The good news is that by identifying your cat's condition, you and your veterinarian can develop a treatment plan for your cat.

A recent peer-reviewed published study demonstrated the initial validity and reliability of a quality of life assessment for chronic diseases, such as osteoarthritis, in cats.[2] Using these questions, you can help your veterinarian assess and monitor how well your cat's chronic pain management treatment is working.

Think about your cat's behavior in the past week and help us determine a starting point by completing the following table.

Is your cat...	My cat couldn't be less						My cat couldn't be more
Energetic & Enthusiastic (Vitality)	0	1	2	3	4	5	6
Active & Comfortable (Comfort)	0	1	2	3	4	5	6
Happy & Content (Emotional well-being)	0	1	2	3	4	5	6

YOUR CAT'S GENERAL BEHAVIOR HISTORY CAN BE HELPFUL

Additional information that can be helpful to your veterinary team is your cat's behavior.

	YES	NO
1. Has your cat's personality and sociability changed?	○	○
2. Has your cat's urination or defecation habits changed?	○	○
3. Is your cat hiding more or does your cat seem to be "slowing down"?	○	○

OA pain can affect cats of any age, and it has been seen in more than 60% of cats that are 6 years or older.[3] If left untreated, the pain can become worse over time. This checklist is designed to help with the recognition of OA pain to help keep your cat happy and active. Your veterinary team will review the results of this checklist with you to identify if your cat might be suffering from OA. This checklist is not a medical diagnostic tool and is not intended to replace discussion with an animal healthcare professional. Discuss medical concerns with your veterinarian.

References: 1. Based on the Musculoskeletal Pain Screening Checklist (MiPSC) ©2019 North Carolina State University. **2.** Reid J., Nolan A.M., Scott E.M, Measuring pain in dogs and cats using structured behavioural observation, *Vet J.* 2018 June; 236: 72-79. **3.** Slingerland LI et al, Cross-sectional study of the prevalence and clinical features of osteoarthritis in 100 cats, *Vet J.* 2011 Mar;187(3):304-9.

zoetis

Figure 53.2 (Continued)

TABLE 53.1 Owner checklist for detecting DJD-associated pain in cats

	YES	NO
Does your cat jump up normally?		
Does your cat jump down normally?		
Does your cat climb up stairs or steps normally?		
Does your cat climb down stairs or steps normally?		
Does your cat run normally?		
Does your cat chase moving objects (e.g., toys)?		

Source: Adapted from Enomoto et al.[1]

DIAGNOSIS

DIFFERENTIAL DIAGNOSIS

- Neoplastic (synovial sarcoma; chondrosarcoma; osteosarcoma).
- Septic or immune-mediated arthritis (erosive vs. nonerosive).
- Other musculoskeletal or neurological conditions that cause lameness or decreased activity/ weakness.

OTHER LABORATORY TESTS

- Coombs' test, antinuclear antibody (ANA), and rheumatoid factor may help to rule out immune-mediated arthritis.
- Serum titers for *Borrelia*, *Ehrlichia*, and *Rickettsia* to evaluate for infectious arthritis.

IMAGING

- Radiographic changes
    - Joint capsular distention, osteophytosis, enthesophytosis, soft-tissue thickening, and narrowed joint spaces.
    - In severely affected patients: subchondral sclerosis and intra-articular calcified bodies (joint mice).
- Radiographic severity often does not correlate with clinical severity.
- Stress radiography may identify underlying instability and accentuate joint incongruity (e.g., distraction index, passive hip laxity of coxofemoral joint is predictive of hip OA).
- Bone nuclear scintigraphy can assist in localizing subtle OA.
- Arthroscopy can allow direct observation of cartilage and characterization by Modified Outerbridge Score.

DIAGNOSTIC PROCEDURES

- Arthrocentesis and synovial fluid analysis—cell counts are normal or slightly increased (<2000–5000 cells/mL) predominantly mononuclear (macrophages) and occasional synovial lining cells.

- Bacterial culture of synovial fluid or synovium—negative.
- Biopsy of synovial tissue to rule out neoplasia or immune-mediated arthropathy (lymphocytic plasmacytic synovitis, systemic lupus erythematosus).

COAST—Canine OsteoArthritis Staging Tool

- Incorporates pet owner and veterinary team evaluations.
- Stages
    - Pre-clinical
        - Stage 0—clinically normal no OA risk factors
        - Stage 1—clinically normal, OA risk factors present
    - Clinical
        - Stage 2—Mild OA
        - Stage 3—Moderate OA
        - Stage 4—Severe OA
- Grade the dog: Clinical Metrology Instrument (CMI), Degree of Dog's discomfort, Static Posture, Motion
- Grade the Joint: pain upon manipulation, passive range of motion, radiography
- Highest "grade" from evaluating the dog or joint determines the final COAST stage.
    - Re-evaluate if there is disparity between the two results.

TREATMENT

Goal—relieve pain, promote overall joint health

SURGICAL CONSIDERATIONS

- Arthroscopy—used to diagnose and remove aggravating causes.
- Arthrotomy—used to remove aggravating causes (e.g., fragmented coronoid process, ununited anconeal process, osteochondral flaps).
- Reconstructive procedures—used to eliminate joint instability and correct anatomic problems (cruciate ligament rupture, patella luxation, angular deformity).
- Joint removal—femoral head and neck ostectomy, temporomandibular joint arthroplasty.
- Joint replacement—total hip replacement is widely used, total elbow and stifle replacement are used with less frequency, total ankle and shoulder replacement are experimental and used infrequently at this time.
- Joint fusion (arthrodesis)—in selected chronic cases and for joint instability, complete or partial; carpus, hock: generally excellent outcome; shoulder, elbow, stifle: less predictable outcome.

MEDICATIONS

DRUG(S) OF CHOICE

Nonsteroidal Anti-inflammatory Drugs (NSAIDs)

- Inhibit prostaglandin synthesis through cyclooxygenase enzymes.
    - Deracoxib (3–4 mg/kg PO q24h, chewable).
    - Carprofen (2.2 mg/kg PO q12h or q24h).
    - Meloxicam (load 0.2 mg/kg PO, then 0.1 mg/kg PO q24h, liquid).

- Tepoxalin (load 20 mg/kg, then 10 mg/kg PO q24h).
- Cats—some caution with chronic kidney disease
  - Meloxicam (0.1 mg/kg PO q24h, liquid) or
    - Retrospective study—no adverse effect on renal CKD (IRIS 1–3).
    - Prospective study 0.02 mg/kg q24h for 6 months—higher protein/creatinine ratio
  - Robenacoxib (1 mg/kg PO q24h for 3 days).
    - Off-label study—28 days IRIS stage 1–2—no adverse effects

- Inhibit prostaglandin synthesis at receptor specific sites (EP4)
  - Grapiprant (2.0 mg/kg PO q24h, chewable).

Disease-Modifying Osteoarthritis Agents (DMOAs)

- Polysulfated glycosaminoglycan (PSGAG) molecules to repair and regenerate cartilage (wide variety of products and quality); early intervention recommended.
  - Adequan®—clinical study in dogs with hip dysplasia; 4.4 mg/kg IM every 3–5 days for 8 injections had positive, temporary effect.
- Glucosamine and chondroitin sulfate – multiple supplements available, many with additional compounds.

ALTERNATIVE DRUG(S) AND THERAPIES

- Monoclonal antibodies—anti-NGF—species-specific
  - NGF is elevated in response to injury, disease, and noxious stimuli and contributes to neurogenic inflammation and increased perception of pain.
  - Should not be used if any inflammation or pain is based on neurological issues or if other neurological issues exist (e.g., GOLPP)
- Amantadine (3–5 mg/kg PO q24h)—best used in combination with another analgesic such as NSAID. Only analgesic (other than NSAID) with scientific evidence for usage with OA.
- Gabapentin (5–10 mg/kg PO q8-12h)—no scientific evidence for usage with OA.
- Opioids—Codeine (1–2 mg/kg PO q8–12h)—no scientific evidence for usage with OA; suggested for short-term use during flare-ups.
- Glucocorticoids—inhibit inflammatory mediators and cytokines; however, chronic use delays healing and initiates damage to articular cartilage; potential systemic side effects documented; goal is low dose (dogs, 0.5–2 mg/kg; cats, 2–4 mg/kg) q48h.
- Prednisone—initial dose 1–2 mg/kg PO q24h for dogs and 4 mg/kg PO q24h for cats.
- Cannabinoids—considered safe, may reduce pain scores, but evidence is uncertain as to clinical efficacy.

Intra-articular Injections

- Triamcinolone hexacetonide—intra-articular injection of 5 mg in dogs showed a protective and therapeutic effect in one model.
- Hyaluronic acid—intra-articular injection (15–30 mg/joint) used as a series of 3 separated by 1 week or in combination with an intra-articular steroid.
- Platelet-rich plasma—intra-articular injection to decrease inflammatory mediators; many patients need more than 1 injection separated by 2 weeks; weak scientific evidence for efficacy.
- 117mSn (tin) colloid (Synovetin OA®)

- Stem cells (also intravenous stem cell investigations)
- Collagen–Elastin Hydrogel Microparticles (CEHM)

SUPPLEMENTS

- The types, formulations, and combinations of supplements that are available for adjunct management of osteoarthritis are too numerous to list in this topic.
- Omega 3 fatty acids have evidence of efficacy in numerous studies.

CONTRAINDICATIONS

- Acetaminophen must not be given to cats.

PRECAUTIONS

- NSAIDs may cause gastric ulceration.
- Cyclooxygenase-2 (COX-2)-selective drugs may interfere with liver function when used outside of dosage range.
- When switching NSAIDs—wait 3 days for washout before starting new drug.

POSSIBLE INTERACTIONS

Steroids with NSAIDS.

DIET

- Weight reduction for obese patients—decreases stress placed on arthritic joints.
- Omega n-3 fatty acids decrease production of certain prostaglandins and modulate inflammation. Dosage should be 150–175 mg/kg DHA/EPA daily.

NURSING CARE

- Physical rehabilitation—very beneficial during periods of flare-ups.
- Maintaining or increasing joint motion—active and passive range-of-motion exercises, stretching, massage, therapeutic exercises, and hydrotherapy.
- Pain management—cold and heat therapy, transcutaneous electrical stimulation (TENS), chiropractic adjustments, and acupuncture.
    - Photobiomodulation—low-level laser therapy—shallow depth but may help decrease pain, increase range of motion and quality of life.
    - Extracorporeal shock wave therapy—penetrate deeper tissues, increase blood flow, decrease swelling.
    - Targeted Pulsed electromagnetic field—decrease inflammation and pain
- Muscle tone/strengthening—
    - Daily leash walking work up to 20 minutes on level ground,
    - Incorporation of inclines/declines, stair ascent and stair descent, walking on uneven terrain and land treadmill.
    - Open water swimming, underwater treadmill.
- Maintenance of a lean body weight through both diet and daily exercise.

ACTIVITY

- During flare-ups, limit daily activity that may aggravate clinical signs (running, chasing, jumping, playing)
- During periods of quiet, see muscle tone/strengthening above

ENVIRONMENT

- Adjust areas that can be difficult to access—stairs, "doggy-doors," high-edged litter boxes.
- Provide orthopedic bedding.
- Ramps for stairs, furniture, car
- Non-slick flooring or mats
- Raised platform for food and water bowls (not in GOLPP)

CLIENT EDUCATION

- Medical therapy is palliative, and the condition is likely to progress.
- Describe identifying signs of flare-ups and importance of getting it under control quickly.
- Discuss management options, daily exercise, activity level, and diet.
- Discuss quality-of-life assessments (QOL)

FOLLOW-UP

PATIENT MONITORING

- During flare-up recheck 2 weeks later; pain should be better controlled at this time; then recheck every 4–6 weeks until flare-up under control.
- Recheck OA patients every 4–6 months for life.
- Any clinical deterioration could indicate a flare-up—need to change drug selection or dosage; may indicate need for intra-articular injection, formal rehabilitation therapy, or surgical intervention.

PREVENTION/AVOIDANCE

Early identification of predisposing causes and prompt treatment to help reduce progression of secondary conditions, e.g., surgical removal of osteochondral lesions.

EXPECTED COURSE AND PROGNOSIS

- Slow progression of disease likely.
- Some form of medical or surgical treatment usually allows a good quality of life when managed appropriately and aggressively.

MISCELLANEOUS

Resources

- CARE
    - Canine Arthritis Resources & Education|Dog arthritis tips and resources

- COAST
    - Canine-OsteoArthritis-Staging-Tool-COAST.pdf (morrisanimalfoundation.org)
- IVAPM—International Academy of Pain Management
    - Home—IVAPM

Abbreviations

- ANA = antinuclear antibody
- COAST = Canine Osteoarthritis Staging Tool
- COX-2 = cyclooxygenase-2.
- DMOA = disease-modifying osteoarthritis agent.
- MSM = methylsulfonylmethane.
- NSAID = nonsteroidal anti-inflammatory drug.
- OA = osteoarthritis.
- OCD = osteochondritis dessicans.
- PSGAG = polysulfated glycosaminoglycan.

Suggested Reading

Aragon CL, Hofmeister EH, Budsberg SC. Systematic review of clinical trials of treatments for osteoarthritis in dogs. *J Am Vet Med Assoc* 2007;230(4):514–521.

Budsberg SC, Bartges JW. Nutrition and osteoarthritis in dogs: does it help? *Vet Clin North Am Small Anim Pract* 2006;36(6):1307–1323.

Cachon T, Frykman O, Innes JF, Lascelles BDX, Okumura M, Sousa P, Staffieri F, Steagall PV, Van Ryssen B. COAST Development Group's international consensus guidelines for the treatment of canine osteoarthritis. *Front Vet Sci* 2023 Aug 3;10:1137888. doi: https://doi.org/10.3389/fvets.2023.1137888. PMID: 37601753; PMCID: PMC10436090.

Enomoto M, Mantyh PW, Murrell J, Innes JF, Lascelles BDX. Anti-nerve growth factor monoclonal antibodies for the control of pain in dogs and cats. *Vet Rec* 2019 Jan 5;184(1):23. doi: https://doi.org/10.1136/vr.104590. Epub 2018 Oct 27. PMID: 30368458; PMCID: PMC6326241.

Hampton T. Efficacy still uncertain for widely used supplements for arthritis. *J Am Med Assoc* 2007;297(4):351–352.

Johnston SJ. Osteoarthritis joint anatomy, physiology and pathobiology. *Vet Clin North Am* 1997;27:699–723.

Mlacnik E, Bockstahler BA, Muller M, et al. Effects of caloric restriction and a moderate or intense physiotherapy program for treatment of lameness in overweight dogs with osteoarthritis. *J Am Vet Med Assoc* 2006;229(11):1756–1760.

Patikorn C, Nerapusee O, Soontornvipart K, Lawonyawut K, Musikpodok K, Waleethanaphan K, Anantachoti P. Efficacy and safety of cannabidiol for the treatment of canine osteoarthritis: a systematic review and meta-analysis of animal intervention studies. *Front Vet Sci* 2023 Sep 15;10:1248417. doi: https://doi.org/10.3389/fvets.2023.1248417. PMID: 37781283; PMCID: PMC10540436.

Van Der Kraan PM, Van Den Berg WB. Osteophytes: relevance and biology. *Osteoarthr Cartil* 2007;15(3):237–244.

Reference

1. Enomoto M, Lascelles BDX, Gruen ME. Development of a checklist for the detection of degenerative joint disease-associated pain in cats. *J Feline Med Surg* 2020 Dec;22(12):1137–1147. doi: https://doi.org/10.1177/1098612X20907424. Epub 2020 Mar 3. PMID: 32122226; PMCID: PMC7736399.

Author/editor: Heidi Lobprise
Topic adapted from Five Minute Veterinary Consultation, 7th edition, 2021
Original Topic: Osteoarthritis

Author: David Dycus
Consulting Editor: Mathieu M. Glassman

Chapter 54

Spondylosis Deformans

BASICS

OVERVIEW

- Degenerative, noninflammatory condition of the vertebral column that occurs in response to intervertebral disc degeneration.
- Often an incidental finding, rarely clinically important.
- Characterized by the production of osteophytes along the ventral, lateral, and dorsolateral aspects of the vertebral endplates. Radiographically, appears as smooth, ventral bridging bone.
- Most common location in dogs is the thoracolumbar spine in the area of the anticlinal vertebra and the upper lumbar vertebrae; in cats, the thoracic vertebrae.

SIGNALMENT

- Dog and cat.
- Females > males.
- Dogs—commonly seen in large breeds, especially German shepherd dog; also boxer, Airedale terrier, and cocker spaniel.
- Occurrence increases with age. Present in 50% of dogs by 6 years and 75% by 9 years. May be radiographically evident in young dogs with an inherited predisposition.
- Boxers—positive correlation between spondylosis deformans and hip dysplasia. Both heritable traits are detectable in predisposed animals by radiographic examination at 1 year.
- Cats—present in 68% of asymptomatic cats.

SIGNS

General Comments

- Patients are typically asymptomatic; lesions are of minor if any clinical importance.
- Pain may follow fracture of bony spurs or bridges.

Historical Findings

- Stiffness.
- Restricted motion.
- Spinal pain.

Blackwell's Five-Minute Veterinary Consult Clinical Companion: Small Animal Senior Care, First Edition. Edited by Heidi B. Lobprise.

Companion website: www.wiley.com/go/lobprise/Senior

Physical Examination Findings

Neurologic deficits are uncommon. If present, referable to compression of the spinal cord or nerve root.

CAUSES AND RISK FACTORS

- Repeated microtrauma.
- Major trauma.
- Inherited predisposition.
- Acromegaly.

DIAGNOSIS

DIFFERENTIAL DIAGNOSIS

- Discospondylitis—differentiated by radiographic evidence of endplate lysis.
- Spinal osteoarthritis—degeneration of articular facet joints.
- Neoplasia—may have irregular, ventral, nonbridging bone.

CBC/BIOCHEMISTRY/URINALYSIS

Normal

Radiographic Findings

Spinal radiography initially shows osteophytes as triangular projections several millimeters from the edge of the vertebral body. With progression, osteophytes appear to bridge the intervertebral space. True ankylosis is rare.

DIAGNOSTIC PROCEDURES

In uncommon presentations, MRI, CT, or CT myelography can be used to demonstrate an atypical dorsal osteophyte compressing the spinal cord or nerve roots or encroaching on critical soft-tissue structures.

TREATMENT

- Typically not needed. Inform client that the condition is usually an asymptomatic, incidental finding, and is likely not responsible for any clinical signs that may be present.
- Treat spondylosis on an outpatient basis with strict rest and analgesia, possibly acupuncture.
- If overconditioned, recommend weight-reduction program.
- Acupuncture—dry needle or electroacupuncture treatment at weekly or biweekly interval and tapered to as-needed basis can be very effective in relief of pain. Useful in animals who do not tolerate medication or when clients prefer an alternative treatment modality.

MEDICATIONS

DRUG(S) OF CHOICE

Use only when the patient is exhibiting signs.

Nonsteroidal Anti-inflammatory Drugs (NSAIDs)

- In dogs, NSAIDs are preferable to steroids (fewer side effects) unless patient has neurologic deficits or concomitant disease prohibits use. Administer with food.
- If gastrointestinal sensitivity, use in combination with an or a gastrointestinal protectant to reduce the possibility of ulceration.

Non-NSAID Analgesics

- Use may enable reduction of dose or frequency of anti-inflammatory medications.
- Gabapentin 10 mg/kg PO q8–12h in dogs or cats.
- Buprenorphine 0.01–0.03 mg/kg PO q8h in cats.
- Acetaminophen 5 mg/kg POq12h in dogs.

Corticosteroids

- Only use in patients with neurologic deficits.
- Prednisone 0.25–0.5 mg/kg PO q12h; or dexamethasone 0.025–0.05 mg/kg PO q12h.
- Taper to alternate-day prednisone or twice-weekly dexamethasone.

CONTRAINDICATIONS/POSSIBLE INTERACTIONS

- Acetaminophen—do not use in cats. Use NSAIDs with caution in cats.
- Avoid prolonged administration of NSAIDs, simultaneous use of NSAIDs and acetaminophen, simultaneous use of NSAIDs and steroids, use of NSAIDs in patients with gastrointestinal (GI) or renal disease. Doing so decreases risk of GI ulceration and renal pathology.

FOLLOW-UP

PATIENT MONITORING

- If signs are present, restrict activity and gradually return the animal to normal activity after signs have subsided for several weeks.
- Relapse can occur with strenuous activity.
- With prolonged use of analgesic medications, periodic biochemistry testing is warranted.

PREVENTION/AVOIDANCE

Boxers—given genetic correlation between spondylosis deformans and hip dysplasia and potential for early radiographic detection, dogs should be screened and selectively bred.

Suggested Reading

Romatowski J. Spondylosis deformans in the dog. *Compend Contin Educ Pract Vet* 1986;8:531–536.

Author/editor: Heidi Lobprise
Topic adapted from Five Minute Veterinary Consultation, 7th edition, 2021
Original Topic: Spondylosis Deformans

Authors: Richard J. Joseph and Anne E. Buglione

Neurological

Chapter 55

Ataxia

BASICS

DEFINITION

- A sign of sensory dysfunction causing loss of coordination of the limbs, head, and/or trunk.
- Three clinical types—sensory (proprioceptive), vestibular, and cerebellar. All cause limb incoordination, but only vestibular and cerebellar ataxia cause head and neck incoordination.

PATHOPHYSIOLOGY

Sensory (Proprioceptive)

- Proprioceptive pathways in the spinal cord (i.e., fasciculus gracilis, fasciculus cuneatus, and spinocerebellar tracts) relay limb and trunk positions to the brain.
- When the spinal cord is slowly compressed, proprioceptive deficits are usually the first signs observed, because these tracts or pathways are located more superficially in the white matter and their larger axons are more susceptible to compression than are other tracts.
- Limb weakness (paresis) will occur if more centrally located motor tracts or pathways become involved; weakness is not always obvious early in the course of the disease.
- Ataxia can occur with spinal cord, brainstem, and cerebral lesions. Ataxia can be mild to absent with unilateral brainstem lesions, and subtle to absent with unilateral cerebral lesions.

Vestibular

- Changes in balance and head and neck positions are detected by vestibular receptors of the inner ear, relayed to the vestibulocochlear nerve, which is connected to vestibular nuclei in the brainstem.
- The inner ear's vestibular receptors and nerve are components of the peripheral nervous system, whereas brainstem vestibular nuclei are components of the central nervous system.
- Vestibular ataxia should be localized to either the peripheral or central vestibular nervous system, because prognosis and rule-outs differ for these two locations.
- Both locations of vestibular disease cause various degrees of vestibular ataxia, often manifested by head tilt and leaning, falling, or even rolling toward the side of the lesion.
- Central vestibular disease usually has vertical nystagmus or changing types of nystagmus; somnolence, stupor, or coma (due to involvement of the nearby ascending reticular activating system); multiple cranial nerve signs (e.g., trigeminal or facial nerve deficits); proprioceptive deficits and quadriparesis or hemiparesis.

Blackwell's Five-Minute Veterinary Consult Clinical Companion: Small Animal Senior Care, First Edition. Edited by Heidi B. Lobprise.

Companion website: www.wiley.com/go/lobprise/Senior

- Peripheral vestibular disease does not typically show changes in mental status, vertical nystagmus, proprioceptive deficits, quadriparesis, or hemiparesis.
- Bilateral vestibular disease is uncommon and most often peripheral in origin. Typical vestibular signs are absent. Wide swinging back and forth head motions and poor-to-absent physiologic nystagmus are characteristic.

Cerebellar

- The cerebellum regulates, coordinates, and modulates motor activity.
- Proprioception is normal because the ascending proprioceptive pathways to the cortex are intact; weakness does not occur because the upper motor neurons are intact.
- While strength is preserved, affected animals have uncoordinated motor activity of limbs, head, and neck manifested by hypermetria; dysmetria; head tremors; intention tremors; and truncal sway. Menace responses may be absent without visual dysfunction.

SYSTEMS AFFECTED

Nervous—spinal cord (and brainstem and cortex), cerebellum, vestibular system.

SIGNALMENT

Any age, breed, or sex.

SIGNS

- Important to define the type of ataxia to localize the problem.
- Only one limb involved—rule out a musculoskeletal problem.
- Only hind limbs affected—likely a spinal cord disorder affecting the spinocerebellar tracts.
- All limbs or ipsilateral limbs affected—cervical spinal cord or cerebellar localization.
- Head tilt and/or nystagmus—vestibular localization.

CAUSES

Cerebellar

- Degenerative—abiotrophy (Kerry blue terrier, Gordon setter, rough-coated collie, Australian kelpie, Airedale, Bernese mountain dog, Finnish harrier, Brittany spaniel, border collie, beagle, Samoyed, wirehaired fox terrier, Labrador retriever, Great Dane, chow chow, Rhodesian ridgeback, domestic shorthair cats); storage diseases often have cerebello-medullary involvement.
- Anomalous—hypoplasia secondary to perinatal infection with panleukopenia virus (cats); malformed cerebellum due to herpesvirus infection (newborn puppies); arachnoid or epidermoid cyst located near fourth ventricle.
- Neoplastic—any CNS tumor (primary or secondary) localized to the cerebellum.
- Infectious—canine distemper virus; feline infectious peritonitis (FIP); and any other CNS infection affecting the cerebellum.
- Inflammatory, idiopathic, immune-mediated—meningoencephalomyelitis of undetermined etiology.
- Toxic—metronidazole.

Vestibular—CNS

- Infectious—FIP; canine distemper virus; rickettsial diseases.
- Inflammatory, idiopathic, immune-mediated—meningoencephalomyelitis of undetermined etiology.
- Nutritional—thiamine deficiency.
- Toxic—metronidazole.

Vestibular—Peripheral Nervous System

- Infectious—otitis media interna; *Cryptococcus* granuloma (cats).
- Inflammatory—nasopharyngeal (middle ear) polyps (cats).
- Idiopathic—geriatric vestibular disease (dogs); idiopathic vestibular syndrome (cats).
- Metabolic—hypothyroidism.
- Neoplastic—squamous cell carcinoma, bone tumors.
- Traumatic.

Spinal Cord

- Degenerative—degenerative myelopathy (old German shepherd, pug, boxer, Welsh corgi, others); degenerative disc disease.
- Vascular—fibrocartilaginous embolic myelopathy.
- Anomalous—hemivertebrae; dens hypoplasia with atlantoaxial subluxation-luxation; Chiari-like malformation; cervical spondylomyelopathy; spinal subarachnoid diverticulum; other spinal cord and vertebral malformation.
- Neoplastic—primary bone tumors; multiple myeloma and metastatic tumors that infiltrate the vertebral body; meningioma; others.
- Infectious—discospondylitis; myelitis.
- Traumatic—intervertebral disc herniation; fracture or luxation; atlantoaxial subluxation-luxation.

Metabolic

- Anemia.
- Polycythemia.
- Electrolyte disturbances—especially hypokalemia, hypocalcemia, and hypoglycemia.

Miscellaneous

- Drugs—acepromazine; antihistamines; antiepileptic drugs; flea and tick products.
- Respiratory compromise.
- Cardiac compromise—reverse patent ductus arteriosus, aortic thromboembolism.

RISK FACTORS

- Intervertebral disc disease—dachshund, poodle, cocker spaniel, beagle, and others.
- Cervical spondylomyelopathy—Doberman pinscher and Great Dane.
- Fibrocartilaginous embolism—young, large-breed dogs and miniature schnauzers.
- Dens hypoplasia and atlantoaxial luxation—small-breed dogs, poodles.
- Chiari-like malformation—cavalier King Charles spaniel, small-breed dogs.

DIAGNOSIS

DIFFERENTIAL DIAGNOSIS

- Differentiate the types of ataxia.
- Differentiate from other disease processes that can affect gait—musculoskeletal, metabolic, cardiovascular, respiratory.
- Musculoskeletal disorders—typically produce lameness, pain, and a reluctance to move; degenerative joint disease signs often improve with increased movements.
- Systemic illness and endocrine, cardiovascular, and metabolic disorders—can cause intermittent ataxia, especially of the pelvic limbs; with fever, weight loss, murmurs, arrhythmias, hair loss, or collapse with exercise, suspect a non-neurologic cause; obtain minimum data from hemogram, biochemistry, and urinalysis.
- Head tilt or nystagmus—likely vestibular localization.
- Intention tremors of the head or hypermetria—likely cerebellar localization.
- All four limbs affected—lesion is in the cervical spinal cord, cerebellum, or is multifocal to diffuse.
- Only pelvic limbs affected—lesion is anywhere below the second thoracic vertebra.

CBC/BIOCHEMISTRY/URINALYSIS

Normal unless metabolic cause (e.g., hypoglycemia, electrolyte imbalance, anemia, polycythemia).

OTHER LABORATORY TESTS

- Hypoglycemia—determine serum insulin concentration on sample that has low glucose value; low glucose and higher than expected insulin value suggest insulin-secreting tumor.
- Anemia—differentiate as nonregenerative or regenerative on the basis of the reticulocyte count.
- Electrolyte imbalance—correct the problem; see if ataxia resolves.
- Antiepileptic drugs—if being administered, evaluate serum concentration for toxicity.

IMAGING

- Spinal radiography, myelography, CT, or MRI—if spinal cord dysfunction suspected.
- Bullae radiography—if peripheral vestibular disease suspected; CT or MRI superior; for inner ear disease, MRI superior to CT.
- Thoracic radiography—for older patients and patients suspected to have neoplasia or systemic fungal infection.
- CT or MRI—if cerebellar disease suspected; MRI superior to CT.
- Abdominal ultrasonography—if hepatic, renal, adrenal, or pancreatic dysfunction suspected.

DIAGNOSTIC PROCEDURES

- Cerebrospinal fluid analysis—helps confirm nervous system etiology.
- Cerebrospinal fluid culture, antibody titer, or polymerase chain reaction—helps confirm nervous system infectious etiology.

TREATMENT

- Usually outpatient, depending on severity and acuteness of clinical signs.
- Exercise—decrease or restrict if ataxia originates from spinal cord disease.
- Client should monitor gait for increasing dysfunction or weakness; if paresis worsens or paralysis develops, other testing is warranted.
- Avoid drugs that could contribute to the problem; may not be possible in patients on antiepileptic drugs for seizures.

MEDICATIONS

DRUG(S) OF CHOICE

Not recommended until the source or cause of the problem is identified.

FOLLOW-UP

PATIENT MONITORING

Periodic neurologic examinations to assess condition.

POSSIBLE COMPLICATIONS

- Spinal cord—progression to weakness and possibly paralysis.
- Hypoglycemia—seizures.
- Cerebellar disease—head tremors and bobbing.
- Brainstem disease—stupor, coma, death.

MISCELLANEOUS

Abbreviations

- FIP = feline infectious peritonitis

Suggested Reading

Cherubini GB, Lowrie M, Anderson J. Pelvic limb ataxia in the older dog. *In Pract* 2008;30:386–391.
Davies C, Shell L. Neurological problems. In: Davies C, Lawrence T, Shell L (eds) *Common Small Animal Medical Diagnoses: An Algorithmic Approach*. Philadelphia, PA: Saunders, 2002; pp. 36–59.
Lowrie M. Vestibular disease: anatomy, physiology, and clinical signs. *Compend Contin Educ Vet* 2012;34:E1–5.
Penderis J. The wobbly cat: diagnostic and therapeutic approach to generalised ataxia. *J Fel Med Surg* 2009;11:349–359.
Rossmeisl JH Jr. Vestibular disease in dogs and cats. *Vet Clin North Am Small Anim Pract* 2010;40:81–100.

Author/editor: Heidi Lobprise
Topic adapted from Five Minute Veterinary Consultation, 7th edition, 2021
Original Topic: Ataxia

Author: Linda G. Shell

Chapter 56

Canine Degenerative Myelopathy

BASICS

DEFINITION

- Progressive adult-onset fatal neurodegenerative disease
- A result of a mutation in the superoxide dismutase 1 gene (*SOD1*); similar mutations known to cause some forms of amyotrophic lateral sclerosis (ALS), or Lou Gehrig's disease.
- Initial signs of progressive upper motor neuron spastic paresis and general proprioceptive ataxia in the pelvic limbs in older dogs.
- Clinical signs progress to flaccid tetraparesis/plegia and other lower motor neuron signs.

PATHOPHYSIOLOGY

- A second *SOD1* missense mutation (*c.52 A>T*) has been seen only in Bernese mountain dogs.
- Lesions may represent a multisystem central-peripheral axonopathy.
- Paucity of vascular supply in thoracic spinal cord may predispose it to damage.

SYSTEMS AFFECTED

- Central and peripheral nervous systems.
- Thoracolumbar spinal cord in early stage.
- Progresses to involve the cervical and lumbar spinal cord and peripheral nervous system later in the course of the disease.
- Neurons in the brainstem also may be affected.
- Disease also involves the sensory nerve roots and dorsal root ganglia.

GENETICS

- Most commonly autosomal recessive inheritance, and a familial inheritance is currently suspected.
- Mutations in *SOD1* are causative for DM but are incompletely penetrant.
- Dogs that are homozygous for the mutant allele are *at highest risk* for developing DM but not all will develop DM.
    - Dogs that test normal (clear) are highly unlikely to develop DM.
    - Dogs that test carrier are less likely to develop DM.

INCIDENCE/PREVALENCE

Prevalence rate of DM reported for all dogs collected from the Veterinary Medical Database (1990–1999) was 0.19%.

SIGNALMENT

Breed Predilections

- The most common mutation is in >150 breeds or varieties.
- A second mutation was found only in Bernese mountain dogs.
- DM has been histopathologically confirmed in many purebred and mixed-breed dogs.

Mean Age and Range

- Mean—9 years of age in large dogs; mean age at onset is 11 years in Pembroke Welsh corgi.
- Range—between 8 and 14 years.

Predominant Sex

No known sex predilection.

SIGNS

- Early:
  - Upper motor neuron paraparesis.
  - Insidious, progressive, asymmetric general proprioceptive ataxia; gait shows long-strided spastic paraparesis.
  - Paw replacement deficits.
  - Spinal reflexes usually present or exaggerated (patellar reflex may be reduced).
  - Presence of crossed-extensor reflex is variable.
  - Lack of paraspinal hyperesthesia is key clinical feature.
- Later:
  - Pelvic limb paresis leading to plegia, eventually progressing to tetraparesis/plegia.
  - Mild-to-moderate loss of muscle mass in pelvic limbs due to neurogenic atrophy.
  - Reduced spinal reflexes in pelvic limbs.
  - ±Urinary and fecal incontinence.
- End stage:
  - Flaccid tetraplegia.
  - Difficulty with swallowing and tongue movements.
  - Absence of spinal reflexes in all limbs.
  - Reduced-to-absent cutaneous trunci reflex.
  - Profound generalized muscle wasting.
  - Urinary and fecal incontinence.

CAUSES

- Hereditary disease and genetic predisposition.
- Other hypothesized causes include immune-mediated, metabolic deficiencies, toxic, and oxidative stress.

RISK FACTORS

- Dogs homozygous for the mutant allele(s) are at highest risk.
- There may be other environmental factors and modifying genes; studies underway.

DIAGNOSIS

DIFFERENTIAL DIAGNOSIS

- Type II intervertebral disc herniation.
- Intramedullary spinal cord neoplasia.
- Degenerative lumbosacral stenosis.
- Hip dysplasia.
- Other coexisting orthopedic disease.

CBC/BIOCHEMISTRY/URINALYSIS

- Usually normal.
- Performed to rule out other underlying metabolic disease.
- Urinalysis may identify secondary urinary tract infection.

OTHER LABORATORY TESTS

- Urine culture and sensitivity testing.
- Thyroid function testing.
- Electrodiagnostic testing results are normal in early diagnosis of DM.
- Genetic testing—test result of at-risk can support a presumptive diagnosis of DM in light of typical clinical signs and normal findings on neuroimaging and cerebrospinal fluid analysis.

IMAGING

- Survey spinal radiography.
- Myelography evaluates for compressive spinal cord disease.
- Myelography combined with CT—more sensitive technique to evaluate suspicious lesions.
- MRI—preferred technique to evaluate for extramedullary compressive and intramedullary lesions.

DIAGNOSTIC PROCEDURES

- CSF analysis evaluates for inflammatory disease.
- Definitive diagnosis is determined by post-mortem histopathology of spinal cord.

PATHOLOGIC FINDINGS

- Spinal cord axons and myelin affected most severely in dorsal and dorsal portion of lateral funiculi.

- Vacuolated axon cylinders/myelin sheaths most extensive in mid-thoracic spinal cord.
- Astroglial proliferation is prominent in severely affected areas of lesion distribution.
- Usually, lesion distribution is described as asymmetric and discontinuous; however, more recent evidence describes lesion distribution as symmetric and continuous in dogs that survive for long periods with DM.
- Neuronal cell body loss in ventral horn is evident at terminal or end-stage disease.
- Nerve specimens show fiber loss resulting from axonal degeneration and secondary demyelination.
- Muscle specimens show large and small groups of atrophic fibers typical of denervation.

TREATMENT

APPROPRIATE HEALTH CARE

- Supportive care.
- Breeds of small size may survive longer with DM because the pet owner is able to more easily give the appropriate care.

NURSING CARE

- When dog becomes non-ambulatory, keep on a well-padded surface to prevent decubitus ulceration over bony prominences.
- Keep hair trimmed, and skin clean and dry to prevent urine scald secondary to incontinence.
- Urine should be monitored for odor and color change, which may indicate urinary tract infection.
- Physical therapy using range-of-motion and active exercises may help maintain limb mobility and muscle strength.

ACTIVITY

- Exercise is encouraged to slow disuse atrophy of pelvic limbs, but fatigue should be monitored and exercise intensity adjusted.
- Hydrotherapy can involve use of an underwater treadmill setup.
- A wheel cart may assist with patient mobility.

DIET

- Maintain balanced diet.
- Prevent weight gain.

CLIENT EDUCATION

- Long-term prognosis is poor.
- Meticulous nursing care is crucial to preventing secondary complications in a recumbent patient.

MEDICATIONS

DRUG(S) OF CHOICE

Clinical trials are underway to determine effectiveness in slowing or halting disease progression.

FOLLOW-UP

PATIENT MONITORING

- Repeat neurologic examinations.
- Urine retention.
- Urinalysis and urine culture to monitor for urinary tract infection.

PREVENTION/AVOIDANCE

- Decubitus ulceration.
- Urine retention.
- Dermatitis from urine scald.
- Weight gain.

POSSIBLE COMPLICATIONS

- Urine retention may predispose to urinary tract infections.
- Local skin infections from decubitus ulceration.

EXPECTED COURSE AND PROGNOSIS

- Nonambulatory paraparesis occurs within 9–12 months from time of onset of signs.
- Tetraparesis may be evident within 3 years from time of onset of signs.
- Long-term prognosis is poor.

MISCELLANEOUS

Associated Conditions

- Other neurologic diseases associated with old-age onset.
- Spinal cord neoplasia.
- Intervertebral disc disease.
- Orthopedic disease.

Abbreviations

- ALS = amyotrophic lateral sclerosis
- DM = degenerative myelopathy.
- *SOD1* = superoxide dismutase 1.

Internet Resources

Accessed 29 June 2024

- www.caninegeneticdiseases.net/dm/maindm.htm
- www.ofa.org/diseases/dna-tested-diseases/dm

Suggested Reading

Awano T, Johnson GS, Wade C, et al. Genome-wide association analysis reveals a *SOD1* missense mutation canine degenerative myelopathy that resembles amyotrophic lateral sclerosis. *Proc Natl Acad Sci USA* 2009;106:2794–2799.

Coates JR, March PA, Ogelsbee M, et al. Clinical characterization of a familial degenerative myelopathy in Pembroke Welsh Corgi dogs. *J Vet Intern Med* 2007;21:1323–1331.

Coates JR, Wininger FA. Canine degenerative myelopathy. *Vet Clin North Am Small Anim Pract* 2010;40:929–950.

March PA, Coates JR, Abyad R, et al. Degenerative myelopathy in 18 Pembroke Welsh Corgi dogs. *Vet Pathol* 2009;46:241–250.

Ogawa M, Uchida K, Yamato O, et al. Neuronal loss and decreased GLT-1 expression observed in the spinal cord of Pembroke Welsh Corgi Dogs with canine degenerative myelopathy. *Vet Pathol* 2014;51:591–602.

Wininger FA, Zeng R, Johnson GS, et al. Degenerative myelopathy in a Bernese Mountain Dog with a novel *SOD1* missense mutation. *J Vet Intern Med* 2011;25:1166–1170.

Zeng R, Coates JR, Johnson GC, et al. Breed distribution of *SOD1* alleles previously associated with canine degenerative myelopathy. *J Vet Intern Med* 2014;28:515–521.

Author/editor: Heidi Lobprise

Topic adapted from Five Minute Veterinary Consultation, 7th edition, 2021

Original Topic: Canine Degenerative Myelopathy

Author: Joan R. Coates

Chapter 57

Cerebrovascular Accidents

BASICS

DEFINITION

- Sudden onset of nonprogressive focal brain signs.
- Signs must remain for >24 hours for a diagnosis of cerebrovascular accident (CVA).
- Permanent brain damage usually ensues.
- Called transient ischemic attack or TIA if clinical signs resolve within 24 hours.

PATHOPHYSIOLOGY

- Cerebrovascular diseases are the underlying cause of CVA.
- Brain abnormality resulting from a pathologic process that compromises the blood supply to the brain.
- Lesions affecting the cerebral blood vessels are divided into two broad categories:
    - Hemorrhagic stroke—ruptured blood vessel with hemorrhage into or around the brain.
    - Ischemic stroke—abrupt disruption of blood flow from blockage of an artery depriving the brain tissue of oxygen and glucose.

SYSTEMS AFFECTED

- Nervous.
- Multisystemic—if underlying cause present.

INCIDENCE/PREVALENCE

Unknown; supposed low compared to human.

SIGNALMENT

Species

Dog and cat.

Blackwell's Five-Minute Veterinary Consult Clinical Companion: Small Animal Senior Care, First Edition. Edited by Heidi B. Lobprise.

Companion website: www.wiley.com/go/lobprise/Senior

Breed Predilections

- Ischemic stroke—cavalier King Charles spaniel and greyhound seem predisposed; small breed (≤15 kg) more likely to have cerebellar infarct; large breed (>15 kg) more likely to have midbrain or thalamic infarct.
- Hemorrhagic stroke—unknown.

SIGNS

Historical Findings

- Ischemic stroke—peracute-to-acute nonprogressive focal brain signs.
- Hemorrhagic stroke—acute-to-subacute focal or multifocal brain signs that can progress over a short period of time.

Physical Examination Findings

- Fundus examination—may reveal tortuous vessels (systemic hypertension), hemorrhage (coagulopathy or systemic hypertension), or papilledema (elevated intracranial pressure [ICP]).
- Coagulation defects—may underlie hemorrhagic stroke and cause hemorrhage in any tissue or organ and anemia.

Neurologic Examination Findings

- Ischemic stroke—signs depend on the localization of the vascular insult (prosencephalon, midbrain, pons, medulla, cerebellum).
- Hemorrhagic stroke—signs relate to increased ICP with nonspecific forebrain and/or brainstem disturbance.

CAUSES

Ischemic Stroke

Dogs

- Unknown in 50% of cases.
- Endocrine diseases—hyperadrenocorticism, hypothyroidism, diabetes.
- Embolism, thromboembolism—neoplastic (hemangiosarcoma, lymphoma), infectious (associated with bacterial endocarditis or other sources of infection), and aortic or cardiac.
- Systemic hypertension—chronic kidney disease, protein losing enteropathy.
- Fibrocartilaginous embolism.
- Intravascular lymphoma.
- Parasite migration (*Cuterebra*) or embolism (*Dirofilaria immitis*).

Cats

- High likelihood of concurrent disease.
- Parasite migration (*Cuterebra* or heartworms).
- Systemic hypertension—hyperthyroidism, chronic kidney disease, heart disease.
- Neoplastic embolism.
- Intracranial telangiectasia.
- Hypertropic cardiomyopathy.
- Hyperthyroidism.

- Pulmonary disease.
- Liver disease.
- Neoplasia elsewhere in the body.

Hemorrhagic Stroke

Dogs

- Ruptured congenital vascular anomalies.
- Primary and secondary brain tumors.
- Inflammatory disease of arteries and veins (vasculitis).
- Intravascular lymphoma.
- Brain hemorrhagic infarction.
- Impaired coagulation.

Cats

- Primary and secondary brain tumors.
- Inflammatory disease of arteries and veins (vasculitis).
- Brain hemorrhagic infarction.
- Impaired coagulation—cerebral amyloid angiopathy.
- Systemic hypertension.

RISK FACTORS

- Ischemic stroke—systemic hypertension, systemic conditions associated with hypercoagulability syndrome.
- Hemorrhagic stroke—systemic hypertension, coagulopathy.

DIAGNOSIS

DIFFERENTIAL DIAGNOSIS

- Head trauma—history and physical findings suggestive of trauma.
- Decompensation from primary or metastatic brain tumor—signs are progressive.
- Infectious and noninfectious encephalitis—acute-to-subacute clinical signs that gradually worsen.
- Neurotoxicity—bilateral, symmetric neurologic deficits.

CBC/BIOCHEMISTRY/URINALYSIS

Most often normal; may show changes reflecting underlying cause.

OTHER LABORATORY TESTS

- Cerebrospinal fluid—unlikely to confirm CVA, may help rule out inflammatory CNS disease. Variable findings; either normal, or mild mononuclear or neutrophilic pleocytosis; protein concentration occasionally elevated.
- Prothrombin time—screening test for extrinsic mechanism defects.
- Activated partial thromboplastin time—screening test for intrinsic mechanism defects.

- Bleeding time—prolonged in patients with von Willebrand's disease; normal with most other coagulation defects, except disseminated intravascular coagulation.
- Thromboelastography, D-dimer assay, and antithrombin III—screening tests for hypercoagulability syndrome as possible cause of ischemic stroke.
- Endocrine testing—hyperadrenocorticism, thyroid disease, and pheochromocytoma.
- Renal disease—urine protein/creatinine ratio.

IMAGING

Ischemic Stroke

- CT—often normal during acute phase.
- MRI—within 12–24 hours of onset to distinguish hemorrhage from infarction; T2-weighted and fluid-attenuated inversion recovery (FLAIR) images particularly useful; T2*-weighted (gradient echo) images to show presence of or exclude intracranial hemorrhage; diffusion-weighted imaging (DWI) sequence: ideal for identification of hyperacute stroke, excluding stroke mimics; perfusion-weighted MRI can be used to depict brain regions of hypoperfusion and derive the tissue at risk by comparing the results with the findings on DWI.
- Time-of-flight magnetic resonance angiography (MRA) and contrast-enhanced MRA can be used to assess intracranial vascular status of stroke patients.

Hemorrhagic Stroke

- CT—very sensitive for detection of acute hemorrhage; hyperdensity due to hyperattenuation of X-ray beam by the globin portion of blood; attenuation decreases until the hematoma is isodense at about 1 month from onset; periphery of hematoma contrast-enhances from 6 days to 6 weeks after onset due to revascularization.
- MRI—signal intensity of intracranial hemorrhage is influenced by several intrinsic (time from ictus, source, size, and location of hemorrhage) and extrinsic (pulse sequence and field strength) factors; as hematoma ages, oxyhemoglobin in blood breaks down sequentially into several paramagnetic products (deoxyhemoglobin, methemoglobin, hemosiderin), each with different MRI signal intensities; compared to other conventional sequences, T2*-weighted (gradient echo) images demonstrate readily detectable hypointensity regardless of time from ictus, source and location of hemorrhage, or field strength.
- Multiple hemorrhagic lesions <5 mm—most often associated with hyperadrenocorticism, hypertension, chronic kidney disease, or hypothyroidism.
- Single hemorrhagic lesion—most often associated with *Angiostrongylus vasorum*.
- Multiple hemorrhagic lesions ≥ 5 mm—most often associated with *Angiostrongylus vasorum*, primary extracranial neoplasia with metastases (hemangiosarcoma).

DIAGNOSTIC PROCEDURES

Diagnosis of potential underlying causes.

Ischemic Stroke

Evaluate for hypertension (and potential underlying causes), endocrine disease (hyperadrenocorticism, hypothyroidism, hyperthyroidism, diabetes mellitus), chronic kidney disease (especially protein-losing nephropathy), protein-losing enteropathy, heart disease, and metastatic diseases (particularly hemangiosarcoma).

Hemorrhagic Stroke

Evaluate for coagulopathy (and potential underlying causes), hypertension (and potential underlying causes), and metastatic diseases (particularly hemangiosarcoma).

TREATMENT

NURSING CARE

Ischemic Stroke

- Monitoring and correction of basic physiologic variables (e.g., oxygen level, fluid balance, blood pressure, body temperature).
- Maintenance of systemic arterial blood pressure within physiologic range; aggressive lowering of blood pressure should be avoided during acute stages unless the patient is at high risk of end-stage organ damage (systolic blood pressures >180 mmHg); hypertension can develop as a physiologic response to a stroke to ensure adequate cerebral perfusion pressure; elevated blood pressure can persist for up to 72 hours after the onset of injury.
- No evidence that glucocorticoid provides beneficial neuroprotection; most neuroprotective agents tested have either failed to prove their efficacy in clinical trials or are awaiting further investigation.

Hemorrhagic Stroke

- Patient stabilization (airway protection, monitoring and correction of vital signs).
- Assessment and monitoring of neurologic status.
- Determination and treatment of potential underlying causes of hemorrhage.
- Assessment for the need of specific treatment measures including management of raised ICP, which revolves around reducing cerebral edema, optimizing cerebral blood volume, and eliminating space-occupying mass.
- Risk of neurologic deterioration and cardiovascular instability highest during the first 24 hours after onset of intracranial hemorrhage, as the space-occupying lesion slowly expands and cerebral vasogenic edema develops.

MEDICATIONS

DRUG(S) OF CHOICE

Ischemic Stroke

- Antihypertensive—consider if systemic BP >180 mmHg on serial evaluation and/or severe ocular manifestations of hypertension.
- Angiotensin-converting enzyme (ACE) inhibitor—enalapril (0.25–0.5 mg/kg q12h) or benazepril (0.25–0.5 mg/kg q12h) and/or calcium channel blockers such as amlodipine (0.1–0.25 mg/kg q24h); amlodipine is more effective in severe hypertension.
- Prevention of clot formation—consider in proven cardiac sources of embolism; antiplatelet therapy with low-dose aspirin (0.5 mg/kg PO q24h) or clopidogrel (2–4 mg/kg PO q24h) and low-molecular-weight heparin can be used prophylactically; low-molecular-weight heparin 80–150 IU/kg SC can be used in suspected or confirmed case of hypercoagulable state; anti-factor Xa activity should be monitored, although this may not be practical.

Hemorrhagic Stroke

Mannitol—if suspected elevated ICP unresponsive to extracranial stabilization measures (0.25–2 g/kg IV over 10–20 minutes up to q4–8h).

FOLLOW-UP

PATIENT MONITORING

Frequent neurologic evaluations in the first 48–72 hours to monitor progress.

EXPECTED COURSE AND PROGNOSIS

- Maximum severity of signs usually reached within 24 hours for ischemic stroke.
- Resolution of signs—gradual within 2–10 weeks; some dogs/cats may be left with permanent neurologic signs due to irreversible brain damage.
- Dogs with causal medical condition significantly more likely to relapse and have significant shorter survival time than dogs with no identifiable medical condition.
- Despite having a high likelihood of concurrent disease, cat with ischemic stroke have been reported to have a favorable short-term outcome, if neither clinical presentation nor concurrent disease was severe.
- Prognosis for global brain ischemia difficult to predict as there are no controlled studies.

MISCELLANEOUS

Abbreviations

- ACE = angiotensin-converting enzyme
- CVA = cerebrovascular accident.
- DWI = diffusion-weighted imaging.
- FLAIR = fluid-attenuated inversion recovery.
- ICP = intracranial pressure.
- MRA = magnetic resonance angiography.
- TIA = transient ischemic attack.

Suggested Reading

Lowrie M, De Risio L, Dennis R, et al. Concurrent medical conditions and long-term outcome in dogs with nontraumatic intracranial hemorrhage. *Vet Radiol Ultrasound* 2012;53:381–388.

Whittaker DE, Drees R, Beltran E. MRI and clinical characteristics of suspected cerebrovascular accident in nine cats. *J Feline Med Surg* 2017;20:674–684.

Author/editor: Heidi Lobprise
Topic adapted from Five Minute Veterinary Consultation, 7th edition, 2021
Original Topic: Cerebrovascular Accidents

Author: Laurent Garosi

Chapter 58

Deafness

BASICS

DEFINITION

- Partial or complete hearing loss.
- Two forms:
  - Sensorineural deafness—caused by damage to receptors in cochlea, cochlear nerve, or auditory pathways in CNS.
  - Conduction deafness—caused by inability to conduct sound vibration through external-to-inner-ear structures.

PATHOPHYSIOLOGY

Sensorineural Deafness

- Acquired—cochlear degeneration due to chronic infection, ototoxicity, neoplasia, chronic exposure to loud noises, anesthesia-associated, or age-related loss of hair cells and spiral ganglion cells (presbycusis).

Conduction Deafness

- Acquired defects resulting in stenosis/obstruction of external ear canal, rupture of tympanic membrane, or fusion of bony ossicles; most commonly associated with chronic otitis or middle ear polyps.

SYSTEMS AFFECTED

Nervous—inner ear.

SIGNALMENT

- Acquired deafness may occur in any breed or age of dog and cat.

SIGNS

- Unilateral deafness often goes unnoticed. Rarely, dogs have difficulty localizing sound.

Blackwell's Five-Minute Veterinary Consult Clinical Companion: Small Animal Senior Care, First Edition. Edited by Heidi B. Lobprise.

Companion website: www.wiley.com/go/lobprise/Senior

- With bilateral disease, animals do not respond to auditory cues such as calling their name or rattling food dish. Often they are easily startled. Commonly have heightened response to vibration and visual cues.

CAUSES

Sensorineural Deafness

- Acquired cochlea and cochlear nerve damage—infectious (otitis interna), neoplasia of bony labyrinth or nerve, trauma (physical or noise), systemic or topically applied drugs or toxins (antibiotics: aminoglycosides, polymyxin, erythromycin, vancomycin, chloramphenicol; antiseptics: ethanol, chlorhexidine, cetrimide; antineoplastics: cisplatin, carboplatin; diuretics: furosemide; heavy metals: arsenic, lead, mercury; miscellaneous: ceruminolytic agents, propylene glycol, salicylates), presbycusis, anesthesia-induced.

Conduction Deafness

- Otitis externa and other external ear canal disease (e.g., stenosis of canal, foreign bodies, neoplasia, or ruptured tympanum).
- Otitis media, middle-ear polyps, primary secretory otitis media.

RISK FACTORS

- Chronic otitis externa, media, or interna.
- Use of ototoxic drugs.
- General anesthesia.

DIAGNOSIS

DIFFERENTIAL DIAGNOSIS

- Use of ototoxic drugs, recent anesthesia, or chronic ear disease—suggests acquired causes.
- Evaluate for brain disease.

CBC/BIOCHEMISTRY/URINALYSIS

Usually normal.

OTHER LABORATORY TESTS

- Bacterial culture and sensitivity of ear canal if otitis externa.
- Myringotomy with culture of aspirates if otitis media.

IMAGING

- Tympanic bullae and skull radiographs—may show soft-tissue opacity and bone remodeling of tympanic bulla; often unremarkable in cases with otitis media/interna.
- Ultrasound of tympanic bullae—may show anechoic content in cases with otitis media/interna, but low sensitivity.

- CT/MRI—higher sensitivity for middle–inner ear disease and intracranial pathology.

DIAGNOSTIC PROCEDURES

- Brainstem auditory-evoked response (BAER)—gold standard test for evaluation of hearing. Measures electrical response of cochlea and auditory pathways in the brain to an auditory stimulus; reliable to identify dogs with unilateral disease or partial hearing loss. Bone conduction stimulation can be useful to distinguish sensorineural from conduction deafness. Can be used to determine the hearing threshold.
- Otoacoustic emissions (OAEs)—low-level sounds produced by inner ear as part of the normal hearing process that can be measured by placing a probe containing a microphone in the external ear canal. Two forms have been used in dogs for assessment of sensorineural deafness—transient-evoked OAEs (TEOAEs) and distortion product OAEs (DPOAEs). OAE is best suited for cases with congenital deafness, as it tests outer hair cell function and is not affected by inner hair cell, synapse, or cochlear nerve deficiencies. DPOAEs may show benefits in assessing age-related and noise-induced hearing loss and may reduce cost and testing times in congenital sensorineural deafness compared to BAER.

TREATMENT

CLIENT EDUCATION

Deaf animals may be functional pets, but require patience, specialized training, and extra protection from traffic.

SURGICAL CONSIDERATIONS

- Directed toward acquired causes; congenital deafness irreversible.
- Otitis externa, media, or interna—medical or surgical approaches depend on culture and sensitivity test results, response to antibiotics, and imaging findings. Conduction may improve as otitis externa or media resolves.
- Cochlear implants can be used in dogs with moderate-to-profound deafness, but only preliminary data available and very expensive.

MEDICATIONS

DRUG(S) OF CHOICE

- Treat otitis based on culture and sensitivity results.

PRECAUTIONS

- Aminoglycosides or other ototoxic drugs—use with caution.
- Topical treatment of external ear canal—avoid if tympanic membrane is ruptured.

FOLLOW-UP

PATIENT MONITORING

As needed for management of otitis.

POSSIBLE COMPLICATIONS

Deaf dogs need protected environments and training to be functional pets.

MISCELLANEOUS

- Hereditary or congenital deafness found in over 90 breeds of dogs, most with a large amount of white pigmentation (merle or piebald genes) with early onset. White cats with blue eyes have a high incidence of deafness as well.

Abbreviations

- BAER = brainstem auditory-evoked response
- DPOAE = distortion product OAE.
- OAE = otoacoustic emission.
- TEOAE = transient-evoked OAE.

Author/editor: Heidi Lobprise
Topic adapted from Five Minute Veterinary Consultation, 7th edition, 2021
Original Topic: Deafness

Author: Rita Gonçalves

Chapter 59

Fibrocartilaginous Embolic Myelopathy

BASICS

DEFINITION

Acute ischemic necrosis of the spinal cord caused when fibrocartilaginous emboli become lodged in the spinal vasculature.

PATHOPHYSIOLOGY

- Emboli—found in spinal cord vasculature; histologically and histochemically identical to nucleus pulposus of the intervertebral disc.
- Exact mechanism of entry into the spinal vasculature unknown.

INCIDENCE/PREVALENCE

- Common cause of spinal cord disease in nonchondrodystrophic breeds of dogs.
- Rarely reported in chondrodystrophic breeds.
- Uncommon in cats.

SIGNALMENT

Species

Dog and cat.

Breed Predilections

- Giant- and large-breed dogs most common but seen in small breeds as well.
- Miniature schnauzers overrepresented.

Mean Age and Range

- Median age 5 years.
- Range: 8 weeks–14.5 years.
    - While the median age of onset is 5 years, this is in the senior life stage rage for giant breeds and many large-breed dogs

Predominant Sex

Males overrepresented.

Blackwell's Five-Minute Veterinary Consult Clinical Companion: Small Animal Senior Care, First Edition. Edited by Heidi B. Lobprise.

Companion website: www.wiley.com/go/lobprise/Senior

SIGNS

Historical Findings

- May be associated with trauma or physical activity at or immediately before onset of signs.
- Sudden onset, generally nonprogressive and nonpainful.
- Discomfort occasionally noted at onset but resolves rapidly (minutes to hours).
- Signs of paresis or paralysis develop over a matter of seconds, minutes, or hours.
- Condition typically stabilizes within 24 hours.

Neurologic Examination Findings

- Localization—any spinal cord segment can be affected; T3–L3 and L4–S3 most common; multifocal lesions may rarely be seen; may see spinal shock with T3–L3 lesions, which can give the appearance of a multifocal spinal cord lesion.
- Deficits—commonly lateralized (due to spinal vascular anatomy) but can be symmetric; contralateral side may be mildly affected or normal.
- Severity of deficits—related to severity of infarction. Most display nonambulatory paresis, or plegia with intact nociception; fewer patients display ambulatory paresis, or plegia with absent nociception.
- Spinal pain—may be present briefly at onset of signs (owner report) and generally resolves by the time patient is examined.

RISK FACTORS

- Trauma/physical activity may precede the incident.
- Hyperlipoproteinemia may be a comorbidity in miniature schnauzers and Shetland sheepdogs.

DIAGNOSIS

DIFFERENTIAL DIAGNOSIS

- Acute noncompressive nucleus pulposus extrusion (ANNPE)—most important clinical difference may be persistent spinal pain beyond 24 hours; differentiate with cross-sectional imaging; may be indistinguishable but treated the same.
- Thrombi/emboli from other sources can cause similar ischemic injury to the spinal cord—consider underlying predisposing conditions (cardiomyopathy, hypothyroidism, hyperthyroidism, hyperadrenocorticism, chronic kidney disease, hypertension, hyperlipidemia; especially in cats).
- Intervertebral disc disease; discospondylitis; neoplasia; fracture and luxation—typically painful with symmetric deficits; survey radiography, MRI, CT, and/or myelography help confirm the diagnosis.
- Intra- and extramedullary hemorrhage secondary to coagulopathy (e.g., anticoagulant rodenticide ingestion, thrombocytopenia, or disseminated intravascular coagulation)—rule out by examining for underlying causes of hemorrhage, performing platelet count, and determining blood clotting times.
- Infectious/immune-mediated focal myelitis—differentiate on progressive history and cerebrospinal fluid (CSF) analysis.
- Acute, nonprogressive, asymmetric, and nonpainful spinal cord disease—presence of these characteristics greatly helps in diagnosis of fibrocartilaginous embolic myelopathy (FCE).

CBC/BIOCHEMISTRY/URINALYSIS

Usually normal.

IMAGING

- Survey spinal radiograph—usually normal, used to rule out other causes of myelopathy such as fracture, neoplasia, or discospondylitis.
- Myelography and CT myelography—in acute stage often demonstrates focal intramedullary swelling at embolic site; later, often normal or shows area of cord atrophy.
- MRI—preferred imaging modality for antemortem diagnosis: may see increased T2 signal intensity within spinal cord at site of lesion; may see mild contrast enhancement.

DIAGNOSTIC PROCEDURES

CSF Analysis

- Normal or nonspecific changes (mild pleocytosis/elevated protein concentration). Profound elevations in cell count can occasionally be observed with severe necrosis.
- Results depend on location (lumbar vs. cerebellomedullary cistern) and time of collection in relation to onset of clinical signs.

PATHOLOGIC FINDINGS

- Gross—focal spinal cord swelling ± hemorrhage.
- Microscopic—emboli of fibrocartilage in arteries and/or veins of spinal cord within or near area of focal spinal cord swelling; gray matter generally more affected than white matter.
- Histologic examination required for definitive diagnosis. Presumptive antemortem diagnosis is based on typical presentation and exclusion of other causes of acute myelopathy.

TREATMENT

APPROPRIATE HEALTH CARE

Inpatient—for immediate medical treatment and diagnostic procedures.

NURSING CARE

- Keep recumbent patients on padded surface; turn frequently to prevent pressure sores.
- Assist and encourage patients to ambulate as soon as possible.
- Assist bladder emptying (catheterize or express) several times daily if needed.
- Physical rehabilitation therapy may improve recovery and reduce residual neurologic deficits.
- Sling or harness support for assisted walking at home.

ACTIVITY

- Restrict until diagnosis is made in case of vertebral column instability from other causes such as intervertebral disc herniation or fracture/luxation.
- Once FCE is confirmed, activity should be encouraged, not restricted.

DIET

Normal unless other general health comorbidities are present.

CLIENT EDUCATION

- Gradual recovery from paresis or paralysis; most will recover ambulation, but residual neurologic deficits are common. Patients who are paraplegic with absent nociception have a more guarded prognosis for return of function.
- Most patients need considerable home care during recovery, including bladder management.

MEDICATIONS

DRUG(S) OF CHOICE

No specific medications are indicated for the treatment of FCE. Use of steroids such as methylprednisolone sodium succinate is controversial and unlikely to be of benefit.

CONTRAINDICATIONS

Nonsteroidal analgesics should not be administered with methylprednisolone sodium succinate.

FOLLOW-UP

PATIENT MONITORING

- Sequential neurologic evaluations—during first 12–24 hours after initial examination.
- Neurologic status—at 2, 3, and 4 weeks after onset of clinical signs.
- Urinary incontinence—manually express bladder in patients who are not voluntarily urinating. Urinalysis and culture/sensitivity to detect urinary tract infection.

PREVENTION/AVOIDANCE

- Recurrence highly unlikely but possible.
- No known method of prevention in most cases.

POSSIBLE COMPLICATIONS

- Fecal and urinary incontinence.
- Urinary tract infection.
- Urine scalding and pressure sores.

EXPECTED COURSE AND PROGNOSIS

- Generally good prognosis for recovery of ambulation.
- Most patients (85%) recover ambulation within 3 weeks (range: 3 days–12 weeks).
- Most patients retain some permanent neurologic deficits despite recovering ambulation.
- Paraplegia with loss of pain perception at presentation implies more guarded prognosis.

MISCELLANEOUS

Associated Conditions

Disorders that lead to compromise in circulatory function may predispose or mimic FCE—hyperadrenocorticism; hypothyroidism; high systemic blood pressure; hyperviscosity syndrome; hyperlipidemia; bleeding diathesis; bacterial endocarditis.

Pregnancy/Fertility/Breeding

High-dose corticosteroid administration—may cause premature delivery.

Abbreviations

- ANNPE = acute noncompressive nucleus pulposus extrusion
- FCE = fibrocartilaginous embolic myelopathy.
- CSF = cerebrospinal fluid.

Suggested Reading

Bartholomew KA, Stover KE, Olby NJ, Moore SA. Clinical characteristics of canine fibrocartilaginous embolic myelopathy (FCE): a systematic review of 393 cases (1973–2013). *Vet Rec* 2016;179:650.

De Risio L, Adams V, Dennis R, et al. Magnetic resonance imaging findings and clinical associations in 52 dogs with suspected ischemic myelopathy. *J Vet Int Med* 2007;21:1290–1298.

De Risio L, Platt SR. Fibrocartilaginous embolic myelopathy in small animals. *Vet Clin North Am Small Anim Pract* 2010;233:129–135.

Gandini G, Cizinauska S, Lang J, et al. Fibrocartilaginous embolism in 75 dogs: clinical findings and factors influencing the recovery rate. *J Small Anim Pract* 2003;44:76–80.

Hawthorne JC, Wallace LJ, Fenner WR, et al. Fibrocartilaginous embolic myelopathy in miniature schnauzers. *J Am Anim Hosp Assoc* 2001;37:374–383.

Mikszewski JS, Van Winkle TJ, Troxel MT. Fibrocartilaginous embolic myelopathy in five cats. *J Am Anim Hosp Assoc* 2006;42:226–233.

Summers BA, Cummings JF, de Lahunta A. *Veterinary Neuropathology*. St Louis, MO: Mosby, 1995; pp. 246–249.

Author/editor: Heidi Lobprise
Topic adapted from Five Minute Veterinary Consultation, 7th edition, 2021
Original Topic: Fibrocartilaginous Emolic Myopathy

Authors: Kristen Bartholomew and Sarah A. Moore

Chapter 60

Geriatric-Onset Laryngeal Paralysis and Polyneuropathy (GOLPP)

BASICS

DEFINITION

- LarPar—laryngeal paralysis; the nerve and muscles that control the opening and closing of the larynx do not function properly, blocking the airway.
- GOLPP—Geriatric-onset laryngeal paralysis and polyneuropathy, a degenerative polyneuropathy, previously described as idiopathic laryngeal paralysis

PATHOPHYSIOLOGY

- Disruption in nerve signals from the recurrent laryngeal nerve (rLN) to the lower laryngeal nerve.
  - May be a spastic paralysis that makes it challenging to intubate
  - If both cranial and recurrent laryngeal nerves are involved, the paralysis is more relaxed.
- Decreased diameter of the laryngeal opening increases resistance to airflow during inspiration and results in stridor on inspiration.
  - The decrease in airflow will lead to hypoxemia, cyanosis, and/or respiratory distress and a decrease in heat exchange (heat intolerance, hyperthermia).
- Inflammation or lesions of the vocal cords can lead to aphonia or change in bark/meow.
- Degeneration of the pararecurrent LN reduces esophageal motility; increases risk for aspiration pneumonia.
- Older dogs with laryngeal paralysis often have geriatric-onset laryngeal paralysis and polyneuropathy (GOLPP), which includes hind-limb weakness.
- Depression, stupor, or coma may occur if severe laryngeal obstruction leads to severe hyperthermia.

INCIDENCE/PREVALENCE

- GOLPP is a common disease of older large-breed dogs, especially Labrador and golden retrievers; exact prevalence unknown.

Blackwell's Five-Minute Veterinary Consult Clinical Companion: Small Animal Senior Care,
First Edition. Edited by Heidi B. Lobprise.

Companion website: www.wiley.com/go/lobprise/Senior

SIGNALMENT

Species

- GOLPP is most often found in large-breed dogs (especially Labrador and golden retrievers).

Mean Age and Range

- Middle-aged-to-older, medium-to-large breeds, males more than females.

SIGNS

Historical Findings

- Change in bark, gagging, throat-clearing, stridor, and dyspnea.
- Exacerbation with exercise, excitement, or hot environments—often presented as an emergency.
- Occasional cough (coughing is more common with tracheal disease)
- Severe cases—inspiratory respiratory distress, collapse, syncope, or even sudden death.
- Polyneuropathy—weakness, abnormal gait (pattern of abnormalities varies) (see Figure 60.1).

Physical Examination Findings

- Panting, polypnea, and inspiratory stridor in canine cases; with esophageal signs of gagging or regurgitation
- Aspiration pneumonia—fever, crackles on respiratory auscultation.
- Polyneuropathy—paraparesis or tetraparesis with decreased spinal reflexes.
  - Gait abnormality, wide stance, difficulties getting up—may be challenging to distinguish from osteoarthritis.

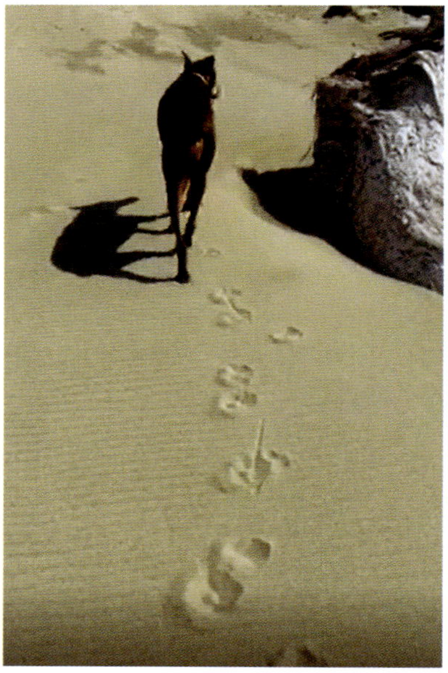

Figure 60.1 This senior Doberman progressed from laryngeal paralysis to hind limb neuropathy, evidenced by the dragging gait pattern in the sand. Source: Photo Courtesy of Dr. Mary Gardner.

- Get a detailed history with onset of signs, the perceived rate of progression, and the frequency and timing of throat-clearing.
  - If there is regurgitation, when does it happen: associated with eating or drinking? in the morning? at random?
- Palpate neck for thyroid carcinoma
- Complete neurological examination
  - If normal at presentation, over half with have signs within 6 months, and almost all will have signs at 12 months
- Need to distinguish from orthopedic issues—do complete orthopedic examination and trial of pain medication.

DIAGNOSIS

DIFFERENTIAL DIAGNOSIS

- Pharyngeal diseases—gagging, stridor, and cough; dysphagia that is not seen with GOLPP
- Tracheal disease—similar signs but with coughing
- Laryngeal paralysis due to other neuropathic, injuries, or iatrogenic causes
  - Thyroid tumors and cranial mediastinal masses may impact nerves

CBC/BIOCHEMISTRY/URINALYSIS

- No specific abnormalities
- Leukocytosis may be present in aspiration pneumonia.
- Mild-to-moderate increase in liver enzymes if chronic hypoxemia.
- Hypercholesterolemia may be present if concurrent hypothyroidism is present.

OTHER LABORATORY TESTS

- Thyroid panel

IMAGING

- Thoracic radiographs—three views and one lateral neck view: to rule out aspiration pneumonia as a complication, other lower airway conditions
- Barium swallow with fluoroscopy to identify esophageal dysfunction.

DIAGNOSTIC PROCEDURES

- Laryngoscopy
  - Method of choice to identify laryngeal paralysis, collapse, mass, trauma, foreign body, or laryngitis.
  - General anesthesia or deep sedation is required; alfaxalone or propofol; administer dopram HCL (1–2 mg/kg) to enhance respiration for evaluation.
- Laryngeal paralysis:
  - Diagnosis confirmed by loss of abduction of arytenoid cartilages during deep inspiration (see Figure 60.2).

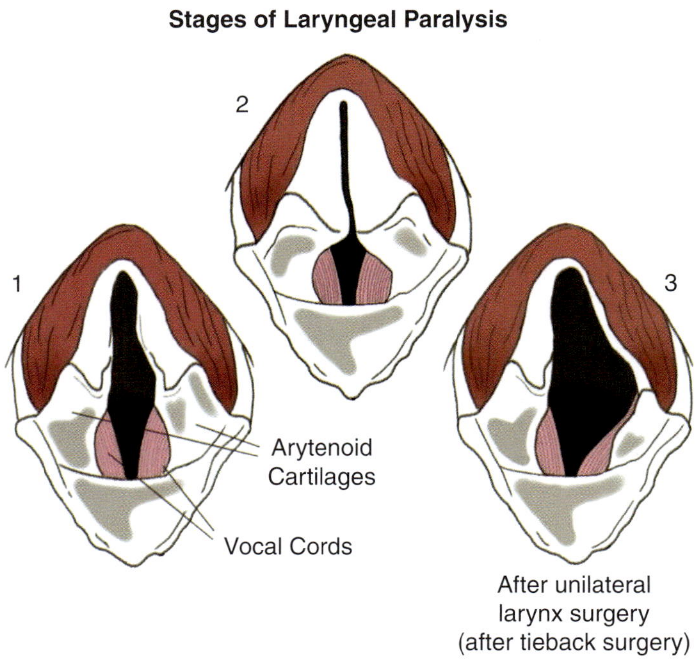

■ **Figure 60.2** Classic Schematic of the stages of laryngeal paralysis with (1) normal arytenoid cartilage position, (2) closed (loss of abduction) arytenoid cartilage position and (3) arytenoid cartilage position (after unilateral tie back surgery).

- Usually bilateral but unilateral paralysis is possible in the early course of the disease.
  - If hemiplegia and not too compromised breathing, re-examine in 3 months
- False-positive result possible because of the influence of general anesthesia on laryngeal function.
- Assess gag reflex, laryngeal sensitivity, epiglottic and hyoepiglottic assessment, palate assessment, piriform recesses, cuneiform and corniculate mucosal exams, vocal folds and ventricles.
- Flexible scope—retroflexed view
- Text flaccidity/spasticity of the paralysis with a soft-tipped probe
  - Thyroid carcinoma—spastic paralysis rLNs
- Repeat laryngoscopy post-operatively to confirm complete abduction

TREATMENT

APPROPRIATE HEALTH CARE

- Laryngeal paralysis
  - Surgical palliation (arytenoid lateralization) is recommended for dogs with clinical signs but may be associated with postoperative aspiration (see Figure 60.2).
  - If signs are mild, avoidance of triggers is advised (e.g., heat, humidity).

NURSING CARE

- Emergency:
  - Sedation/anesthesia; supplemental oxygen; cooling therapy.
- Laryngeal Paralysis
  - Avoid warm, poorly ventilated environments, stress, and intense excitation as these further compromise normal cooling mechanisms and proper air exchange.
  - Avoid cervical collars.
  - Avoid weight gain.
- Esophageal dysfunction
  - Feeding angle—recommendations unclear; use what is best for that patient
  - Minimize acid reflux—cisapride or sildenafil (metoclopramide not as effective)
- Polyneuropathy
  - Physical therapy—prioritize muscle strengthening, balance, and coordination
    - Can slow progression and enhance overall well-being and longevity of affected dogs
    - Water treadmill physiotherapy, balancing and coordinating exercise long-term for all dogs!!
    - Maintain muscle mass and minimized proprioceptive loss
    - Backwards walking, figure of eights, cavaletti exercises.
    - Home exercise with long, slow walks daily
    - Acupuncture benefits in some
    - tPEMF to help decrease laryngeal swelling

ACTIVITY

Exercise should be severely restricted in animals suffering from laryngeal paralysis, especially in warm temperatures.

DIET

Loss of weight is advocated in overweight patients with any upper airway disorder.

CLIENT EDUCATION

- The diagnosis and care for a GOLPP patient can be overwhelming
- Laryngeal paralysis
  - Discuss the importance of surgery and the risk of not performing surgery (chronic hypoxemia, heat stroke, risk of suffocation, and death) in moderately to severely affected dogs.
  - Discuss potential complications of surgery including aspiration pneumonia.
- The client needs to be able to identify early signs of aspiration pneumonia—inappetance, lethargy, fever.
  - Early and aggressive treatment will improve outcome
- As condition progresses—hind-limb supports can be used, occasionally cars
- Euthanasia typically when non-ambulatory or repeated episodes of aspiration pneumonia

SURGICAL CONSIDERATIONS

- Surgery (unilateral crico- (or thyro-)arytenoid lateralization—tie back—left side) is the treatment of choice; asymmetrically widens the rima glottidis.
  - Immediate alleviation of sx, improves QoL
  - Some gagging and throat clearing may persist for months
  - Aspiration pneumonia is seen in 10–20% of the cases, from months to years after surgery
  - Alternative surgery—ventral laryngotomy with resection of vocal folds, no distinct benefit shown.
- Bilateral surgical correction is not advised because it increases the risk of aspiration pneumonia

MEDICATIONS

DRUG(S) OF CHOICE

- Anti-emetics during upper airway examination
- Pre-operative pantoprazole or omeprazole to decrease gastric pH
- Post-operative and maintenance—cisapride and sildenafil
  - Famotidine
- Anxiolytics—trazodone, alprazolam

FOLLOW-UP

PATIENT MONITORING

- Needs thorough evaluation every 6 months until EOL (end-of-life)—usually 2–4 years.
- While this progresses at a steady rate, patient may succumb to other diseases.
- Monitor for aspiration pneumonia (short and long term).
- If surgery is successful, breathing, stridor, exercise, and heat tolerance should improve.

POSSIBLE COMPLICATIONS

LarPar—recurrence of clinical signs is uncommon if surgery is correctly performed; aspiration pneumonia is possible as the larynx is placed in a fixed open position; risk of aspiration pneumonia increased if bilateral arytenoid lateralization is performed or if dysphagia due to pharyngeal and/or esophageal dysfunction coexists.

EXPECTED COURSE AND PROGNOSIS

- Paralysis associated with esophageal dysfunction—poor.
- Descending paresis.

Abbreviations

- GOLPP = Geriatric-onset laryngeal paralysis and polyneuropathy
- LarPar = laryngeal paralysis
- LN = laryngeal nerve
- tPEMF = targeted pulsed electromagnetic field

Internet Resources

Accessed 29 June 2024
HOME | GOLPP (allaboutgolpp.com)

Authors: Heidi Lobprise
Thanks to: Sheilah Robertson and Mary Gardner for resources

Author/editor: Heidi Lobprise
Topic adapted from Five Minute Veterinary Consultation, 7th edition, 2021
Original Topic: Laryngeal Diseases

Author: Elizabeth Rozanski
Consulting Editor: Elizabeth Rozanski

Chapter 61

Incontinence, Fecal

BASICS

DEFINITION

Inability to retain feces or generate a coordinated and appropriate act of defecation.

PATHOPHYSIOLOGY

- The colon, rectum, and anus are primary sites of function in normal defecation.
- Coordinated contractions of the circular and longitudinal smooth muscle of the colon result in orderly accumulation of fecal matter, which is stored in the descending colon.
- Intense propulsive activity down the length of the colon, called mass movement, is stimulated by the autonomic nervous system and moves fecal matter toward the anus.
- The internal anal sphincter is composed of smooth muscles, while the external anal sphincter is composed of striated muscle; parasympathetic innervation to the internal sphincter is provided by the pelvic nerves via the sacral segments (S1–S3); sympathetic innervation is provided by the hypogastric nerves via the lumbar segments (L1–L4); parasympathetic stimulation leads to relaxation of the internal sphincter and contraction of the rectum, whereas sympathetic stimulation leads to contraction of the internal sphincter and relaxation of the rectum; the striated muscles of the external anal sphincter are under conscious control via the caudal rectal nerve (a branch of the pudendal nerve).
- Neurogenic sphincter incompetence can be caused by damage or denervation of the pudendal nerve, lesions that cause lumbar or sacral spinal segment dysfunction, autonomic dysfunction, or generalized peripheral neuropathy or myopathy.
- Non-neurogenic sphincter incompetence is caused by damage to the anal sphincters.
- Damage to, or degeneration of, the levator ani and coccygeus muscles may also contribute to fecal incontinence.
- Reservoir fecal incontinence develops when disease processes reduce the capacity or compliance of the rectum; the patient is aware of the need to defecate, but sphincter control is overwhelmed by fecal volume or spastic colorectal/anal disease.

SYSTEMS AFFECTED

- Gastrointestinal (GI).
- Neurologic.

Blackwell's Five-Minute Veterinary Consult Clinical Companion: Small Animal Senior Care,
First Edition. Edited by Heidi B. Lobprise.

Companion website: www.wiley.com/go/lobprise/Senior

SIGNALMENT

Species

Dog and cat.

Mean Age and Range

Increased incidence in older patients.

SIGNS

Historical Findings

- Reservoir incontinence—urge to defecate; frequent, conscious defecation; defecation may be associated with tenesmus or dyschezia.
- Sphincter incontinence—involuntary expulsion or dribbling of fecal material, especially during excitement or barking and coughing.
- History of neurologic signs, anorectal surgery, and/or trauma.
- Concurrent urinary incontinence suggests neurogenic sphincter incontinence.

Physical Examination Findings

- Reservoir incontinence—anorectal sensitivity or pain on digital palpation, rectal mass or thickening of rectal mucosa; external anal sphincter tone and perineal reflex are normal.
- Non-neurogenic sphincter incontinence—evidence of perineal trauma or perianal fistulae; anal reflex is present, but external anal sphincter may not be completely closed if sphincter has been anatomically disrupted.
- Neurogenic sphincter incontinence—loss of tone to external anal sphincter; perineal reflex is absent or diminished.
- Neurologic examination findings may include lumbosacral pain, paraparesis, paraplegia, decreased postural reactions, hopping, paw placements, normal-to-decreased reflexes (patellar, withdrawal, perineal reflex), or absent nociception in perineum or tail.
- Diffuse lower motor neuron (LMN) signs suggest generalized peripheral neuropathy or myopathy; these are rare causes of fecal incontinence in small animals.

CAUSES

Reservoir Incontinence

- Colorectal disease—colitis, irritable bowel syndrome, and neoplasia.
- Diarrhea—large volumes of feces from any cause can overwhelm the absorptive and storage capacity of the colon.

Non-neurogenic Sphincter Incontinence

- Traumatic anal injuries.
- Neoplasia.
- Iatrogenic—complication of anorectal surgery.
- Anorectal or perianal diseases—e.g., perianal fistulae.
- Mucocutaneous diseases—e.g., immune-mediated, infectious.

Neurogenic Sphincter Incontinence

- Iatrogenic—traumatic nerve injury as postoperative complication.
- Diseases affecting dorsal funiculus (L4 and cranial).
- Spinal cord—arachnoid diverticulum, arachnoid cysts, spinal malformations, syringomyelia, trauma, intervertebral disc disease, neoplasia, infectious or inflammatory meningomyelitis, fibrocartilaginous embolism, myelomalacia.
- Degenerative lumbosacral stenosis—L6–L7 or L7–S1, intervertebral disc disease, severe spondylosis deformans, synovial cysts, ligamentous hypertrophy, lumbosacral instability, neoplasia.
- Peripheral neuropathy—infectious, endocrine/metabolic, immune-mediated, drug-induced (e.g., vincristine), dysautonomia, idiopathic.
- Diffuse neuromuscular diseases—neuropathies, junctionopathies, myopathies (LMN unit).
- Degeneration (aging)—multiple factors likely involved, including atrophy of muscles involved in fecal continence, weakness, degenerative neuropathy, cognitive dysfunction.

RISK FACTORS

- Colonic disease.
- Anorectal disease and surgery.
- Neurologic disease.

DIAGNOSIS

DIFFERENTIAL DIAGNOSIS

- Primary GI disease can increase urge to defecate; these animals typically attempt to go outside to defecate, or posture to defecate.
- Behavioral disorders (e.g., separation anxiety) often associated with destructive activities or excessive vocalization.

CBC/BIOCHEMISTRY/URINALYSIS

Usually unremarkable.

OTHER LABORATORY TESTS

- Thyroid testing.
- If junctionopathy suspected, consider submitting acetylcholine receptor antibody titers.
- If polymyositis suspected, submit *Toxoplasma* and *Neospora* titers.
- Rectal scraping for cytology is indicated in regions where *Heterobilharzia*, histoplasmosis, or pythiosis is endemic; rectal cytology may also indicate presence of neoplasia.
- Zinc sulfate flotation tests and fecal PCR, ELISA, or culture to detect *Giardia* sp., *Tritrichomonas* (cats), and other parasitic, bacterial, viral, and protozoal infections.
- Serum-trypsin-like immunoreactivity to rule out exocrine pancreatic insufficiency.
- Serum cobalamin and folate concentrations to investigate small intestinal malabsorptive disease.

IMAGING

- Lateral and ventrodorsal survey radiography of lumbosacral spine may show evidence of intervertebral disc extrusion, spondylosis deformans, discospondylitis, vertebral neoplasia, lumbosacral trauma, or vertebral malformations.
- Abdominal ultrasound, barium radiographic studies, and CT may help identify masses or intestinal lining abnormalities.
- MRI is optimum diagnostic tool to demonstrate specific spinal cord and brain lesions.
- CT with IV contrast or CT with myelography may also demonstrate compressive lesions within spinal canal.

DIAGNOSTIC PROCEDURES

- Full-thickness or endoscopic GI biopsies if diarrhea present.
- Colonoscopy and colorectal mucosal biopsy if reservoir incontinence suspected.
- Electromyography/nerve conduction studies.
- Muscle and nerve biopsy for myopathy and peripheral neuropathy.
- Analysis of cerebrospinal fluid (CSF) may reveal evidence of CNS infectious or inflammatory process, neoplasia, or trauma.

PATHOLOGIC FINDINGS

Dependent on underlying disease.

TREATMENT

APPROPRIATE HEALTH CARE

Inpatient vs. outpatient depends on underlying disease.

NURSING CARE

- In recumbent patients or patients with difficulty ambulating and fecal incontinence, nursing care is of paramount importance.
- To prevent decubital ulcers, rotate recumbency every 2–4 hours and utilize a water bed.
- Soiled bed should be changed immediately, and soiled hair coat and skin should be washed with gentle soap and warm water and dried thoroughly.
- Occasional warm water enemas will diminish volume of feces in colon and may decrease incidence of inappropriate defecation.
- Reflex defecation may be stimulated by applying warm washcloth to anus or perineum.
- Physical therapy options include massage, passive range of motion exercises, and assisted walking; hydrotherapy, thermal therapies, and acupuncture may be considered when appropriate.

ACTIVITY

Animal should be encouraged to go outside to urinate and defecate every 4–6 hours. Sling walking may be necessary.

DIET

Fecal volume can be reduced by feeding low-residue commercial diets or foods such as cottage cheese and rice. Feed pet at established times to better control times needed to defecate.

CLIENT EDUCATION

- Prognosis for recovery of function is poor if underlying cause cannot be identified and successfully corrected; discuss prognosis with client early in evaluation to avoid unrealistic expectations.
- Environmental changes (e.g., providing designated area that is easy to clean) may increase client satisfaction and thus avoid euthanasia of otherwise healthy animal.

SURGICAL CONSIDERATIONS

Fascial slings, silicone elastomer slings, and other surgical techniques to repair external anal sphincter or improve anorectal angulation have been attempted with low success rates.

MEDICATIONS

DRUG(S) OF CHOICE

- Diphenoxylate (0.1–0.2 mg/kg PO q12h) and loperamide (0.1–0.2 mg/kg PO q8–12h) are opiate motility-modifying drugs; they inhibit GI motility, thus increasing the amount of water absorbed from the feces.
- Anti-inflammatory agents, such as glucocorticoids, metronidazole, and sulfasalazine (dogs only), may benefit patients with suspected reservoir incontinence due to inflammatory bowel disease or colitis.
- Improvement in signs may be achieved if specific therapy for perianal fistulae, colitis, or other reservoir or non-neurogenic causes of incontinence can be given, but there are no specific drugs effective in patients with neurogenic incontinence.

CONTRAINDICATIONS

- Do not use motility-modifying drugs in patients if infectious or toxigenic cause of diarrhea is suspected.
- Do not use opiate motility modifiers in debilitated patients, or patients with impaired liver or renal function.
- Do not use diets containing high concentrations of insoluble fibers as this will produce large, bulky stool that is difficult to pass or may cause obstipation.

PRECAUTIONS

- Opiate motility-modifying drugs may cause sedation.
- Use loperamide with caution in patients with p-glycoprotein defects.

POSSIBLE INTERACTIONS

Increased sedation and respiratory depression are possible when opiates are used concurrently with other CNS depressants (e.g., barbiturates, tranquilizers).

FOLLOW-UP

PATIENT MONITORING

- If fecal incontinence is due to underlying neurologic cause, use serial neurologic examinations to monitor patient progress.
- Radiographic procedures, electromyography, CSF analysis, and MRI can also be used to follow progress.
- Check fecal consistency and volume and make sure pet does not become constipated or obstipated.
- Examine perianal skin and hair coat to ensure there is no fecal matter and secondary inflammation or infection.
- Adjust diet to find appropriate therapy for each individual patient.

POSSIBLE COMPLICATIONS

Neurogenic sphincter incontinence is often unresponsive despite appropriate dietary, medical, and surgical treatment.

EXPECTED COURSE AND PROGNOSIS

50% of pets with fecal incontinence were euthanized in a recent study.

MISCELLANEOUS

Zoonotic Potential

- Exposure to animal feces increases risk of exposure to zoonotic parasites.
- Advise clients about zoonotic diseases (e.g., salmonellosis, cutaneous and visceral larval migrans, and toxoplasmosis).

Abbreviations

- CSF = cerebrospinal fluid
- GI = gastrointestinal.
- LMN = lower motor neuron.

Suggested Reading

de Lahunta A, Glass E, Kent M. Lower motor neuron: spinal nerve general somatic efferent system. In: de Lahunta A, Glass E, Kent M (eds) *Veterinary Neuroanatomy and Clinical Neurology*, 4th edn. St. Louis, MO: Elsevier Saunders, 2015; pp. 102–161.

Foley P. Constipation, tenesmus, dyschezia, and fecal incontinence. In: Ettinger SJ, Feldman EC, Côté E (eds) *Textbook of Veterinary Internal Medicine*, 8th edn. St. Louis, MO: Elsevier Saunders, 2017; pp. 171–174.

Schermerhorn T. Gastrointestinal endocrinology. In: Ettinger SJ, Feldman EC, Côté E (eds) *Textbook of Veterinary Internal Medicine*, 8th edn. St. Louis, MO: Elsevier Saunders, 2017; pp. 1833–1838.

Washabau RJ. Dysmotility/fecal incontinence. In: Washabau RJ, Day MJ (eds) *Canine and Feline Gastroenterology*. St. Louis, MO: Elsevier Saunders, 2013; pp. 791–798.

Author/editor: Heidi Lobprise
Topic adapted from Five Minute Veterinary Consultation, 7th edition, 2021
Original Topic: Incontinence—Fecal

Author: Andrea W. Munk
Consulting Editor: Mark P. Rondeau

Chapter 62

Lumbosacral Stenosis and Cauda Equina Syndrome

BASICS

DEFINITION

- Lumbosacral stenosis refers to narrowing of the lumbosacral vertebral canal and/or L7–sacral intervertebral foramina, causing compression of L7, sacral, or caudal nerves.
- Cauda equina syndrome implies pain or other clinical signs related to dysfunction of these nerves.

PATHOPHYSIOLOGY

Acquired—bony and soft-tissue degenerative changes, most commonly affecting the L7 intervertebral disc, that cause stenosis of the vertebral canal and/or intervertebral foramina. Specific syndrome of sacral osteochondrosis dissecans is recognized in young German shepherd dogs and other breeds.

SIGNALMENT

Species

- Reasonably common in dogs.
- Uncommonly reported in cats but suspected with increasing frequency.

Breed Predilections

- Acquired—any medium–large dog; often suspected in working dogs, so frequently German shepherd dogs and Malinois but also common in boxers, Rottweilers.

Mean Age and Range

- Acquired—mean age at onset 6–7 years. Sacral osteochondrosis signs often appear ~1 year old.

Predominant Sex

- Acquired—male.

Blackwell's Five-Minute Veterinary Consult Clinical Companion: Small Animal Senior Care, First Edition. Edited by Heidi B. Lobprise.

Companion website: www.wiley.com/go/lobprise/Senior

SIGNS

- Lumbosacral pain—salient feature; may be the only clinical sign; may be evident in reluctance to jump or climb stairs. Pain on pressure on, or dorsiflexion of, the lumbosacral vertebral column (often also induced during extension of hip joints).
- Pelvic limb lameness—caused by lumbar 7th and/or sacral nerve dysfunction; may progress to pelvic limb weakness, muscle wasting, and postural reaction deficits.
- Urinary and/or fecal incontinence—caused by S1–S3 nerve dysfunction.
- Abnormal tail carriage, tail weakness, or paralysis—results from dysfunction of caudal nerves.
- Self-inflicted lesions—most often associated with congenital lesions or cauda equina inflammation.

CAUSES

- Intervertebral disc herniation (types I and II).
- Hypertrophy or hyperplasia of the interarcuate ligament.
- Proliferation of the articular facets and/or periarticular soft tissues.
- Subluxation at the lumbosacral junction.
- Inflammatory or neoplastic disease of the vertebral canal can produce identical clinical signs (hence "cauda equina syndrome").

RISK FACTORS

Dogs with lumbosacral transitional vertebrae, especially German shepherd dogs, have increased risk to develop the syndrome.

DIAGNOSIS

DIFFERENTIAL DIAGNOSIS

- Hip dysplasia or other orthopedic disease (notably iliopsoas injury)—distinguish via thorough orthopedic examination ± imaging.
- Chronic discospondylitis, osteomyelitis, neoplastic disease—cannot be differentiated by clinical signs alone.
- Vertebral fractures and subluxations—acute; characterized by more bilateral signs.
- Localized meningomyelitis or radiculoneuritis—usually more diffuse pain.

CBC/BIOCHEMISTRY/URINALYSIS

- Usually normal.
- Urinalysis—may reveal lower urinary tract infection secondary to urinary incontinence or associated with discospondylitis.

OTHER LABORATORY TESTS

If images suggest the need, cerebrospinal fluid (CSF) analysis may aid in diagnosing inflammatory (or infectious or neoplastic) disease.

IMAGING

- Radiology—commonly exhibit spondylosis at the lumbosacral junction; narrowing of the L7–S1 disc space; ventral displacement of the sacrum relative to the lumbar vertebrae; *but* interpret with caution because all these can be observed in clinically normal animals.
- CT and MRI—modalities of choice. Apparent abnormalities must be interpreted with regard to the whole clinical picture because many are also observed in normal animals.

DIAGNOSTIC PROCEDURES

- Electromyography—denervation may be detected in muscles innervated by the nerves L7 to caudal; denervation confirms localization of the lesion but is not specific for compressive lesions.
- Slowed sciatic–tibial nerve conduction or prolongation of F wave latencies may be detected.

PATHOLOGIC FINDINGS

- May see one or more of the following features:
    - Type II disc disease with bulging of dorsal annulus.
    - Hypertrophy of the interarcuate ligament.
    - Stenosis of the intervertebral foramen by soft tissue or bony proliferation compressing L7 nerve(s) or as a congenital lesion.
    - Ventral displacement of the sacrum in relation to lumbar vertebrae.
    - Proliferation of articular facets and hypertrophy of joint capsule.
    - Congenitally shortened pedicles.
    - Thickened and sclerotic laminae and articular processes.
    - Various vertebral malformations (not only transitional vertebrae).
- Cauda equina syndrome can also be associated with neoplasia, inflammation, infection.

TREATMENT

APPROPRIATE HEALTH CARE

Urinary incontinence—inpatient for initial management.

NURSING CARE

Urinary incontinence—manual expression or catheterize the bladder until adequate voluntary contrcl returns; monitor for urinary tract infection and administer appropriate antibiotics following culture and sensitivity.

ACTIVITY

- Nonsurgical treatment—confinement and restricted leash walks, alone or combined with systemic anti-inflammatory drugs or analgesics, or epidural injection of corticosteroids, frequently alleviate pain; clinical signs may return with increasing levels of exercise.
- If treated surgically, restrict for 6–12 weeks; then gradual return to athletic function.

DIET

Avoid obesity; excess weight increases biomechanical stress on the spine.

CLIENT EDUCATION

- Inform client that there may be progressive neurologic impairment of the pelvic limbs, urinary and fecal incontinence, and paralysis of the tail.
- Inform client that pelvic limb lameness and self-inflicted lesions result from pain associated with nerve root irritation and/or compression.
- Discuss surgical treatment, which is appropriate for cases with severe pain and may be suitable for cases with neurologic deficits (especially incontinence, which may be difficult to reverse).
- Medical management is frequently successful for animals with mild pain and/or mild neurologic deficits only.

SURGICAL CONSIDERATIONS

Several options, each focused on alleviating the specific source of the problems defined by imaging; dorsal laminectomy, lateral foraminotomy, or fixation–fusion may all be effective in specifically selected cases.

MEDICATIONS

DRUG(S) OF CHOICE

- NSAIDs—e.g., carprofen 2 mg/kg q12h for 5–7 days then reducing doses until PRN.
- Gabapentin—frequently used at ~20–30 mg/kg q8h and may be effective (side effect: sedation; dizziness reported in humans).
- Epidural corticosteroid—methylprednisolone acetate 1 mg/kg (<0.5 mL total volume).

FOLLOW-UP

POSSIBLE COMPLICATIONS

- Syndrome progression, increasingly severe neurologic signs.
- Seroma formation—frequent sequela to surgery; can be effectively managed by cage rest and surgical drainage. Prevent by careful soft-tissue closure.
- Adhesions between nerves and surrounding soft tissues after surgery.
- Recurrence of clinical signs following medical (commonly) or surgical (less commonly) intervention.
- Failure of fixation–fusion implant.
- Fracture of articular process after excessive lateral bone excision at surgery.
- Infection (especially if an implant is used for surgery).

EXPECTED COURSE AND PROGNOSIS

- Vary with the severity of neurologic injury.
- Majority are successfully managed medically, but need to ensure outcome matches requirements for dog's way of life; surgery remains an option.

- If low lumbar pain and mild neurologic deficits—good prognosis after surgery; 70–80% have an excellent or good outcome.
- If fecal and urinary incontinence—guarded prognosis.

MISCELLANEOUS

Associated Conditions

Lower urinary tract infections frequently accompany urinary incontinence.

Age-Related Factors

- If a lumbosacral transitional vertebra is present, syndrome may develop 1–2 years earlier than the average dog.
- Older large-breed dogs may have concomitant diseases that also cause neurologic deficits: type II disc protrusions at other sites, degenerative peripheral nerve disease (especially Labrador retrievers), degenerative myelopathy (especially German shepherd dogs).

Abbreviations

- CSF = cerebrospinal fluid
- NSAID = nonsteroidal anti-inflammatory drug.

Suggested Reading

De Risio L, Sharp NJ, Olby NJ, et al. Predictors of outcome after dorsal decompressive laminectomy for degenerative lumbosacral stenosis in dogs: 69 cases (1987–1997). *J Am Vet Med Assoc* 2001;219(5):624–628.

Janssens L, Beosier Y, Daems R. Lumbosacral degenerative stenosis in the dog. The results of epidural infiltration with methylprednisolone acetate: a retrospective study. *Vet Comp Orthop Traumatol* 2009;22(6):486–491.

Jeffery ND, Barker A, Harcourt-Brown T. What progress has been made in the understanding and treatment of degenerative lumbosacral stenosis in dogs during the past 30 years? *Vet J* 2014;201(1):9–14.

Jones JC, Banfield CM, Ward DL. Association between postoperative outcome and results of magnetic resonance imaging and computed tomography in working dogs with degenerative lumbosacral stenosis. *J Am Vet Med Assoc* 2000;216(11):1769–1774.

Linn L, Bartels K, Rochat M, et al. Lumbosacral stenosis in 29 military working dogs: Epidemiologic findings and outcome after surgical intervention (1990–1999). *Vet Surg* 2003;32:21–29.

Meij BP, Bergknut N. Degenerative lumbosacral stenosis in dogs. *Vet Clin North Am Small Anim Pract* 2010;40(5):983–1009.

Suwankong N, Voorhout G, Hazewinkle HA, Meij BP. Agreement between computed tomography, magnetic resonance imaging, and surgical findings in dogs with degenerative lumbosacral stenosis. *J Am Vet Med Assoc* 2006;229(12):1924–1929.

Author/editor: Heidi Lobprise
Topic adapted from Five Minute Veterinary Consultation, 7th edition, 2021
Original Topic: Lumbosacral Syndrome—Cauda Equina

Author: Nick D. Jeffery

Chapter 63

Myasthenia Gravis—Acquired

BASICS

DEFINITION

A disorder of neuromuscular transmission characterized by muscular weakness and excessive fatigability.

PATHOPHYSIOLOGY

Transmission failure at the neuromuscular junction—results from structural or functional abnormalities of the nicotinic acetylcholine receptors (AChRs) or other end-plate proteins and enzymes (congenital form) and from autoantibody-mediated destruction of AChRs and post-synaptic membranes (acquired form).

SYSTEMS AFFECTED

- Neuromuscular—result of abnormalities or destruction of AChRs, choline acetyltransferase, or end-plate cholinesterase.
- Respiratory—may find aspiration pneumonia secondary to megaesophagus.

GENETICS

- Congenital familial forms
- Acquired—as with other autoimmune diseases, requires appropriate genetic background for disease to occur; multifactorial, involving environmental, infectious, and hormonal influences.
- Familial forms of acquired myasthenia gravis (MG) occur in the Newfoundland and Great Dane breeds.

INCIDENCE/PREVALENCE

- Congenital—rare.
- Acquired—not uncommon in dogs; uncommon in cats.

Blackwell's Five-Minute Veterinary Consult Clinical Companion: Small Animal Senior Care, First Edition. Edited by Heidi B. Lobprise.

Companion website: www.wiley.com/go/lobprise/Senior

SIGNALMENT

Species

Dogs and cats.

Breed Predilections

- Acquired—several breeds: golden retrievers; German shepherd dogs; Labrador retrievers; dachshunds; Scottish terriers; Akitas; and Abyssinian and Somali cats.

Mean Age and Range

- Acquired—bimodal age of onset; dogs: 1–4 years of age and 9–13 years of age.

Predominant Sex

- Acquired—may be a slight predilection for females in the young age group; none in the old age group.

SIGNS

General Comments

- Acquired—may have several clinical presentations ranging from focal involvement of the esophageal, pharyngeal, and extraocular muscles to acute generalized collapse.
- Should be on the differential diagnosis of any dog with acquired megaesophagus, lower motor neuron weakness, or a cranial mediastinal mass.

Historical Findings

- Regurgitation—common; important to differentiate between vomiting and regurgitation.
- Voice change.
- Exercise-related weakness.
- Acute collapse.
- Progressive weakness.
- Sleep with eyes open.

Physical Examination Findings

- Patient may look normal at rest.
- Excessive drooling, regurgitation, and repeated attempts at swallowing.
- Muscle atrophy—usually not found.
- Dyspnea—with aspiration pneumonia.
- Fatigue or cramping—with mild exercise.
- Careful neurologic examination—subtle findings: decreased or absent palpebral reflex (may be fatigable); may note a poor or absent gag reflex; spinal reflexes usually normal but fatigable (rarely absent and dog unable to support its weight).
- Ventroflexion of the neck (cats, uncommon in dogs).

CAUSES

- Congenital.
- Immune-mediated.
- Paraneoplastic.

RISK FACTORS

- Appropriate genetic background.
- Neoplasia—particularly thymoma.
- Methimazole treatment (cats)—may result in reversible disease.
- Vaccination can exacerbate active MG.
- Intact female.

DIAGNOSIS

DIFFERENTIAL DIAGNOSIS

- Other disorders of neuromuscular transmission—tick paralysis; botulism; cholinesterase toxicity.
- Acute or chronic polyneuropathies.
- Polymyopathies—including polymyositis.
- Diagnosis depends upon a careful history, thorough physical and neurologic examinations, and specialized laboratory testing.

CBC/BIOCHEMISTRY/URINALYSIS

- Normal.
- Serum creatine kinase activity—usually normal; may be elevated if MG is associated with polymyositis and concurrent thymoma.

OTHER LABORATORY TESTS

- Serum AChR antibody titer—diagnostic for acquired form.
- Thyroid and adrenal function—may see abnormalities associated with acquired form.

IMAGING

Thoracic radiographs—megaesophagus; cranial mediastinal mass, aspiration pneumonia.

DIAGNOSTIC PROCEDURES

- Ultrasound-guided biopsy of cranial mediastinal mass—may support diagnosis of thymoma.
- Dramatic increase in muscle strength after administration of edrophonium chloride 0.1 mg/kg IV—may see false-negative and false-positive responses.
- Decreased or absent palpebral reflex—may return after edrophonium chloride administration.
- Electrophysiologic evaluation—necessity questionable with increased availability of AChR antibody testing; many patients with acquired form are poor anesthetic risks.
- Electrocardiogram—with bradycardia; third-degree heart block has been documented in some patients with acquired disease.

PATHOLOGIC FINDINGS

Biopsy of a cranial mediastinal mass may reveal thymoma, thymic hyperplasia, or thymic atrophy.

TREATMENT

APPROPRIATE HEALTH CARE

- Inpatient—until adequate dosages of anticholinesterase drugs are achieved.
- Aspiration pneumonia—may require intensive care.
- Gastrostomy tube—may be required if patient is unable to eat or drink without significant regurgitation.

NURSING CARE

- Oxygen therapy, intensive antibiotic therapy, IV fluid therapy, and supportive care—generally required for aspiration pneumonia.
- Nutritional maintenance with a gastrostomy tube—multiple feedings of a high-caloric diet; good hygiene care.
- Elevation of food and water.

ACTIVITY

Self-limited owing to the severity of muscle weakness and extent of aspiration pneumonia.

DIET

May try different consistencies of food—gruel; hard food; soft food; evaluate what is best tolerated.

CLIENT EDUCATION

- Warn client that, although the acquired disease is treatable, most patients require months of special feeding and medication.
- Inform client that a dedicated owner is important to a favorable outcome for acquired myasthenia.
- Prognosis is poor for congenital myasthenic syndrome.

SURGICAL CONSIDERATIONS

- Cranial mediastinal mass—thymoma.
- Before attempting surgical removal, stabilize patient with anticholinesterase drugs and treat aspiration pneumonia.
- Weakness may not be clinically evident initially.
- Suspected thymoma—test all patients for acquired MG before surgery.

MEDICATIONS

DRUG(S) OF CHOICE

- Anticholinesterase drugs—prolong the action of acetylcholine at the neuromuscular junction; pyridostigmine bromide tablets or syrup (Mestinon syrup, diluted half and half in water) at 1–3 mg/kg PO q8–12h.
- Corticosteroids 0.5 mg/kg q24h; initiated if there is a poor response to pyridostigmine or if there is no response to the edrophonium chloride challenge.

CONTRAINDICATIONS

Avoid drugs that may reduce the safety margin of neuromuscular transmission—aminoglycoside antibiotics; antiarrhythmic agents; phenothiazines; anesthetics; narcotics; muscle relaxants; magnesium.

PRECAUTIONS

- Avoid large volumes of barium for evaluating megaesophagus.
- Large air-filled esophagus seen on survey radiographs—barium study not indicated.
- Avoid immunosuppressive dosages of prednisone—may worsen muscle weakness.
- Avoid unnecessary vaccinations.

ALTERNATIVE DRUG(S)

- Azathioprine 2 mg/kg PO through gastrostomy tube q24h. Taper to q48h when clinical remission of the disease.
- Mycophenolate 20 mg/kg PO q12h. Reduce dosage by 50% once significant improvement or resolution of clinical signs is noted.

FOLLOW-UP

PATIENT MONITORING

- Return of muscle strength should be evident.
- Thoracic radiographs—evaluated every 4–6 weeks for resolution of megaesophagus.
- AChR antibody titers—evaluated every 8–12 weeks; decrease to the normal range with immune remission.

POSSIBLE COMPLICATIONS

- Aspiration pneumonia.
- Respiratory arrest.

EXPECTED COURSE AND PROGNOSIS

- No severe aspiration pneumonia or pharyngeal weakness—good prognosis for complete recovery; resolution usually within 6–8 months.

- Thymoma present—guarded prognosis unless complete surgical removal and control of myasthenic signs are achieved.

MISCELLANEOUS

Associated Conditions

- Other autoimmune disorders—thyroiditis; skin disorders; hypoadrenocorticism, thrombocytopenia, hemolytic anemia, inflammatory bowel disease.
- Disorders of the thymus—thymoma; thymic hyperplasia.
- Other neoplasias.

Age-Related Factors

Bimodal age of onset—1–4 years of age and 9–13 years of age.

Abbreviations

- AChR = acetylcholine receptor
- MG = myasthenia gravis.

Internet Resources

Accessed 29 June 2024
Comparative Neuromuscular Laboratory: http://vetneuromuscular.ucsd.edu

Suggested Reading

Khorzad R, Whelan M, Sisson A, Shelton GD. Myasthenia gravis in dogs with an emphasis on treatment and critical care management. *Vet Emerg Crit Care* 2011;21:193–208.

Mace S, Shelton GD, Eddlestone S. Megaesophagus. *Compend Contin Edu Vet* 2012;34:E1–E8.

Shelton GD. Myasthenia gravis and disorders of neuromuscular transmission. *Vet Clin North Am* 2002;31:189–200.

Shelton GD. Routine and specialized laboratory testing for the diagnosis of neuromuscular diseases in dogs and cats. *Vet Clin Pathol* 2010;39:278–295.

Shelton GD. Treatment of autoimmune myasthenia gravis. In: Bonagura JD, Twedt DC (eds) *Current Veterinary Therapy XIV*. Philadelphia, PA: Saunders, 2009; pp. 1108–1111.

Shelton GD, Lindstrom JM. Spontaneous remission in canine myasthenia gravis: implications for assessing human MG therapies. *Neurology* 2001;57:2139–2141.

Author/editor: Heidi Lobprise
Topic adapted from Five Minute Veterinary Consultation, 7th edition, 2021
Original Topic: Myasthenia Gravis—Acquired

Author: Lauren Talarico
Consulting Editor: Mathieu M. Glassman

Chapter 64

Nystagmus

BASICS

DEFINITION

- Involuntary, rhythmic oscillation of the eyeballs.
- Jerk nystagmus—most common; slow eye movements in one direction with a rapid recovery phase in the opposite direction.
- Pendular nystagmus—seen less frequently; characterized by slow oscillations of the eyes in a trajectory that resembles that of a pendulum, with no fast phase.

PATHOPHYSIOLOGY

- Neural projections traverse in the brainstem from the vestibular nuclei to cranial nerve (CN) III, IV, and VI nuclei, which innervate the extraocular muscles. This pathway is part of the vestibular system and provides coordinated conjugate eye movements in association with changes in head position.
- Physiologic nystagmus (ocular–vestibular reflex)—normal finding, induced by rotating the head from side to side; characterized by a jerk nystagmus with a slow drifting of the eye in the opposite direction of the head rotation followed by a fast compensatory phase in the same direction as the head movement. Decreased-to-absent physiologic nystagmus is indicative of vestibular disease.
- Pathologic nystagmus—a sign of vestibular dysfunction; characterized by a jerk nystagmus that develops independent of head movement. The nystagmus is described according to the axis of movement of the globe (horizontal, rotary, or vertical), and the direction of the fast phase of movement.
- Spontaneous or resting nystagmus—pathologic nystagmus that occurs when the head is in a normal position and not moving; frequently resolves after several days.
- Positional nystagmus—pathologic nystagmus, elicited only when the head is placed in unusual position; can often be seen in more chronic conditions.
- Jerk nystagmus must be differentiated from pendular nystagmus and from opsoclonus.
- Pendular nystagmus—congenital abnormality in which a larger-than-usual portion of the optic nerve fibers crosses in the chiasm; most often observed as an incidental finding in Siamese, Birman, and Himalayan cats but can also be seen with cerebellar disease and with visual deficits.
- Opsoclonus—involuntary, rapid, random eye movements in multiple directions that can be seen with cerebellar disease; can be differentiated from jerk nystagmus by the lack of a slow phase and its chaotic nature.

Blackwell's Five-Minute Veterinary Consult Clinical Companion: Small Animal Senior Care, First Edition. Edited by Heidi B. Lobprise.

Companion website: www.wiley.com/go/lobprise/Senior

SYSTEMS AFFECTED

Nervous

INCIDENCE/PREVALENCE

Nystagmus, as a sign of vestibular disease, is a relatively common clinical presentation in dogs and cats.

SIGNALMENT

Species

Dog and cat.

Breed Predilections

None

Mean Age and Range

Varies, depending on underlying cause; neoplastic and vascular conditions and canine geriatric vestibular disease more common in older animals.

Predominant Sex

None

CAUSES

Peripheral Vestibular Disease

- Metabolic—hypothyroidism.
- Neoplastic—nerve sheath tumor or tumor involving surrounding bone or soft tissues.
- Inflammatory—otitis media-interna; nasopharyngeal polyps (cats).
- Idiopathic—canine geriatric vestibular disease; feline idiopathic vestibular disease.
- Toxic—e.g., aminoglycosides, topical iodophors, topical chlorhexidine.
- Trauma.

Central Vestibular Disease

- Degenerative—storage disorders; neuronal degeneration; demyelinating disease.
- Neoplastic—primary or metastatic tumors.
- Nutritional—thiamine deficiency.
- Inflammatory/infectious—viral (canine distemper, feline infectious peritonitis); bacterial; protozoal (toxoplasmosis, neosporosis); fungal (cryptococcosis, blastomycosis, histoplasmosis, coccidioidomycosis, aspergillosis); rickettsial (ehrlichiosis, Rocky Mountain spotted fever); inflammatory, noninfectious (meningoencephalitis of unknown etiology; includes granulomatous meningoencephalomyelitis and the necrotizing meningoencephalitides).
- Toxic—lead; hexachlorophene; metronidazole.
- Trauma.
- Vascular—cerebrovascular disease (hemorrhage, infarction).

RISK FACTORS

Systemic administration of certain antibiotics (metronidazole, aminoglycoside), otic administration of iodophors and chlorhexidine solutions.

DIAGNOSIS

DIFFERENTIAL DIAGNOSIS

Peripheral Vestibular Disease

- Nystagmus—either rotary or horizontal in character, with the fast phase directed away from the side of the lesion; does not change direction with different head positions.
- Other signs of vestibular disease—head tilt, ataxia, circling, falling or rolling, and vestibular strabismus often present and occur ipsilateral to the lesion.
- Ipsilateral facial nerve deficits and/or Horner's syndrome—can be seen due to the close association of CN VII and sympathetic nerve to CN VIII as they course through the petrous temporal bone.

Central Vestibular Disease

- Nystagmus—horizontal, rotary, or vertical; can change direction with different head positions.
- Other signs of vestibular disease—head tilt, ataxia, circling, falling or rolling, and vestibular strabismus often present.
- Involvement of other brainstem structures—alterations in level of consciousness, paresis, postural reaction deficits, and other CN deficits (V and VII most common); deficits are typically ipsilateral to the lesion.
- Paradoxical vestibular disease—with certain lesions of the cerebellum; in these cases, postural reaction deficits occur ipsilateral to the lesion whereas the head tilt and other vestibular signs are contralateral to the lesion.

CBC/BIOCHEMISTRY/URINALYSIS

Results usually normal

OTHER LABORATORY TESTS

- Thyroid profile—if hypothyroidism is suspected.
- Bacterial culture of sample obtained via myringotomy—if otitis media-interna is likely.
- Serologic testing—for potential infectious agents.

IMAGING

- Imaging of the tympanic bullae to assess for otitis media-interna—survey radiographs of limited value; CT and MRI are more sensitive.
- Brain imaging (CT or MRI)—indicated in animals with central vestibular disease to evaluate for structural brain abnormalities. MRI is superior to CT for imaging the brain.

DIAGNOSTIC PROCEDURES

CSF—if central disease, to evaluate for inflammation.

TREATMENT

APPROPRIATE HEALTH CARE

- The cause of the disease and the severity of signs determine whether the animal is best treated on an inpatient or an outpatient basis.
- In general, animals with central disease require more intensive care than those with peripheral disease.

NURSING CARE

- Fluid therapy is indicated in the acute stages of disease for animals that experience anorexia and vomiting.
- Animals with severe vestibular dysfunction should be confined to a well-padded area in the acute stage of the disease to minimize self-trauma secondary to disorientation.

ACTIVITY

- Animals should be housed on nonslippery surfaces; stairs should be avoided.
- Exercise should be supervised, with assistance provided until signs of imbalance resolve.

CLIENT EDUCATION

- Many animals show improvement over the first several days; the nervous system is able to compensate for vestibular disturbances that remain static or are slowly progressive regardless of cause.
- Compensation involves visual and somatosensory (tactile) cues and is dependent on feedback from vestibular pathways; return to normal activity should be encouraged to enhance compensatory mechanisms.

SURGICAL CONSIDERATIONS

Signs of vestibular dysfunction can transiently worsen after an anesthetic episode; most likely reflects a loss of compensation.

MEDICATIONS

DRUG(S) OF CHOICE

- Meclizine (dogs: 4 mg/kg PO q24h) or maropitant (dogs: 1 mg/kg SC or 2 mg/kg PO q24h; cats: 1 mg/kg SC q24h)—used to treat motion sickness; can alleviate nausea and vomiting associated with acute disease.

- Diazepam (dogs: 0.5 mg/kg PO q8h)—recommended in cases of metronidazole toxicity; can help decrease acute vestibular signs from other causes by decreasing the resting activity of vestibular neurons and alleviating the imbalance in vestibular input to the brain.
- Specific medical therapy is directed at the underlying cause, if one can be identified.

CONTRAINDICATIONS

- Avoid potential ototoxic drugs, such as aminoglycosides. Toxicity is more likely in animals with renal impairment.
- Avoid instilling topical medications into the ear of an animal with suspected otitis media-interna, especially if the tympanic membrane cannot be visualized or is not intact. Such agents can exacerbate vestibular signs and cause deafness.

PRECAUTIONS

- Avoid the use of metronidazole at daily doses greater than 60 mg/kg, as this has been associated with vestibular dysfunction in dogs.
- Vestibular dysfunction can develop after administration of metronidazole at lower dosages but is less likely.

FOLLOW-UP

PATIENT MONITORING

Repeat neurologic examination—perform 2 weeks after initial diagnosis to monitor for improvement or progression of disease.

POSSIBLE COMPLICATIONS

- Dehydration and electrolyte imbalance associated with anorexia and vomiting.
- Rare extension of otitis media-interna into the adjacent brainstem.

EXPECTED COURSE AND PROGNOSIS

- Prognosis varies, depending on the cause of the vestibular disturbance.
- In general, animals with peripheral vestibular disease have a better prognosis than those with central involvement.
- Residual deficits can remain after resolution of the underlying disease process due to irreversible damage to the neural structures.
- Recurrence is possible with some of the conditions (otitis media-interna, canine geriatric vestibular disease, feline idiopathic vestibular disease).

MISCELLANEOUS

Abbreviations

- CN = cranial nerve

Internet Resources

Accessed June 29, 2024

- http://www.vetfolio.com/neurology/vestibular-disease-diseases-causing-vestibular-signs-compendium
- https://vestibular.org/sites/default/files/page_files/Vestibular%20disease%20in%20dogs%20and%20cats.pdf

Suggested Reading

Lowrie M. Vestibular disease: anatomy, physiology, and clinical signs. *Compend Contin Educ Vet* 2012;34(7):E1–E5.

Rossmeisl JH Jr. Vestibular disease in dogs and cats. *Vet Clin North Am Small Anim Pract* 2010;40:81–100.

Author/editor: Heidi Lobprise
Topic adapted from Five Minute Veterinary Consultation, 7th edition, 2021
Original Topic: Nystagmus

Author: Karen R. Muñana

Chapter 65

Paralysis

BASICS

DEFINITION

- Paresis—weakness of voluntary movement.
- Paralysis—lack of voluntary movement.
- Quadriparesis (tetraparesis)—weakness of voluntary movements in all limbs.
- Quadriplegia (tetraplegia)—absence of all voluntary limb movement.
- Paraparesis—weakness of voluntary movements in pelvic limbs.
- Paraplegia—absence of all voluntary pelvic limb movement.
- Schiff–Sherrington syndrome—may occur with severe spinal cord trauma below T2. Patient presents paraplegic, in lateral recumbency with extension of front limbs and neck. However front limb function is normal on neurologic examination. Prognosis based on presence or absence of pain perception in pelvic limbs.
- Spinal shock—may occur with severe spinal cord trauma, usually near the thoracolumbar spine. Initially the paralyzed pelvic limbs are areflexic but become hyperreflexic (and more indicative of a T3–L3 lesion localization) within minutes to a few hours after the trauma.

PATHOPHYSIOLOGY

- Weakness—caused by lesions in the upper motor neuron (UMN) or lower motor neuron (LMN) systems.
- UMN system—cell bodies or nuclei located within the brain are responsible for initiating voluntary movement; axons from these cell bodies form tracts (rubrospinal, corticospinal, vestibulospinal, reticulospinal) that descend from the brain to synapse on the interneurons in the spinal cord. Interneuronal axons synapse on large alpha motor neurons in the ventral gray matter of the spinal cord; these are cell bodies of origin for the LMN system, which is responsible for spinal reflexes.
- LMN system—collections of lower motor neurons in the cervical and lumbar intumescences give rise to axons that form the ventral nerve roots, spinal nerves, and (ultimately) the peripheral nerves that innervate limb muscles.
- Evaluation of limb reflexes—determines which system (UMN or LMN) is involved.
- UMN and their axons—have inhibitory influence on the large alpha motor neurons of the LMN system; maintain normal muscle tone and normal spinal reflexes.
- If UMN is injured, spinal reflexes are no longer inhibited or controlled and spinal reflexes become exaggerated or hyperreflexic.

Blackwell's Five-Minute Veterinary Consult Clinical Companion: Small Animal Senior Care,
First Edition. Edited by Heidi B. Lobprise.

Companion website: www.wiley.com/go/lobprise/Senior

- If LMN system is injured, spinal reflexes cannot be elicited (areflexic) or are reduced (hyporeflexic). Large alpha motor neurons or their processes (peripheral nerves) also maintain normal muscle tone. With LMN injury, muscle wasting is usually severe and within 5–7 days of injury.

SYSTEMS AFFECTED

Nervous

SIGNALMENT

Dog and cat.

SIGNS

General Comments

Limb weakness—acute or gradual onset.

Historical Findings

- Owner may describe the patient as being “down,” unable to move, walk, or get up.
- Many focal compressive spinal cord diseases begin with ataxia and progress to weakness, then to paralysis.

Physical Examination Findings

- Usually normal, unless the disease is systemic.
- If in pain, patient may resent handling and manipulation.
- Aortic emboli (ischemic neuromyopathy)—patient may be paraplegic and areflexic or hyporeflexic; femoral pulses absent; limbs often cold; nail beds often blue.

Neurologic Examination Findings

- Confirm that the problem is weakness or paralysis.
- If limbs are paralyzed—likely bladder is also paralyzed, negating voluntary urination.
- Localize problem to either LMN or UMN system.
- Tetraparesis with exaggerated spinal reflexes in all limbs—lesion located at C1–C5 spinal segments or in the brain.
- Tetraparesis with normal or depressed front limb spinal reflexes and exaggerated pelvic limb spinal reflexes—lesion located at C6–T2 spinal segments.
- Tetraparesis with depressed spinal reflexes and decreased muscle tone in all limbs—lesion is diffuse involving muscles or peripheral nerves, or both intumescences (cervical C6–T2 spinal cord segments and lumbar L4–S2 spinal segments).
- Normal front limbs but paraparesis/paraplegia with exaggerated pelvic limb spinal reflexes—lesion located at T3–L3 spinal segments.
- Normal front limbs but paraparesis/paraplegia with depressed to absent pelvic limb spinal reflexes—lesion located at L4 spinal segment and caudally.
- Normal front limb and pelvic limb motor activity but flaccid tail/anus and urinary and/or fecal incontinence—lesion located at S2 spinal segment and caudally.
- Normal front limbs but paraparesis/paraplegia and depressed patellar reflexes—lesion involves spinal segments L4–L6, located in vertebral bodies L3–L4.

- Normal front limbs but paraparesis/paraplegia, exaggerated patellar reflexes, and weak flexor and sciatic reflexes—if only the spinal cord is affected (no root involvement), lesion involves spinal segments L6–S2, located in vertebral bodies L4–L6.

CAUSES

Quadriplegia

- If LMN system—acute onset: acute idiopathic polyradiculoneuritis (coonhound paralysis), botulism, tick paralysis, fulminating form of myasthenia gravis, protozoal myoneuritis.
- If LMN system—more gradual onset: polyneuropathies and polymyopathies from toxicity, infection, inflammation, endocrinopathy, metabolic disease, or congenital/inherited disease.
- If UMN system—acute onset: disc herniation; fibrocartilaginous embolism; trauma; neoplasia; myelitis of many causes.
- If UMN system—gradual onset: disc herniation; discospondylitis; neoplasia; myelitis of many causes; malformations of the spine or spinal cord.

Paraplegia

- If UMN or LMN system—acute onset: disc herniation; fibrocartilaginous embolism; neoplasia; trauma.
- If UMN or LMN system—gradual onset: disc herniation; congenital malformations of spine or spinal cord; degenerative myelopathy; lumbosacral instability; discospondylitis; neoplasia.

Quadriplegia with Cranial Nerve Deficits, Seizures, or Stupor

- UMN system—diseases of the brainstem: encephalitis; neoplasia; trauma; vascular accidents; congenital or inherited disorders.

RISK FACTORS

- Degenerative disc disease—dachshunds, poodles, cocker spaniels, beagles, others.
- Hunting dogs—acute idiopathic polyradiculoneuritis (coonhound paralysis).
- Roaming animals—spinal cord and vertebral trauma, tick paralysis, botulism.
- Atlantoaxial luxation—toy and small breeds.
- Lumbosacral instability—large breeds, working breeds, German shepherd dogs.
- Cervical spondylomyelopathy (wobbler syndrome)—large breeds, Doberman pinschers, Great Danes.
- Syringomyelia—cavalier King Charles spaniels, brachycephalic toy breeds and others.
- Spinal arachnoid diverticulum: Rottweilers, pugs, small breeds.

DIAGNOSIS

DIFFERENTIAL DIAGNOSIS

- Weak or paralyzed pelvic limbs—ensure femoral pulses are present and normal; aortic or femoral artery emboli may lead to LMN paraparesis or paraplegia.
- Spinal reflexes—localize weakness to the cervical, thoracolumbar, or lower lumbar cord segments.
- Acute onset—be careful when moving patient if possibility of trauma.

CBC/BIOCHEMISTRY/URINALYSIS

Usually normal, unless inflammatory diseases involved.

OTHER LABORATORY TESTS

- Urinary tract inflammation—urine culture may be positive in discospondylitis or in any dog that has had chronic bladder paralysis or repeated urinary catheterizations.
- Discospondylitis—diagnose by spinal radiography (intervertebral disc space lysis); perform *Brucella* titer; consider blood and urine bacterial cultures.
- Exercise-induced weakness—determine acetylcholine receptor antibody titers (test for myasthenia gravis); check serum creatine kinase concentration (polymyositis or polymyopathy), red blood cell count (anemia or polycythemia), and blood glucose concentration (hypoglycemia); check for cardiac arrhythmia/hypoxia via electrocardiogram, thoracic radiography, Holter monitoring, echocardiography; muscle biopsy.
- LMN weakness or muscle pain, muscle atrophy, or hypertrophy—determine creatine kinase concentration (polymyositis or polymyopathy); evaluate *Neospora caninum* and *Toxoplasma gondii* serum titers; perform electromyography, nerve conduction, muscle and nerve biopsies.
- Myelitis or meningitis—Dog: perform titers for *N. caninum*, *T. gondii*, canine distemper virus and/or fungal diseases; perform PCR for Rocky Mountain spotted fever, *Ehrlichia* spp., and canine distemper virus; evaluate spinal fluid for infectious diseases. Cat: evaluate for feline leukemia virus and feline immunodeficiency virus; perform serum titers for *T. gondii* and *Cryptococcus* spp.; evaluate spinal fluid for signs of feline infectious peritonitis virus and *Cryptococcus* spp.

IMAGING

- Spinal radiography—may reveal disc herniation, discospondylitis, bony tumor, congenital vertebral malformation, and fracture or luxation.
- Myelography—required if survey radiography not diagnostic and if CT or MRI unavailable.
- CT or MRI—has replaced myelography where technology is available.

DIAGNOSTIC PROCEDURES

- CSF—before myelography to detect myelitis and meningitis; if high protein value or inflammatory cells, consider infectious disease diagnostics (titers, PCR).
- Needle electromyography and motor nerve conduction velocity—may help with diagnosis and characterization of generalized LMN.
- Muscle and nerve biopsy—generalized LMN weakness.
- Aspiration of intervertebral disc space under fluoroscopy if discospondylitis observed on imaging studies—perform cytology and culture to isolate an infectious agent.

TREATMENT

- Inpatient—with severe weakness or paralysis until bladder function can be ascertained.
- Hand feeding if necessary—with diffuse LMN, swallowing can be affected.
- Feeding from an elevated platform or installation of a feeding tube if necessary—recommended for animals with megaesophagus.

- Activity—restrict until spinal trauma and disc herniation can be ruled out.
- Physical therapy—important for paralyzed patients; tone muscles and keep joints flexible.
- Bedding—check and clean frequently to prevent urine scalding and superficial pyoderma; use padded bedding or waterbed to help prevent decubital ulcer formation.
- Turn quadriplegic patients from side to side 4–8 times daily to prevent hypostatic lung congestion and decubital ulcer formation.
- Surgery—for disc herniation, fracture, and some neoplasias and congenital conditions; often the quickest and most effective method to improve neurologic status.

MEDICATIONS

DRUG(S) OF CHOICE

- Medications depend on underlying cause of weakness.
- NSAIDs for spinal diseases associated with bone discomfort or pain.
- Corticosteroid use, even in known diseases like spinal trauma or disc herniation, is controversial. May help to allay pain associated with some causes of paralysis, but does not expedite spinal cord recovery.
- Dexamethasone 0.1–0.2 mg/kg q48h for pain relief for 2–3 doses. Prednisolone 0.5–1 mg/kg q12–24h for pain relief for 3–5 days.
- Antibiotics or antifungals—used for discospondylitis, protozoal myelitis/meningitis.
- Pyridostigmine bromide 0.5–3 mg/kg PO q8–12h for suspected myasthenia gravis; administer cautiously at low dose while waiting for titer results.
- If acute generalized LMN signs—check for ticks; use appropriate insecticides.

CONTRAINDICATIONS

Corticosteroids—do not use with discospondylitis or fungal or protozoal myelitis/meningitis; do not use with myasthenia gravis if aspiration pneumonia is present.

PRECAUTIONS

Corticosteroids—associated with GI ulceration and hemorrhage, delayed wound healing, and heightened susceptibility to infection.

ALTERNATIVE DRUG(S)

- Gabapentin 3–10 mg/kg q12h PO for neuropathic pain.
- Butorphanol 0.2–0.6 mg/kg q2–4h for pain control.
- Tramadol has been prescribed in the past; but effectiveness in most dogs is likely insufficient for pain management.

FOLLOW-UP

PATIENT MONITORING

- Neurologic examinations—daily to monitor status.

- Bladder—evacuate (via manual expression or catheterization) 3–4 times a day to prevent overdistension and subsequent bladder atony; once bladder function has returned, patient can be managed at home.

POSSIBLE COMPLICATIONS

- Urinary tract infection, bladder atony, urine scalding and pyoderma, constipation, decubital ulcer formation.
- Aspiration pneumonia—with generalized LMN disease or in any quadriplegic patient.
- Myelomalacia—with severe spinal cord trauma or disc herniations.
- Respiratory compromise or paralysis—with myelomalacia or generalized LMN disease.

MISCELLANEOUS

See Also

- Fibrocartilaginous Embolic Myelopathy.
- Lumbosacral Stenosis and Cauda Equine Syndrome.
- Myelopathy—Paresis/Paralysis—Cats.
- Polyneuropathies (Peripheral Neuropathies).

Abbreviations

- LMN = lower motor neuron
- NSAID = nonsteroidal anti-inflammatory drug.
- UMN = upper motor neuron.

Suggested Reading

de Lahunta A, Glass EN, Kent M. *Veterinary Neuroanatomy and Clinical Neurology*, 4th edn. St. Louis, MO: Elsevier-Saunders, 2015.

Negrin A, Schatzberg S, Platt SR. The paralyzed cat: neuroanatomic diagnosis and specific spinal cord diseases. *J Feline Med Surg* 2009;11:361–372.

Author/editor: Heidi Lobprise
Topic adapted from Five Minute Veterinary Consultation, 7th edition, 2021
Original Topic: Paralysis

Author: Linda G. Shell
<web/> Client Education Handout available online

Chapter 66

Vestibular Disease, Geriatric—Dogs

BASICS

DEFINITION

Acute-onset nonprogressive disturbance of the peripheral vestibular system in older dogs.

PATHOPHYSIOLOGY

- Unknown.
- Suspected abnormal flow of the endolymphatic fluid in the semicircular canals of the inner ear secondary to disturbance in production, circulation, or absorption of the fluid.
- Possible intoxication of the vestibular receptors or inflammation of the vestibular portion of the vestibulocochlear nerve (cranial nerve VIII).
- Often incorrectly referred to as a stroke, geriatric vestibular disease is neither central in location nor suspected to be vascular or ischemic in origin.

INCIDENCE/PREVALENCE

Common, sporadic, acquired disease of older dogs.

SIGNALMENT

Species

Dog

Breed Predilections

- None reported.
- Seems to occur more frequently in medium-to-large breeds.

Mean Age and Range

Geriatric; patients usually >8 years old, no predominant Sex.

Blackwell's Five-Minute Veterinary Consult Clinical Companion: Small Animal Senior Care, First Edition. Edited by Heidi B. Lobprise.

Companion website: www.wiley.com/go/lobprise/Senior

SIGNS

General Comments

- Signs of acute-onset peripheral vestibular dysfunction usually unilateral but occasionally bilateral.
- If vestibular signs are severe, do not incorrectly attribute the signs (especially the gait) to a central (i.e., CNS) location.

Historical Findings

- Sudden onset of imbalance, disorientation, reluctance to stand, and (usually) head tilt and irregular eye movements.
- May be preceded or accompanied by nausea and vomiting.

Physical Examination Findings

- Head tilt—mild to marked; directed toward the side of the lesion; occasionally disease is bilateral with erratic side-to-side head movements either without a head tilt or with a mild tilt in direction of the more severely affected side.
- Abnormal (resting) nystagmus common in early stages; either horizontal or rotatory with the fast phase always in the direction opposite to the head tilt; with bilateral disease, abnormal nystagmus usually mild or not present and physiologic nystagmus or conjugate eye movements diminished to absent.
- Mild-to-marked disorientation and vestibular ataxia with tendency to lean or fall in the direction of the head tilt.
- Strength and proprioception normal; with severe disease, patient may be reluctant/unable to stand and may have other issues (e.g., hip dysplasia), making assessment of gait difficult; with bilateral disease, may have base-wide stance.

CAUSES

Unknown

DIAGNOSIS

DIFFERENTIAL DIAGNOSIS

- Primarily distinguished from other causes of vestibular deficits by the acute onset and usually rapid improvement without specific treatment.
- Otitis media and interna—may have concurrent ipsilateral facial nerve (cranial nerve VII) paresis or paralysis, deafness, and/or Horner's syndrome; otitis externa with ruptured tympanic membrane may be present with otitis media and interna.
- Ototoxic drugs—eliminated by history.
- Trauma—may cause similar acute changes; differentiated by history, results of physical examination.
- Hypothyroid neuropathy—usually not as acute in onset or as severe; may be associated with clinical signs of hypothyroidism and possible cranial nerve VII deficit.
- Neoplasia—either affecting CN VIII peripherally or in a central location; signs usually not as acute in onset as geriatric vestibular disease and signs persistent and usually progressive in nature.

CBC/BIOCHEMISTRY/URINALYSIS

- Generally normal.
- Hemoconcentration secondary to dehydration may be present.
- Unrelated concurrent disorders (e.g., renal and hepatic disease) associated with geriatric state may cause laboratory abnormalities.

IMAGING

- Usually none required.
- Radiographs of tympanic bullae: normal radiographs do not rule out bulla disease.
- CT or MRI (preferred over radiographs)—may be required to rule out other causes such as otitis media and interna, central causes (e.g., ischemic event, neoplasia, inflammatory disease).

DIAGNOSTIC PROCEDURES

- Brainstem auditory-evoked response—to assess cochlear portion of cranial nerve VIII; may help to evaluate for otitis media and interna since only the vestibular portion of cranial nerve VIII is affected with geriatric vestibular disease.
- Deafness may, however, be present as an unrelated aging change.

TREATMENT

APPROPRIATE HEALTH CARE

- Mild disease—usually can manage as outpatient.
- Severe disease—patients that cannot ambulate or require IV fluid support should be hospitalized during the initial stages.

NURSING CARE

- Treatment supportive, including rehydration by IV fluids if required.
- Keep recumbent patients warm and dry using soft, absorbent bedding and, if required, urinary catheter.
- Severe disease—physical therapy, including passive manipulation of limbs and moving body to alternate sides, may be required initially.

ACTIVITY

Restrict activity as required by the degree of disorientation and vestibular ataxia.

DIET

- No modification usually required.
- Nausea, vomiting, and severe disorientation—initially withhold oral intake, then supervised feeding.

CLIENT EDUCATION

Reassure client that although the initial signs can be alarming and incapacitating, the prognosis for rapid improvement and recovery is excellent.

MEDICATIONS

DRUG(S) OF CHOICE

- Sedatives—for severe disorientation and ataxia; diazepam 2–10 mg/dog PO or IV q8h, acepromazine 0.02–0.05 mg/kg IM, SC, IV to maximum of 2 mg, dexmedetomidine 1–2 μg/kg IV.
- Antianxiety—trazodone approximately 5 mg/kg PO q8–24h.
- Antiemetic drugs or drugs against motion sickness—questionable benefit; dimenhydrinate 4–8 mg/kg PO, IM, IV q8h, meclizine HCl 25 mg PO q24h, maropitant 1 mg/kg SC q24h for up to 5 days or 2 mg/kg PO q24h for up to 5 days.
- Glucocorticoids—not recommended since do not alter course of the disease; may exacerbate concurrent issues (e.g., dehydration).
- Antibiotics—recommended when otitis media and interna cannot be ruled out; trimethoprim-sulfa 15 mg/kg PO q12h or 30 mg/kg PO q12–24h; first-generation cephalosporin (e.g., cephalexin 10–30 mg/kg PO q12h); amoxicillin–clavulanic acid 12.5 mg/kg PO q12h, enrofloxacin 5–20 mg/kg PO q24h or divided q12h.

FOLLOW-UP

PATIENT MONITORING

- Neurologic examination of outpatient—repeat 2–3 days later to confirm stabilization and initial improvement.
- Discharge inpatient when able to ambulate and resume eating and drinking.

POSSIBLE COMPLICATIONS

- Fluid and electrolyte imbalances and decompensation of preexistent renal insufficiency may follow vomiting and/or insufficient fluid and food intake.
- Pressure sores/abrasions.

EXPECTED COURSE AND PROGNOSIS

- Improvement of clinical signs usually starts within 72 hours with gradual resolution of vomiting and improvement of nystagmus and vestibular ataxia.
- Head tilt and ataxia—significant improvement usually occurs over 7–10 days; if no improvement other causes of peripheral vestibular disease should be pursued; mild head tilt may persist.
- Most patients return to normal within 2–3 weeks.
- Recurrence—repeat episodes of geriatric vestibular disease can occur on the same or opposite side but are uncommon; brief return of signs may occur with stress (e.g., anesthesia).

MISCELLANEOUS

Age-Related Factors

Geriatric dogs affected (mean age suggested 12.5 years).

Suggested Reading

de Lahunta A, Glass EN, Kent M. *Veterinary Neuroanatomy and Clinical Neurology*, 4th edn. St. Louis, MO: Saunders Elsevier, 2015; pp. 348–349.

Dewey CW. *A Practical Guide to Canine and Feline Neurology*, 2nd edn. Ames, IA: Wiley-Blackwell, 2008; pp. 272–273.

Garosi L. Head tilt and nystagmus. In: Platt SR, Garosi LS (eds) *Small Animal Neurological Emergencies*. London: Manson Publishing, 2012; pp. 253–263.

Author/editor: Heidi Lobprise
Topic adapted from Five Minute Veterinary Consultation, 7th edition, 2021
Original Topic: Vestibular Disease—Geriatric Dogs

Author: Susan M. Cochrane

Ophthalmic

Chapter 67

Cataracts

BASICS

DEFINITION

Opacification of the lens (focal or diffuse).

PATHOPHYSIOLOGY

- The normal lens is composed of perfectly aligned lens fibers that create a transparent structure. A clear capsule surrounds the cortex and nucleus. New lens fibers are continually produced at the equator of the lens cortex throughout life. The aqueous humor provides nutrition to the lens.
- A cataract occurs when there is derangement of lens fibers due to changes in lens nutrition, energy metabolism, protein synthesis or metabolism, or osmotic balance.
- Anterior uveitis is a common cause of altered lens nutrition.
- Genetics can result in altered protein and energy metabolism, or protein synthesis, in the lens.
- Diabetes mellitus affects the osmotic balance in the lens. Hyperglycemia increases glucose in the aqueous and lens overwhelming the glycolysis pathway; glucose is shunted to the sorbitol pathway; sorbitol creates an osmotic gradient that draws water into the lens and rapid cataract formation. The sorbitol pathway requires aldose reductase enzyme and dogs have more aldose reductase than cats, making cats more resistant to developing diabetic cataracts. The enzyme levels vary between individuals, which may explain dogs that are resistant to cataract development.

SYSTEMS AFFECTED

Ophthalmic

GENETICS

- Inheritance has been established for many dog breeds; the most common mode of inheritance is autosomal recessive.
- Inheritance has been established in the Himalayan cat (autosomal recessive).

Blackwell's Five-Minute Veterinary Consult Clinical Companion: Small Animal Senior Care,
First Edition. Edited by Heidi B. Lobprise.

Companion website: www.wiley.com/go/lobprise/Senior

INCIDENCE/PREVALENCE

- One of the leading causes of blindness in dogs.
- The prevalence of genetic cataracts varies significantly; up to 10% in some breeds.
- Most diabetic dogs will develop cataracts regardless of their diabetic control.
- Cataracts are rare in cats.

SIGNALMENT

Species

Dogs and cats.

Breed Predilections

Over 135 dog breeds are suspected as being predisposed to hereditary cataracts.

Mean Age and Range

Cataracts can develop at any age; genetic cataracts can develop as early as 6 months of age.

SIGNS

Historical Findings

- Cloudy/white appearance of the lens.
- Vision loss when the cataracts are bilateral and diabetic cataracts with a rapid, bilateral onset.
- Polyuria/polydipsia is noticed prior to cataract development in diabetic dogs.

Physical Examination Findings

- General physical examination findings—unremarkable unless the dog is an undiagnosed diabetic.
- Ophthalmic examination findings—opacification in one or both lenses.
  - Incipient stage—small, focal opacity/opacities in the lens that does not interfere with the view of the fundus; no vision deficits.
  - Immature stage—diffusely cloudy appearance to the lens with the tapetal reflection still visible and some portions of the fundus visible through a dilated pupil; the menace reflex is positive.
  - Mature stage—completely opaque lens with no tapetal reflection visible; blind.
  - Hypermature stage—wrinkled lens capsule, areas of dense white mineralization, may have portions of liquefied cortex (white, sparkly to clear); deep anterior chamber; blind unless there is a large area of clear liquefied cortex.
  - Intumescent mature cataract—opaque, swollen lens usually due to the hyperosmotic effect of diabetes; shallow anterior chamber.

CAUSES

- Hereditary—most common cause in dogs.
- Diabetes mellitus.
- Anterior uveitis—either by altered nutrition of the lens from the abnormal aqueous, or by posterior synechia and inflammatory debris causing opacification of the anterior lens capsule.

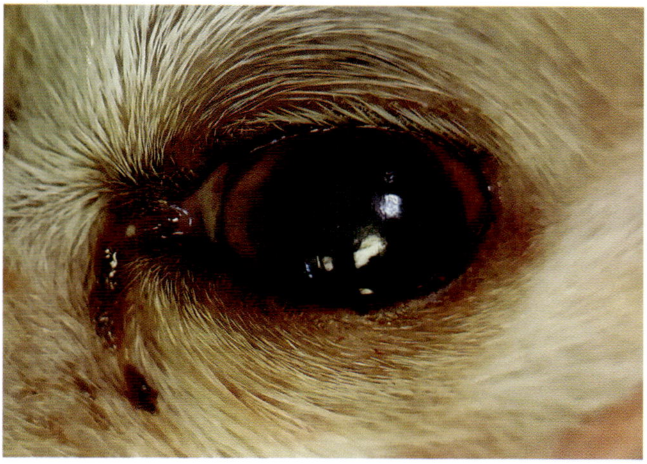

Figure 67.1 Lenticular sclerosis in an aging dog.

- Trauma—perforating injury that disrupts the anterior lens capsule, most commonly a cat claw injury, especially in puppies and kittens.
- Senile—slowly progressive cataract in geriatric animals, usually beginning as dense nuclear sclerosis followed by gradual spoke-like opacities extending into the cortex (see Figure 67.1).
- Congenital—due to heredity, in utero insult, or associated with other congenital ocular anomalies.
- Surgery—transpupillary laser energy, intraocular instrument trauma.
- Toxic—long-term ketoconazole therapy; suspected secondary to toxic by-products of degenerating photoreceptors in dogs with progressive retinal atrophy.
- Radiation—when the eye is in the radiation treatment field for neoplasia of the mouth or head.
- Hypocalcemia—can cause bilateral, diffuse punctate or incipient cataracts.
- Electrical shock—chewing electrical cords or lightning strike.

RISK FACTORS

- Diabetes mellitus (dogs).
- Chronic anterior uveitis.
- Progressive retinal atrophy.

DIAGNOSIS

DIFFERENTIAL DIAGNOSIS

Lenticular nuclear sclerosis—normal aging change in the lens of dogs and cats starting at 6 years of age due to compression of older lens fibers in the center of the lens; gradually becomes more visible with age and can be mistaken for a cataract in geriatric patients; definitive diagnosis can be made using mydriasis (1% tropicamide) and the observation of a perfectly round, bilaterally symmetric, homogeneous nucleus in the center of each lens, and the ability to view the fundus through the lens; vision is rarely affected and treatment is not indicated.

CBC/BIOCHEMISTRY/URINALYSIS

Dogs with diabetic cataracts may have hyperglycemia and glucosuria.

IMAGING

Ocular ultrasound can be used to evaluate the posterior lens capsule for any sign of rupture and can evaluate for retinal detachment prior to cataract surgery.

DIAGNOSTIC PROCEDURES

ERG is performed prior to cataract surgery to evaluate for retinal degeneration when the fundus is not visible due to the cataract.

TREATMENT

ACTIVITY

For safety, blind animals should not be allowed access to an in-ground swimming pool or elevated decks with open railings; use caution near stairs; restrict outside activity to fenced yards or leash walks.

CLIENT EDUCATION

- Cataract surgery is routinely performed, with an overall 80–90% success rate.
- Once the cataracts are removed they cannot return.
- Artificial lens implants will restore essentially normal vision.
- Evaluation for surgery should be done early in the course of cataract development to avoid complications that may result in the cataract becoming inoperable, to allow time to plan for the surgery, and in some cases to eliminate the need and extra cost for an ocular ultrasound and ERG.

SURGICAL CONSIDERATIONS

- Phacoemulsification (removal of the cataract through a corneal incision using ultrasonic waves to emulsify and aspirate the lens) is the most common technique for cataract removal.
- The ideal time for cataract surgery is the immature/early mature stage.
- Inherited, diabetic, and senile cataracts are potentially good candidates for surgery; cataracts secondary to anterior uveitis are normally poor surgical candidates.
- Artificial intraocular lenses are routinely placed inside the patient's lens capsule; lens implants restore normal focus and help minimize posterior capsular fibrosis; if a lens cannot be implanted (e.g., due to an unstable lens capsule or luxated lens), the dog or cat will still have functional vision.
- Traumatic lens perforation with release of lens cortex into the anterior chamber may require surgery to remove the lens, depending on the size of the capsular tear.

MEDICATIONS

DRUG(S) OF CHOICE

- Topical anti-inflammatory medication is recommended q6–24h to help prevent or treat lens-induced uveitis with immature, mature, and hypermature cataracts; this can be a topical nonsteroidal anti-inflammatory drug (NSAID) such as flurbiprofen, diclofenac, or ketorolac, or a topical steroid such as prednisolone acetate 1% or dexamethasone 0.1%; topical NSAIDs may be preferable in diabetic patients.
- Topical atropine q8–24h is indicated for lens-induced uveitis; *contraindicated with glaucoma*.
- Oral NSAIDs (carprofen, meloxicam, deracoxib) are also used to treat lens-induced uveitis.
- Topical antioxidants are advertised as able to reverse cataract changes; to date there have been no published data conclusively showing a significant reversal, or delay in progression; time spent trying medical therapy will delay evaluation for surgery, resulting in surgery being performed at a suboptimal stage, or complications from the cataract making it inoperable.
- A topical aldose reductase inhibitor, Kinostat®, is in the final stage of FDA approval. When made available, it may prove helpful in delaying the onset of diabetic cataracts in dogs.

FOLLOW-UP

PATIENT MONITORING

- Incipient or early immature cataracts should be monitored regularly for progression in order to select the ideal time for surgery and to avoid complications associated with cataracts.
- Postoperative monitoring by the surgeon is critical for the success of surgery and should be clearly discussed with the owner prior to surgery.

POSSIBLE COMPLICATIONS

- Lens-induced uveitis—associated with hypermature cataracts and cataracts that progress rapidly; caused by antigenic lens proteins leaking through the lens capsule. Clinical signs can be subtle (e.g., low intraocular pressure) to extreme (granulomatous uveitis with aqueous flare, miosis, synechia, keratic precipitates); preoperative uveitis increases postoperative complications.
- Secondary glaucoma—impaired aqueous outflow from intraocular changes associated with lens-induced uveitis, or from an intumescent cataract causing a forward displacement of the iris, narrowing the iridocorneal angle.
- Retinal detachment—associated with hypermature cataracts and cataracts in young dogs with a rapid onset and cortical liquefaction.
- Lens luxation—associated with hypermature cataracts in which the lens and capsule shrink, causing the zonules to stretch and break, resulting in a lens subluxation or luxation.

EXPECTED COURSE AND PROGNOSIS

- Most cataracts are progressive, although the rate of progression can vary widely depending on age, breed, and location of the cataract.
- Long-term prognosis following cataract surgery is very good; however, some patients have increased risk for postoperative complications.
- Those that do not pursue surgery should be monitored for uveitis and glaucoma.

MISCELLANEOUS

Associated Conditions

- Retinal detachment.
- Lens-induced uveitis.
- Congenital ocular anomalies.

Age-Related Factors

- Nuclear sclerosis is prominent in geriatric animals; a dilated exam may be necessary to definitively distinguish nuclear sclerosis from cataract.

Abbreviation

- NSAID = nonsteroidal anti-inflammatory drug

Author/editor: Heidi Lobprise
Topic adapted from Five Minute Veterinary Consultation, 7th edition, 2021
Original Topic: Cataracts

Author: Margi A. Gilmour
Consulting Editor: Kathern E. Myrna

Chapter 68

Corneal Opacities

BASICS

OVERVIEW

Acquired corneal disorder characterized by lipid or calcium deposition. May be unilateral or bilateral, have distinct margins, and occur secondary to other ocular or systemic disorders.

SIGNALMENT

Primarily in dogs, uncommon in cats. Lipid deposition most common in geriatric dogs. May be associated with systemic hyperlipoproteinemia.

SIGNS

- Lipid deposits—gray-white or crystalline; band-shaped, irregular, or circular.
- Calcium deposits—dense white to crystalline; irregular, punctate to band-shaped lesions in the superficial stroma.
- Frequently associated with inflammatory disorders such as keratitis or uveitis.
- Corneal vascularization, edema, and pigmentation often present.
- With progression the cornea may develop a roughened appearance; disruption of epithelium can lead to ulceration.
- Associated ocular conditions that may lead to corneal degeneration—corneal scars, keratoconjunctivitis sicca (KCS), exposure keratitis, chronic uveitis, episcleritis, phthisis bulbi, chronic topical steroid therapy, limbal neoplasia.
- When lipid deposition occurs secondary to hyperlipoproteinemia, perilimbal annular ring may form with clear zone between affected cornea and limbus; often bilateral but may be asymmetric; vascularization is variable.

CAUSES AND RISK FACTORS

- Lipid—hyperlipoproteinemia may increase risk or worsen existing deposits; can be secondary to hypothyroidism, diabetes mellitus, hyperadrenocorticism, diet, pancreatitis, nephrotic syndrome, liver disease, hyperlipidemia of miniature schnauzers.
- Calcium—hypercalcemia, hyperphosphatemia, hypervitaminosis D, hyperadrenocorticism, uremia.
- Lipid and calcium deposits are frequently seen together.

Blackwell's Five-Minute Veterinary Consult Clinical Companion: Small Animal Senior Care,
First Edition. Edited by Heidi B. Lobprise.

Companion website: www.wiley.com/go/lobprise/Senior

DIAGNOSIS

DIFFERENTIAL DIAGNOSIS

- Corneal scar—nonpainful lesion, gray to white; fluorescein negative; relatively smooth corneal surface; distinct margins.
- Corneal stromal dystrophies—bilateral, often symmetric foci of gray to white deposition, distinct margins; heritable, not associated with ocular inflammation; do not retain fluorescein stain; often occur away from the limbus.
- Edema—bluish to gray; usually homogeneous; varies in size depending on severity; indistinct margins; can retain fluorescein stain if corneal erosion/ulceration present (see Figure 68.1).
- Corneal ulcer—ocular pain, retains fluorescein stain, varying degrees of edema around the lesion.
- Inflammatory cell infiltrates—ocular pain, gray to tan to yellow with indistinct margins; cytologic examination of cornea reveals white blood cells, microorganisms.

CBC/BIOCHEMISTRY/URINALYSIS

- Systemic tests only necessary if hyperlipidemia is suspected; no systemic tests necessary for most cases.
- Lipid—evaluate fasting cholesterol, triglyceride, blood glucose concentrations.
- Calcium—evaluate ionized calcium concentration.

OTHER LABORATORY TESTS

Endocrinopathy testing—thyroid function, adrenocorticotropic hormone (ACTH) stimulation test.

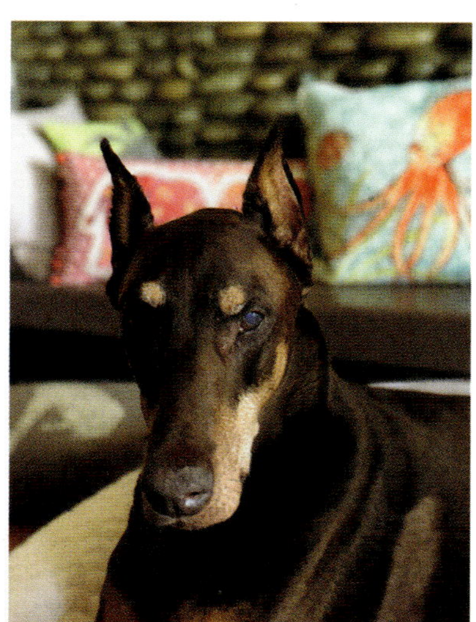

Figure 68.1 A senior Doberman with corneal edema. Source: Photo Courtesy of Dr. Mary Gardner.

DIAGNOSTIC PROCEDURES

Fluorescein staining—may retain dye around margins of deposit if raised.

TREATMENT

- Treat primary ocular disease if present.
- Corneal deposits causing patient discomfort or impaired vision may benefit from corneal debridement or superficial keratectomy followed by medical treatment; deposits likely to recur if underlying cause not corrected.
- Hyperlipoproteinemia may resolve with low-fat diet and treatment of systemic disease if present; both may slow or stop progression of ocular disease.

MEDICATIONS

DRUG(S) OF CHOICE

- Topical broad-spectrum antibiotics (i.e., triple antibiotic) for ulcerated cornea; frequency depends on severity; usually uncomplicated ulcers treated q8–12h.
- Topical nonsteroidal anti-inflammatory drug q8–12h—indicated if uveitis noted.
- Topical 0.2% cyclosporine—to improve tear film quality, reduce inflammation.
- Topical 1% atropine q8–24h—indicated to reduce pain if uveitis or ulceration is present.
- Topical ethylene diamine tetra-acetate (EDTA) solution 0.5–3% q6h; may help minimize calcium deposits; usually used following debulking procedure to improve efficacy.
- Artificial tear ointment q6–12h; may prevent or reduce frequency of secondary corneal ulceration; provides lubrication and improves comfort when corneal surface is irregular.

CONTRAINDICATIONS/POSSIBLE COMPLICATIONS

- Topical corticosteroids—not recommended, may worsen severity; contraindicated with corneal ulceration.
- Topical atropine—contraindicated with KCS, glaucoma, lens luxations.

FOLLOW-UP

PATIENT MONITORING

Monitor serum cholesterol and triglycerides to assess efficacy of dietary management in hyperlipidemic patients; monitor treatment of primary disease if present.

EXPECTED COURSE AND PROGNOSIS

- Corneal ulceration—associated with worsening of disease.
- Vision—may be affected in advanced disease; may be severe if primary ocular disease (e.g., uveitis) present.
- Deposits may recur following superficial keratectomy.

MISCELLANEOUS

Abbreviations

- ACTH = adrenocorticotropic hormone
- EDTA = ethylene diamine tetra-acetate.
- KCS = keratoconjunctivitis sicca.

Internet Resources

Accessed 29 June 2024

- https://www.columbiaeye.org/education/digital-reference-of-ophthalmology/cornea-external-diseases/degenerations

Suggested Reading

Crispin SM, Barnett KC. Dystrophy, degeneration and infiltration of the canine cornea. *J Small Anim Pract* 1983;24:63–83.

Author/editor: Heidi Lobprise
Topic adapted from Five Minute Veterinary Consultation, 7th edition, 2021
Original Topic: Corneal Opacities—Degenerations and Infiltrates

Author: Kathern E. Myrna
Consulting Editor: Kathern E. Myrna

Chapter 69

Glaucoma

BASICS

DEFINITION

- A group of diseases where elevated intraocular pressure (IOP) causes optic nerve and retinal degeneration with subsequent loss of vision.
- Diagnosis—IOP >20 mmHg (dogs) or >25 mmHg (cats) as determined by tonometry, with changes in vision or the appearance of the globe, optic nerve, and/or retina.

PATHOPHYSIOLOGY

- Multifactorial disease where obstruction of aqueous humor outflow leads to increased IOP and optic nerve degeneration.
- Elevated IOP induces mechanical changes (stretching of sclera in lamina cribosa damages optic nerve axons) and vascular changes (decreased ocular perfusion causes ischemic damage to retina), resulting in ganglion cell death and optic nerve atrophy.

SYSTEMS AFFECTED

- Ophthalmic.
- Nervous.

GENETICS

PRIMARY CAUSES OFTEN NOT SEEN UNTIL MIDDLE AGE, PROGRESSING WITH AGE

- Primary angle-closure glaucoma (PACG; dogs)—complex trait with multiple genetic risk factors and uncertain mode of inheritance.
- Primary open-angle glaucoma (POAG; dogs)—monogenic (*ADAMTS10*) and autosomal recessive.
- Primary congenital glaucoma (PCG; cats)—monogenic (*LTBP2*) and autosomal recessive.

Blackwell's Five-Minute Veterinary Consult Clinical Companion: Small Animal Senior Care,
First Edition. Edited by Heidi B. Lobprise.

Companion website: www.wiley.com/go/lobprise/Senior

INCIDENCE/PREVALENCE

- Dogs—prevalence depends on breed; primary and secondary glaucoma are each listed as approximately 0.8% of all hospital admissions in the North American Veterinary Medical Database (NAVMDB).
- Cats—relatively uncommon; less than 0.3% of diagnoses in NAVMDB.

SIGNALMENT

Species

- Dog—primary and secondary common.
- Cat—primary rare; secondary more common (due to intraocular neoplasia or chronic uveitis).

Breed Predilections

- PACG—Alaskan Malamute, American cocker spaniel, Australian cattle dog, basset hound, Boston terrier, bouvier des Flandres, bullmastiff, Chinese Shar-Pei, chow chow, Dalmatian, Dandie Dinmont terrier, English cocker spaniel, English springer spaniel, flat-coated retriever, golden retriever, Great Dane, Labrador retriever, Newfoundland, poodle, Samoyed, Shiba Inu, shih tzu, Siberian husky, Welsh springer spaniel.
- POAG—beagle, Norwegian elkhound, petit basset griffon Vendéen.
- PCG—Siamese cats.
- Other forms of primary glaucoma—Burmese, Persian, Siamese cats.

Mean Age and Range

- Primary (dogs)—any age; predominantly affects middle-aged (4–9 years).
- Secondary (cats)—usually affects older cats (>6 years).

Predominant Sex

Females suffer PACG compared to males at a ratio of 2 : 1.

SIGNS

General Comments

All well-equipped small animal hospitals should have a tonometer.

Historical Findings

- Dogs—owners may note pain (blepharospasm, tenderness about the head), serous to seromucoid ocular discharge, red or cloudy eye, dilated pupil, or altered vision; in chronic cases, globe enlargement may be apparent.
- Cats—signs are more subtle; eye may not appear painful, red, or cloudy; owners may note dilated pupil, vision changes, or enlarged globe.

Physical Examination Findings

Acute Primary

- High IOP (often >30 mmHg).
- Blepharospasm.
- Enophthalmos with elevated third eyelid.

- Episcleral injection.
- Diffuse corneal edema.
- Mydriasis.
- Vision loss—may be detected by lack of menace response, dazzle reflex, and/or direct or consensual pupillary light reflex.
- Optic nerve may be normal or swollen and hyperemic.

Chronic (End Stage)

- High or normal IOP.
- Buphthalmos.
- Descemet's streaks (Haab's striae).
- Subluxated lens with an aphakic crescent.
- Optic nerve head atrophy will appear dark and cupped.
- Retinal atrophy detected by peripapillary or generalized tapetal hyper-reflectivity.

Secondary

- High IOP.
- Episcleral injection.
- Corneal edema.
- Aqueous flare.
- Iris changes (miosis or mydriasis, posterior synechia, iris bombé).
- Hyphema.
- Anterior lens luxation.
- Intumescent cataracts.
- Intraocular mass.

CAUSES

- Congenital—severe dysgenesis/lack of formation of the iridocorneal angle.
- Primary—developmental iridocorneal angle anomalies that impede aqueous humor outflow.
- Secondary—obstruction of aqueous humor outflow by various mechanisms, e.g., uveitis (inflammatory cells or debris), anterior lens luxation (lens or attached vitreous), red blood cells, or neoplastic cells.

RISK FACTORS

- Age.
- Breed.
- Chronic uveitis.
- Goniodysgenesis—developmental defect of iridocorneal angle.
- Lens luxation.
- Hypermature or intumescent cataracts.
- Hyphema.
- Intraocular neoplasia.
- Topically applied mydriatics—may precipitate acute glaucoma in predisposed animals.
- Primary glaucoma is bilateral and often asymmetric; the unaffected fellow eye is at risk for developing glaucoma.

DIAGNOSIS

DIFFERENTIAL DIAGNOSIS

- Conjunctivitis—normal IOP and pupil size with conjunctival hyperemia (diffuse, red discoloration) instead of episcleral vessel engorgement.
- Uveitis—initially low IOP with miotic pupil.

IMAGING

Ocular ultrasound—facilitates evaluation of eye with opaque ocular media; may identify cause of secondary glaucoma (lens luxation, intraocular tumor).

DIAGNOSTIC PROCEDURES

- Rebound or applanation tonometry—essential for diagnosis of glaucoma.
- Gonioscopy—referral procedure that allows for evaluation of iridocorneal angle and assists with diagnosis of primary vs. secondary glaucoma.
- Systemic workup may be indicated in cases of secondary glaucoma due to chronic uveitis, hyphema, or intraocular neoplasia.

PATHOLOGIC FINDINGS

- Histopathologic evaluation is required for all eyes enucleated due to intractable glaucoma.
- Iridocorneal angle morphology assists diagnosis of primary vs. secondary glaucoma.
- Loss of retinal ganglion cells.
- Gliosis and "cupping" of optic nerve head.

TREATMENT

APPROPRIATE HEALTH CARE

- Acute—outpatient medical management vs. referral.
- Chronic—outpatient medical management vs. salvage surgical management.

CLIENT EDUCATION

- Warn client that primary glaucoma is a bilateral disease; more than 50% of dogs develop glaucoma in the other eye within 8 months without prophylactic therapy.
- Warn client that up to 50% of dogs will be blind in the affected eye within the first year regardless of therapy.

SURGICAL CONSIDERATIONS

- Acute, visual eyes (dogs)—referral surgical procedures aim to control IOP by decreasing aqueous humor production (transscleral or endoscopic cyclophotocoagulation), increasing outflow (gonioimplants), or both; medical treatment is still required long term to control IOP and inflammation.

- Blind, painful eyes (dogs and cats)—salvage procedures include enucleation, evisceration with intrascleral prosthesis (if no intraocular infection or neoplasia), and intravitreal gentamicin or cidofovir injection to minimize long-term medical therapy.

MEDICATIONS

DRUG(S) OF CHOICE

Use multiple agents to lower IOP into the normal range as quickly as possible in an attempt to salvage vision and maintain comfort. Topical hypotensive drugs have largely replaced systemic therapy due to higher efficacy and fewer side effects.

Acute Primary (Dogs)

- Prostaglandin analog—latanoprost 0.005% q12h. In emergency, apply one drop to affected eye, followed by another drop in 30 min. Recheck IOP in 1–2 hours.
- Carbonic anhydrase inhibitor—dorzolamide 2% q8h. Use in combination with latanoprost for long-term therapy.
- Topical corticosteroids—0.1% dexamethasone or 1% prednisolone acetate q12h. Use to control intraocular inflammation from initial hypertensive episode.
- ±Topical beta blocker—timolol maleate 0.5% q12h. Minimal effect on lowering IOP in companion animals. Use as auxiliary or prophylactic medication.
- ±Hyperosmotic agent—mannitol 1–2 g/kg IV over 20 minutes. In emergency, use to dehydrate vitreous humor and lower IOP if topical medications ineffective.

Secondary (Dogs and Cats)

- Identify and treat primary disease.
- Topical corticosteroids—to reduce inflammation if no ulcerative keratitis.
- Topical carbonic anhydrase inhibitors.
- ±Topical beta blockers.

CONTRAINDICATIONS

- Topical atropine—do not use with glaucoma.
- Prostaglandin analogs/miotic agents—do not use with primary anterior lens luxation or uveitis; mostly ineffective in cats.

PRECAUTIONS

- Systemic absorption of topical beta blockers may cause bronchoconstriction and bradycardia in small dogs and cats.
- Hyperosmotic agents may initiate acute pulmonary edema in patients with cardiovascular disease or hypervolemia.

POSSIBLE INTERACTIONS

Concurrent administration of latanoprost with a topical nonsteroidal anti-inflammatory drug such as flurbiprofen 0.03% may decrease its hypotensive effect.

ALTERNATIVE DRUG(S)

- Prostaglandin analogs—travoprost 0.004% q12h, bimatoprost 0.03% q12h.
- Carbonic anhydrase inhibitor—brinzolamide 1% q8h.
- Beta blockers—levobunalol 0.5% q12h, betaxolol 0.5% q12h.
- Osmotic agents—hypertonic hydroxyethyl starch 6–7.5% (4 mL/kg IV over 15–20 minutes).

FOLLOW-UP

PATIENT MONITORING

- IOP—monitored often (weekly to monthly) after starting initial therapy, then q3–4 months long term. Client's daily observation of comfort and vision is most important.
- Monitor for drug reactions.

PREVENTION/AVOIDANCE

- Primary—bilateral disease; recommend that a veterinary ophthalmologist examine the unaffected eye to determine its risk of developing glaucoma.
- Prophylactic therapy for the predisposed, unaffected eye delays onset of glaucoma—0.25% demecarium bromide (miotic) q12h, or 0.5% timolol maleate q12h, or 2% dorzolamide q8–12h

POSSIBLE COMPLICATIONS

- Blindness.
- Chronic ocular pain.

EXPECTED COURSE AND PROGNOSIS

- Chronic disease that requires constant medical treatment (even with surgical intervention).
- With medical treatment only—most patients ultimately become blind.
- Referral surgical treatment—better chance of retaining vision longer; most patients do not remain visual for more than 2 years after initial diagnosis.
- Secondary to lens luxation—may carry fair prognosis with referral for successful removal of luxated lens and postoperative medical therapy.
- Secondary to anterior uveitis—may carry fair prognosis with control of uveitis.

MISCELLANEOUS

Pregnancy/Fertility/Breeding

- All listed drugs may affect pregnancy.
- Primary and lens luxation cases—inherited; do not breed affected animals.

Abbreviations

- IOP = intraocular pressure
- PACG = Primary angle-closure glaucoma.
- POAG = Primary open-angle glaucoma.
- PCG = Primary congenital glaucoma.
- NAVMDB = North American Veterinary Medical Database.

Suggested Reading

Miller PE. The glaucomas. In: Maggs DJ, Miller PE, Ofri R (eds) *Slatter's Fundamentals of Veterinary Ophthalmology*, 6th edn. St. Louis, MO: Elsevier, 2018; pp. 279–305.
Pizzirani S (ed.) Glaucoma. *Vet Clin Small Anim* 2015;45(6): 1102–1378.

Author/editor: Heidi Lobprise
Topic adapted from Five Minute Veterinary Consultation, 7th edition, 2021
Original Topic: Glaucoma

Author: Erin M. Scott
Consulting Editor: Kathern E. Myrna

Chapter 70

Iris Atrophy

BASICS

OVERVIEW

- Degeneration of iris tissues; both the iris stroma and posterior iris epithelium can be affected, resulting in loss of iris sphincter and dilator muscle function, atrophy of iris vessels, and loss of iris pigment.
- Both the pupillary margin and more peripheral portions of the iris can be affected, resulting in an iris that is thin or has areas of full-thickness tissue loss.
- Senile or secondary change.
- Secondary iris atrophy is usually a result of chronic inflammation (uveitis).
- Iris sphincter muscle is frequently affected by atrophy, resulting in incomplete pupillary constriction, unequal pupil size (anisocoria), and possibly abnormal pupil shape (dyscoria).
- Irregular scalloped, moth-eaten pupil margin is a common manifestation.
- Pupil margin may remain unaffected; peripheral loss of iris tissue can cause large holes in the iris that resemble multiple pupillary openings.
- Vision largely unaffected.

SIGNALMENT

- Dog—common aging change; all breeds, but affects small breeds (e.g., miniature and toy poodles, miniature schnauzers, Chihuahuas) more commonly.
- Cat—uncommon; most common with blue irides.
- Secondary—any breed of dog or cat.

SIGNS

Historical Findings

- Large or dyscoric pupil in one or both eyes.
- Photophobia.
- Previous episodes of uveitis.

Physical Examination Findings

- Incomplete or absent pupillary light reflex accompanied by normal menace response and dazzle reflex.
- Anisocoria may be present with unilateral or asymmetric presentation.

Blackwell's Five-Minute Veterinary Consult Clinical Companion: Small Animal Senior Care, First Edition. Edited by Heidi B. Lobprise.

Companion website: www.wiley.com/go/lobprise/Senior

- Irregular, scalloped edge to pupillary margin; dyscoria.
- Tapetal reflex visible through thin or absent areas of the iris on transillumination—translucent patches or holes within the iris stroma: may resemble additional pupils.
- Strands of iris arising from free pupillary margin occasionally remain, spanning across portions of the pupil.
- Secondary—may be accompanied by any sign associated with chronic uveitis.

CAUSES AND RISK FACTORS

- Normal aging.
- Uveitis.
- Glaucoma.

DIAGNOSIS

DIFFERENTIAL DIAGNOSIS

- Must differentiate from congenital iris anomalies:
- Pupil dilation due to glaucoma—elevated intraocular pressure (IOP), corneal edema, conjunctival ± episcleral vascular injection, enlargement of globe may also be present; may also be blind.
- Adhesions of iris to lens or cornea (posterior or anterior synechia) as a result of uveitis or trauma—differentiate based on associated abnormalities consistent with uveitis or perforating trauma (e.g., full-thickness corneal scar).

DIAGNOSTIC PROCEDURES

Tonometry—low IOP possible if secondary to uveitis; high IOP if secondary to glaucoma or if uveitis has also caused secondary glaucoma; normal IOP if primary senile iris atrophy.

TREATMENT

- Irreversible.
- Secondary—successful treatment aimed at controlling the underlying disease may halt progression of the condition.
- Patient may exhibit photophobia because of inability to constrict the pupil; provide adequate shade and consider using eye protection/sunglasses.

MEDICATIONS

DRUG(S) OF CHOICE

- Senile—none.
- Secondary—depending on underlying disease.

CONTRAINDICATIONS/POSSIBLE INTERACTIONS

Topical atropine—exacerbates pupillary dilation and photophobia.

FOLLOW-UP

- Senile—may continue to progress with age.
- Secondary—usually does not progress once primary disease is controlled.

MISCELLANEOUS

Abbreviations

- IOP = intraocular pressure

Suggested Reading

Hendrix DVH. Diseases and surgery of the canine anterior uvea. In: Gelatt KN, Gilger BC, Kern TJ (eds) *Veterinary Ophthalmology*, 5th edn. Ames, IA: Wiley-Blackwell, 2013; pp. 1146–1198.

Author/editor: Heidi Lobprise
Topic adapted from Five Minute Veterinary Consultation, 7th edition, 2021
Original Topic: Iris Atrophy

Author: Simon A. Pot
Consulting Editor: Kathern E. Myrna

Chapter 71

Keratitis, Ulcerative

BASICS

DEFINITION

Inflammation of the cornea associated with loss of corneal epithelium (corneal erosion) or loss of variable amounts of underlying corneal stroma (corneal ulcer).

PATHOPHYSIOLOGY

- May be caused by any condition (traumatic or nontraumatic) that disrupts corneal epithelium or stroma.
- Ulcers—superficial or deep, uncomplicated or complicated:
    - Superficial—involves epithelium and possibly superficial stroma.
    - Deep—involves a greater thickness of stroma and may extend to Descemet's membrane (descemetocele), possibly leading to rupture of globe.
    - Complicated—persistence of underlying/inciting cause, microbial infection, or production of degradative enzymes (melting).
- Epithelial wound healing—adjacent corneal epithelial cells loosen and begin migration over the defect within a few hours; mitosis occurs within a few days to restore normal epithelial thickness; healing process complete in 5–7 days in uncomplicated, superficial ulcers.
- Stromal wound healing—slower, more complex; can be in an avascular or vascular manner; in shallow wounds, epithelial migration may be sufficient to fill defect; epithelium may cover some deeper ulcers even when epithelium and stromal regeneration are insufficient to restore normal corneal thickness (nonulcerated divot defect is called a facet); stroma usually heals by fibrovascular infiltration, resulting in scarring.
- Stromal ulcers—often complicated by microbial infection or enzymatic destruction initiated by microbial organisms, host inflammatory cells, or corneal epithelial or stromal cells; enzymatic destruction may result in gelatinous appearance of corneal stroma ("melting" or "malacic" ulcer).

SYSTEMS AFFECTED

Ophthalmic

Blackwell's Five-Minute Veterinary Consult Clinical Companion: Small Animal Senior Care, First Edition. Edited by Heidi B. Lobprise.

Companion website: www.wiley.com/go/lobprise/Senior

GENETICS

- No proven basis; breed predilections exist.
- May be secondary to other corneal diseases with breed predispositions and genetic basis.

INCIDENCE/PREVALENCE

Common

SIGNALMENT

Species

Dog and cat.

Breed Predilections

- Dogs—brachycephalic breeds predisposed.
- Spontaneous chronic corneal epithelial defects (SCCED)/indolent erosion—any breed.
- Cats—Persian, Himalayans, Siamese, and Burmese predisposed to corneal sequestrums (see Corneal Sequestrum—Cats).

Mean Age and Range

- Age of onset—variable; determined by cause.
- SCCED—middle-aged and older dogs.

SIGNS

Historical Findings

- May be acute or chronic (SCCED).
- Tearing, squinting, rubbing at eyes.
- Owners may report a "film" over the eye (often corneal edema); prolapsed third eyelid.
- Herpetic ulcers (cats)—may have history of respiratory disease.

Physical Examination Findings

- Nonspecific—serous-to-mucopurulent ocular discharge, blepharospasm, nictitans prolapse, conjunctival hyperemia.
- Superficial—may note one or more circumscribed, linear, or geographic defects in cornea.
- Deep stromal ulcer or descemetocele—may appear as a crater-like defect.
- Depending on cause and duration—may see neovascularization, pigmentation, scarring, inflammatory cell infiltrate (yellow-to-cream-colored opacity with indistinct margins, often surrounded by corneal edema), collagenolytic activity (melting) of corneal stroma.
- SCCED—loose or redundant epithelial edges; may demonstrate fluorescein stain extending into areas with seemingly intact epithelium (ring of less intense staining).
- Reflex anterior uveitis—mild or severe, secondary to ulceration; severe may result in hypopyon; severe suggests concurrent bacterial infection.

CAUSES

- Trauma—blunt; penetrating; perforating.
- Adnexal disease—ectopic cilia, entropion, ectropion, eyelid mass, distichiasis.
- Lagophthalmos (inability to close eyelids completely)—results in exposure keratitis; may be breed-related in brachycephalic dogs and cats; may be caused by exophthalmos, buphthalmos, or may be neuroparalytic from facial nerve paralysis.
- Tear-film abnormality—quantitative tear deficiency (keratoconjunctivitis sicca [KCS]); qualitative tear film deficiency caused by mucin deficiency or some other unidentified tear abnormality.
- Infection—usually secondary in dogs; can be primary herpesvirus infection in cats.
- Miscellaneous—foreign body (corneal or conjunctival), chemical burns, neurotrophic keratitis (loss of trigeminal sensation), immune-mediated disease.

DIAGNOSIS

DIFFERENTIAL DIAGNOSIS

- Other causes of a red and painful eye—conjunctivitis, uveitis, KCS, glaucoma (see Red Eye).
- May develop concurrently with other causes of a red eye (e.g., secondary to KCS).

OTHER LABORATORY TESTS

- Corneal culture and sensitivity—aerobic culture; particularly for complicated, deep, or rapidly progressive corneal ulcers.
- Herpesvirus (cats)—PCR or immunofluorescent antibody test (IFA) for herpesvirus available; negative test does not rule out herpesvirus infection.

DIAGNOSTIC PROCEDURES

Fluorescein Staining

- Homogeneous stain uptake—superficial or stromal ulcer; may be circular to geographic, linear, or combination; location and shape may help determine cause (e.g., linear may indicate foreign body or rubbing of ectopic cilia); interpretation of depth subjective.
- SCCED—may have leakage of stain under surrounding loose epithelium.
- Descemetocele—crater-like defect that retains stain at periphery but is clear at center; may see Descemet's membrane bulging if large defect.
- Previous stromal ulcer that has epithelialized (facet)—crater-like defect with transient pooling of stain that is easily rinsed; must distinguish from descemetocele.

Other

- Cytologic evaluation of cornea and Gram, Giemsa, or Wright staining may reveal microbial or fungal organisms and help direct initial antimicrobial therapy.
- Schirmer tear test may identify ulceration associated with KCS; contraindicated in very deep ulcers or descemetoceles.

PATHOLOGIC FINDINGS

- Ulcers—suppurative inflammation, possibly neovascularization, loss of epithelium and basement membrane; possibly organisms.
- SCCEDs—superficial hylanized zone in stroma; epithelial lipping around erosions; varying degrees and types of leukocytic infiltrate and fibrosis.

TREATMENT

APPROPRIATE HEALTH CARE

Hospitalize deep or rapidly progressive ulcers; these may require surgery and/or frequent medical treatments.

NURSING CARE

Keep facial hair out of eyes and clean.

ACTIVITY

- Restrict with deep stromal ulcer or descemetocele to prevent rupture.
- Prevent self-trauma with Elizabethan collar.

CLIENT EDUCATION

- Instruct client to wait at least 5 minutes between medications if more than one ophthalmic drop is prescribed; wait longer between ointments.
- Advise client to contact veterinarian if patient appears more painful or the eye markedly changes in appearance.
- SCCED—discuss protracted course with client; usually achieve healing within 2–6 weeks but may require weekly rechecks and multiple procedures.

SURGICAL CONSIDERATIONS

- Superficial ulcers do not usually require surgery if inciting cause has been eliminated.
- Ulcer that extends one-half or greater corneal thickness and particularly to Descemet's membrane may benefit from surgery.
- Descemetocele or full-thickness corneal laceration—surgical emergency, possible referral.

Procedures

- SCCED—debridement of loose epithelium with a dry, sterile, cotton-tipped swab after application of topical anesthesia (50% success rate); punctate or grid keratotomy easily performed after epithelial debridement with topical anesthesia (80% success rate); superficial keratectomy is more invasive and may cause more scarring but has 100% success rate; application of a contact lens or nictitans flap after any of these procedures may improve comfort and aid healing.
- Diamond burr keratotomy for SCCED/indolent erosion only; use gently over surface of erosion; may be associated with increased risk of infection.
- Rotational pedicle conjunctival flap, corneoscleral transposition, corneal transplant—surgical procedures for ulcers >50% stromal thickness and descemetoceles.

- Cyanoacrylate repair (corneal glue)—can be used for deep ulcers; promotes corneal vascularization and stabilizes cornea, but has lower success rate compared to other corneal surgeries.

MEDICATIONS

DRUG(S) OF CHOICE

Antibiotics

- Topical agents—indicated for all patients.
- Frequency of application—determined by severity and preparation; ointments have relatively long contact time and are applied q6–12h; solutions are applied more frequently (q2–6h) in initial treatment of complicated ulcers; solutions probably more appropriate in deep ulcers.
- Commonly used agents—erythromycin (cats); triple antibiotic, gentamicin, and tobramycin.
- Uncomplicated ulcers or superficial erosions—combination of neomycin, polymyxin B, and bacitracin an excellent first choice; broad spectrum of antimicrobial activity; often used 2–3 times/day for prophylactic therapy.
- Complicated ulcers—often use combination therapy of cefazolin (use IV solution to make 33–50 mg solution in saline or artificial tears for topical use) with a fluoroquinolone (ciprofloxacin, ofloxacin); particularly in rapidly progressive, deep, or melting ulcers; frequency depends on severity but usually a minimum of q3–4h.

Atropine

- 1% ointment or solution.
- Indicated for reflex anterior uveitis; frequency—usually q8–24h to effect (mydriasis).

Antiviral Agents

- Indicated for herpetic ulcers in cats.
- Trifluridine (Viroptic) solution—q4–6h until clinical response is observed; then reduce for 1–2 weeks after clinical signs have subsided.
- Famciclovir—90 mg/kg PO q12h for 2–4 weeks.

Nonsteroidal Anti-inflammatory Drugs (NSAIDs)

- Flurbiprofen, diclofenac.
- For anti-inflammatory and analgesic properties.

CONTRAINDICATIONS

- Topical corticosteroids—contraindicated with any corneal erosion or ulcer.
- Topical NSAIDs—contraindicated with herpetic ulcers.
- Topical atropine—contraindicated with glaucoma, KCS.

PRECAUTIONS

- Topical NSAIDs may delay corneal healing, may potentiate corneal melting.
- Trifluridine, neomycin—may be irritating.
- Topical cyclosporine can be used safely in KCS patients with uncomplicated ulcers.

POSSIBLE INTERACTIONS

Combining antibiotics in solution may inactivate some antibiotics.

ALTERNATIVE DRUG(S)

- Acetylcysteine—anticollagenolytic agent used for treatment of melting ulcers; efficacy is controversial; dilute 20% stock solution to 5–10% with artificial tears; apply q2–4h.
- Serum—anticollagenolytic agent; keep refrigerated; avoid contamination; discard after 48 hours.

FOLLOW-UP

PATIENT MONITORING

- Superficial ulcers—repeat fluorescein stain in 3–6 days; if it persists 7 days or longer, either inciting cause has not been eliminated or patient has an SCCED.
- Deep stromal or rapidly progressive ulcers—assess every 24 hours initially if outpatient until improvement is seen; many of these patients are hospitalized or undergo surgery; decrease frequency of antibiotic therapy as condition improves.

PREVENTION/AVOIDANCE

- Brachycephalic dogs—lubricant ointment administration, permanent partial tarsorrhaphy surgery, or both may prevent recurrent ulceration.
- KCS-related ulcers—lifelong treatment of KCS (cyclosporine) or parotid duct transposition surgery.
- Herpesvirus (cats)—oral lysine (250 mg PO q12h) may prevent viral replication; may decrease severity and/or frequency of outbreaks.

POSSIBLE COMPLICATIONS

Progressive corneal ulceration—rupture of globe, endophthalmitis, secondary glaucoma, phthisis bulbi, blindness, blind and painful eye (may require enucleation).

EXPECTED COURSE AND PROGNOSIS

- Uncomplicated superficial ulcer—usually heals in 5–7 days.
- SCCED—may persist for weeks to months; may require multiple procedures.
- Deep corneal ulcer treated medically—may require several weeks for fibrovascular repair of defect; does not always granulate satisfactorily; continued deterioration of ulcer and globe rupture are possible.
- Deep ulcer treated with conjunctival flap—frequently results in more comfort within a few days after surgery; blood supply to flap can be cut in 4–6 weeks to decrease scarring.

MISCELLANEOUS

Abbreviations

- IFA = immunofluorescent antibody test
- KCS = keratoconjunctivitis sicca.
- NSAID = nonsteroidal anti-inflammatory drug.
- SCCED = spontaneous chronic corneal epithelial defect.

Author/editor: Heidi Lobprise
Topic adapted from Five Minute Veterinary Consultation, 7th edition, 2021
Original Topic: Keratitis—Ulcerative

Author: Ellison Bentley
Consulting Editor: Kathern E. Myrna

Chapter 72

Keratoconjunctivitis Sicca

BASICS

OVERVIEW

- Deficiency of the aqueous layer of precorneal tear film.
- Causes corneal/conjunctival drying and resultant surface inflammation.

SIGNALMENT

- Common in dog; rare in cat.
- Predisposed dog breeds—many brachycephalic and spaniel breeds, miniature schnauzers, poodles, bloodhounds, Samoyeds, West Highland white terriers, and Yorkshire terriers.
- Inheritance—undefined.
- Age of onset—variable and depends on inciting cause but tends to intensify with age.

SIGNS

- Conjunctival hyperemia.
- Mucoid-to-mucopurulent ocular discharge—intermittent to persistent depending on severity.
- Blepharospasm.
- Corneal changes—dryness, superficial vascularization, pigmentation, fibrosis, ulceration.
- Blepharitis due to ocular exudates.
- Severe disease—impaired vision or blindness.
- Cats are less symptomatic than dogs.

CAUSES AND RISK FACTORS

- Immune-mediated/idiopathic—most common, possibly associated with other immune-mediated diseases (e.g., atopy).
- Infectious—canine distemper virus; leishmaniasis; chronic blepharoconjunctivitis (e.g., feline herpesvirus).
- Iatrogenic—removal of third eyelid gland (especially in at-risk breeds), radiation therapy.
- Congenital—Yorkshire terriers overrepresented.
- Neurologic—loss of parasympathetic innervation to lacrimal gland, trigeminal nerve deficit, or dysautonomia; neurogenic parasympathetic loss may have ipsilateral dry nose.

Blackwell's Five-Minute Veterinary Consult Clinical Companion: Small Animal Senior Care, First Edition. Edited by Heidi B. Lobprise.

Companion website: www.wiley.com/go/lobprise/Senior

- Traumatic—after ocular proptosis or orbit inflammation.
- Systemic disease—diabetes mellitus, hyperadrenocorticism, hypothyroidism, or any debilitating disease.
- Drug-induced—systemic sulfonamides (e.g., trimethoprim-sulfadiazine).
- Transient—general anesthesia and atropine.

DIAGNOSIS

DIFFERENTIAL DIAGNOSIS

- Often confused with allergic or bacterial conjunctivitis.
- Dogs with keratoconjunctivitis sicca (KCS) may have concurrent bacterial overgrowth.
- Differentiate with Schirmer tear test.

DIAGNOSTIC PROCEDURES

- Schirmer tear test—normal value at least 9 mm/min (cat) or 15 mm/min (dog) of wetting; symptomatic patients usually <10 mm/min of wetting; lower values combined with clinical signs suggest KCS.
- Fluorescein staining—may show corneal ulcers.
- Conjunctival cytology—may demonstrate bacterial overgrowth.

TREATMENT

- Outpatient—unless severe corneal ulceration.
- Instruct client to use solution(s) before ointment(s) and wait 5 minutes between treatments.
- Advise client to call at once if ocular pain increases (patients are predisposed to corneal ulceration).
- Parotid duct transposition—surgical option for dogs and cats that reroutes parotid duct to deliver saliva to ocular surface if KCS is refractory to lacrimostimulant therapy.
  - More common with congenital KCS.
  - Saliva can irritate cornea and result in mineral deposits; some patients require ongoing topical therapy.
- Episcleral cyclosporine implant—for dogs responsive to topical cyclosporine but with poor owner compliance.

MEDICATIONS

DRUG(S) OF CHOICE

- Lacrimostimulants—cyclosporine 0.2% ointment or 1–2% solution; tacrolimus 0.02–0.03% solution or ointment—therapy q12h recommended (q8h if severe or refractory).
- For neurogenic KCS—pilocarpine 0.1–0.2% topically q8h or very careful oral pilocarpine (narrow therapeutic window; see Suggested Reading).
- For feline KCS—antiviral therapy (see Conjunctivitis—Cats); hyaluronate-based artificial tear in short term; consider lacrimostimulant therapy.

- Lacrimomimetics—artificial tears to moisten ocular surface to improve comfort; use viscous solutions or gels q2–12h depending on severity and ointment before bedtime; can reduce frequency once patient responds to lacrimostimulants.
- Broad-spectrum antibiotics—topical ointment q6–8h for 3–4 weeks; indicated for secondary bacterial overgrowth or concurrent corneal ulceration.
- Ocular cleansing—use eye wash to remove discharge and debris prior to administering medications; if mucoid discharge is very tenacious, 5% *N*-acetylcysteine can be used q6–12h as a mucinolytic agent prior to eye rinsing.
- Corticosteroids—topical; minimize inflammation; can reduce corneal vascularization and pigmentation once aqueous tears improve; not commonly used (corneal ulcer risk).

CONTRAINDICATIONS/POSSIBLE INTERACTIONS

- Topical cyclosporine or tacrolimus—rarely irritating, but if noted consider compounded aqueous preparation.
- Pilocarpine—initially irritating topically; systemic side effect risk.
- Topical corticosteroids—avoid with ulcerative keratitis or severe KCS (corneal ulcer risk).

FOLLOW-UP

- Regular rechecks—monitor response and progress.
- Schirmer tear test—4–6 weeks after initiating cyclosporine or tacrolimus (patient should receive drug as prescribed on day of visit).
- Usually requires life-long treatment.
- Good prognosis but refractory cases may require more aggressive therapy (e.g., up to 1% tacrolimus) or surgery (e.g., parotid duct transposition).

MISCELLANEOUS

Abbreviations

- KCS = keratoconjunctivitis sicca

Suggested Reading

Leiva M, Gimenez TP. Diseases of the lacrimal system. In: Maggs DJ, Miller PE, Ofri R (eds) *Slatter's Fundamentals of Veterinary Ophthalmology*, 6th edn. St. Louis, MO: Elsevier, 2018; pp. 186–212.

Author/editor: Heidi Lobprise
Topic adapted from Five Minute Veterinary Consultation, 7th edition, 2021
Original Topic: Keratoconjunctivitis Sicca

Author: Rachel A. Allbaugh
Consulting Editor: Kathern E. Myrna

Chapter 73

Lens Luxation—Secondary

BASICS

OVERVIEW

- Lens luxation—total dislocation of lens from its normal location; occurs when lens capsule separates 360° from the zonules that hold lens in place.
- Anterior—forward displacement through the pupil into anterior chamber.
- Posterior—backward displacement into vitreous.
- Subluxation—partial separation of lens from its zonular attachments; lens remains in a normal or near-normal position in pupil.
- Secondary luxation—due to chronic inflammation, buphthalmia, intraocular neoplasia, senile zonular degeneration, or trauma.

SIGNALMENT

- Secondary—dog and cat; any age/breed.

SIGNS

- Fibrils of liquefied vitreous in anterior chamber.
- Abnormally shallow (anterior luxation) or deep anterior chamber (posterior luxation).
- Abnormal iris curvature secondary to tilting of lens.
- Phacodonesis (tremor of lens with globe movement).
- Iridodonesis (tremor of iris with globe movement).
- Aphakic crescent (crescent-shaped area of pupil lacking lens).
- Acute or chronic painful eye, episcleral injection, diffuse or central corneal edema.
- Glaucoma more common in anterior lens luxation but can be detected in any stage.
- Uveitis.
- Cataracts.
- Retinal detachment.

CAUSES AND RISK FACTORS

- Chronic uveitis.
- Intraocular neoplasia—secondary to physical luxation or chronic inflammation.

Blackwell's Five-Minute Veterinary Consult Clinical Companion: Small Animal Senior Care, First Edition. Edited by Heidi B. Lobprise.

Companion website: www.wiley.com/go/lobprise/Senior

- Trauma—rarely causes a normal lens to luxate without severe ocular injury.
- Cataracts—can cause tension and breakage of lens zonules.

DIAGNOSIS

DIFFERENTIAL DIAGNOSIS

- Uveitis, glaucoma—painful, red eyes with corneal edema; may be concurrent.
- Buphthalmia may cause lens luxation.
- Corneal endothelial dystrophy or degeneration may also cause corneal edema.
- Diagnosis made by careful ophthalmic examination and history.

CBC/BIOCHEMISTRY/URINALYSIS

Normal, unless systemic disease present.

IMAGING

- Thoracic radiographs, abdominal ultrasonography—may be indicated if intraocular neoplasia.
- Ocular ultrasonography—useful if corneal edema or cloudy ocular media preclude examination.

DIAGNOSTIC PROCEDURES

- Complete ophthalmic examination, including tonometry.
- Genetic test available for some predisposed breeds.

TREATMENT

- Potentially visual eyes—immediate referral to a veterinary ophthalmologist for possible intracapsular lens extraction is indicated.
- Manual trans-corneal reduction of anterior lens luxation and medical management of posterior luxation has been described.
- Topical miotic therapy may be used to keep a posteriorly luxated lens behind pupil and avoid surgery in some cases.
- Irreversibly blind eyes can be enucleated or eviscerated with intrascleral prosthesis; if secondary to neoplasia, enucleation is the best choice (therapeutic and diagnostic).

MEDICATIONS

DRUG(S) OF CHOICE

- Topical miotics—demecarium bromide or prostaglandin analogs (latanoprost) q12h indicated if the lens is primarily subluxated or posteriorly luxated.
- If the pupil is blocked due to anterior lens luxation, tropicamide may allow the pupil to dilate, releasing lens and decreasing risk for pupillary block glaucoma.
- Mannitol: 1 g/kg IV over 20 minutes indicated for intraocular pressure (IOP) >40 mmHg.

- Carbonic anhydrase inhibitors—topical dorzolamide q8h for high IOP.
- Topical anti-inflammatory—0.1% dexamethasone sodium phosphate or 1% prednisolone acetate (q6–24h) if inflammation present.

CONTRAINDICATIONS/POSSIBLE INTERACTIONS

- Topical miotics—contraindicated if lens in anterior chamber.
- Client must verify location of lens prior to applying a miotic
- Mannitol—contraindicated in patients with cardiac disease, dehydration, pulmonary edema, anuria, and intracranial bleeding.

FOLLOW-UP

- Medically treated primary posterior luxation—recheck IOP 24 hours after starting treatment and frequently thereafter; once IOP is stable, re-examine patient 3 or 4 times/year.
- Monitor for secondary glaucoma and retinal detachment.
- If only one lens is involved at the time of examination, the other lens may eventually luxate as well; the ophthalmologist may choose to perform prophylactic phacoemulsification in the contralateral eye if not yet luxated.

MISCELLANEOUS

Abbreviations

- IOP = intraocular pressure

Suggested Reading

Davidson MG, Nelms SR. Diseases of the lens and cataract formation. In: Gelatt KN (ed.) Veterinary Ophthalmology, 5th edn. Ames, IA: Wiley Blackwell, 2013, pp. 1199–1233.

Maggs DJ, Miller PE, Ofri R. Diseases of the lens. In: Slatter's Fundamentals of Veterinary Ophthalmology, 6th edn. St. Louis, MO: Saunders, 2018, pp. 306–333.

Author/editor: Heidi Lobprise
Topic adapted from Five Minute Veterinary Consultation, 7th edition, 2021
Original Topic: Lens Luxation—Secondary

Author: Renee T. Carter
Consulting Editor: Kathern E. Myrna

Chapter 74

Retinal Degeneration

BASICS

DEFINITION

- Degeneration of the retina from inherited or acquired causes.
- Inherited—generalized progressive retinal atrophy (PRA); a group of progressive retinal diseases.

PATHOPHYSIOLOGY

- A number of genetic defects in photoreceptor metabolism have been identified.
- May be secondary to retinal pigment epithelial or choroidal disease; amino acid metabolic disorders, and storage diseases.
- Central PRA: genetic defect in vitamin E metabolism, or acquired with vitamin E deficiency.
- May be idiopathic, secondary to diffuse or focal inflammation and scarring (e.g., chorioretinitis), toxin exposure, nutritional deficiency, or previous retinal detachment.
- Sudden acquired retinal degeneration syndrome (SARDS): idiopathic, may be immune-mediated retinitis.

SYSTEMS AFFECTED

- Nervous.
- Ophthalmic.

GENETICS

Dogs

- PRA—generally autosomal recessive, dominant in mastiffs.
- Inheritance in many breeds not determined.

Cats

- Early onset—mixed breed, Persians and Abyssinian.
- Late onset—Abyssinian rod-cone degeneration, autosomal recessive; PRA in many breeds including Siamese.

Blackwell's Five-Minute Veterinary Consult Clinical Companion: Small Animal Senior Care, First Edition. Edited by Heidi B. Lobprise.

Companion website: www.wiley.com/go/lobprise/Senior

INCIDENCE/PREVALENCE

- Hereditary—prevalence greater in dogs than cats.
- Taurine deficiency—uncommon with nutritionally complete cat foods.

SIGNALMENT

Species

Dog and cat.

Breed Predilections

Hereditary—Dogs (Senior Impact Variants)

- Late-onset PRA—miniature and toy poodle, American and English cocker spaniel, basenji, Labrador retriever, Tibetan terrier, dachshund, Akita, Samoyed, Siberian husky.
- SARDS—Brittany spaniel, miniature schnauzer, dachshund, others.

Hereditary—Cats

- Abyssinian, Somali, Persian; Siamese breed group.

Mean Age and Range

- Late PRA—clinical signs >4–6 years.
- SARDS—middle-aged to old.
- Older cats are often affected by systemic hypertension and may have retinal hemorrhage

Predominant Sex

- PRA—X-linked recessive condition in Siberian husky and Samoyed, therefore primarily males.
- SARDS—70% female.

SIGNS

Historical Findings

- PRA (dog)—gradually progressing nyctalopia that ultimately affects vision in bright light; may note dilated pupils or bright tapetal reflex; may appear acutely blind. Dysplasias have early onset and blindness by 2 years. Degenerations are later onset and blind in later life.
- SARDS—vision lost in 1–4 weeks; polyuria, polydipsia, and polyphagia common.

Physical Examination Findings

- If severe—direct and consensual pupillary light reflexes impaired or nearly abolished.
- Tapetal hyperreflectivity and nontapetal depigmentation or mottled hyperpigmentation; retinal blood vessel attenuation and optic nerve atrophy.
- PRA (dogs)—cataracts and vitreous degeneration can occur.
- SARDS (dogs)—obesity; may note slow or absent pupillary light reflexes (PLR). Chromatic PLR testing (melan 100), reduced or no red PLR, normal blue PLR.
- Borzoi chorioretinopathy—multifocal chorioretinal lesions (hyperpigmented and hyperreflective).
- Taurine-deficient retinopathy (cats)—begins as a spot in area centralis; then horizontal band forms superior to optic nerve; finally, diffuse degeneration and hyperreflectivity.
- Storage diseases—may have cloudy corneas and possibly neurologic signs.

CAUSES

Degenerative

- PRA—affects both eyes symmetrically.
- Chronic or uncontrolled glaucoma—retinal and optic nerve atrophy.
- Secondary to scarring from previous multifocal or diffuse retinal detachment or inflammation.

Metabolic

- Storage disease—mucopolysaccharidosis, gangliosidosis, mannosidosis, fucosidisis (English springer spaniel).
- Ornithine aminotransferase deficiency—progressive and total atrophy of choroid and retina; older cats.

Neoplastic

Neoplastic infiltrate may lead to scars from previous retinal detachment if treated.

Nutritional

- Severe deficiency of vitamin E or A (dogs and cats)—may cause partial or complete degeneration.
- Taurine deficiency (cats)—retinal degeneration, dilated cardiomyopathy.

Infectious/Immune

- Retina will degenerate from inflammation; may be focal, multifocal, or generalized. SARDS—some cases are immune-mediated retinitis.

Idiopathic

SARDS—dogs; post-inflammatory—dogs and cats.

Toxic

- Idiosyncratic reaction to griseofulvin or enrofloxacin (cats).
- Radiation—dogs or cats treated for nasal or CNS neoplasia.
- Phototoxicity—operating microscopes, welding light exposure.

RISK FACTORS

- Ocular disease—cataracts, panuveitis, chorioretinitis, retinal detachment, glaucoma.
- Cats—enrofloxacin dose should not exceed 5 mg/kg/day. Toxicity noted at lower doses in compromised animals (i.e., renal disease).

DIAGNOSIS

DIFFERENTIAL DIAGNOSIS

- Acute vision loss, PLR slow or absent—SARDS, optic neuritis, retinal detachment, unrecognized PRA, or glaucoma; PLR normal—rapidly developing diabetic cataracts or visual cortex disease.

- Slowly progressive visual loss—PRA, cataracts, severe corneal disease (e.g., pigmentation, scarring, or edema), chronic retinitis, chorioretinitis, vitreal inflammation.

CBC/BIOCHEMISTRY/URINALYSIS

- Usually normal, unless systemic disease.
- SARDS (dogs)—may suggest hyperadrenocorticism.

OTHER LABORATORY TESTS

- Test for hyperadrenocorticism, evaluate sex hormone levels, check blood pressure, evaluate for proteinuria with SARDS.
- Taurine concentration (cats)—especially with dilated cardiomyopathy.
- Serum and urine ornithine concentrations (cats)—elevated with ornithine aminotransferase deficiency.

IMAGING

- Thoracic radiographs and cardiac ultrasound—in cats with suspected taurine deficiency.
- CT or MRI—investigate causes of central blindness.

DIAGNOSTIC PROCEDURES

- Ophthalmic examination.
- Electroretinography—localizes cause of blindness when retina not visible or appears normal.
- Chromatic PLR (Melan 100)—differentiates outer retinal layer problems (red reduced) vs. inner retina layers (absent blue). Definitive diagnosis requires electroretinogram as interpretation can be confounded by iris atrophy and stress-induced mydriasis.
- Cerebrospinal fluid tap—for cases of suspected optic neuritis.

PATHOLOGIC FINDINGS

- Thin retina.
- Edges of focal retinal scars—sharply delineated.
- Hyperpigmented areas—associated with postinflammatory scars or central PRA.
- End-stage degenerations—marked photoreceptor atrophy and reduction in retinal cell density.
- Lysosome storage diseases—accumulation in neuronal/retinal layers/cornea.

TREATMENT

DIET

- Cats—food should contain 500–750 ppm taurine.
- Dogs—balanced diet, avoid those high in polyunsaturated fats.

CLIENT EDUCATION

- Most blind animals function well in stable environment.
- Blind dogs should be supervised if outside, in unfenced yards, or in an area with a pool.
- Suggest playing with toys that make sounds.
- Older blind animals with hearing loss or senility may not adapt well.
- Some blind animals experience behavioral changes such as aggression or reduced activity.
- Animals with only one blind eye can function normally.
- Blind cats should be kept indoors.

SURGICAL CONSIDERATIONS

Not indicated unless painful.

MEDICATIONS

DRUG(S) OF CHOICE

- None currently effective.
- Pyridoxine—for ornithine aminotransferase deficiency (cats).
- Adequate dietary taurine—halt progression of taurine-deficient retinopathy.
- SARDS—if autoimmune retinitis, immune suppressive treatment may preserve/restore some vision.

GENE THERAPY

Experimental—retinal pigment epithelium dystrophy in briard.

PRECAUTIONS

Cataract surgery—not recommended if retinal degeneration is severe; perform preoperative electroretinogram.

FOLLOW-UP

PATIENT MONITORING

- Serial fundic examinations—signs of degeneration over weeks with SARDS; months with PRA.
- Cataract formation—with PRA or SARDS.

PREVENTION/AVOIDANCE

- Do not breed known or suspected carriers of PRA or other heritable diseases.
- Genetic testing on breeding animals.

POSSIBLE COMPLICATIONS

- Cataracts.
- Glaucoma.
- Uveitis.
- Ocular trauma (result of visual impairment).
- Obesity (reduced activity).

EXPECTED COURSE AND PROGNOSIS

- Inherited PRA—progresses to blindness; slow progression allows patient to adapt to visual loss.
- Degeneration from inflammation—usually does not progress unless persistent or recurrent inflammation.
- SARDS—irreversible blindness.
- Taurine deficiency (cats)—degeneration may halt at any stage.

MISCELLANEOUS

Associated Conditions

SARDS—hyperadrenocorticism, proteinuria, hypertension, elevated sex hormones.

Abbreviations

- PLR = pupillary light reflex
- PRA = progressive retinal atrophy.
- SARDS = sudden acquired retinal degeneration syndrome.

Suggested Reading

Narfström K, Petersen-Jones S. Diseases of the canine ocular fundus. In: Gelatt KN, Gilger BC Kern TJ (eds) *Veterinary Ophthalmology*, 5th edn. Ames, IA: Blackwell, 2013; pp. 2087–2235.

Author/editor: Heidi Lobprise
Topic adapted from Five Minute Veterinary Consultation, 7th edition, 2021
Original Topic: Retinal Degeneration

Author: Patricia J. Smith
Consulting Editor: Kathern E. Myrna

Chapter 75

Retinal Detachment

BASICS

DEFINITION

Separation of the neural retina from the retinal pigment epithelium (RPE).

PATHOPHYSIOLOGY

- Subretinal space—a potential space between RPE and neural retina in which fluid or exudates accumulate.
- Etiopathogenesis is one or a combination of rhegmatogenous (retinal tear), subretinal exudation, or traction.

Rhegmatogenous Retinal Detachment (RRD)

A tear or hole in retina related to age, cataracts, traction from inflammatory debris or vitreal degeneration, trauma, or retinal degeneration. Vitreous fluid moves into the subretinal space, resulting in detachment. Probably the predominant type occurring in association with cataracts and after cataract or lens surgery.

Exudative

- Fluid accumulates in the subretinal space because of breakdown of blood–retinal barrier.
- Subretinal fluid—serous, hemorrhagic, or exudative.
- Hematogenous/systemic pathogenetic factors—common.
- Vasculitis, hypertension, and hyperviscosity—may cause serous detachment with or without hemorrhage.

Traction

- Fibrous or fibrovascular tissue; detaches retina and/or may cause retinal tear.
- Associated with trauma, intraocular foreign bodies, or any cause of severe vitreal inflammation.

SYSTEMS AFFECTED

- Nervous.
- Ophthalmic.
- May be manifestation of systemic disease or neoplasia.

Blackwell's Five-Minute Veterinary Consult Clinical Companion: Small Animal Senior Care, First Edition. Edited by Heidi B. Lobprise.

Companion website: www.wiley.com/go/lobprise/Senior

GENETICS

- Depends on cause—dogs with hereditary cataracts or lens luxation may develop RRD.
- Some breeds may develop RRD from primary vitreous abnormalities (shih tzu), colobomas of optic nerve (collie), or severe retinal dysplasia inducing retinal tears or traction.

INCIDENCE/PREVALENCE

- Exudative—most common in dogs and cats.
- RRD—uncommon. More common in dogs because of the greater prevalence of severe vitreal degeneration, cataracts, and cataract surgery.

GEOGRAPHIC DISTRIBUTION

Varies with the distribution of infectious etiologies.

SIGNALMENT

Species

Dog and cat.

Breed Predilections

- Depends on cause.
- Terrier breeds—predisposed to primary lens luxation, may contribute to RRD.
- Breeds that develop cataracts.
- Shih-tzu, Boston terrier, Italian greyhound, Chihuahua, corgi—predisposed to spontaneous RRD owing to abnormal liquefied vitreous.
- Dogs with merle coat color (Australian shepherd dog, Shetland sheepdog, Great Dane, collie) may have severe retinal dysplasia and optic nerve or scleral colobomas, leading to RRD.
- Breeds with severe retinal dysplasia: English springer spaniel, Labrador retriever, Bedlington terrier.
- Breeds with serous retinopathy (also known as RPE dysplasia, canine multifocal retinopathy): Great Pyrenees, mastiff, coton de Tulear.

Mean Age and Range

- Depends on cause.
- Older patients—cataracts and systemic diseases (e.g., hypertension, neoplasia, immune-mediated disease).

SIGNS

- Blindness or reduced vision in affected eye.
- Dilated pupil with slow or no pupillary light response (PLR). PLR may be near normal if detachment is acute.
- Blood vessels or a "membrane" may be observed easily through the pupil just behind the lens.
- Vitreous abnormalities—floaters, hemorrhage, or syneresis (liquefaction); common.
- Interruption or alteration of course of blood vessels due to retinal elevation.

- With clear subretinal fluid—vessels may cast shadows.
- With exudative fluid or blood, tapetum/RPE may not be visible.
- Other signs related to underlying systemic disease or inflammation (see Chorioretinitis)

CAUSES

Bilateral—suggests a systemic problem, except in breeds with a predisposition to severe vitreal degeneration (e.g., shih tzu).

Degenerative

End-stage progressive retinal degeneration—may lead to RRD if retina tears.

Anomalous

- Colobomas—collie eye anomaly; abnormal retina around colobomatous optic nerve or large choroidal staphylomas may lead to RRD (merle ocular dysgenesis).
- Severe retinal dysplasia, or oculoskeletal dysplasia (Labrador retrievers, Samoyeds).
- Multiple ocular anomalies.

Metabolic

- Hyperviscosity (e.g., due to hyperproteinemia from multiple myeloma or other causes).
- Polycythemia.
- Shock.
- Dogs—systemic hypertension, hypothyroidism, hypercholesterolemia.
- Cats—systemic hypertension (usually related to hyperthyroidism, chronic renal disease).

Neoplastic

- Primary or metastatic.
- Multiple myeloma, lymphoma, and intraocular masses (e.g., ciliary body adenocarcinoma or melanoma).
- Pheochromocytoma may cause hypertension.

Infectious

- Infectious retinitis or chorioretinitis may cause focal or diffuse detachment. • Infection may extend from or to the CNS.

Immune-Mediated/Inflammatory

- Immune complex disease—vasculitis or inflammation can result in exudative detachment:
    - Dogs—systemic lupus erythematosus (SLE); uveodermatologic syndrome, meningoencephalitis of unknown etiology.
    - Cats—periarteritis nodosa; SLE.

Idiopathic

- If all other causes are ruled out, including retinal tears.
- Idiopathic steroid-responsive detachment—reported in giant-breed dogs; may occur in any breed.

Trauma and Toxic

- Penetrating injury or foreign body.
- Severe blunt trauma with inflammation or hemorrhage, usually unilateral.

- Surgical trauma—if lens or vitreous disturbed (e.g., cataract surgery), can lead to RRD.
- Toxic—drug reactions (e.g., trimethoprim-sulfa, ethyelene glycol, griseofulvin [cats]).

RISK FACTORS

- Systemic hypertension.
- Old age—retinal thinning, severe vitreal degeneration.
- Hypermature, intumescent cataracts that may rupture (e.g., diabetic cataracts).
- Luxated lenses.
- Lens extraction.

DIAGNOSIS

DIFFERENTIAL DIAGNOSIS

- Blindness or impaired vision—optic neuritis, glaucoma, cataracts, progressive retinal atrophy, sudden acquired retinal degeneration syndrome (SARDS; see Retinal Degeneration), CNS disease.
- Dilated pupil with slow or absent pupillary light reflexes—glaucoma, oculomotor nerve lesion, optic neuritis, progressive retinal atrophy, SARDS.
- Membrane or vessels associated with or behind lens—persistent tunica vasculosa lentis, persistent pupillary membranes, fibrovascular membrane due to intraocular neoplasia or inflammation.

CBC/BIOCHEMISTRY/URINALYSIS

Typically normal, unless systemic disease present.

OTHER LABORATORY TESTS

- Depends on suspected systemic problem.
- Protein electrophoresis or documentation of Bence Jones proteinuria.
- Coagulation profile.
- Bacterial culture of ocular or body fluids.
- Thyroid hormone measurement.
- Serologic or PCR testing for infectious diseases.

IMAGING

- Thoracic and abdominal radiographs, ultrasound, and/or CT.
- Spinal radiographs may reveal bony changes consistent with multiple myeloma.
- Ocular ultrasound—if ocular media is opaque, can identify retinal detachments or intraocular masses.

DIAGNOSTIC PROCEDURES

- Ophthalmic examination.
- Serial blood pressure measurement—normal systolic arterial pressure <160 mmHg.
- Cerebral spinal fluid tap—indicated if CNS disease or optic neuritis.

- Vitreocentesis or subretinal fluid aspirate—if other testing fails to determine cause and infection or neoplasia is suspected; may aggravate inflammation or induce hemorrhage.

TREATMENT

APPROPRIATE HEALTH CARE

- Usually outpatient; depends on condition of patient.
- Vision may be restored if underlying cause is rapidly identified and treated, but degeneration occurs quickly.

CLIENT EDUCATION

- May be a sign of systemic disease.
- If associated with vitreal degeneration, lens luxation, or cataract surgery, fellow eye at risk for same condition.
- Blind pets can adapt remarkably well and live a good-quality life.

SURGICAL CONSIDERATIONS

- RRD—may be surgically repaired by an ophthalmologist.
- Laser retinopexy—may reverse detachments associated with optic disc colobomas; may stabilize partial/small detachments. May prevent detachment in predisposed fellow eye.

MEDICATIONS

DRUG(S) OF CHOICE

- Depends on underlying systemic cause.
- Prednisone for immunosuppression (for immune-mediated causes) 2–4 mg/kg PO, divided q12 for 3–10 days (dog, cat), then taper slowly over months (do not exceed 80 mg/day). Rule out systemic mycosis prior to use; may facilitate retinal reattachment.
- Corticosteroids at anti-inflammatory doses—prednisone 0.5–1 mg/kg PO q24h (dog), prednisolone 1–2 mg/kg PO q24h (cat), then taper; may be useful for exudative detachments of an infectious nature as long as the underlying disease is being definitively treated.
- Antihypertensive agents—amlodipine 0.1–0.5 mg/kg PO q12–24h (dog); 0.625–1.25 mg/cat PO q12–24h (cat). Consult with internist or cardiologist if persistent hypertension.

CONTRAINDICATIONS

Systemic corticosteroids—do not use unless systemic mycosis is ruled out or is being definitively treated.

ALTERNATIVE DRUG(S)

Adjunctive immunosuppressive therapy (azathioprine, cyclosporine, mycophenolate, leflunomide) may be needed in some immune-mediated retinal detachment if prednisone is not effective or tolerated long term.

FOLLOW-UP

PATIENT MONITORING

- Some immunosuppressive therapy (e.g., azathioprine) requires regular CBC and serum biochemistry analysis to monitor for bone marrow suppression or hepatotoxicity.
- Serial blood pressure monitoring in hypertensive patients.

POSSIBLE COMPLICATIONS

- Permanent blindness.
- Cataracts.
- Glaucoma—if eye becomes blind and painful enucleation may be necessary.
- Chronic ocular pain.
- Death secondary to systemic disease/neoplastic process.

EXPECTED COURSE AND PROGNOSIS

- Prognosis for vision with complete detachment—guarded. Exception is hypertensive retinopathy that is diagnosed and treated promptly.
- Surgical reattachment of retina is about 72% successful at restoring vision for up to 1.5 years.
- Vision may return if underlying cause is removed and reattachment occurs.
- Blindness—may develop in days to weeks even with reattachment (more likely and rapid with exudative than serous detachments).

MISCELLANEOUS

Associated Conditions

- Cataracts.
- Trauma.
- Vitreous abnormalities.
- Primary neurologic disease or systemic disease affecting CNS.

Abbreviations

- PLR = pupillary light reflex
- RPE = retinal pigment epithelium.
- RRD = rhegmatogenous retinal detachment.
- SARDS = sudden acquired retinal degeneration syndrome.
- SLE = systemic lupus erythematosus.

Suggested Reading

Maggs DJ, Miller PE, Ofri R. *Slatter's Fundamentals of Veterinary Ophthalmology*, 5th edn. St. Louis, MO: Saunders, 2013.

Author/editor: Heidi Lobprise
Topic adapted from Five Minute Veterinary Consultation, 7th edition, 2021
Original Topic: Retinal Detachment

Author: Patricia J. Smith
Consulting Editor: Kathern E. Myrna

Renal

Chapter 76

Chronic Kidney Disease

BASICS

DEFINITION

Chronic kidney disease (CKD)

- Functional or structural lesions (in one or both kidneys).
- Detected by blood or urine tests, imaging studies, or kidney biopsy.
- Present for >3 months.
- IRIS CKD stages 1–4
    - Based on >2 serum creatinine values obtained over several weeks when the patient is fasted and well hydrated.
- Azotemia is an excess of urea, creatinine, or other nonprotein nitrogenous substances in blood, plasma, or serum.
- Uremia is the polysystemic toxic syndrome resulting from marked loss in kidney functions. Uremia occurs simultaneously in animals with increased quantities of urine constituents in blood (azotemia), but azotemia may occur in the absence of uremia.

PATHOPHYSIOLOGY

- With more than ~67–75% reduction in renal function, impaired urine-concentrating ability leads to polyuria/polydipsia (PU/PD) and retention of nitrogenous waste products of protein catabolism (azotemia).
- CKD is progressive; more advanced CKD results in uremia.
- Decreased renal erythropoietin and calcitriol production results in hypoproliferative anemia and renal secondary hyperparathyroidism, respectively.

SYSTEMS AFFECTED

- Cardiovascular—hypertension; uremic pericarditis.
- Endocrine/metabolic—renal secondary hyperparathyroidism, activation of renin–angiotensin–aldosterone system, erythropoietin deficiency.
- Gastrointestinal—uremic stomatitis and halitosis, nausea, vomiting, anorexia, gastrointestinal bleeding, diarrhea.
- Hemic/lymphatic/immune—anemia; hemorrhagic diathesis.

Blackwell's Five-Minute Veterinary Consult Clinical Companion: Small Animal Senior Care, First Edition. Edited by Heidi B. Lobprise.

Companion website: www.wiley.com/go/lobprise/Senior

INCIDENCE/PREVALENCE

- 9 cases per 1000 dogs and 16 cases per 1000 cats examined.
- Prevalence increases with age—age >15 years, reportedly 57 cases per 1000 dogs and 153 cases per 1000 cats examined.

Mean Age and Range

Mean age at diagnosis is 7 years in dogs and 9 years in cats. Animals of any age can be affected; prevalence increases with age.

SIGNS

General Comments

- Clinical signs related to stage of CKD and complications such as proteinuria and hypertension.
- CKD stages 1 and 2 may be asymptomatic; overt clinical signs typically become apparent in stages 3 and 4.
- Animals with stable CKD (particularly stages 3 and 4) may decompensate, resulting in uremic crisis.

Historical Findings

- PU/PD.
- Polyuria—increased frequency and volume of urine >2 mL/kg/h and urine specific gravity <1.025.
- Anorexia; weight loss.
- Lethargy.
- Vomiting; constipation or diarrhea
- Nocturia.
- Acute blindness.
- Seizures or coma.
- Cats may have ptyalism and muscle weakness with cervical ventroflexion.

Physical Examination Findings

- Kidneys may be small, irregular, enlarged (secondary to polycystic kidney disease or lymphoma), or normal in size.
- Dehydration.
- Cachexia.
- Weakness.
- Pale mucous membranes, oral ulceration and/or uremic halitosis
- Hypertensive retinopathy.
- Renal osteodystrophy may manifest as bone pain, particularly in skull.
- Reduced body temperature with uremia.

CAUSES

- Unknown in most cases due to late diagnosis.
- Familial and congenital renal disease, nephrotoxins, hypercalcemia, hypokalemic nephropathy, glomerulopathies, amyloidosis, pyelonephritis, polycystic kidney disease, nephroliths, chronic urinary obstruction, drugs, lymphoma, leptospirosis (following acute kidney injury [AKI]), feline infectious peritonitis.

RISK FACTORS

Age, proteinuria, hypercalcemia, hypokalemia, hypertension, urinary tract infection (UTI).

DIAGNOSIS

DIFFERENTIAL DIAGNOSIS

- Polyuria and Polydipsia—multiple differential diagnosis.
- Azotemia
  - Prerenal azotemia—azotemia with urine specific gravity (USG) >1.030 in dogs and >1.035 in cats; rapid reduction in azotemia after correcting hypoperfusion; commonly occurs with primary renal azotemia when gastrointestinal signs of uremia are present.
  - Postrenal azotemia—obstruction or rupture of excretory system; rapid correction of azotemia following elimination of obstruction or resolution of leakage from urinary tract.
- AKI (see below)—differentiated by normal-to-large renal size, cylindruria, lack of indications of chronicity, and history of recent nephrotoxin exposure or hypotensive episode; AKI can also occur in patients with CKD where rapid developing increase in serum creatinine concentration and uremic signs suggests acute-on-chronic CKD.
- Glomerulonephritis (see below)—immune-mediated, more in middle-aged dogs.

CBC/BIOCHEMISTRY/URINALYSIS

- Hypoproliferative anemia.
- High blood urea nitrogen (BUN), creatinine, and symmetric dimethylarginine (SDMA).
- With marked muscle loss, base staging on SDMA, as creatinine may decrease

IRIS	Stage 1	Stage 2	Stage 3	Stage 4
Creatinine dog (mg/dL)	<1.4	1.4–2.8	2.9–5.0	>5.0
Creatinine cat (mg/dL)	<1.6	1.6–2.8	2.9–5.0	>5.0
SDMA (μg/dL) dog	<18	18–35	36–54	>54
SDMA (μg/dL) cat	<18	18–25	26–38	>38

- UPC Ratio—substage
  - Nonproteinuric < 0.2 (dog and cat)
  - Borderline proteinuric 0.2–0.5 (dog and cat)
  - Proteinuric >0.5 (dog): >0.4 (cat)
- Systolic blood pressure (mm Hg)—substage—dog and cat
  - Normotensive <140
  - Prehypertensive 140–159
  - Hypertensive 160–179
  - Severely hypertensive ≥180
- Hyperphosphatemia.
  - Metabolic acidosis (normal or high anion gap).
  - Hypokalemia or hyperkalemia.

- Hypercalcemia or hypocalcemia.
- USG <1.030 in dogs and <1.035 in cats, in the presence of azotemia.
- Proteinuria. To Diagnose Stage 1 and early Stage 2 (one or more of these) (IRIS)
  - Creatinine or SDMA increasing with no prerenal cause apparent
  - Persistently elevated SDMA >14 µg/dL—monitor closely
  - Abnormal kidney imaging
  - Persistent renal proteinuria
    - UPC >0.5 in dogs
    - UPC >0.4 in cats

OTHER LABORATORY TESTS

Urinary protein: creatinine ratio to assess proteinuria.

- FGF-23 (fibroblast growth factor)—in cats
  - Measure in IRIS CDK stages 1 and 2 with serum phosphorous <4.6 mg/dL (not later stages).
  - Delineate which cats would potentially benefit from phosphate reduction therapy and decrease risk of hypercalcemia when renal diets are introduced.
  - Can identify mineral disruption and phosphorus overload earlier than total serum phosphorous elevations.

IMAGING

- Abdominal radiographs may demonstrate small kidneys, or large kidneys secondary to polycystic kidney disease, uroliths, or lymphoma.
- Ultrasound demonstrates small kidneys and hyperechoic renal parenchyma with less apparent distinction between cortex and medulla in some animals. Animals with lymphoma often have renomegaly with hypoechoic renal parenchyma.

DIAGNOSTIC PROCEDURES

- Blood pressure measurement to detect hypertension.
- Measurement of glomerular filtration rate may be useful for detection of loss of kidney function before onset of azotemia.
- Renal biopsy may be indicated in proteinuric patients with normal to large kidneys.

TREATMENT

APPROPRIATE HEALTH CARE

Patients with compensated CKD may be managed as outpatients; patients in uremic crisis should be managed as inpatients.

NURSING CARE

- Uremic crisis
  - Correct fluid and electrolyte deficits with IV fluids, providing 25% of calculated fluid deficit in first hour;
  - Then, serially monitor perfusion, blood pressure, and urine output to assess adequacy of fluid therapy.

- If perfusion not improved, additional fluid should cautiously be administered.
- Provide remaining fluid deficit over next 12–24 hours.
- Overhydration can result in anuria; once patient has been hydrated, only sufficient fluid to sustain hydration should be administered.

- Subcutaneous fluid therapy may benefit patients with moderate to severe CKD. Continue therapy only if clinical improvement noted.

ACTIVITY

Unrestricted

DIET

- Diets designed for CKD delay onset of uremic crisis and extend survival in dogs and cats with CKD stages 2–4; they are standard of care for these patients.
    - Consider starting them prior to periods of inappetence.
- Important components of renal foods—reduced protein, phosphorus, sodium, and net acid content, supplementation of n-3 fatty acids and antioxidants.
    - AST-120 (Azodyl)—oral adsorbent to reduce uptake of uremic toxins.
- Free access to fresh water.
    - Nutrient-enriched water to promote adequate fluid intake (Hydracare)
- Feeding tube may be needed in Stage 4 patients for feeding, fluids and medications.

CLIENT EDUCATION

- CKD typically progresses to terminal kidney failure over months to years, but may not be progressive in some cats, which may live for years.
- Higher levels of proteinuria associated with shorter survival; may be mitigated by anti-proteinuria therapy.
- Heritability of familial renal diseases.

SURGICAL CONSIDERATIONS

- Avoid hypotension during anesthesia.
- Renal transplantation has been successfully performed in cats with CKD; controversial due to ethical issues.

MEDICATIONS

DRUG(S) OF CHOICE

Uremic Crisis

- Antiemetics (maropitant 1 mg/kg q24h; or ondansetron 0.2–1 mg/kg IV q12h) to minimize vomiting and hyporexia due to nausea.
- Potassium chloride in IV fluids or potassium gluconate PO (2–6 mEq/cat/day) as needed to correct hypokalemia.

- Stage 2–4 hypokalemia in cats
- Sodium bicarbonate to correct metabolic acidosis (IV to raise blood pH >7.1).
    - Stage 3 and 4

Compensated CKD

- Antiemetic (maropitant) and potassium gluconate as above.
- Appetite stimulants (Stages 2–4)
    - Mirtazapine (cats, 1.88 mg PO q 24–48h) to promote appetite.
    - Capromelin—ghrelin receptor agonist (dog and cat)
- Intestinal phosphate binders as needed to correct hyperphosphatemia if renal diet not sufficient:
    - Aluminum hydroxide, aluminum carbonate, calcium carbonate, calcium acetate, lanthanum carbonate; 30–60 mg/kg/day in divided doses in meal, to effect
    - Monitor for aluminum toxicity (muscle weakness and neurological signs) in dogs
    - Keep below 4.6 mg/dL (Stages 1 and 2); 5.0 mg/dL (Stage 3); 6.0 mg/dL (Stage 4)
- Anemia (PCV <20) (Stages 3 and 4)
    - Darbepoetin less antigenic than epoetin alfa; anabolic steroids may be detrimental.
    - Conditional approval—molidustat—increase erythropoetin.
- Hypertension
    - Amlodipine (dogs, 0.1–0.6 mg/kg PO q24h; cats, 0.625–1.25 mg/cat PO q24h)
        - IRIS 0.12–0.25 mg/kg or
    - Angiotensin-converting enzyme (ACE) inhibitors (0.5 mg/kg PO q24h) or
    - Angiotensin receptor blockers (ARB; e.g., telmisartan 1–3 mg/kg PO q24h) as needed for hypertension
    - Amlodipine and telmisartan are more effective than ACE inhibitors for CKD-induced hypertension
    - If refractory to monotherapy, consider combination of amlodipine and ACE inhibitor or ARB, with frequent monitoring of blood pressure and electrolytes
        - IRIS—increase amlodipine to 0.25–0.5 mg/kg if used with telmisartan
- Proteinuria
    - ACE inhibitor (start at 0.5 mg/kg PO q24h; increase to 1 mg/kg PO q12h) or ARB (telmisartan 1–3 mg/kg PO q24h) for proteinuria.
    - Thromboembolic therapy if needed: clopidogrel (10–18.75 mg/day).
    - Appropriate maintenance fluids parenterally as needed to maintain hydration (Stages 3 and 4).

CONTRAINDICATIONS

- Avoid nephrotoxic drugs (aminoglycosides, cisplatin, amphotericin B), NSAIDs, and corticosteroids.
    - Long-term treatment of cats with oral meloxicam did not appear to reduce the lifespan of cats with pre-existent stable CKD.
- RAAS inhibitor should not be used in dehydrated or hypovolemic cats.

PRECAUTIONS

- Drug dosage or dosing interval may need to be modified for some drugs eliminated by the kidneys.
- Use ACE inhibitors and ARB cautiously; monitor for worsening of azotemia,
- Generally avoid nonsteroidal anti-inflammatory drugs.

POSSIBLE INTERACTIONS

Cimetidine or trimethoprim may cause artifactual increases in serum creatinine concentration by reducing tubular secretion in dogs with CKD.

ALTERNATIVE DRUG(S)

- Hemodialysis units are available at selected referral hospitals.

FOLLOW-UP

PATIENT MONITORING

- Monitor at regular intervals; initially weekly for patients receiving erythropoietin; every 1–3 months for stable patients with CKD stages 3 and 4.
- Proteinuric patients—monitor at least every 3–4 months (minimum: serum creatinine and urine protein: creatine ratio).

PREVENTION/AVOIDANCE

- Do not breed animals with familial renal disease.
- Include urinalysis and serum creatinine in yearly examination for older pets; if serum creatinine is elevated (even within the normal range, but trending upward), increase frequency to every 4–6 months.

POSSIBLE COMPLICATIONS

- Systemic hypertension.
- Uremia.
- Anemia.
- UTI.
- Nephroureterolithiasis.

EXPECTED COURSE AND PROGNOSIS

- Short term—depends on severity.
- Long term—guarded to poor in dogs (CKD tends to be progressive over months to years); poor to good in cats, some with slower progression.

MISCELLANEOUS

Acute Kidney Injury (AKI)

- IRIS—grades represent a moment in the course of the disease and often changes
  - Grade I—<1.6 mg/dL; <140 μmol/L creatinine
    - Progressive nonazotemic increase in blood creatinine: >0.3 mg/dL; 26.4 μmol/L within 48 hours
    - Measured oliguria (<1 mL/kg/h) or anuria over 6 hours
    - Urine volume is readily fluid-volume responsive
  - Grade II—1.7–2.5 mg/dL; 141–220 μmol/L creatinine
    - Progressive azotemic increase in blood creatinine: >0.3 mg/dL; 26.4 μmol/L within 48 hours
    - Measured oliguria (<1 mL/kg/h) or anuria over 6 hours
    - Urine volume is readily fluid-volume responsive
  - Grade III—2.6–5.0 mg/dL; 221–439 μmol/L creatinine
  - Grade IV—5.1–10.0 mg/dL; 440–880 μmol/L creatinine
  - Grade V—>10.0 mg/dL; >880 μmol/L creatinine
  - Grades III, IV, and V are also subgraded:
    - Urine production
      - O—oliguic; <1 mL/kg/h
      - A—anuric; no urine produced
      - NO—nonoliguric; >1 mL/kg/h
    - Requirement for renal replacement therapy—established on the need to correct life-threatening consequences
- Patients with (CKD) are very predisposed to the development of clinical AKI.
  - 6–8 years of age peak prevalence.
  - Older animals at greater risk due to decreased renal reserve (AKI on CKD).
- Sudden onset—anorexia, listlessness, depression, V/d
- Causes—lepto, toxins, ureteral obstruction (cat)
  - Hemodynamic—hypoperfusion, shock trauma
  - Nephrotoxic—grapes, raisin, ethylene glycol, medications (NSAIDs, aminoglycoside antibiotics)
  - Leptospirosis, pancreatitis, pyelonephritis, lymphoma.
- Prerenal, intrinsic renal, or postrenal
- Differential diagnoses
  - Prerenal azotemia—oliguria correctible with fluids
  - Postrenal azotemia—stranguria, obstruction
- Diagnostics—monitor urine output and creatinine levels during therapy
- Treatment—eliminate causes, correct fluids, diet,
  - Continuous renal replacement therapy (CRRT)
    - Dialysis not available at many facilities, peritoneal dialysis possible
  - Avoid overhydration;
  - Manage acid–base disorders—bicarbonate replacement
  - Manage hyperkalemia—loop diuretics; dextrose ± insulin
  - Manage vomiting
- Outcome assessment
  - Patients with grades I and II AKI may regain renal function within 2–5 days
  - Patients with higher AKI grades or those with progression may require weeks of supportive care before the onset of renal repair.

- Patients with severe AKI (grades IV and V) may die within 5–10 days despite appropriate conventional management unless supported with RRT for an indefinite time.

- Anticipate AKI in aged patients or those with systemic disease, sepsis, trauma, hemodynamic instability, receiving nephrotoxic drugs, multiple organ failure, or undergoing prolonged anesthesia, particularly with hypotension.

Glomerulonephritis

- Glomerulonephritis—immune complex (ICGN): immune-mediated inflammation in the glomerulus with antigens or antigen–antibody complexes (due to infection such as Lyme disease or inflammation) entrapped within the glomerular basement membrane.
    - Proteinuria as initial symptom
    - Middle-age range but can occur at any time
    - Can progress to chronic renal failure
    - Requires immunosuppressive therapy

Associated Conditions

- Renal secondary hyperparathyroidism.
- Systemic hypertension.
- Nephroureterolithiasis.

Age-Related Factors

Renal function may decrease with aging.

Abbreviations

- ACE = angiotensin-converting enzyme
- AKI = acute kidney injury.
- ARB = angiotensin receptor blocker.
- BUN = blood urea nitrogen.
- CKD = chronic kidney disease.
- PU/PD = polyuria/polydipsia.
- RRT = renal replacement therapy
- SDMA = symmetric dimethylarginine.
- USG = urine-specific gravity.
- UTI = urinary tract infection.

Internet Resources

Accessed 29 June 2024

- www.iris-kidney.com

Suggested Reading

Polzin DJ. Chronic kidney disease. In: Ettinger SJ, Feldman EC (eds) *Textbook of Veterinary Internal Medicine*, 7th edn. St. Louis, MO: Elsevier, 2010; pp. 1990–2021.

Ross SJ, Polzin DJ, Osborne CA. Clinical progression of early chronic renal failure and implications for management. In: August JR (ed.) *Consultations in Feline Internal Medicine*. St. Louis, MO: Elsevier, 2006; pp. 389–398.

Gowan RA, Baral RM, Lingard AE, Catt MJ, Stansen W, Johnston L, Malik R. A retrospective study of the effects of meloxicam on the longevity of aged cats with and without overt chronic kidney disease. *J Fel Med Surg* 2012;14(12):876–881.

Chen H, Klainbart S, Kelmer E, Segev G. Continuous renal replacement therapy is a safe and effective modality for the initial management of dogs with acute kidney injury. *J Am Vet Med Assoc* 2022;261(1):87–96. doi: 10.2460/javma.22.07.0294. PMID: 36288204.

Author/editor: Heidi Lobprise
Thanks to: Elizabeth Settles for review
Topic adapted from Five Minute Veterinary Consultation, 7th edition, 2021
Original Topic: Chronic Kidney Disease

Author: David J. Polzin
Consulting Editor: J.D. Foster

Chapter 77

Lower Urinary Tract Infection and Pyelonephritis, Bacterial

BASICS

DEFINITION

- Urinary tract infection (lower) LUTI—bacterial adherence, replication, and persistence within the urinary tract associated with clinical signs and/or inflammation.
- Pyelonephritis—microbial colonization of the upper urinary tract, including the renal pelvis, collecting diverticula, renal parenchyma, and ureters.

PATHOPHYSIOLOGY

- UTI development is dependent on the interplay between bacterial virulence factors and impairment of the anatomical, functional, environmental, and immunologic competency of the host. Most commonly, uropathogenic bacteria originate from the enteric flora and ascend from the distal urogenital tract into the proximal urethra and urinary bladder. Colonization may elicit a mucosal inflammatory response resulting in dysuria, pollakiuria, pyuria, and hematuria.
- Pyelonephritis usually occurs by ascension of microbes causing lower UTI, though it can develop secondarily to infected nephroliths.
    - Obstruction of an infected kidney or ureter can rapidly cause septicemia (urosepsis).

INCIDENCE/PREVALENCE

- Bacteriuria is not equivalent to UTI. Current data identifies UTI prevalence given predisposing conditions.
- Prevalence of bacteriuria in dogs:
    - With subclinical bacteriuria: 2.1–8.9%.
    - With diabetes mellitus: 37%.
    - With hyperadrenocorticism, at diagnosis: 46%.
    - With thoracolumbar intervertebral disc extrusion: 20.0–38.5%.
    - With indwelling urinary catheters: 63.8%.
- Prevalence of bacteriuria in cats:
    - With subclinical bacteriuria: 0.9–28.8%.
    - With lower urinary-tract-associated clinical signs: 3.4–12.0%.
    - With ureteral calculi: 8.4%.
    - With chronic kidney disease: 16.9–29.1%.

Blackwell's Five-Minute Veterinary Consult Clinical Companion: Small Animal Senior Care, First Edition. Edited by Heidi B. Lobprise.

Companion website: www.wiley.com/go/lobprise/Senior

- With diabetes mellitus: 12.2–12.8%.
- With perineal urethrostomies: 22%.

- Prevalence of pyelonephritis is unknown, but probably more common than is recognized clinically, because many animals with pyelonephritis are asymptomatic or have signs limited to lower UTI.

SIGNALMENT

Species

UTI and pyelonephritis—More common in dogs than cats.

Breed Predilections

Breed-associated conditions (hyperadrenocorticism, urolithiasis, etc.) may promote bacteriuria.

Mean Age and Range

- UTIs occur at any age, but are more common in older dogs and cats.
  - Dogs—female: mean 7.7 ± 0.1 years; male: mean 8.0 ± 0.1 years.
  - Cats—female: mean 11.8 ± 4.4 years; male: mean 9.8 ± 4.8 years.

Predominant Sex

- Dogs—female dogs more commonly affected.
- Cats—female cats are slightly overrepresented.

SIGNS

General Comments

Differentiation between pyelonephritis, subclinical bacteriuria, and lower UTI may be difficult in some patients.

Historical Findings

- Patients may be asymptomatic.
- Pollakiuria, dysuria, hematuria, stranguria, inappropriate elimination, and excessive licking at or discharge from the genitalia may be present.
- Systemic clinical signs (anorexia, fever) are infrequent and suggest complicating factors (e.g., pyelonephritis).

Physical Examination Findings

- Unremarkable in most animals.
- Abnormalities occasionally noted with urinary bladder palpation in LUTI:
  - Stimulation of micturition.
  - Pain reactions.
- Pyelonephritis—reduction or increase in kidney size; pain upon palpation

CAUSES

- Uropathogenic bacteria commonly originate from enteric flora with rare hematogenous origins.
- *Escherichia coli* is the most common bacterial isolate in dogs (45–55%) and cats (37.3%).

- Eight species of bacteria (*E. coli*, *Staphylococcus*, *Proteus*, *Streptococcus*, *Klebsiella*, *Enterococcus*, *Pseudomonas*, and *Corynebacterium*) account for approximately 95% of UTIs.

RISK FACTORS

- Immune dysfunction/suppression (e.g., hyperadrenocorticism, feline leukemia virus [FeLV], feline immunodeficiency virus [FIV]).
- Nidus for bacterial adherence and harboring (e.g., indwelling urinary catheters, uroliths).
- Altered urine composition (e.g., persistently dilute urine, glucosuria).
- Abnormal micturition/urine retention (e.g., loss of urethral tone, neurologic disease, urethral obstruction).
- Abnormal anatomy (e.g., ectopic ureters, hooded vulva).
- Disrupted urinary tract mucosal defenses (e.g., mucosal trauma).

DIAGNOSIS

DIFFERENTIAL DIAGNOSIS

- UTI cannot be diagnosed or excluded based on the presence/absence of clinical signs.
- Dysuria, pollakiuria, hematuria, and stranguria occur with lower urinary tract diseases including cystolithiasis, urinary tract neoplasia, prostatitis, obstructive uropathy, and feline idiopathic cystitis.
- Consider pyelonephritis as a rule-out for fever of unknown origin, polyuria/polydipsia, acute decline in renal function, and/or lumbar/abdominal pain.

CBC/BIOCHEMISTRY/URINALYSIS

- CBC and biochemistry are often unremarkable.
- With chronic pyelonephritis; leukocytosis and immature neutrophilia may be detected in some patients; indicators of CKD;
- Urinalysis:
  - Proteinuria and hematuria indicate inflammation.
  - Urine pH >7.5 may indicate the presence of urease-producing bacteria (*Proteus* spp., *Staphylococcus* spp., *Ureaplasma* spp., or *Corynebacterium* spp.).
  - Pyuria is present in most animals with UTI but is not synonymous with infection.
  - Bacteriuria identification increases UTI suspicion. Using a modified Wright–Giemsa stain (Diff-Quik) or Gram stain can improve bacterial detection.
- Leukocyte casts are diagnostic for renal inflammation in pyelonephritis, but unfortunately are very uncommon.

OTHER LABORATORY TESTS

Urine Culture

- Definitive diagnosis requires aerobic urine culture.
- In female dogs with limited antibiotic exposure forgoing a urine culture can be justified for uncomplicated UTI if the pathogen and local susceptibility patterns are known. In male dogs, cats, and animals with recurrent UTI urine culture is recommended.

- Cystocentesis is the gold standard method for collecting urine culture specimens. Bacterial growth $>10^3$ cfu/mL is diagnostic.
- Urine samples obtained by catheterization are often contaminated by the normal flora of the distal urethra. Bacterial growth $>10^4$ cfu/mL in male dogs, $>10^5$ cfu/mL in female dogs, and $>10^3$ cfu/mL in cats is diagnostic. Indwelling catheters may be colonized without concurrent UTI; therefore, sample collection from indwelling urinary catheters should be avoided.
- Culturing voided midstream urine samples should be avoided unless other urine collection techniques are contraindicated or not possible.
- Urine collected from nonsterile surfaces should not be cultured.

Antibiotic Sensitivity Testing

Antibiotic sensitivity is accurately predicted by use of the isolate's "susceptible" vs. "resistant" profiles.

IMAGING

- Rarely is imaging necessary for uncomplicated LUTIs. Radiographs, contrast studies, and ultrasound may help to identify recurrent UTI-predisposing causes.
- Ultrasonography and excretory urography are the best methods for presumptively differentiating between upper and lower UTI.

DIAGNOSTIC PROCEDURES

- Cystoscopy is used in patients with recurrent UTI to visualize abnormalities within the urinary bladder and urethra including uroliths, masses, polyps, ectopic ureters, etc.
- For pyelonephritis, definitive diagnosis requires urine cultures obtained from the renal pelvis by pyelocentesis; though cultures are usually similar to bladder cultures unless obstruction is present.

TREATMENT

APPROPRIATE HEALTH CARE

Outpatient treatment is appropriate; inpatient treatment may be necessary with UTI complications or associated conditions (e.g., acute pyelonephritis).

Diet

- Applicable with concomitant CKD or nephro/uroliths.

Surgical Considerations

- LUTI—Management of uroliths, polypoid cystitis, and infection niduses may require surgical intervention.
- Pyelonephritis—
  - Complete obstruction of the upper urinary tract of a patient with pyelonephritis may rapidly progress to septicemia and therefore should be regarded as a medical emergency.
  - Infected nephroliths—dissolve medically or remove surgically

MEDICATIONS

DRUG(S) OF CHOICE

LUTI considerations

- Given the morbidity associated with sporadic cystitis, empiric antimicrobial treatment is commonly started before receiving urine culture results.
- When susceptibility data is available, the lowest tier antimicrobial should be selected.
- "First-line" antimicrobials—should be selected when possible:
  - Amoxicillin (11–15 mg/kg PO q8h).
  - Trimethoprim-sulfadiazine (TMS) (15 mg/kg PO q12h).
  - Amoxicillin/clavulanic acid (12–25 mg/kg PO q12h).
- "Second-line" antimicrobials—reserved for resistant isolates based on culture and sensitivity or when patient factors prohibit the use of "first-line" therapies:
  - Fluoroquinolones (e.g., marbofloxacin 2.7–5.5 mg/kg PO q24h; enrofloxacin; ciprofloxacin).
  - Cefovecin (8 mg/kg SC).
  - Nitrofurantoin (4.4–5.0 mg/kg PO q8h).
- "Third-line" antimicrobials—reserved for multidrug resistant infections necessitating therapeutic intervention:
  - Amikacin (dogs 15–30 mg/kg IV or SC q24h; cats 10–14 mg/kg IV or SC q24h).
  - Chloramphenicol (dogs 40–50 mg/kg PO q8h; cats 12.5–20 mg/kg [not exceeding 50 mg/cat] PO q12h).
- Antibiotic treatment of uncomplicated infections is recommended for 3–10 days.
- Recurrent UTI treatment requires a urine culture and sensitivity.
- Treatment durations are extended for persistent and relapse infections (up to 4 weeks).
- Reinfections are treated as multiple uncomplicated infections; however, an attempt to identify an abnormality in host defenses should be pursued.

Pyelonephritis considerations

- If systemically ill or azotemic, administer IV antibiotics for initial 48 hours.
- Give orally administered antibiotics at full therapeutic dosages for 2–6 weeks. Duration of antibiotics required for resolution of pyelonephritis is not definitively known.
- Do not use drugs that achieve good concentrations in urine but poor concentrations in serum (e.g., nitrofurantoin).

CONTRAINDICATIONS

Do not use aminoglycosides unless no other alternatives exist on the basis of urine culture and susceptibility testing.

PRECAUTIONS

- Pyelonephritis or prostatitis necessitates therapies able to penetrate the respective tissues
- Trimethoprim-sulfa combinations can cause side effects (keratoconjunctivitis sicca, blood dyscrasias, and polyarthritis) when administered for more than 4 weeks.

ALTERNATE DRUGS

LUTI: Nonsteroidal anti-inflammatory drugs (NSAIDs) may be used cautiously to reduce clinical signs in dogs with cystitis while awaiting urine culture results. They should not be used in dehydrated patients.

FOLLOW-UP

Patient Monitoring

- For uncomplicated UTIs clinical improvement should occur within 48 hours. If clinical signs remain for >48 hours, complicating factors should be investigated.
- Complicated UTIs—continue therapy for 7–10 days beyond resolution of clinical signs, pyuria, and bacteriuria. Confirm resolution via urine culture 7–10 days after end of therapy.
- Pyelonephritis—Perform urine cultures and urinalysis during antibiotic administration (~5–7 days into treatment) and 1 and 4 weeks after antibiotics are finished.

Prevention/Avoidance

LUTI

- Diagnosis and control of predisposing conditions is the most effective method for preventing UTIs.
- Ancillary therapies can be considered to prevent recurrence:
    - Cranberry extract may inhibit *E. coli* attachment to the bladder mucosa.
    - Methenamine—converted into formalin when urine pH is <7.0. Concurrent administration of ascorbic acid (vitamin C) promotes urinary acidification.
    - Prophylactic antibiotics—once-daily administration of antibiotics may lengthen infection-free intervals; however, multidrug resistance is likely in subsequent isolates.

Possible Complications

- UTIs may lead to pyelonephritis, struvite urolith formation, or polypoid cystitis.
- Pyelonephritis may lead to progressive CKD, recurrent pyelonephritis, struvite nephroliths, septicemia, septic shock, metastatic infection (e.g., endocarditis, polyarthritis).

EXPECTED COURSE AND PROGNOSIS

LUTI:

- Prognosis for patients with uncomplicated UTIs is excellent. The prognosis for patients with complicated infections is determined by successful control or resolution of predisposing conditions.

Pyelonephritis

- Patients with acute or subacute pyelonephritis—fair to good, with a return to normal health unless the patient also has nephroliths, CKD, or some other underlying cause for UTI (e.g., obstruction or neoplasia).
- Established chronic infection of the renal medulla may be difficult to resolve because of poor tissue penetration of antibiotics.
- Patients with CKD caused by pyelonephritis—prognosis determined by the severity and rate of progression of the CKD.
- Recurrent pyelonephritis is likely if infected nephroliths are not removed.

MISCELLANEOUS

See Also

- Prostatitis and Prostatic Abscess.
- Urolithiasis, Struvite—Dogs.

Abbreviations

- FeLV = feline leukemia virus
- FIV = feline infectious virus.
- NSAID = nonsteroidal anti-inflammatory drug.
- TMS = trimethoprim-sulfadiazine.
- UTI = urinary tract infection.

Suggested Reading

Bouillon J, Snead E, Casswell J, et al. Pyelonephritis in dogs: retrospective study of 47 histologically diagnosed cases (2005–2015). *J Vet Intern Med* 2018;32:249–259.

Etedali NM, Reetz JA, Foster JD. Complications and clinical utility of ultrasonographically guided pyelocentesis and antegrade pyelography in cats and dogs: 49 cases (2007–2015). *J Am Vet Med Assoc* 2019;254:826–834.

Foster JD, Krishnan H, Cole S. Characterization of subclinical bacteriuria, bacterial cystitis and pyelonephritis in dogs with chronic kidney disease. *J Am Vet Med Assoc* 2018;252:1257–1262.

Weese JS, Blondeau JM, Boothe D, et al. International Society for Companion Animal Infectious Diseases (ISCAID) guidelines for the diagnosis and management of bacterial urinary tract infections in dogs and cats. *Vet J* 2019;247:8–25.

Wood MW. Lower urinary tract infections. In: Ettinger SJ, Feldman EC, Cote E (eds) *Textbook of Veterinary Internal Medicine*, 8th edn. St. Louis, MO: Saunders, 2016; pp. 1992–1996.

Author/editor: Heidi Lobprise
Topic adapted from Five Minute Veterinary Consultation, 7th edition, 2021
Original Topic: Lower Urinary Tract Infections and Pyelonephritis, Bacterial

Author: Michael W. Wood—LUTI

Author: Larry G Adams—Pyelonephritis
Consulting Editor: J.D. Foster

Chapter 78

Nephrolithiasis

BASICS

DEFINITION

- Nephroliths—uroliths located in the renal pelvis or collecting diverticula of the kidney.
- Nephroliths or nephrolith fragments may pass into the ureters (ureteroliths).
- Nephroliths that are not infected, causing obstruction or clinical signs, or progressively enlarging are termed *incidental* nephroliths.

PATHOPHYSIOLOGY

Nephroliths can obstruct the renal pelvis or ureter, predispose to pyelonephritis, and lead to compressive injury of the renal parenchyma and chronic kidney disease (CKD).

SYSTEMS AFFECTED

- Renal/urologic—affects the urinary tract, with potential for obstruction, recurrent urinary tract infection (UTI), or progressive CKD.
- Obstruction of the renal pelvis or ureter with pyelonephritis may result in septicemia and affect any body system.

INCIDENCE/PREVALENCE

- Nephroliths comprise 1–1.5% of uroliths submitted to the Minnesota Urolith Center for analysis. The true incidence of nephroliths is likely higher. Many animals with nephroliths are asymptomatic or are not treated by methods that allow retrieval of uroliths for analysis.
- Composition of canine nephroliths submitted for analysis, in descending frequency: calcium oxalate, struvite, compound, purines, calcium phosphate, cystine, and silica. Composition of nephroliths in cats (descending frequency): calcium oxalate, dried solidified blood calculi, compound, struvite, calcium phosphate, and purine.

SIGNALMENT

Species

Dog and cat.

Blackwell's Five-Minute Veterinary Consult Clinical Companion: Small Animal Senior Care, First Edition. Edited by Heidi B. Lobprise.

Companion website: www.wiley.com/go/lobprise/Senior

Breed Predilections

Dogs

- Calcium oxalate—shih tzu, Yorkshire terrier, bichon frise, miniature schnauzer, and Maltese.
- Struvite—miniature schnauzer, shih tzu, pug, and miniature poodle, related to urinary tract infection.
- Purine—English bulldog, Dalmatian, Yorkshire terrier, and shih tzu.
- Cystine—Newfoundland, English bulldog, and French bulldog.

Cats

Domestic shorthair, European and American shorthair, domestic longhair, Persian, Siamese, and Scottish fold.

Mean Age and Range

- Dogs—mean age 10 years (range 2 months–21.5 years).
- Cats—mean age 7.7 years (range 5 months–19.5 years).

Predominant Sex

- Dogs—nephroliths slightly more common in females than males; struvite nephroliths, females > males; however, calcium oxalate, cystine, and urate nephroliths, males > females.
- Cat—nephroliths slightly more common in females than males; for calcium oxalate, females > males; however, non-crystalline matrix (includes dried blood), and urate nephroliths, males > females.

SIGNS

General Comments

Many patients are asymptomatic, and the nephroliths are diagnosed during evaluation of other problems.

Historical Findings

- None or hematuria, vomiting, and recurrent UTI; dysuria and pollakiuria in animals with UTI or concomitant urocystoliths.
- Uremia in animals with bilateral obstruction or nonfunctional contralateral kidney.
- Signs referable to lower urinary tract urolithiasis if uroliths are present in the upper and lower urinary tract.
- Renal colic with acute abdominal/lumbar pain and vomiting is possible.

Physical Examination Findings

Abdominal or lumbar pain upon palpation of kidneys or no significant findings.

CAUSES

Oversaturation of the urine with calculogenic minerals is a risk factor for urolithiasis.

RISK FACTORS

- Alkaluria—struvite and calcium phosphate uroliths.
- Aciduria—calcium oxalate, cystine, urate, and xanthine uroliths.
- Urine retention and formation of highly concentrated urine.

- Lower UTI—ascending infection and pyelonephritis.
- Conditions that predispose to UTI.

DIAGNOSIS

DIFFERENTIAL DIAGNOSIS

- Consider nephroliths in any patient with CKD, recurrent UTI, acute vomiting (pancreatitis, gastroenteritis, intestinal or gastric obstruction, etc.), or abdominal or lumbar pain (e.g., intervertebral disc protrusion, peritonitis).
- Nephroliths are usually confirmed by radiographs or ultrasonography; differentiate mineralization of the renal pelvis or collecting diverticula from true nephrolithiasis.

CBC/BIOCHEMISTRY/URINALYSIS

- CBC—usually normal; patients with pyelonephritis may have leukocytosis, immature neutrophilia, and thrombocytopenia.
- Serum biochemistry—usually normal unless bilateral obstruction, pyelonephritis, or compressive renal injury leads to acute kidney injury (AKI) or CKD; hypercalcemia may contribute to formation of calcium oxalate or calcium phosphate nephroliths.
- Urinalysis—may reveal hematuria and crystalluria; crystal type may suggest mineral composition; pyuria, proteinuria, and bacteriuria may also be seen with UTI.

OTHER LABORATORY TESTS

- Submit nephroliths or nephrolith fragments for quantitative analysis.
- Urine culture may confirm UTI or concurrent pyelonephritis.

IMAGING

- Can detect radiopaque nephroliths (e.g., calcium phosphate, calcium oxalate, struvite) by survey radiography; cystine and silica are slightly radiopaque.
- Purines (urate or xanthine) are often radiolucent or faintly radiopaque when large unless they contain other radiodense minerals.
- Use ultrasonography or contrast CT to confirm, size, and number of nephroliths or ureteroliths.

DIAGNOSTIC PROCEDURES

After extracorporeal shock wave lithotripsy (ESWL), fragments can be retrieved for quantitative analysis by voiding, cystoscopic basket retrieval, or voiding urohydropropulsion.

TREATMENT

APPROPRIATE HEALTH CARE

Manage patients with incidental nephroliths as outpatients. When appropriate, medical dissolution protocols can be administered to outpatients. Removal of nephroliths by surgery or ESWL requires hospitalization.

DIET

Medical dissolution of nephroliths requires a diet appropriate for the specific nephrolith type. See Medications.

CLIENT EDUCATION

- Incidental nephroliths—may not require removal but should be monitored periodically by urinalysis, urine culture, and imaging. Nephroliths may cause obstruction at any time, which can result in hydronephrosis without clinical signs. Conservative management and monitoring carry a risk of undetected and potentially irreversible renal damage, which must be weighed against the potential renal damage from nephrotomy.
- Nephroliths often recur after removal; monitor the patient every 3–6 months.

SURGICAL CONSIDERATIONS

- Indications for removal of canine nephroliths—obstruction, recurrent infection, progressive nephrolith enlargement, and a nonfunctional contralateral kidney. In cats, only obstructive uroliths in the renal pelvis or ureters are treated.
- Treatment options for nephroliths—medical dissolution, surgery, and ESWL. Calcium oxalate is the most common nephrolith in dogs and cats and is not amenable to medical dissolution. Medical dissolution of nephroliths causing outflow obstruction requires endoscopic or surgical placement of a ureteral stent, or subcutaneous ureteral bypass system (SUB).
- Surgical options—nephrotomy, percutaneous endoscopic nephrolithotomy, or surgically assisted endoscopic nephrolithotomy. Endoscopic nephrolithotomy may be preferred over ESWL for nephroliths >1.5 cm in diameter.
- ESWL—safe and effective method of treating canine nephroliths and ureteroliths; nephrolith fragments pass down the ureter into the bladder and are voided with urine or removed by voiding urohydropropulsion. Large (1–1.5 cm) nephroliths may be managed by endoscopic placement of ureteral stent to induce ureteral dilatation followed by ESWL 2–4 weeks later.
- ESWL is not safe or effective for treatment of nephroureteroliths in cats.

MEDICATIONS

DRUG(S) OF CHOICE

- Antibiotics selected on the basis of urine culture and sensitivity testing as needed; periprocedural antibiotics are recommended when infected nephroliths are treated by ESWL or surgical removal.
- Medical dissolution protocols are limited to struvite, purine, and cystine uroliths.
- When feasible, consumption of water in high moisture (canned) foods should be incorporated into dissolution protocol. Target urine-specific gravity <1.020 (dogs), <1.025 (cats).
- Medical dissolution protocols for canine struvite nephroliths include struvite-preventative or -dissolution diets and culture-guided antibiotic therapy for the duration of dissolution.
- Medical dissolution of canine purine nephroliths can be attempted by a purine-restricted diet, allopurinol 15 mg/kg PO q12h, and supplemental potassium citrate as needed to maintain urine pH ~7.0.
- Medical dissolution of canine cystine nephrolithiasis can be attempted using a therapeutic diet, 2-mercaptopropionylglycine (2-MPG, tiopronin) 15 mg/kg PO q12h, and supplemental potassium citrate as needed to maintain urine pH ~7.5.

CONTRAINDICATIONS

- Do not use allopurinol without dietary purine restriction; this combination may cause xanthine nephrolithiasis in dogs predisposed to urate urolithiasis.
- Do not give acidifying diets to azotemic patients unless blood pH and total CO_2 are monitored for development of metabolic acidosis.

FOLLOW-UP

PATIENT MONITORING

Abdominal radiographs or ultrasonography, urinalysis, and urine culture every 3–6 months to detect nephrolith recurrence. Dogs treated with ESWL—check every 2–4 weeks by radiographs and ultrasonography until nephrolith fragments have passed.

PREVENTION/AVOIDANCE

Eliminate factors predisposing to individual urolith type, augment urine volume, and correct factors contributing to urine retention. Dietary therapy is indicated for prevention of urate and cystine nephroliths; dietary therapy is still unproven for calcium oxalate uroliths. Castration of male dogs with cystine uroliths aids in prevention.

POSSIBLE COMPLICATIONS

Hydronephrosis, AKI, CKD, recurrent UTI, and pyelonephritis.

EXPECTED COURSE AND PROGNOSIS

- Highly variable; depends on nephrolith type, location, and size, secondary complications (e.g., obstruction, infection, CKD), and owner compliance with treatment and prevention protocol.
- Incidental nephroliths may remain inactive for years, resulting in an excellent prognosis.
- Return to normal health and good prognosis have been observed with ESWL for treatment of dogs with nephroliths.
- The prognosis for patients with CKD caused by nephrolithiasis depends on the severity and rate of progression of CKD.
- Nephroliths causing outflow obstruction should not be dissolved medically without placement of a ureteral stent.

MISCELLANEOUS

Associated Conditions

- Hyperadrenocorticism and glucocorticoid administration are associated with calcium oxalate uroliths, and UTI resulting in struvite urolithiasis.
- Portosystemic vascular malformations and genetic mutations in certain breeds predispose to urate uroliths.

Pregnancy/Fertility/Breeding

ESWL is contraindicated in pregnant animals.

Abbreviations

- 2-MPG = 2-mercaptopropionylglycine
- AKI = acute kidney injury.
- CKD = chronic kidney disease.
- ESWL = extracorporeal shock wave lithotripsy.
- UTI = urinary tract infection.
- SUB = subcutaneous ureteral bypass system

Suggested Reading

Adams LG, Goldman CK. Extracorporeal shock wave lithotripsy. In: Polzin DJ, Bartges JB (eds) *Nephrology and Urology of Small Animals*. Ames, IA: Blackwell Publishing, 2011; pp. 340–348.

Berent AC, Adams LG. Interventional management of complicated nephrolithiasis. In: Weisse CW, Berent AC (eds) *Veterinary Imaging-Guided Interventions*. Ames, IA: Wiley-Blackwell, 2015; pp. 289–300.

Author/editor: Heidi Lobprise
Thanks to: Julie Byron for review
Topic adapted from Five Minute Veterinary Consultation, 7th edition, 2021
Original Topic: Nephrolithiasis

Author: Larry G. Adams
Consulting Editor: J.D. Foster

Chapter 79

Perirenal Pseudocysts

BASICS

OVERVIEW

- Renomegaly caused by accumulation of fluid between the kidney and its surrounding capsule. One or both kidneys are affected.
- It is not lined with secretory epithelium; the name "pseudo"-cyst is appropriate.

SIGNALMENT

- Primarily older male cats (>8 years), rare in dogs

SIGNS

- May be asymptomatic.
- Nonpainful, enlarged abdomen is common.
- Signs of concomitant renal failure in some patients.

CAUSES AND RISK FACTORS

- Cause is often not understood and the accumulation of pseudocyst fluid is a dynamic, not a static, process.
- Cytologic and biochemical evaluation of pseudocyst fluid may aid understanding of pathophysiologic mechanisms.
- Transudate—due to high capillary hydrostatic pressure, lymphatic obstruction, or rupture of renal cysts.
- Renal fibrosis in some cats with progressive renal parenchymal contraction may occlude lymphatics and blood vessels, promoting transudation of fluid.
- Perirenal urine—disruption of the renal pelvis or the proximal ureter.
- Blood from external trauma, surgery, neoplastic erosion of blood vessels, rupture of aneurysms, coagulopathies, or paracentesis of the urinary tract.

Blackwell's Five-Minute Veterinary Consult Clinical Companion: Small Animal Senior Care, First Edition. Edited by Heidi B. Lobprise.

Companion website: www.wiley.com/go/lobprise/Senior

DIAGNOSIS

DIFFERENTIAL DIAGNOSIS

- Causes of renomegaly include renal neoplasia, hydronephrosis, polycystic kidney disease (common), feline infectious peritonitis, and mycotic or bacterial nephritis (less common).
- Ascites and enlargement of other abdominal organs can cause nonpainful distension of the abdomen.

CBC/BIOCHEMISTRY/URINALYSIS

- Results unremarkable until patient develops renal insufficiency.
- Azotemia and inappropriately low urinary-specific gravity (<1.035) indicate concomitant chronic kidney disease (CKD).

OTHER LABORATORY TESTS

N/A

IMAGING

- Renomegaly is commonly detected by abdominal radiography.
- Excretory urography and ultrasonography can be used to determine whether the underlying renal parenchyma is normal or abnormal. Small kidneys beneath an abnormally wide fluid-filled intracapsular space is a common finding.

DIAGNOSTIC PROCEDURES

Cytologic examination of pseudocyst fluid may provide evidence of the underlying disease process resulting in fluid accumulation (e.g., transudation, hemorrhage, lymphatic obstruction, inflammation, and urine) or secondary complications (e.g., infection). Creatinine concentrations that are higher in pseudocyst fluid compared to serum are consistent with urinary tract rupture.

TREATMENT

- Perirenal pseudocysts are not immediately life-threatening.
- Some patients need no treatment.
- Many patients require further diagnostic evaluation and treatment of concomitant CKD.
- Capsulectomy or pseudocyst fenestration (remove greater than 1 × 1 cm section of capsule to minimize spontaneous closure of the fenestration) is generally associated with amelioration of abdominal distention and abdominal organ displacement. Early stages of CKD may resolve; however, progression of CKD commonly occurs.
- Long-term response is unknown.
- Avoid nephrectomy to maximize remaining kidney function.
- Decompression by paracentesis with a needle and syringe provides temporary relief.
- If pseudocysts refill with fluid (often in 1–2 weeks), paracentesis can then be repeated.

MEDICATIONS

DRUG(S) OF CHOICE

Consider appropriate antimicrobic (i.e., lipid-soluble antibiotic chosen on the basis of antimicrobial susceptibility) if pseudocysts become infected.

FOLLOW-UP

- Monitor patients periodically (every 2–6 months) for development and progression of CKD.
- Short-term prognosis appears favorable with or without pseudocyst decompression in patients with no evidence of CKD.
- Long-term prognosis is unknown because it has not been determined whether perirenal pseudocysts are associated with underlying lesions in the renal parenchyma that may be progressive. It is also unknown whether perirenal pseudocysts are associated with hypertension.
- Survival is related to the severity and progression of CKD.

MISCELLANEOUS

Abbreviations

- CKD = chronic kidney disease

Suggested Reading

Beck JA, Bellenger CR, Lamb WA, et al. Perirenal pseudocysts in 26 cats. *Aust Vet J* 2000;78:166–171.

Lulich JP, Osborne CA, Polzin DJ. Cystic diseases of the kidney. In: Osborne CA, Finco DR (eds) *Canine and Feline Nephrology and Urology*. Philadelphia, PA: Williams & Wilkins, 1995; pp. 460–483.

Ochoa VB, DiBartola SP, Chew DJ, et al. Perinephric pseudocysts in the cat: a retrospective study and review of the literature. *J Vet Intern Med* 1999;13:47–55.

Author/editor: Heidi Lobprise
Topic adapted from Five Minute Veterinary Consultation, 7th edition, 2021
Original Topic: Perirenal Pseudocysts

Author: Jody P. Lulich
Consulting Editor: J.D. Foster

Chapter 80

Urolithiasis—Overview

This overview of urolithiasis will include specific information on calcium oxalate, calcium phosphate, and struvite (cat and dog) uroliths as they pertain (somewhat) to senior patients. Other uroliths that are more prevalent in younger pets will be briefly mentioned in the miscellaneous section.

BASICS

DEFINITION

- Calcium Oxalate (CaOx)—Formation of CO uroliths within the urinary tract and associated clinical conditions (e.g., urinary obstruction, idiopathic hypercalcemia, chronic kidney disease).
- Calcium phosphate (CaPh) uroliths within the urinary tract and associated clinical conditions, including calcium phosphate apatite (CAP), calcium phosphate carbonate (CPC), calcium hydrogen phosphate dihydrate (brushite), and uncommon minerals—tricalcium phosphate (whitlockite) and octacalcium phosphate.
- Cat—Struvite
    - Struvite uroliths are polycrystalline concretions composed primarily of magnesium ammonium phosphate (MAP) and small quantities of matrix.
    - Struvite urethral plugs are composed of large quantities of matrix mixed with crystals (especially MAP), while others are composed primarily of organic matrix, sloughed tissue, blood, and/or inflammatory reactants.
- Dog—Struvite—Formation of polycrystalline concretions composed of magnesium ammonium phosphate hexahydrate (MAP, struvite) in the urinary tract.

PATHOPHYSIOLOGY

- CaOx—Presence of hypercalciuria, hyperoxaluria, hypocitraturia, and defective crystal growth inhibitors. (see causes and risk factors)
- Struvite—cat and dog
    - Infection-Induced Struvite
        - MAP supersaturation of urine (needed for struvite formation) is often associated with urinary tract infections (UTIs) with urease-producing microbes (*Staphylococcus*, *Proteus*, and *Ureaplasma*).
        - Excess dietary proteins result in additional urea accumulation in urine, favoring formation struvite, carbonate apatite, and calcium apatite uroliths.

Blackwell's Five-Minute Veterinary Consult Clinical Companion: Small Animal Senior Care, First Edition. Edited by Heidi B. Lobprise.

Companion website: www.wiley.com/go/lobprise/Senior

- Sterile Struvite
  - Uncommon in dogs; may involve dietary or metabolic factors.
  - Microbial urease is not involved in formation of sterile struvite uroliths.
  - In cats, most urethral plugs contain large quantities of matrix in addition to minerals, especially struvite. Risk factors associated with formation of MAP crystals contained in urethral plugs are similar to those associated with formation of struvite uroliths. Prevention or control of these risk factors should minimize the recurrence of the struvite component of urethral plugs.

GENETICS

- The high incidence of struvite uroliths in some breeds such as miniature schnauzers suggests a familial tendency. Susceptible miniature schnauzers may inherit an abnormality of local host defenses of the urinary tract that increases their susceptibility to UTI.
- Sterile struvite uroliths were found in a family of English cocker spaniels.

INCIDENCE/PREVALENCE

- CaOx
  - Dogs—40% of lower urinary tract uroliths; 45% of upper urinary tract uroliths
  - Cats—40% of lower urinary tract uroliths; 90% or upper urinary tract uroliths
- CaPh
  - Dog <1.0%, Cats <0.5%)—more in upper tract than lower
- Stuvite—cat
  - Currently about 50% in lower urinary tract, 95% are sterile (decreasing numbers from 1982 to 2002; more CaOx)
  - In 8% of feline nephroliths but 90% in matrix-crystalline urethral plugs
- Struvite—dog
  - Approximately 40% of lower urinary tract uroliths; 23% of upper urinary tract uroliths.

SIGNALMENT

Breed Predilections

- CaOx—Six breeds represent 60% of canine cases: miniature schnauzer, Lhasa apso, Yorkshire terrier, bichon frisé, shih tzu, and miniature poodle. Cat—Himalayan, Scottish fold, Persian, ragdoll, and Burmese are at greater risk.
- Struvite—dogs: Miniature schnauzer, shih tzu, bichon frise, miniature poodle, cocker spaniel, and Lhasa apso.

Mean Age and Range

- CaOx
  - Dogs—8.5 ± 3 years; 60%, 6–11 years.
  - Cats—97% >2 years; 53%, 7–15 years.
- CaPh—rarely detected in animals <1 year old
- Struvite—cat
  - Mean age at time of diagnosis is 7 years (range, <1–22 years).
  - Sterile struvite uroliths do not affect immature cats; infection-induced struvite may occur in immature (<1 year) and senior cats (>10 years).

- Struvite—dog
  - Mean age, 6 years (range <1 to >19 years).
  - Most uroliths in immature (<12 months old) dogs are infection-induced struvite.

Predominant Sex

- CaOx—Mostly male dogs (73%) and male cats (55%).
- CaPh—primarily in female dogs (72%)
- Struvite—cats
  - Struvite uroliths are more common in female cats (55%) than in males.
  - Struvite urethral plugs primarily affect males.
- Struvite—dogs
  - More common in females (~85%) than males (~15%), which may be related to the greater propensity for females to develop bacterial UTI.

SIGNS

General Comments

- Asymptomatic in some animals.
- Depend on location, size, cause, and number of uroliths.
- Animals with nephroureteroliths are typically asymptomatic but may have persistent hematuria.
- Ureteral obstruction associated with contralateral microrenale, ipsilateral hydronephrosis, and acute onset of uremia occurs frequently in cats with chronic kidney disease.

Historical Findings

- For all types: Typical signs of urocystoliths or urethroliths include pollakiuria, dysuria, and hematuria. Some may present for urethral obstruction.
- Nephroureteroliths common (45%) in cats with chronic kidney disease.
- Struvite—cat:
  - Signs of renal dysfunction (PU/PD)
  - Signs of outflow obstruction (e.g., dysuria, large painful urinary bladder, and postrenal azotemia) are found with struvite urethral plugs.
  - Sometimes will void small, smooth urolith.
- Struvite—dogs
  - Sometimes small, smooth uroliths are voided.
  - Some medium-size uroliths are associated with urethral obstruction.
  - Nephroliths may be associated with manifestations of renal insufficiency. Obstruction to urine outflow with bacterial UTI may result in generalized pyelonephritis and septicemia.

Physical Examination Findings

- CaOX
  - Detection of urocystoliths is by abdominal or urethral palpation; failure to palpate uroliths does not exclude them from consideration.
  - Large urinary bladder with complete urethral obstruction (more common in cats).
  - Urocystoliths with irregular contours rarely cause complete urethral obstruction.

- CaPh
- Struvite—cats
  - A thickened, firm, contracted bladder wall may be appreciated.
  - Palpation is insensitive and unreliable for detection of urocystoliths.
  - Urethral plugs or urethroliths may be detected by examination of the distal penis.
  - Outflow obstruction results in an enlarged urinary bladder and signs of postrenal azotemia.
- Struvite—dogs
  - Uroliths may be palpated in the urinary bladder and urethra (by rectal exam).
  - Urethral obstruction may cause enlargement of the urinary bladder.
  - Ureteral obstruction may cause enlargement and pain of the associated kidney.
  - Complete urine outflow obstruction combined with bacterial infection may cause ascending UTI and signs of renal failure and septicemia.

CAUSES

- CaOx
  - Hypercalciuria
    - Normocalcemic—intestinal hyperabsorption of calcium or reduced renal tubular reabsorption of calcium.
    - Hypercalcemic—excessive glomerular filtration of mobilized calcium
  - Hyperoxaluria—inherited abnormalities in humans, excessive consumption or fat malabsorption.
  - Hypocitraturia—urine citrate inhibits CaOx (competes with calcium); acidosis is associated with low urinary citrate excretion
  - Defective crystal growth inhibitors—decrease ability to enhance solubility of CaOx.
  - Feeding diets to promote aciduria, associated with hypercalciuria (bone mobilization of calcium) and hypocitraturia.
- CaPh
  - CPC—commonly a minor component of struvite and calcium oxalate uroliths.
  - Pure CP uroliths—usually associated with metabolic disorders, e.g., primary hyperparathyroidism, renal tubular acidosis, and excessive dietary calcium and phosphorus.
  - Urinary tract infections—increased calcium excretion in combination with urinary tract infection with urease producing bacteria may be risk factors favoring CPC.
  - Nephroliths, urocystoliths, and urethroliths composed of blood clots mineralized with CP suggest dystrophic mineralization of tissue, in contrast to metastatic mineralization reflecting abnormal calcium and phosphorus metabolism.
- Struvite
  - Cats (see Pathophysiology)
    - Diet Related (seldom infection-induced): MAP saturation and increased urea in urine
    - Formation of MAP in urethral plugs.
  - Dogs
    - Urinary tract disorders that predispose to infections with urease-producing bacteria, fungal pathogens, or ureaplasma in patients whose urine contains a large quantity of urea.
    - Specific causes of sterile struvite uroliths are unknown.

RISK FACTORS

- CaOx
  - Oral calcium supplements given independent of meals.
  - Feeding acidifying foods
    - Aciduria was a risk factor for first-time CaOx urolith formation in dogs.
    - By inducing alkaluria via dietary formulation with potassium citrate in healthy cats, urinary undersaturation for CaOx was achieved.
  - Hypercalciuria
    - Excessive dietary protein, sodium, and vitamin D.
    - Glucocorticoids and furosemide administration.
  - Hyperoxaluria
    - Additional dietary oxalate (e.g., chocolate and peanuts) and ascorbic acid promote hyperoxaluria.
    - Vitamin B6-deficient diets
  - Consumption of dry diets has a higher risk for CaOx urolith formation than consumption of high-moisture canned diets.
- Struvite—cat
  - Sterile struvite uroliths—mineral composition, energy content, and moisture content of diets; urine-alkalinizing metabolites in diets; quantity of diet consumed; *ad libitum* vs. meal-feeding schedules; formation of concentrated urine; and retention of urine.
  - Infection-induced struvite urolithiasis—urinary tract infection (UTI) with urease-producing bacteria, abnormalities in local host defenses that allow bacterial UTIs, and the quantity of urea excreted in urine.
  - The small diameter of the male distal urethra predisposes to obstruction with plugs and urethroliths.
- Struvite—dog
  - Exogenous or endogenous exposure to high concentrations of glucocorticoids predispose to bacteriuria.
  - Abnormal retention of urine.
  - Alkaline urine decreases the solubility of struvite.
  - Females more than dogs because of increased risks of UTI

DIAGNOSIS

DIFFERENTIAL DIAGNOSIS—IN GENERAL

- Other causes of pollakiuria, dysuria, periuria, hematuria, and/or outflow obstruction.
  - Urethral obstruction, urinary tract infection, urinary tract neoplasia, and idiopathic feline lower urinary tract disease.
- Differentiate between radiodense uroliths
- Metastatic or dystrophic mineralization of urinary tract parenchyma may resemble uroliths.

CBC/BIOCHEMISTRY/URINALYSIS

- Hematological and serum profile results are usually unremarkable.
  - CaOx—Hypercalcemia (rare in dogs, more common in cats) should be further evaluated to determine its cause and contribution to urolith formation.

- CaPh—Hypercalcemia or azotemia rarely detected; postrenal azotemia in some animals with complete urinary outflow obstruction
- Struvite—Complete outflow obstruction may cause postrenal azotemia in cats and dogs, hyperphosphatemia in dogs.

■ Urinalysis (absence of crystalluria does not exclude uroliths)
- CaOX crystals
- CaPh—amorphous crystals in some; Brushite crystals: elongated, rectangular, lath-shaped.
- MAP crystals typically appear as colorless, orthorhombic (having three unequal axes intersecting at right angles), coffin-like prisms. They often have 3–8 sides.

OTHER LABORATORY TESTS

■ All types: Quantitative mineral analysis of uroliths (and plugs) is necessary to confirm their mineral composition.

■ CaPh
- Parathyroid hormone, parathyroid hormone–related peptide, and hydroxycholecalciferol values may help establish underlying causes.

■ Struvite—cat
- Pretreatment urine cultures (preferably obtained by cystocentesis) to detect primary urease-producing microbes to differentiate them from infections acquired as a sequelae to urolithiasis.
- Bacterial culture of inner portions of uroliths with urease-positive UTI.

■ Struvite—dog
- Quantitative bacterial culture of urine, preferably collected by cystocentesis.
- Bacterial culture of inner portions of infection-induced struvite uroliths.

IMAGING

■ CaOx uroliths $\geq$2 mm in diameter are radio-opaque and easily detected by survey radiography.
- IV urography, contrast pyelography, or ultrasonography may be needed to verify ureteral obstruction.
- Urinary tract mineralization may resemble uroliths.

■ CaP
- Radiodense (as dense as bone) and are often detected by survey radiography and may be detected by ultrasonography.
- Most do not have a characteristic shape, except brushite uroliths (round and smooth).
- CP uroliths are usually cream or tan in color. Blood clots mineralized with CP are typically black (in appearance).

■ Struvite—cat
- Struvite uroliths—radiodense, single or multiple, rough or smooth, round or faceted, sometimes disc-shaped; some struvite urethral plugs may be detected by survey radiography.
- The size and number of uroliths are not a reliable index of probable efficacy of dissolution therapy.
- Contrast urethrocystography helps identify the site of urethral obstruction and strictures.
- Ultrasonography detects location and approximate size and number of uroliths. Tends to overestimate stone size and underestimate stone number.
  - Does not indicate degree of radiodensity or shape of uroliths.

- Struvite—dog
  - Radiodense and may be detected by survey radiography.
  - Ultrasonography can detect uroliths, but provides no information about their density, shape, or size.
  - Determine precise location, size, and number of uroliths; the size and number are not a reliable index of probable efficacy of dissolution therapy.

DIAGNOSTIC PROCEDURES

- Uroliths and urocystoliths in the urethra and bladder may be detected by cystoscopy.

PATHOLOGIC FINDINGS

- Struvite—cat: Urethral plugs may contain red blood cells, white cells, transitional epithelial cells, bacteria, and/or viruses in addition to matrix and minerals.

TREATMENT

APPROPRIATE HEALTH CARE

- CaOx
  - CaOx uroliths are not amenable to medical dissolution.
  - Voiding urohydropropulsion or basket retrieval to remove small stones that can pass through the urethra (<3 mm in most dogs >5 kg).
  - Percutaneous cystolithotomy or routine cystotomy can be used to remove stones in smaller dogs and male cats.
  - Consider laser lithotripsy, percutaneous cystolithotomy, or routine cystotomy to remove larger stones from the urinary bladder.
  - Urethral surgery is discouraged. Flush urethral stones back into the urinary bladder by retrograde urohydropropulsion then remove by cystotomy.
  - Persistently obstructed ureters require urgent intervention to minimize progressive kidney damage.
  - Removal of unobstructing nephroliths is usually unnecessary.
- CaPh
  - Medical dissolution of CP uroliths remains a goal for the future.
  - Use basket retrieval to remove urethroliths, retrograde urohydropropulsion to flush urethroliths into the bladder or using lithotripsy to fragment urethroliths.
    - Shock wave lithotripsy is an alternative to surgery for removal of nephroliths, ureteroliths, and urocystoliths in dogs.
  - Consider surgical removal of lower tract uroliths that cannot be removed by minimally invasive procedures.
  - Correction of hyperparathyroidism or other causes of hypercalcemia should minimize further urolith formation.
- Struvite—cat
  - Retrograde urohydropropulsion to eliminate urethral stones; lavage to remove urethral plugs.
  - Voiding urohydropropulsion to eliminate small bladder and urethral stones in females.
  - Medical dissolution of struvite uroliths is an outpatient strategy.

- Struvite—dog
  - Medical dissolution with antimicrobials and therapeutic food is preferred treatment for non-obstructing struvite uroliths.
  - Ureteral stenting facilitates medical dissolution of obstructing nephroureteroliths.
  - Appropriate antimicrobic administration is the cornerstone of treatment for infection-induced struvite dissolution and prevention.
  - Voiding urohydropropulsion, laser lithotripsy, percutaneous cystolithotomy, and/or surgery require short periods of hospitalization.

ACTIVITY

Reduce during the period of tissue repair after surgery.

DIET

- CaOx
  - Feed high-moisture foods that promote formation of less acidic urine (pH >6.3–6.6).
  - In hypercalcemia cats without evidence of hyperparathyroidism or malignancy feed Hill's Prescription Diet Feline w/d.
- CaPh
  - A high-moisture (canned) diet formulated to prevent formation of calcium oxalate uroliths may help prevent recurrence.
  - Foods for older dogs that are lower in protein, phosphorus, and calcium, and which do not promote acidic urine are usually associated with decreased calcium and phosphorus excretion. Hill's Prescription Diet canned g/d is one example.
- Struvite—cat
  - Medical dissolution is the standard of practice.
  - Treatment with a dedicated struvite calculolytic diet (e.g., Hill's Prescription Diet Feline s/d) results in dissolution within 2–4 weeks of therapy.
  - Treatment with urinary therapeutic foods designed for struvite dissolution and CaOx prevention are effective but may require longer treatment times.
  - Infection-induced struvite urocystoliths may be dissolved by feeding a calculolytic diet and an appropriate antimicrobic.
  - Continue diet therapy for 1 month after radiographic evidence of urolith dissolution.
  - Struvite crystalluria may be minimized by feeding magnesium-restricted urine-acidifying diets.
  - Canned foods help to reduce urine concentration of calculogenic metabolites and promote increased frequency of voiding.
- Struvite—dog
  - Infection-induced and sterile struvite urocystoliths and nephroliths may be dissolved by feeding a calculolytic food (Hill's Prescription Diet Canine c/d, s/d, Royal Canin® and others).
  - Continue calculolytic diet therapy for 1 month beyond survey radiographic evidence of urolith dissolution.
  - Avoid use of protein-restricted diet in patients with protein-calorie malnutrition. Some diets are designed for short-term (weeks to months) dissolution therapy, some for long-term (months to years) prophylactic therapy. Monitor the patient for evidence of

protein malnutrition. Consider dissolution diets meeting maintenance nutritional requirements in immature dogs. Avoid high-sodium foods in dogs with cardiac valvular disease or heart failure.

CLIENT EDUCATION

- CaOx
  - Urolith removal does not alter the factors responsible for urolith formation; eliminating or minimizing risk factors is necessary to minimize recurrence.
  - 50% of dogs reform uroliths within 2–3 years; 1/3 of cats reform uroliths in 2 years.
  - Patients with hypercalcemia typically reform uroliths at a faster rate.
  - Diet may help delay reformation of uroliths, but will not prevent it
- CaPh
- Struvite—cat—see Diet
  - Short-term (weeks to months) treatment with a calculolytic diet and antibiotics as needed is effective in dissolving infection-induced struvite uroliths.
  - Owners of cats with infection-induced struvite urocystoliths must comply with dosage schedule of antibiotics.
- Struvite—dog
  - If dietary management is used, limit access to other foods and treats.
  - Short-term (2–3 months) treatment with a calculolytic food and administration of antibiotics is effective in dissolving struvite uroliths.
  - Comply with dosage schedule for antibiotic and diet therapy.

SURGICAL CONSIDERATIONS

- CaOx
  - Consider surgical removal of lower tract uroliths that cannot be removed by minimally invasive procedures (see above).
  - Avoid performing disfiguring urethrostomies and urethrotomies by using retrograde urohydropropulsion to flush urethroliths into the bladder or using lithotripsy to fragment urethroliths.
  - To minimize urolith reformation over suture nidus, minimize surgical procedures to remove uroliths and use absorbable suture and patterns that minimize suture exposure in the lumen of the urinary tract.
  - Only surgeons trained in ureteral surgery should attempt ureterolithotomy. Ureteral stents in dogs and subcutaneous ureteral access devices or stents in cats should be considered.
  - Consider parathyroidectomy for patients with primary hyperparathyroidism.
- CaPh
  - Avoid performing disfiguring urethrostomies
- Struvite—cat
  - Ureteroliths cannot be dissolved. If severe, consider subcutaneous ureteral bypass, ureteral stents, or traditional surgery.
  - Urethroliths cannot be medically dissolved. Consider voiding urohydropropulsion or retrograde urohydropropulsion.
  - Immovable urethroliths, recurrent urethral plugs, or strictures of the distal urethra may require perineal urethrostomy.
  - Consider laser lithotripsy for urocystoliths and/or urethroliths.

- Consider surgical correction if uroliths are obstructing urine outflow and/or if correctable abnormalities predisposing to recurrent UTI are identified by radiography or other means.
- Radiographs should be obtained immediately following surgery to verify that all uroliths were removed.

■ Struvite—dog
- Ureteroliths and urethroliths may be difficult to medically dissolve because they are minimally immersed in urine.
- Consider ureteral stenting (allow time for decompression and stone dissolution) or shock-wave lithotripsy for persistent ureteroliths associated with morbidity.
- Consider voiding urohydropropulsion if urethroliths are likely to pass, laser lithotripsy or retrograde urohydropropulsion.
- Consider surgical correction if uroliths are obstructing urine outflow and minimally invasive procedures are ineffective or not available. Immovable urethroliths may require urethrotomy or urethrostomy.

MEDICATIONS

DRUG(S) OF CHOICE

■ CaOx
- No available drugs effectively dissolve CaOx uroliths in the urinary tract. *In vitro* dissolution is seen with alkaline solutions (pH ≥8) of 2% or greater EDTA.
- Potassium citrate used to promote alkaluria should not contain cranberry supplements.
- Hydrochlorothiazide may be used to reduce calciuresis

■ CaPh
- No effective medications available for dissolving CP uroliths

■ Struvite—cat
- Appropriate antibiotics, chosen on the basis of bacterial culture and antimicrobial susceptibility tests. Give antibiotics at therapeutic dosages until the UTI is eradicated and there is no radiographic evidence of uroliths.
- Buprenorphine to alleviate discomfort (15 μg/kg via buccal transmucosal administration q8–12h).
- Tolteridine as an anticholinergic and antispasmodic to minimize hyperactivity of the bladder detrusor muscle and urge incontinence (0.05 mg/kg PO q12h).

■ Struvite—dog
- Appropriate antibiotics, chosen on the basis of quantitative bacterial culture and antimicrobial susceptibility tests. Give antibiotics until there is no radiographic evidence of uroliths and there is eradication of UTI.
- In most cases, antimicrobics need to be administered for the entire dissolution period. Shorter duration may be successful if they sterilize the urolith (e.g., small uroliths).

PRECAUTIONS

■ CaOx—Steroids and furosemide promote calciuria.

■ CaPh—avoid vitamin D supplements, other mineral supplements, glucocorticoids.

- Struvite—cat—Azotemic patients are at increased risk for adverse drug events.
- Struvite—dog—Diet-induced polyuria will reduce the concentration of antimicrobial drugs in urine; consider this fact when calculating antimicrobic dosages.

FOLLOW-UP

PATIENT MONITORING

- CaOx
  - Postsurgical radiographs are essential to verify complete urolith removal.
  - Evaluate abdominal radiography every 3–5 months to detect urolith recurrence early. Small uroliths are easily removed by voiding urohydropropulsion or stone basket retrieval.
- CaPh
  - Radiography after surgery to verify complete urolith removal is a standard of practice.
  - Abdominal radiography or ultrasonography every 3–5 months to enhance early detection of urolith recurrence and prevention of the need for repeated surgery.
  - Small uroliths are easily removed by voiding urohydropropulsion or catheter retrieval.
- Struvite—cat
  - Check rate of urolith dissolution monthly by urinalysis, urine culture, survey or contrast radiography, or ultrasonography.
- Struvite—dog
  - Monitor rate of urolith dissolution at 4–6 weeks intervals by urinalysis, urine culture, and imaging (ultrasonography, and/or survey or contrast radiography).

PREVENTION/AVOIDANCE

- CaOx
  - Even with therapy, CaOx urolith recurrence is common (up to 50% in dogs and 33% in cats in 2–3 years). Regular monitoring and compliance check-ins are key.
  - Only recommend high-moisture foods (e.g., can, loaf, gravies).
    - Feeding dry foods, combining dry and wet foods, or adding water to dry food is not effective in maintaining low urinary concentrations (specific gravity <1.020 in dogs and <1.030 in cats) of calculogenic minerals.
    - Feeding high-sodium foods (≥300 mg/100 kcal) should not be recommended as a substitute for feeding high-moisture foods. Their efficacy to promote low urine-specific gravity appears to be short-lived (3–6 months), and their use is contraindicated in kidney or heart disease.
  - Avoid feeding diets that promote urine acidification. A linear increase in urine pH was associated with a linear decrease in urine CaOx saturation in normal cats.
    - If urine is acidic, consider administration of potassium citrate 75 mg/kg PO q12h; adjust dosage to achieve a pH between 6.5 and 7.5.
  - Commercially manufactured diets have been designed to prevent CaOx recurrence, but they may not be ideal for all patients.
    - Hill's Prescription Diet c/d multicare has been shown to decrease calcium and oxalate excretion in dogs with CaOx urolithiasis. This food has lower levels of sodium and protein.
    - Hill's Prescription Diet i/d Low Fat and has been recommended for dogs with CaOx urolithiasis and fat/lipid intolerance or fat/lipid responsive diseases (e.g., dogs with

a history of pancreatitis). Because this diet promotes formation of acidic urine, administer potassium citrate to promote a more favorable urine pH >6.5.
    - Royal Canin SO has been shown to decrease CaOx relative supersaturation in urine of urolith-forming dogs collected by owners. Because this diet promotes acidic urine, concomitant administration of potassium citrate is necessary to achieve a more favorable urine pH (>6.5). Because of its high sodium, this food may be inappropriate for small breeds at risk for degenerative mitral valve disease.
  - Avoid supplements with vitamins D and C (cranberry source, Vit C can increase urine oxalate).
  - Vitamin B6 2–4 mg/kg PO q24–48h may help minimize oxalate excretion, especially for animals fed homemade or pyridoxine-deficient diets.
  - Reevaluate patients in 2–4 weeks to verify reduction in specific gravity (<1.020 for dogs and <1.030 for cats), urine pH (≥6.5), and amelioration of crystalluria.
    - Do not use inappropriately collected or stored urine samples (e.g., urine collected by owners, refrigerated, or contaminated with debris) to monitor therapeutic efficacy.
  - If dietary changes are inadequate at slowing the rate of recurrence, consider hydrochlorothiazide diuretics (dog, 2 mg/kg and cat, 1 mg/kg q12–24h).
  - If the patient is hypercalcemic, correct underlying cause.
  - *Oxalobacter formigenes* is an intestinal bacterium that ingests oxalate as its sole nutrient. By metabolizing dietary oxalate in the intestine, less oxalic acid is available for absorption and less is excreted in urine. To preserve healthy populations of intestinal *Oxalobacter*, avoid indiscriminant or prolonged use of antimicrobics.
- CaPh
  - Canned diets are more effective than dry diets in preventing recurrence.
  - Avoid excessive acidification or alkalinization of urine.
- Struvite—see treatment
  - If dietary management is used, limit access to other foods and treats.
  - Short-term (weeks to months) treatment with a calculolytic diet and antibiotics as needed is effective in dissolving infection-induced struvite uroliths.
  - Avoid feeding calculolytic diets to immature cats.
- Struvite—dog
  - Infection-induced struvite urolithiasis may be prevented by eradicating and controlling infections by urease-producing bacteria.
  - Recurrent sterile struvite uroliths may be prevented by use of acidifying, magnesium-restricted diets (Hill's Prescription Diet Canine c/d and others) or urine acidifiers.
  - Monitor patients whose urine has been acidified for calcium oxalate crystalluria. Change management protocol if persistent calcium oxalate crystalluria develops.
  - In patients at risk for both struvite and other urolith types, focus dietary prevention of metabolic uroliths (e.g., calcium oxalate, urate, cystine)—and UTI prevention for struvite uroliths.

POSSIBLE COMPLICATIONS

- CaOx
  - Urocystoliths can pass into and obstruct the urethra.
  - Dogs that do not consume their daily requirement of some urolith prevention foods may develop various degrees of protein calorie malnutrition.

- Diet-associated hyperlipidemia develops in some patients consuming foods with higher fat content. Miniature schnauzers with hereditary hyperlipidemia are predisposed to pancreatitis when consuming some prevention foods.
- When treating multiple conditions (obesity, diarrhea, etc.) consider diets that are indexed to also prevent CaOx.

■ CaPh
■ Struvite—cat
- Urocystoliths may pass into and obstruct the urethra, especially if the patient is persistently dysuric. Urethral obstruction may be managed by retrograde urohydropropulsion.
- An indwelling transurethral catheter increases the risk for iatrogenic bacterial UTI and urethral stricture.

■ Struvite—dog
- With low protein-high fat struvitolytic diets, potential contraindications include (1) abnormal fluid accumulation, (2) chronic kidney disease, and (3) predispositions to pancreatitis (especially miniature schnauzers with hyperlipidemia).
- Urocystoliths may pass into and obstruct the urethra. Urethral obstruction can be managed by retrograde urohydropropulsion or lithotripsy.
- Dysuria may be minimized by antimicrobic treatment of bacterial UTIs and oral administration of anticholinergic drugs.
- Diet-associated polyuria and increased urine volume (PU) may be associated with varying degrees of urinary incontinence (see Urinary Incontinence). Allow frequent opportunity to urinate to minimize inappropriate housesoiling.

EXPECTED COURSE AND PROGNOSIS

■ CaOx
- Approximately 50% of dogs and 33% of cats reform uroliths in 2–3 years. Treatment to minimize recurrence is helpful.
- Patients with persistent hypercalcemia typically reform uroliths at a faster rate.

■ CaPh
■ Struvite—cat
- Mean times for dissolution of sterile urocystoliths ranged from 13 to 36 days.
- Mean times for dissolution of infection-induced struvite urocystoliths ranged from 21 to 44 days.
- Most struvite uroliths located in the urinary bladder can be safely dissolved with a low risk of adverse effects, including urethral obstruction.

■ Struvite—dog
- Mean time for dissolution of all infection-induced urocystoliths was 3 months (range: 2 weeks–7 months), whereas nephroliths took 6 months (range: 2–10 months). The mean dissolution time of sterile struvite urocystoliths was 6 weeks (range: 4–12 weeks).
- Compliance with dietary recommendations (Hill's s/d) is verified by a reduced concentration of urea in serum (approximately 10 mg/dL) and a low urine-specific gravity (1.004–1.014).
- If uroliths increase or fail to decrease in size after 6–8 months, alternative methods should be considered. Consider:
    - That the wrong mineral component was identified

    - That the nucleus of the uroliths has a different mineral composition than other portions of the urolith
    - The owner is not complying with therapeutic recommendations.
  - With high-sodium dissolution foods lacking protein reduction, the proportion of calcium phosphate carbonate associated with infection-induced struvite has increased and are less amenable to medical dissolution.

MISCELLANEOUS

Associated Conditions

- CaOx: Conditions predisposing to hypercalciuria: hyperadrenocorticism, acidemia, hypervitaminosis D, and hyperparathyroidism; or hyperoxaluria: vitamin B6 deficiency, hereditary hyperoxaluria, and ingestion of chocolate and peanuts.
- Struvite—cat or dog: Any disease that predisposes to bacterial UTI.

Age-Related Factors

- CaOx—Rare in young (<1 year old) animals.
- Struvite—cat—Infection-induced struvite is the most common urolith in immature cats. Sterile struvite is rare in immature cats.
- Struvite—dog: Infection-induced struvite is the most common form of urolith in immature dogs. The uroliths develop as a result of microbial UTI.

Other Uroliths (Not Related To Senior Care)

- Cystine—found in dogs and cats with cystinuria, an inborn error of metabolism caused by defective tubular resorption of cystine (and other compounds)
  - Primarily found in adult dogs and cats
  - Signs depend on location
  - Radiodense, similar to struvite, less than calcium oxalate and phosphate
  - Six-sided, insoluble in acetic acid
  - Management—diet to reduce cystine excretion, diluting and alkalinizing urine.
    - Dogs—Medical dissolution—N-2-MPG (thiol-containing) and u/d
    - Cats—renal insufficiency and geriatric diets
- Urate—uric acid in serum due to impaired conversion of uric acid to allantoin.
  - With (<1 year) or without (mean age: 3.5 years) portosystemic shunts
  - Hepatic function should be evaluated.
  - May be radiolucent.
  - Manage—high moisture, low-purine, alkalinizing diet.
    - Allopurinol for dissolution (not in PSS or Renal failure)
- Xanthine—product of purine degradation; defect in xanthine oxidase—xanthinuria
  - Complication of allopurinol therapy
  - Similar appearance to urate crystals

Synonyms

- Oxalate urolithiasis.
- Apatite uroliths.
- Feline lower urinary tract disease.
- Phosphate calculi.
- Infection stone.
- Urease stone.
- Triple-phosphate stone.

See Also

Nephrolithiasis

Abbreviations

- AAFCO = Association of American Feed Control Officials
- CaOx = calcium oxalate.
- CAP = calcium phosphate apatite.
- CP = calcium phosphate.
- CPC = calcium phosphate carbonate.
- MUC = Minnesota Urolith Center.
- MAP = magnesium ammonium phosphate.
- UTI = urinary tract infection.

Suggested Reading

Appel S, Lefebvre SL, Houston DM, et al. Evaluation of risk factors associated with suture-nidus cystoliths in dogs and cats. *J Am Vet Med Assoc* 2008;233:1889–1895.

Kyles AE, Hardie EM, Wooden BG, et al. Management and outcome of cats with ureteral obstruction: 153 cases (1984–2002). *J Am Vet Med Assoc* 2005;226:937–944.

Lulich JP, Adams LG, Grant D, et al. Changing paradigms in the treatment of uroliths by lithotripsy. *Vet Clin North Am Small Anim Pract* 2009;39:143–160.

Lulich JP, Berent AC, Adams LG, et al. ACVIM Small Animal Consensus recommendations on the treatment and prevention of uroliths in dogs and cats. *J Vet Intern Med* 2016;30:1564–1574.

Lulich JP, Osborne CA. Upper tract urolith: questions, answers, questions. In: August JR (ed.) *Consultations in Feline Internal Medicine*, Volume 5. St. Louis, MO: Elsevier Saunders, 2006; pp. 399–406.

Okafor CC, Lefebvre SL, Pearl DL, et al. Risk factors associated with calcium oxalate urolithiasis in dogs evaluated at general care veterinary hospitals in the United States. *Prevent Vet Med* 2014;115:217–228.

Author/editor: Heidi Lobprise
Thanks to: Julie Byron for review
Topics adapted from Five Minute Veterinary Consultation, 7th edition, 2021
Original Topic: Urolithiasis, Calcium Oxalate

Author: Jody P. Lulich
Original Topic: Urolithiasis, Calcium Phosphate

Authors: Hasan Albasan and Jody P. Lulich
Original Topic: Urolithiasis, Struvite—Cats

Author: John M. Kruger
Original Topic: Urolithiasis, Struvite—Dogs

Author: Jody P. Lulich
Consulting Editor: J.D. Foster

Respiratory

Chapter 81

Bronchitis, Chronic

BASICS

DEFINITION

- Chronic coughing for longer than 2 months that is not attributable to another cause (e.g., neoplasia, congestive heart failure, eosinophilic pneumonia, or infectious bronchitis).
- Partly nonreversible and often slowly progressive condition owing to accompanying pathologic airway changes.

PATHOPHYSIOLOGY

- Recurrent airway inflammation suspected, but a specific cause is rarely determined.
- Persistent tracheobronchial irritation—causes chronic coughing; leads to changes in tracheobronchial epithelium and submucosa.
- Airway inflammation, epithelial edema, and thickening prominent.
- Excess production of thickened mucus is a hallmark.
- In severe, very chronic cases—probable increased lung resistance; decreased expiratory airflow, especially in cats; in dogs, possible sequelae such as broncholamacia and bronchiectasis.

SYSTEMS AFFECTED

- Respiratory
- Cardiovascular—pulmonary hypertension, cor pulmonale.
- Nervous—syncope (infrequent).

SIGNALMENT

Species

Dogs and cats.

Breed Predilections

- Dogs—small and toy breeds common; also observed in large breeds.
- Siamese cats and domestic shorthairs affected.

Mean Age and Range

Most often affects middle-aged and old animals.

Blackwell's Five-Minute Veterinary Consult Clinical Companion: Small Animal Senior Care, First Edition. Edited by Heidi B. Lobprise.

Companion website: www.wiley.com/go/lobprise/Senior

Predominant Sex

N/A, although spayed females are often overrepresented (might be due to weight gain).

SIGNS

Historical Findings

- Coughing—hallmark of tracheobronchial irritation; usually harsh and dry; post-tussive gagging common (owners often misinterpret this as vomiting, especially in dogs).
- Exercise intolerance, difficult breathing, wheezing (in cats).
- Cyanosis and even syncope may be noted in severe cases.

Physical Examination Findings

- Patients usually bright, alert, and afebrile.
- Tracheal palpation—typically results in coughing because of increased tracheal sensitivity.
- Small airway disease—assumed when expiratory abdominal push (during quiet breathing) or end-expiratory wheezing is detected.
- Bronchovesicular lung sounds, end-inspiratory crackles, and wheezing (result of airflow into obstructed airways) may be heard.
- Loud end-expiratory snap is suggestive of concurrent airway collapse.
- Cardiac auscultation—murmurs secondary to valvular insufficiency common in dogs, but not always associated with congestive heart failure; chronic bronchitis usually results in normal or slower-than-normal resting heart rate and pronounced sinus arrhythmia; in cats, tachycardia is possible.
- Obesity—common; important complicating factor.
- Severe dental disease may predispose to lower airway colonization and possible infection (dogs).

CAUSES

Chronic airway inflammation initiated by multiple causes, although specific cause rarely identified.

RISK FACTORS

- Long-term exposure to inhaled irritants.
- Obesity.
- Recurrent bacterial infection.
- Dental disease and laryngeal disease—result in bacterial showering of lower airways.

DIAGNOSIS

DIFFERENTIAL DIAGNOSIS

- Bronchiectasis.
- Eosinophilic bronchopneumopathy.
- Foreign bodies.

- Heartworm disease.
- Bacterial, pneumonia.
- Neoplasia—metastatic more than primary.
- Pulmonary parasites or parasitic larval migration.
- Pulmonary fibrosis—cats and dogs.
- Pulmonary granulomatosis.
- Congestive heart failure—typically associated with high resting heart rate and left atrial enlargement, which may lead to collapse of left principal bronchus.

CBC/BIOCHEMISTRY/URINALYSIS

- Rarely diagnostic.
- Neutrophilic leukocytosis common.
- Absolute eosinophilia—suggests but not diagnostic for allergic bronchitis.
- Polycythemia secondary to chronic hypoxia—may be seen.
- Liver enzymes and bile acids may be elevated due to passive congestion.

OTHER LABORATORY TESTS

- Fecal and heartworm tests—rule out pulmonary parasites.
- Pulse oximetry—useful for detecting hemoglobin desaturation.
- Arterial blood gas analysis—collect, ice, and have analyzed at a local hospital; mild-to-moderately low partial pressure of oxygen (PaO_2) seen with severe condition; aids in prognosis and monitoring treatment.
- As hyperadrenocorticism could be responsible for obesity and/or enlarged liver/abdomen, testing should be considered if clinically indicated.

IMAGING

Thoracic Radiography (High-Resolution Computed Topography)

Common features (in descending order of frequency)—bronchial thickening; interstitial pattern; middle lung lobe consolidation (cats); atelectasis; hyperinflation and diaphragmatic flattening (primarily cats).

Echocardiography

- May reveal right heart enlargement with pulmonary hypertension.
- Helps rule out cardiac disease as a cause of coughing.
- Check for pulmonary hypertension via Doppler echocardiography.

DIAGNOSTIC PROCEDURES

Bronchoscopy

Preferred test for assessing the lower airways.

- Allows direct visualization of structural as well as functional (dynamic) changes; allows selected airway sampling (e.g., biopsy and lavage).
- Gross changes—excess mucoid to mucopurulent secretions; epithelial edema or thickening with blunting of bronchial bifurcations; irregular or granular mucosa; mucosal polypoid proliferations can indicate chronic bronchitis or chronic eosinophilic pneumonia.

- Large airway caliber changes (e.g., static or dynamic airway collapse and bronchiectasis)—may be detected as complicating problems.

Evaluation of Airway Secretions

- Must collect from lower airways—helps to establish underlying cause if present or to determine the severity of inflammation.
- Throat swab cultures are not representative of lower airway flora
- Tracheal aspiration or bronchoalveolar lavage—collect specimens for cytologic examination and bacterial/mycoplasmal culture or qPRC assessment.
- Quantitated aerobic bronchoalveolar lavage (BAL) cultures help differentiate infection versus airway colonization; reported cutoff is $>1.7 \times 10^3$ colony-forming units (CFU) for infection in dogs. Anaerobic and *Mycoplasma* cultures recommended as well.
- Cytology—inflammation primary finding; most cells are neutrophils, eosinophils, or macrophages; evaluate for bacteria, parasites, neoplastic cells, and contamination with foreign material.
- Recurrent infections—implicated in pathogenesis of bronchitis; however, positive cultures are not frequently reported; *Mycoplasma* infection discussed but rarely confirmed as a cause.

TREATMENT

APPROPRIATE HEALTH CARE

- Usually outpatient—oxygen can be given at home in chronic cases.
- Inpatient—if requires oxygen therapy, parenteral medication, or aerosol therapy; patients that owners cannot keep calm at home during initial stages of therapy.

NURSING CARE

Consider saline nebulization followed by coupage and/or gentle exercise to encourage removal of airway secretions.

ACTIVITY

- Exercise—moderate (not forced) useful in clearing secretions; assists with weight loss.
- Limit if exertion causes excessive coughing.
- Use a harness instead of a collar.

DIET

Weight loss critical—improves PaO_2, attitude, and exercise tolerance in obese patients; reduces cough frequency.

CLIENT EDUCATION

- Warn client that chronic bronchitis is an incurable disease and complete suppression of all coughing is an unattainable goal.
- Stress that aggressive treatment (including weight control, avoiding risk factors, and medical treatment) minimizes the severity of the coughing and slows disease progression in most patients.

SURGICAL CONSIDERATIONS

Treat severe dental disease to minimize secondary bacterial complications.

MEDICATIONS

DRUG(S) OF CHOICE

Corticosteroids

- Diminish airway inflammation and coughing regardless of the underlying cause.
- Indicated for noninfectious conditions.
- With allergic or hypersensitivity reactions—require long-term administration; attempt to wean off steroids or determine lowest effective dosage.
- Prednisolone preferred in cats.
- Prednisone or prednisolone usually initiated at 0.5–1 mg/kg PO q12h for a variable time, with tapering of the dosage based on clinical signs.
- Inhaled agents (e.g., budenoside or fluticasone 1–3 puffs using metered dose inhalers [variable concentrations exist] a day) are often effective and can be used to reduce systemic side effects of corticosteroids; they are delivered via a spacer chamber and face mask (e.g., AeroDawg); however, the most adequate dose is not clearly established.

Bronchodilators

Commonly prescribed, although limited evidence of efficacy.

Antibiotics

- Select on basis of quantitated culture and sensitivity test results.

Antitussives

- Indicated for nonproductive, paroxysmal, continuous, or debilitating cough.
- Dogs—butorphanol (0.55 mg/kg PO q6–12h; 0.055–0.11 mg/kg SC); hydrocodone (0.1–0.3 mg/kg q6–8h PO). Over-the-counter cough suppressants are rarely effective; gabapentin 2–5 mg/kg by mouth every eight hours (but unestablished efficacy).

CONTRAINDICATIONS

Lasix and atropine—do not use because of drying effects on tracheobronchial secretions.

PRECAUTIONS

- Beta agonists (e.g., terbutaline and albuterol)—may cause tachycardia, nervousness, and muscle tremors; typically transient.
- Theophylline—may cause tachycardia, restlessness, excitability, vomiting, and diarrhea; evaluate ethylene diamine tetra-acetate (EDTA) plasma sample for peak plasma concentration (ideally 5–20 μg/mL); toxicity may be more common with generic formulations.

POSSIBLE INTERACTIONS

Fluoroquinolones decrease theophylline clearance in dogs and can result in theophylline toxicity.

ALTERNATIVE DRUG(S)

Maropitant (some antitussive properties suggested, but not advised yet).

FOLLOW-UP

PATIENT MONITORING

- Follow abnormalities revealed by physical examination and selected diagnostic tests—determine response to treatment.
- Monitor weight; arterial blood gases usually improve after significant weight loss.

PREVENTION/AVOIDANCE

Avoid and address risk factors (see Risk Factors).

POSSIBLE COMPLICATIONS

- Syncope—possible complication of chronic coughing, particularly in toy-breed dogs.
- Pulmonary hypertension and cor pulmonale—most serious complications.
- Bronchectasis and airway remodeling.

EXPECTED COURSE AND PROGNOSIS

- Progressive airway changes—syncopal episodes, chronic hypoxia, right ventricular hypertrophy, and pulmonary hypertension.
- Acute exacerbations—common with seasonal changes, air quality changes, worsened inflammation, and potentially development of secondary infection.

MISCELLANEOUS

Associated Conditions

- Syncope—secondary to chronic coughing or development of pulmonary hypertension.
- Increased susceptibility to airway infection, chronic hypoxia, pulmonary hypertension, and cor pulmonale.

Abbreviations

- BAL = bronchoalveolar lavage
- CFU = colony-forming unit.
- EDTA = ethylene diamine tetra-acetate.
- PaO_2 = partial pressure of oxygen.

Suggested Reading

Grotheer M, Hirschberger J, Hartmann K, et al. Comparison of signalment, clinical, laboratory and radiographic parameters in cats with feline asthma and chronic bronchitis. *J Feline Med Surg* 2020;22(7):649–655.

Reinero CR, Masseau I, Grobman M, et al. Perspectives in veterinary medicine: description and classification of bronchiolar disorders in cats. *J Vet Intern Med* 2019;33(3):1201–1221.

Rozanski E. Canine chronic bronchitis. An update. *Vet Clin N Am Small Anim Pract* 2020;50:393–404.

Author/editor: Heidi Lobprise
Topic adapted from Five Minute Veterinary Consultation, 7th edition, 2021
Original Topic: Bronchitis, Chronic

Author: Cécile Clercx
Consulting Editor: Elizabeth Rozanski

Chapter 82

Chylothorax

BASICS

DEFINITION

- Accumulation of chyle in the pleural space.
- Chyle—triglyceride-rich fluid from the intestinal lymphatics that empties into the venous system (usually cranial cava/jugular vein) in the thorax.
- Pseudochylous effusion—effusion that contains less triglycerides and more cholesterol compared to serum, but appears fatty grossly.
- Thoracic lymphangiectasia—tortuous, dilated lymphatics found in many animals with chylothorax.
- Fibrosing pleuritis—condition in which pleural thickening leads to constriction of lung lobes; when severe, results in marked restriction of ventilation; can be caused by any chronic pleural exudate, but is most commonly associated with chylothorax and pyothorax.

PATHOPHYSIOLOGY

- Alteration of flow-through thoracic duct (TD) leading to leakage of chyle—can be related to increased pressure or permeability in TD or venous obstruction downstream.
- Can be caused by any disease or process that increases systemic venous pressure at the entrance of the TD to the venous system.
- Cardiac causes—pericardial disease, cardiomyopathy, heartworm disease, other causes of right-sided heart failure; thrombosis around pacing lead wire.
- Noncardiac causes—neoplasia (especially mediastinal lymphoma in cats), lung lobe torsion, diaphragmatic hernia, venous granuloma, venous thrombus.
- Rare TD rupture/trauma—surgical (thoracotomy), nonsurgical (e.g., hit by car).
- Idiopathic considered most common.

SYSTEMS AFFECTED

- Respiratory—due to reduced lung expansion.
- Systemic signs can be present secondary to the respiratory distress (e.g., decreased appetite, weight loss).

Blackwell's Five-Minute Veterinary Consult Clinical Companion: Small Animal Senior Care, First Edition. Edited by Heidi B. Lobprise.

Companion website: www.wiley.com/go/lobprise/Senior

SIGNALMENT

Species

Dog and cat.

Breed Predilections

- Dogs—Afghan hound and Shiba Inu.
- Cats—oriental breeds (e.g., Siamese and Himalayan).

Mean Age and Range

- Any age affected.
- Cats—more common in older cats; could indicate an association with neoplasia.
- Afghan hound—develop when middle-aged.
- Shiba Inu—develop when young (<1–2 years of age).

SIGNS

General Comments

- Signs will depend on the rate of fluid accumulation and volume of pleural effusion.
- Usually not exhibited until there is marked impairment of ventilation.
- Many patients appear to have the condition for prolonged periods before diagnosis.

Historical Findings

- Tachypnea and respiratory difficulty.
- Coughing—can be present for months before examination, likely due to lung compression associated with pleural effusion.
- Lethargy.
- Anorexia and weight loss.
- Exercise intolerance.

Physical Examination Findings

- Vary with cause of effusion.
- Muffled heart and lung sounds ventrally.
- Increased bronchovesicular sounds, particularly in dorsal lung fields.
- Pale mucous membranes or cyanosis.
- Arrhythmia.
- Heart murmur.
- Signs of right-sided heart failure (e.g., jugular pulses, ascites, hepatomegaly).
- Decreased compressibility of anterior chest—common in cats with a cranial mediastinal mass.

CAUSES

- Cranial mediastinal masses—lymphoma, thymoma.
- Cardiac disease—heartworm, cardiomyopathy, pericardial disease, congenital diseases.
- Lung lobe torsion.
- Venous obstruction—granuloma, thrombi.

- Cardiac or thoracic surgery.
- Idiopathic—most common cause.

DIAGNOSIS

DIFFERENTIAL DIAGNOSIS

Other causes of pleural effusion—neoplasia, pyothorax, heart failure, feline infectious peritonitis (FIP).

CBC/BIOCHEMISTRY/URINALYSIS

- Often normal.
- Lymphopenia and hypoalbuminemia—can be found; hyponatremia and hyperkalemia sometimes noted due to fluid shifts with repeat thoracocentesis.

OTHER LABORATORY TESTS

Heartworm testing.

Fluid Analysis

- Classified as an exudate.
- Color will depend on fat content from diet and presence of concurrent hemorrhage—usually milky white and opaque, but can appear serosanguinous and range from yellow to pink.
- Protein content varies, and high lipid content will make refractive index inaccurate.
- Total nucleated cell count—usually <10,000 cells/μL.
- Fluid triglycerides—higher compared to serum.
- Fluid cholesterol—lower compared to serum.

Cytology

- Place sample in an EDTA tube to allow cell count to be performed.
- Initially, cytology comprises primarily small lymphocytes, neutrophils, and macrophages containing lipid.
- Chronic effusions contain fewer lymphocytes due to continued loss and more nondegenerate neutrophils due to inflammation from multiple thoracocenteses or irritation of pleural lining by chyle.
- Atypical lymphocytes—suggestive of underlying neoplasia.

IMAGING

Thoracic Radiography

- Two to four views if patient is stable—pleural effusion.
- Dorsoventral view associated with less stress than ventrodorsal view in animal with respiratory difficulty.
- Repeat radiographs after thoracocentesis to assess for underlying causes of effusion or evidence of fibrosing pleuritis; if collapsed lung lobes do not appear to reexpand after pleural fluid is removed or if respiratory distress persists with only minimal fluid present, suspect underlying pulmonary parenchymal or pleural disease (e.g., fibrosing pleuritis).

Ultrasonography/Echocardiography

- Should be performed before thoracocentesis if patient is stable—fluid acts as an acoustic window, enhancing visualization of thoracic structures.
- Assess for underlying causes—detect abnormal cardiac structure and function, pericardial disease, and mediastinal masses.

CT Lymphangiography

- Can quantify TD branches more accurately than standard radiographic lymphangiography.
- In dogs, percutaneously inject 1–2 mL of nonionic contrast material into mesenteric lymph nodes using ultrasound or CT guidance.
- Acquire helical thoracic CT images before and after injection of contrast media.
- Can document location and character of TD and its tributary lymphatics; likely useful for surgical planning.

TREATMENT

APPROPRIATE HEALTH CARE

- Dyspneic animal—immediate thoracocentesis; removal of even small amounts of pleural effusion can markedly improve ventilation.
- Identify and treat the underlying cause, if possible.
- Medical management—usually treated on outpatient basis with intermittent thoracocentesis as needed based on clinical signs (see Medications).
- Chest tubes—place *only* in patients with suspected chylothorax secondary to trauma (very rare), in cases with rapid fluid accumulation, or after surgery.
- Surgery if medical management does not resolve the problem in 2–3 months (see Surgical Considerations); some clinicians believe earlier intervention is better to avoid potential for development of restrictive pleuritis.

NURSING CARE

- Patients undergoing multiple thoracocenteses can rarely develop electrolyte abnormalities (hyponatremia, hyperkalemia) that may need to be corrected with fluid therapy.
- Thoracocentesis—perform under aseptic conditions to reduce risk of iatrogenic infection; antibiotic prophylaxis generally unnecessary if proper technique is used.

ACTIVITY

Patients will usually restrict their own exercise as pleural fluid volume increases or if they develop fibrosing pleuritis.

DIET

- Low fat—potentially decreases the amount of fat in the effusion, which would improve the patient's ability to resorb fluid from the thoracic cavity; not a cure; may help in management by facilitating reabsorption.
- Medium-chain triglycerides are transported via the TD in dogs and are no longer recommended.

CLIENT EDUCATION

- Inform client that no specific treatment will stop the effusion in all patients with the idiopathic form of the disease.
- Inform client that the condition can spontaneously resolve in some patients after several weeks or months.

SURGICAL CONSIDERATIONS

TD Ligation and Pericardiectomy

- Recommended in patients that do not respond to medical management.
- The duct usually has multiple branches in the caudal thorax where ligation is performed; failure to occlude all branches results in continued pleural effusion.
- Always perform in conjunction with lymphangiography; methylene blue injected in the mesenteric lymph node greatly facilitates visualization and complete occlusion of all branches.
- Thickening of the pericardium can prevent formation of lymphaticovenous communications—perform pericardiectomy simultaneously with TD ligation; reports of up to 100% success rate when both techniques are performed; second surgery can be necessary if all branches are not occluded.
- Video-assisted thorascopic surgery for thoracic duct ligation and pericardiectomy is reported to have similar success rates to thoracotomy (86%).

Other

- Success rates of 83–88% reported for cysterna chyli ablation in combination with TD ligation.
- Salvage procedures for recurrence after TD ligation include cisterna chyli and TD glue embolization, pleuroperitoneal or pleurovenous shunts, or placement of a PleuralPort®.

MEDICATIONS

DRUG(S) OF CHOICE

- Rutin 50–100 mg/kg PO q8h; believed to increase macrophage removal of proteins, which promotes absorption of fluid; complete resolution of effusion appears to occur in some patients; further study is required to determine whether resolution occurs spontaneously or in response to this therapy.
- Somatostatin analog (octreotide)—a naturally occurring substance that inhibits gastric, pancreatic, and biliary secretions and prolongs gastrointestinal transit time, decreases jejunal secretion, and stimulates gastrointestinal water absorption; in traumatic chylothorax, reduction of gastrointestinal secretions may aid healing of the TD by decreasing TD lymphatic flows; resolution of pleural fluid has occurred in dogs and cats with idiopathic chylothorax in which octreotide has been administered, but the mechanism is unknown; octreotide (Sandostatin®; 10 μg/kg SC q8h for 2–3 weeks) is a synthetic analog of somatostatin that has a prolonged half-life and minimal side effects.

CONTRAINDICATIONS

Cardiac disease or neoplasia—treat the underlying disease rather than the effusion (other than heartworm disease in cats where TD ligation may be beneficial while the heartworm infection clears).

FOLLOW-UP

PATIENT MONITORING

- Monitor for signs of recurrence of pleural effusion (tachypnea, labored breathing, respiratory distress)—perform thoracentesis as needed.
- Periodically reevaluate for several years to detect recurrence.

POSSIBLE COMPLICATIONS

- Fibrosing pleuritis.
- Iatrogenic infection with repeated thoracocentesis—important to use aseptic technique.

EXPECTED COURSE AND PROGNOSIS

- Can resolve spontaneously or after surgery.
- Untreated or chronic disease—can result in severe fibrosing pleuritis and persistent dyspnea.
- Euthanasia—frequently performed in patients that do not respond to surgery or medical management.

MISCELLANEOUS

Associated Conditions

Diffuse lymphatic abnormalities (e.g., intestinal lymphangiectasia, hepatic lymphangiectasia, pulmonary lymphangiectasia, and chylous ascites)—may be noted; may worsen the prognosis.

Age-Related Factors

Young patients may have a better prognosis than old animals because of the association of neoplasia with advanced age.

Abbreviations

- FIP = feline infectious peritonitis
- TD = thoracic duct.

Suggested Reading

Allman DA, Radlinsky MG, Ralph AG, Rawlings CA. Thoracoscopic thoracic duct ligation and thoracoscopic pericardiectomy for treatment of chylothorax in dogs. *Vet Surg* 2010;39(1):21–27.

Fossum TW, Mertens MM, Miller MW, et al. Thoracic duct ligation and pericardectomy for treatment of idiopathic chylothorax. *J Vet Intern Med* 2004;18:307–310.

Johnson EG, Wisner ER, Kyles A, et al. Computed tomographic lymphography of the thoracic duct by mesenteric lymph node injection. *Vet Surg* 2009;38(3):361–367.

Author/editor: Heidi Lobprise
Topic adapted from Five Minute Veterinary Consultation, 7th edition, 2021
Original Topic: Chylothorax

Author: Elizabeth Rozanski
Consulting Editor: Elizabeth Rozanski

Chapter 83

Pleural Effusion

BASICS

DEFINITION

Abnormal accumulation of fluid within the pleural cavity.

PATHOPHYSIOLOGY

- More than normal production or less than normal resorption of fluid.
- Alterations in hydrostatic and oncotic pressures or vascular permeability and lymphatic function may contribute to fluid accumulation.

SYSTEMS AFFECTED

- Cardiovascular.
- Respiratory.

SIGNALMENT

Species

Dog and cat.

Breed Predilections

Varies with underlying cause.

Mean Age and Range

- Young animals—more commonly infection.
- Old animals—more commonly cardiac or neoplastic.

Predominant Sex

Varies with underlying cause.

Blackwell's Five-Minute Veterinary Consult Clinical Companion: Small Animal Senior Care, First Edition. Edited by Heidi B. Lobprise.

Companion website: www.wiley.com/go/lobprise/Senior

SIGNS

General Comments

Depend on the fluid volume, rapidity of fluid accumulation, and the underlying cause.

Historical Findings

- Dyspnea, tachypnea, orthopnea, open-mouth breathing.
- Cyanosis.
- Exercise intolerance.
- Lethargy.
- Inappetence.
- Cough.

Physical Examination Findings

- Dyspnea—respirations often shallow and rapid.
- Muffled or inaudible heart and lung sounds ventrally.
- Preservation of breath sounds dorsally.
- Dullness ventrally on thoracic percussion.

CAUSES

High Hydrostatic Pressure

- Congestive heart failure (CHF).
- Overhydration.
- Intrathoracic neoplasia.

Low Oncotic Pressure

Hypoalbuminemia—occurs in protein-losing enteropathy, protein-losing nephropathy, and liver disease.

Vascular or Lymphatic Abnormality

- Infectious—bacterial, viral, or fungal.
- Neoplasia (e.g., mediastinal lymphoma, thymoma, mesothelioma, primary lung tumor, and metastatic disease).
- Chylothorax (e.g., from lymphangiectasia, CHF, cranial vena caval obstruction [sometimes associated with transvenous pacemaker implantation], neoplasia, fungal infections, heartworms, diaphragmatic hernia, lung lobe torsion, trauma).
- Diaphragmatic hernia.
- Hemothorax (e.g., from trauma, neoplasia, coagulopathy, *Angiostrongylus vasorum*).
- Lung lobe torsion.
- Pulmonary thromboembolism.
- Pancreatitis.

DIAGNOSIS

DIFFERENTIAL DIAGNOSIS

- Historical or physical evidence of external trauma—consider hemothorax or diaphragmatic hernia.
- Fever suggests an inflammatory, infectious, or neoplastic cause.

- Murmurs, gallops, or arrhythmias combined with jugular venous distension or pulsation suggest an underlying cardiac cause.
- Concurrent ascites suggests feline infectious peritonitis (FIP), CHF (mainly dogs), severe hypoalbuminemia, diaphragmatic hernia, disseminated neoplasia, or pancreatitis.
- In cats, decreased compressibility of the cranial thorax suggests a cranial mediastinal mass.
- Concurrent ocular changes (e.g., chorioretinitis and uveitis) suggest FIP or fungal disease.
- Hypothermia often associated with cardiac cause.

CBC/BIOCHEMISTRY/URINALYSIS

- Hemogram results may be abnormal in patients with pyothorax, FIP, neoplasia, or lung lobe torsion.
- Severe hypoalbuminemia (generally <1 g/dL to cause effusion) suggests protein-losing enteropathy, protein-losing nephropathy, or liver disease.
- Hyperglobulinemia (polyclonal) suggests FIP.

OTHER LABORATORY TESTS

- Fluid analysis should include physical characteristics (i.e., color, clarity, odor, clots), pH, glucose, total protein, total nucleated cell count, and cytologic examination; Table 83.1 provides characteristics of various pleural fluid types and their disease associations.
- In cats the lactate dehydrogenase concentration in transudates is <200 IU/L and in exudates it is >200 IU/L.
- Pleural fluid pH <6.9 suggests pyothorax in cats.
- Glucose concentration in pleural fluid usually parallels levels in serum. In cats, pyothorax and malignancy lower pleural fluid glucose concentration relative to serum glucose concentration; thus, pleural fluid with a normal pH and low glucose concentration suggests malignancy in cats.
- Serologic tests for feline leukemia virus (if patient has mediastinal lymphoma), feline immunodeficiency virus (if patient has pyothorax), and coronavirus (if FIP is suspected) are available.
- Cardiac disease suspected—consider a heartworm test in dogs and cats; NT-proBNP and thyroid evaluation in cats.
- Infection suspected—obtain aerobic and anaerobic bacterial culture and sensitivity tests and consider special stains (e.g., Gram and acid-fast stains) of the fluid.
- FIP suspected—consider protein electrophoresis of the fluid; gamma-globulin level >32% of total protein strongly suggests a diagnosis of FIP.
- Chyle suspected—do an ether clearance test or Sudan stain of the pleural fluid, and triglyceride and cholesterol evaluations of the fluid and serum.

IMAGING

Radiographic Findings

- Used to confirm pleural effusion; should not be performed until after thoracocentesis in dyspneic patients with evidence of pleural effusion on physical examination.
- Evidence of pleural effusion includes separation of lung borders away from the thoracic wall and sternum by fluid density in the pleural space, fluid-filled interlobar fissure lines, loss or blurring of the cardiac and diaphragmatic borders, blunting of the lung

TABLE 83.1 Characterization of pleural fluid.

	Transudate	Modified transudate	Nonseptic exudate	Septic exudate	Chyle	Hemorrhage
Color	Colorless to pale yellow	Yellow or pink	Yellow or pink	Yellow to red-brown	Milky white	Red
Turbidity	Clear	Clear to cloudy	Clear to cloudy; fibrin	Cloudy to opaque;	Opaque fibrin	Opaque
Protein (g/dL)	<1.5	2.5–5.0	3.0–8.0	3.0–7.0	2.5–6.0	3.0
Nucleated cells/μL	<1000	1000–7000 (LSA up to 100,000)	5000–20,000 (LSA up to 100,000)	5000–300,000	1000–20,000	Similar to peripheral blood
Cytology	Mostly mesothelial cells and macrophages	Mostly macrophages and mesothelial cells; few nondegenerate PMNs; neoplastic cells in some cases	Mostly nondegenerate PMNs and macrophages; neoplastic cells in some cases	Mostly degenerate PMNs; also macrophages; bacteria	Small lymphocytes, PMNs, and macrophages	Mostly RBCs; with erythrophagocytosis
Disease associations	Hypoalbuminemia (protein-losing nephropathy, protein-losing enteropathy, or liver disease); early CHF	CHF; neoplasia; diaphragmatic hernia; pancreatitis	FIP; neoplasia; diaphragmatic hernia; lung lobe torsion	Pyothorax	Lymphangiectasia, CHF, cranial vena cava obstruction, neoplasia, fungal, dirofilariasias, diaphragmatic hernia, lung lobe torsion, trauma	Trauma, coagulopathy, neoplasia, lung lobe torsion

Source: Modified from Sherding RG. Diseases of the pleural cavity. In: Sherding RG (ed.) *The Cat: Diseases and Clinical Management*, 2nd edn. New York: Churchill Livingstone, 1994; p. 1061.

margins at the costophrenic angles (ventrodorsal view), and widening of the mediastinum (ventrodorsal view).
- Rounding of the caudal lung lobe borders (lateral view)—most common in patients with fibrosing pleuritis caused by chylothorax, pyothorax, or FIP.
- Unilateral effusion—most common in patients with chylothorax and pyothorax; hemothorax, pulmonary neoplasia, diaphragmatic hernia, and lung lobe torsion.
- Evaluate post-thoracocentesis radiographs carefully for cardiomegaly, intrapulmonary lesions, mediastinal masses, diaphragmatic hernia, lung lobe torsion, and evidence of trauma (e.g., rib fractures).
- Can diagnose a diaphragmatic hernia with positive-contrast peritoneography.
- Can evaluate the thoracic duct by positive-contrast lymphangiography.
- CT imaging may help differentiate malignant from inflammatory effusions.

Echocardiographic Findings

- Ultrasonographic evaluation of the thorax is recommended whenever cardiac disease, diaphragmatic hernia, or cranial mediastinal mass is suspected.
- Echocardiography is easiest to perform before thoracocentesis, provided the patient is stable.

DIAGNOSTIC PROCEDURES

- Thoracocentesis—allows characterization of the fluid type and determination of potential underlying cause.
- Exploratory thoracotomy or thoracoscopy—to obtain biopsy specimens of lung, lymph nodes, or pleura, if indicated.

TREATMENT

- First, thoracocentesis to relieve respiratory distress; if the patient is stable after thoracocentesis, outpatient treatment may be possible for some diseases. Most patients are hospitalized because they require intensive management such as indwelling chest tubes (e.g., patients with pyothorax) or thoracic surgery.
- Preventing fluid reaccumulation requires treatment based on a definitive diagnosis.
- Surgery is indicated for management of some neoplasias, diaphragmatic hernia repair, lymphangiectasia (i.e., thoracic duct ligation), foreign body removal, and lung lobe torsion (i.e., lung lobectomy).
- Pleuroperitoneal shunts may relieve clinical signs in animals with intractable pleural effusion.
- Vascular access ports attached to intrathoracic Jackson–Pratt drains can be tried for chronic effusions that are not responsive to the therapy of the underlying disorder.

MEDICATIONS

DRUG(S) OF CHOICE

- Treatment varies with specific disease.
- Diuretics generally reserved for patients with diseases causing fluid retention and volume overload (e.g., CHF).

PRECAUTIONS

- Avoid drugs that depress respiration or decrease blood pressure.
- Inappropriate use of diuretics predisposes the patient to dehydration and electrolyte disturbances without eliminating the effusion.

FOLLOW-UP

PATIENT MONITORING

Radiographic evaluation is key to assessment of treatment in most patients.

POSSIBLE COMPLICATIONS

- Death due to respiratory compromise.
- Reexpansion pulmonary edema may develop after pleural effusion is manually removed.

EXPECTED COURSE AND PROGNOSIS

Varies with underlying cause, but usually guarded to poor. In a study of 81 cases of pleural effusion in dogs, 25% recovered completely and 33% died during or were euthanized immediately after completing diagnostic evaluation.

MISCELLANEOUS

Synonyms

- Hydrothorax = transudates and modified transudates.
- Pyothorax = empyema, septic pleuritis.

Abbreviations

- CHF = congestive heart failure
- FIP = feline infectious peritonitis.
- LSA = lymphoma.
- PMN = polymorphonuclear cell.
- RBC = red blood cell.

Suggested Reading

Epstein SE. Exudative pleural diseases in small animals. *Vet Clin North Am Small Anim Pract* 2014;44(1):161–180.

König A, Hartmann K, Mueller RS, et al. Retrospective analysis of pleural effusion in cats. *J Feline Med Surg* 2019;21(12):1102–1110.

Mellanby RJ, Villiers E, Herrtage ME. Canine pleural effusions: a retrospective study of 81 cases. *J Small Anim Pract* 2002;43(10):447–451.

Ruiz MD, Vessieres F, Ragetly GR, Hernandez JL. Characterization of and factors associated with causes of pleural effusion in cats. *J Am Vet Med Assoc* 2018;253(2):181–187.

Smeak DD, Birchard SJ, McLoughlin MA, et al. Treatment of chronic pleural effusion with pleuroperitoneal shunts in dogs: 14 cases (1985–1999). *J Am Vet Med Assoc* 2001;219(11):1590–1597.

Author/editor: Heidi Lobprise
Topic adapted from Five Minute Veterinary Consultation, 7th edition, 2021
Original Topic: Pleural Effusion

Author: Francis W.K. Smith, Jr.
Consulting Editor: Michael Aherne

Chapter 84

Pulmonary Edema, Noncardiogenic

BASICS

DEFINITION

Accumulation of edema fluid in the pulmonary interstitium and alveoli, in the absence of heart disease.

PATHOPHYSIOLOGY

- Associated with increased pulmonary vascular permeability and leakage of fluid into the interstitium and alveoli; if severe, can be accompanied by an inflammatory response and accumulation of neutrophils and macrophages.
- Several mechanisms contribute to changes in pulmonary vascular permeability.
- Stimulation of brainstem (medulla) vasomotor centers can lead to a reflex systemic release of catecholamines resulting in systemic vasoconstriction and temporary shunting of blood into the pulmonary circulation resulting in transient pulmonary circulatory overload and endothelial damage—likely pathogenesis in patients with neurogenic edema, electrocution, and upper airway obstruction.
- In patients with upper airway obstruction, negative intrathoracic pressure from inspiratory attempts against an airway obstruction also contributes to edema formation.
- Increased vascular permeability can be part of a generalized inflammatory response that develops in patients with systemic inflammatory response syndrome (SIRS), sepsis, or pancreatitis.
- The inciting insult can trigger a cascade inflammatory response that often worsens over 24 hours following the initial episode.
- Severity of clinical manifestation varies, ranging from mild to severe; the most seriously affected patients can progress from normal to death rapidly after the incident.

SYSTEMS AFFECTED

- Respiratory.
- Cardiovascular—hypotension, tachycardia, and shock.
- Hemic/lymphatic/immune—if severe and causing respiratory failure, can be associated with disseminated intravascular coagulation (DIC).
- Renal/urologic—acute renal failure.

Blackwell's Five-Minute Veterinary Consult Clinical Companion: Small Animal Senior Care,
First Edition. Edited by Heidi B. Lobprise.

Companion website: www.wiley.com/go/lobprise/Senior

SIGNALMENT

Species

Dog and cat.

Breed Predilections

None specific; brachycephalic dogs are more prone to airway obstruction, older large-breed dogs—laryngeal paralysis, small-breed dogs—tracheal collapse.

Mean Age and Range

- Older—associated with laryngeal obstruction and neoplasia.
- Higher incidence in pediatrics—associated with strangulation, head trauma, and electric cord bites.

SIGNS

General Comments

Vary, depending on underlying cause and severity.

Historical Findings

- Predisposing causes—airway obstruction; electric cord bite; seizures; head trauma; near drowning; smoke exposure; adverse drug effects.
- Acute onset of dyspnea.

Physical Examination Findings

- Mild-to-severe dyspnea.
- Increased respiratory rate and effort; open-mouthed breathing.
- Postural adaptations to respiratory distress (if severe) - orthopnea, unwillingness to lie down.
- Pale or cyanotic mucous membranes (severe).
- Harsh lung sounds (early, mild) or generalized crackles (late, severe) on auscultation.
- Expectoration of pink froth or bubbles; can have large volumes of bloody fluid flowing out of endotracheal tube in severely affected intubated animals.
- Normal cardiac auscultation; can detect arrhythmias; tachycardia common.
- Oral ulceration or burns if electrocution.
- Cranial nervous system abnormalities or other indications of neurologic disease.
- Stridor over the upper airway in cases of brachycephalic syndrome, airway masses/abscesses, or foreign bodies.
- Smokey odor or burns indicative of smoke exposure.

CAUSES

- Upper airway obstruction—laryngeal paralysis; choke-chain injury; mass; abscess.
- Electrocution.
- Acute neurologic disease—head trauma; intra-cranial hypertension, prolonged seizures.
- Smoke inhalation.
- Aspiration pneumonia.

- Systemic inflammatory response syndrome—sepsis; endotoxemia; pancreatitis.
- Anaphylaxis (cats).
- Near drowning.
- Adverse drug reactions including certain anesthetic drugs (ketamine), thiazides, or certain antineoplastics (vincristine, cisplatin in cats).
- Transfusion-related acute lung injury—limited evidence in veterinary medicine.
- Vasculitis.

RISK FACTORS

- Hypoproteinemia.
- Crystalloid fluid resuscitation.

DIAGNOSIS

DIFFERENTIAL DIAGNOSIS

- Cardiogenic pulmonary edema.
- Pulmonary infection—bacterial, viral, or fungal pneumonia.
- Pulmonary neoplasia.
- Pulmonary hemorrhage (e.g., anticoagulant rodenticide exposure).
- Pulmonary thromboembolism.

CBC/BIOCHEMISTRY/URINALYSIS

- Leukocytosis common, leukopenia, and thrombocytopenia possible due to neutrophil sequestration in the lung and platelet consumption.
- Biochemistries—usually normal; may note hypoalbuminemia owing to pulmonary protein loss; mild stress-related hyperglycemia.
- Urinalysis—usually normal.

OTHER LABORATORY TESTS

Coagulation testing—mild-to-moderate prolongation of prothrombin time/partial thromboplastin time (PT/PTT) in animals with consumption and DIC. Severe coagulopathy may indicate hemorrhage as true cause for respiratory signs.

IMAGING

- Thoracic radiographs—vital; can reveal prominent interstitial pattern with mild or early disease; alveolar infiltrates with moderate or severe disease; infiltrates commonly but not always in dorsocaudal lung, sometimes asymmetrical and predominantly right-sided. Cardiac silhouette generally normal.
- Echocardiography—rule out cardiogenic pulmonary edema.
- Point-of-care thoracic ultrasound—increased lung rockets (B-lines) may indicate pulmonary edema, increased left atrial:aortic ratio more indicative of cardiogenic edema and underlying heart disease.

DIAGNOSTIC PROCEDURES

- Cytology of airway fluid—inflammatory: neutrophils and some alveolar macrophages. Fluid tends to have high protein values >3 g/dL. Culture negative unless concurrent bacterial pneumonia.
- Edema-fluid-to-plasma ratio (EF:PL) compares protein in the edema fluid to plasma protein. An increased ratio (>0.65) is indicative of noncardiogenic pulmonary edema.
- Pulse oximetry—noninvasive, continuous monitoring of arterial hemoglobin saturation with oxygen and arterial blood gas analysis. Demonstrates mild-to-severe hypoxemia and hypocapnia; not specific but indicates the severity of pulmonary dysfunction.
- B-type natriuretic peptide (NT-proBNP) testing in cats and dogs can suggest underlying heart disease and supports a diagnosis of cardiogenic edema.

TREATMENT

APPROPRIATE HEALTH CARE

- Inpatient vs. outpatient—depends on the severity of respiratory dysfunction and the underlying cause (e.g., airway obstruction or seizures generally require hospitalization).
- Make every effort to resolve and treat the underlying cause.
- Mild to moderate—patients generally improve within 24–48 hours; cardiovascular and respiratory support while the lung repairs.
- Severe—difficult to treat; usually requires positive-pressure ventilation (PPV) due to respiratory failure; many patients die despite treatment.

NURSING CARE

- Oxygen therapy—vital in moderate-to-severe disease; administer via mask or hood, nasal catheter, or oxygen cage; inspired oxygen concentration depends on the severity of disease; most patients do well on 40–50% oxygen, but severe disease can require 80–100% to maintain stability.
- Severe—can require PPV and positive end-expiratory pressure (PEEP).
- Judicious fluid therapy with a balanced electrolyte solution as replacement solution for dehydration or shock; use cautious fluid administration and avoid fluid overload.
- Plasma, albumin, or synthetic colloids—consider with severe hypoproteinemia or low colloid osmotic pressure; improved oncotic pressure may minimize movement of fluid into lungs.

ACTIVITY

Exercise restriction and minimal stress to decrease oxygen requirements.

CLIENT EDUCATION

- Warn client that the condition can worsen before improving.
- Inform client that severe disease progressing rapidly to fulminant pulmonary edema and respiratory failure is associated with a very poor prognosis.

SURGICAL CONSIDERATIONS

Relevant only for treating the underlying cause.

MEDICATIONS

DRUG(S) OF CHOICE

- Damaged endothelium in the pulmonary vasculature—no specific treatment available.
- Inflammatory response—generated by a variety of mediators and cascades; cannot effectively be blocked by anti-inflammatory drugs.
- Furosemide—diuresis not indicated as edema due to permeability changes, not high hydrostatic pressure. May act as bronchodilator and decrease pulmonary shunting, though evidence is limited. Can consider cautious boluses (0.5–2 mg/kg IV, IM) or nebulization, particularly early in course of disease.
- Corticosteroids—for reduction of airway swelling in patients with upper airway obstruction; generally ineffective for pulmonary inflammatory response; if used, recommend anti-inflammatory dosage (e.g., dexamethasone SP at 0.05–0.1 mg/kg IV).
- The use of beta-adrenergic agonists such as terbutaline may increase clearance of alveolar fluid.
- Sedatives—use cautiously if anxiety is contributing to respiratory distress or airway obstruction. Sedation can decrease central respiratory drive, contributing to progression of respiratory failure.
- Additional therapy as indicated by underlying cause—anticonvulsants, analgesia for oral ulcerations.

PRECAUTIONS

- Diuretics (e.g., furosemide)—can cause dehydration and decrease in intravascular volume, exacerbating cardiovascular collapse or shock with minimal effect on edema.
- Corticosteroids—can predispose patients to infectious complications (e.g., pneumonia).

FOLLOW-UP

PATIENT MONITORING

- Monitor respiratory rate, pattern, and auscultation (every 2–4 hours) for the first 24–48 hours, depending on severity of disease.
- Assess pulmonary function by pulse oximetry or arterial blood gas analysis (initially every 2–4 hours), depending on severity of disease.
- Assess packed call volume (PCV) and total solids. Evaluate mucous membranes, pulse quality, heart rate, blood pressure, and urine output every 2–4 hours to assess cardiovascular status and possible progression to shock.

PREVENTION/AVOIDANCE

- Avoid contact with electric wire.
- Correct and avoid airway obstruction.
- Manage seizures and neurologic disease.

POSSIBLE COMPLICATIONS

Usually none if patient recovers from the acute crisis.

EXPECTED COURSE AND PROGNOSIS

- Mild to moderate—resolution of signs in 24–72 hours with supportive care.
- Severe—difficult to treat; can require PPV if respiratory failure.
- Overall survival rates—80–90%.
- Long-term prognosis—excellent if responsive to therapy.

MISCELLANEOUS

Abbreviations

- DIC = disseminated intravascular coagulation
- NT-ProBNP = B-type natriuretic peptide.
- PCV = packed cell volume.
- PEEP = positive end-expiratory pressure.
- PPV = positive-pressure ventilation.
- PT = prothrombin time.
- PTT = partial thromboplastin time.
- SIRS = systemic inflammatory response syndrome.

Suggested Reading

Drobatz KJ, Saunders HM, Pugh C, Hendricks JC. Noncardiogenic pulmonary edema: 26 cases (1987–1993). *J Am Vet Med Assoc* 1995;206:1732–1736.

Kerr LY. Pulmonary edema secondary to upper airway obstruction in the dog: A review of nine cases. *J Am Anim Hosp Assoc* 1989;25:207–212.

Kolata RJ, Burrows CF. The clinical features of injury by chewing electrical cords in dogs and cats. *J Am Anim Hosp Assoc* 1981;17:219–222.

Rozanski EA, Dhupa N, Rush JR, Murtaugh RJ. Differentiation of the etiology of pulmonary edema by measurement of the protein content. *Proc Int Vet Emerg Crit Care Symp VI* 1998:844.

Ward JL, Lisciandro GR, Ware WA, Viall AK, et al. Evaluation of point-of-care thoracic ultrasound and NT-proBNP for the diagnosis of congestive heart failure in cats with respiratory distress. *J Vet Intern Med* 2018;32:1530–1540.

Author/editor: Heidi Lobprise
Topic adapted from Five Minute Veterinary Consultation, 7th edition, 2021
Original Topic: Pulmonary Edema, Non-Cardiogenic

Author: Cassandra O. Janson
Consulting Editors: Elizabeth Rozanski

Chapter 85

Tracheal Collapse

BASICS

DEFINITION

- Static or dynamic reduction in the luminal diameter of the large conducting airway with respiration.
- Can involve the cervical trachea, the intrathoracic trachea, or both segments.
- Airway collapse (bronchomalacia) refers to collapse of lobar bronchi and smaller airways, which can be seen in conjunction with tracheal collapse (tracheobronchomalacia) or alone.
- Compression of the trachea or bronchi due to hilar lymphadenopathy or external mass lesions—not considered part of this condition.

PATHOPHYSIOLOGY

- Hypocellular tracheal cartilage in the cervical region identified historically in some small-breed dogs.
- Lack of chondroitin sulfate and/or decreased glycoproteins within the cartilage matrix results in a reduction in bound water and loss of rigidity in the cartilage.
- Causes of bronchomalacia not established—cartilage abnormalities could include a mechanism similar to cervical tracheal collapse, defects in chondrogenesis, nutritional deficiencies, or degenerative changes caused by chronic airway disease.
- Collapse—weak tracheal cartilage allows flattening of the normal ring structure; trachea collapses in a dorsoventral direction when pressure fluctuates within the airway lumen. During inspiration, intrapleural pressure becomes more negative leading to a drop in intra-airway pressure. Atmospheric pressure exceeds airway pressure in the cervical region and lack of cartilage support results in cervical collapse. During forced expiration, intrapleural pressure becomes positive and exceeds intrathoracic intra-airway pressure. When cartilaginous airway walls are weakened by bronchomalacia, intrathoracic airway collapse occurs, on expiration.
- Increased tension on the trachealis dorsalis muscle or neurogenic atrophy of the muscle causes stretching of the dorsal tracheal membrane with protrusion into the airway lumen.
- Coughing—mechanical trauma to the tracheal mucosa from collapse of the dorsal tracheal membrane exacerbates airway edema and inflammation.
- Upper airway obstruction worsens clinical signs, and chronic increases in respiratory effort could lead to secondary abnormalities in laryngeal structure and function.
- Small airway disease augments the trans-airway pressure gradient and potentiates collapse in the intrathoracic region.

Blackwell's Five-Minute Veterinary Consult Clinical Companion: Small Animal Senior Care, First Edition. Edited by Heidi B. Lobprise.

Companion website: www.wiley.com/go/lobprise/Senior

SYSTEMS AFFECTED

- Respiratory—chronic airway irritation.
- Cardiovascular—pulmonary hypertension.
- Nervous—can be involved when syncope develops from hypoxia or a vasovagal reflex associated with cough.

GENETICS

Under investigation. Tracheal collapse common in small toy breed dogs. Bronchomalacia seen in large and small breeds.

INCIDENCE/PREVALENCE

Common clinical entity.

SIGNALMENT

Species

Primarily dog, rarely cat.

Breed Predilections

- Tracheal collapse—miniature poodles, Yorkshire terriers, Chihuahuas, Pomeranians, other small and toy breeds.
- Bronchomalacia—all breeds.

Mean Age and Range

- Middle-aged to elderly—onset of signs at 2–14 years of age.
- Severely affected animals <1 year of age.

SIGNS

Historical Findings

- Usually worsened by excitement, heat, humidity, exercise, or obesity.
- Dry honking cough.
- Often have a chronic history of intermittent coughing or difficulty breathing.
- Retching—often seen due to attempts to clear respiratory secretions from the larynx.
- Tachypnea, exercise intolerance, and/or respiratory distress—common.
- Cyanosis or syncope—seen in severely affected individuals.

Physical Examination Findings

- Increased tracheal sensitivity—virtually always seen.
- Respiratory distress—inspiratory with cervical collapse; expiratory with intrathoracic collapse.
- Stridor or musical sounds ausculted over narrowed cervical trachea.
- An end-expiratory snap—heard when a large intrathoracic airway collapses during forceful expiration then reopens.
- Crackles—due to small airway collapse (inspiratory or expiratory) or chronic bronchitis.
- Expiratory wheezes suggest concurrent bronchitis.

- Mitral insufficiency murmurs—often found concurrently in small-breed dogs.
- • Normal-to-low heart rate and/or marked respiratory arrhythmia.
- Loud second heart sound—suggests pulmonary hypertension.
- Hepatomegaly—cause unknown.

CAUSES

- Unknown etiology—congenital, nutritional, or familial defects of chondrogenesis suspected.
- Chronic airway inflammation suggested to contribute to bronchomalacia but relationship not clearly established. Seen with chronic bronchitis or eosinophilic bronchopneumopathy.

RISK FACTORS

- Obesity.
- Airway infection or inflammation.
- Upper airway obstruction.
- Endotracheal intubation.

DIAGNOSIS

DIFFERENTIAL DIAGNOSIS

- Infectious tracheobronchitis.
- Tracheal or laryngeal obstruction or foreign body.
- Chronic bronchitis.
- Pneumonia—viral, bacterial, fungal, parasitic, eosinophilic.
- Bronchiectasis.

CBC/BIOCHEMISTRY/URINALYSIS

- CBC—can show an inflammatory leukogram secondary to chronic stress or concurrent infection.
- Increased liver enzymes common.

OTHER LABORATORY TESTS

Elevated bile acids—mechanism unclear.

IMAGING

Thoracic Radiography

- Airway collapse evident on a lateral thoracic radiographic in a large percentage of dogs with airway collapse; however, the location of collapse on static radiographs agreed with the site determined by fluoroscopy in <50% of cases.
- Inspiratory radiographs—show primarily cervical collapse and collapse at the thoracic inlet.
- Expiratory radiographs—show intrathoracic tracheal collapse; can also note collapse at the carina, ballooning of the cervical trachea, and cranial herniation of the lung lobe through the thoracic inlet.

- Right-sided heart enlargement—can be seen secondary to chronic pulmonary disease and cor pulmonale, or heart can be artifactually enlarged due to obesity or breed conformation.

Fluoroscopy

Dynamic collapse of the cervical or intrathoracic trachea and/or dorsal tracheal membrane can be visible during tidal respirations—usually more easily identified after induction of cough. Cranial lung herniation through the thoracic inlet is common.

DIAGNOSTIC PROCEDURES

Caution is warranted in anesthetizing and intubating dogs with tracheal collapse because endotracheal tube irritation can worsen clinical signs. Loss of respiratory drive from anesthetic drugs or excess excitement on recovery can precipitate airway obstruction.

Tracheal Wash

Use oral intubation (rather than the transtracheal approach) with a small endotracheal tube and a sterile catheter when obtaining samples for cytologic examination and bacterial culture/susceptibility.

Bronchoscopy

- Grade the severity of collapse:
  - Grade I—slight protrusion of the dorsal tracheal membrane into the airway lumen; diameter reduced by <25%,
  - Grade II—reduction of the tracheal lumen by 50%,
  - Grade III—reduction of the tracheal lumen by 75%,
  - Grade IV—tracheal rings flattened; <10% of the tracheal lumen can be seen; in some cases (particularly Yorkies), a double lumen trachea is observed, where tracheal rings have bowed dorsally to contact the trachealis muscle.
- Identify small airway disease—collapse or inflammation. Submit airway samples for cytologic examination and bacterial/susceptibility; specific culture for *Mycoplasma* is recommended.

Cytology

- Unremarkable in uncomplicated tracheal or bronchial collapse.
- Neutrophilia without intracellular bacteria or marked bacterial growth—indicates airway inflammation.
- Lymphocytic inflammation is also common.
- Sepsis and suppuration along with marked bacterial growth of a pathogen—suggests pulmonary infection.

TREATMENT

APPROPRIATE HEALTH CARE

- Outpatient—stable patients.
- Inpatient—oxygen therapy and sedation for severe respiratory distress. Sedation and cough suppression—butorphanol 0.1–0.4 mg/kg SC or IV; addition of acepromazine 0.01–0.04 mg/kg SC or IV can enhance sedative effects and further reduce the cough reflex.

NURSING CARE

Monitor respiratory effort.

ACTIVITY

- Severely limited until patient is stable.
- During management of disease—gentle exercise recommended to encourage weight loss.

DIET

- Many affected dogs improve after losing weight.
- Institute weight-loss program with restriction of caloric intake; use a gradual weight-loss program (1–2% weight loss/week).

CLIENT EDUCATION

- Warn client that weight gain, overexcitement, and humid conditions can precipitate a crisis.
- Advise client to use a harness instead of a collar.
- Advise owners that tracheal collapse is irreversible and that treatment strategies are designed to lessen triggers of cough.
- For surgical candidates, advise owner of the likelihood of complications after surgery (e.g., persistent cough, respiratory distress, or laryngeal paralysis); some patients can require a permanent tracheostomy. For stent candidates, advise owners of need for extensive follow-up to avoid stent fracture, migration, or granulation tissue formation.

SURGICAL CONSIDERATIONS

- Treatment of upper airway obstructive disorders (elongated soft palate, everted laryngeal saccules)—can reduce signs due to tracheal collapse.
- The presence of mainstem bronchial collapse worsens prognosis.
- Placement of extraluminal C-shaped rings by a skilled surgeon in selected patients with cervical collapse will enhance quality of life and reduce clinical signs when adequate stabilization of the airway can be achieved and when bronchomalacia does not limit resolution of clinical signs. Postoperative laryngeal paralysis is a potential complication.
- Intraluminal stents are life-saving in selected cases with intrathoracic airway collapse that fail aggressive medical management. Aspiration pneumonia is common after placement.

MEDICATIONS

DRUG(S) OF CHOICE

- Narcotic cough suppressants (butorphanol 0.5–1 mg/kg PO q4–8h or hydrocodone 0.22 mg/kg PO q4–8h) used to break the cycle of cough; reduce dose rate to the least frequent administration that controls signs. Use after infection or inflammation has been managed.

- Reduction of tracheal inflammation—prednisone 0.5 mg/kg PO q12h then 0.25 mg/kg q12h for a total of 5–7 days may help. Inhaled steroids given via facemask and spacing chamber are preferred to avoid systemic effects of panting and weight gain.
- Sustained-release theophylline 10 mg/kg PO q12h—thought to reduce the pressure gradient in small airways and decrease cough in dogs with intrathoracic airway collapse or bronchomalacia—bronchodilators have no effect on tracheal diameter.
- Bacterial infection uncommon but doxycycline 3–5 mg/kg PO q12h is sometimes beneficial, perhaps through reduction in bacteria within the airway or reduction of inflammation.

PRECAUTIONS

Avoid long-term steroid use because of the propensity for weight gain and diseases associated with immunosuppression.

POSSIBLE INTERACTIONS

Theophylline metabolism—increased by concurrent treatment with ketoconazole or phenobarbital, which results in inadequate plasma concentration; decreased by fluoroquinolones (e.g., enrofloxacin), erythromycin, cimetidine, steroids, beta-blockers, mexiletine, and thiabendazole, which results in toxic plasma concentration and gastrointestinal upset, nervousness, or tachycardia; adjust dosages when concurrent use is necessary.

ALTERNATIVE DRUG(S)

Over-the-counter cough suppressants—rarely reduce cough.

FOLLOW-UP

PATIENT MONITORING

- Body weight.
- Exercise tolerance.
- Pattern of respiration.
- Incidence of cough.

PREVENTION/AVOIDANCE

- Avoid obesity in breeds commonly afflicted.
- Avoid heat and humidity.
- Use harness rather than leash.

POSSIBLE COMPLICATIONS

Intractable respiratory distress leading to respiratory failure or euthanasia.

EXPECTED COURSE AND PROGNOSIS

- Combinations of medications along with weight control can reduce clinical signs, but dogs will likely cough throughout life and can suffer recurrent exacerbations of disease.
- Surgery—benefits dogs severely affected with cervical collapse.
- Stent placement—benefits some dogs, primarily those with respiratory difficulty rather than cough and those with intrathoracic collapse. Medications usually required post procedure.
- Prognosis—based on bronchoscopic evidence of airway obstruction and development of complications.

MISCELLANEOUS

Associated Conditions

- Chronic bronchitis.
- Laryngeal paralysis.
- Pulmonary hypertension.
- Breeds of dogs that develop tracheal collapse also commonly have mitral insufficiency.

Author/editor: Heidi Lobprise
Topic adapted from Five Minute Veterinary Consultation, 7th edition, 2021
Original Topic: Tracheal Collapse

Author: Lynelle R. Johnson
Consulting Editor: Elizabeth Rozanski

Urogenital

Chapter 86

Benign Prostatic Hyperplasia and Prostate Disease

BASICS

OVERVIEW

- Age-related pathologic change in prostate gland, making it non-painfully large.
- Occurs in two phases, glandular and complex.
- Glandular phase characterized by high number of large prostatic cells and symmetrically large prostate gland.
- Complex phase characterized by glandular hyperplasia and atrophy, small cyst formation, chronic inflammation, and squamous metaplasia of epithelium.

SIGNALMENT

Prevalence increases with age; 60% of intact male dogs affected by 6 years and 95% of intact male dogs affected by 9 years of age.

SIGNS

Historical Findings

- None in most dogs.
- Serosanguinous urethral discharge.
- Hemospermia.
- Hematuria.
- Dysuria.
- Dyschezia.
- Ribbon-like stools.

Physical Examination Findings

- Symmetric, non-painfully enlarged prostate gland.
- Prostatic pain in dogs with complication of bacterial infection or prostatic carcinoma.

CAUSES AND RISK FACTORS

- Dihydrotestosterone (DHT; strongly) and testosterone (weakly).
- Estrogens.

Blackwell's Five-Minute Veterinary Consult Clinical Companion: Small Animal Senior Care, First Edition. Edited by Heidi B. Lobprise.

Companion website: www.wiley.com/go/lobprise/Senior

- Aging as intact male.
- Risk eliminated by castration.

DIAGNOSIS

DIFFERENTIAL DIAGNOSIS

- Acute bacterial prostatitis—fever, depression, pain on rectal palpation, neutrophilia, pyuria, and bacteriuria; occurs concurrently with and secondary to benign prostatic hyperplasia (BPH).
- Chronic bacterial prostatitis—recurrent lower urinary tract infections and subfertility; occurs concurrently with and secondary to BPH.
- Prostatic adenocarcinoma—poor appetite, weight loss, hind limb weakness, dysuria, hematuria and dyschezia; may see carcinoma cells in urine sediment.
- Prostatic and paraprostatic cysts—can cause palpable abdominal cystic mass filled with yellow to orange fluid.

CBC/BIOCHEMISTRY/URINALYSIS

- CBC and biochemistry—normal in BPH.
- Urinalysis—may be normal or reveal hematuria; pyuria and bacteriuria absent unless concurrent bacterial infection.

OTHER LABORATORY TESTS

Elevated serum concentration of canine prostate-specific arginine esterase correlates with histologic evidence of BPH.

IMAGING

- Radiography—abdominal radiographs reveal prostatomegaly.
- Ultrasonography—reveals enlarged prostate gland with uniform prostatic parenchymal echogenicity; small, fluid-filled cysts.

DIAGNOSTIC PROCEDURES

Prostatic fluid obtained by ejaculation or prostatic massage may be clear or hemorrhagic; red blood cell count high; white blood cell count normal; culture reveals <100,000 colony-forming units of bacteria/mL unless dog has concurrent bacterial infection.

TREATMENT

- Not required if asymptomatic.
- Castration—most effective and prevents recurrence; if BPH complicated by acute bacterial prostatitis, delay surgery until infection resolved.
- Finasteride, if castration not desired, as long as dog is to remain intact.

MEDICATIONS

DRUG(S) OF CHOICE

If castration not acceptable, the following are the most available and clinically useful:

- Finasteride (0.1 mg/kg/day, not to exceed 5 mg/dog/day) for as long as dog remains intact—inhibits conversion of testosterone to DHT by enzyme 5-α-reductase.
- Osaterone acetate (0.25 mg/kg PO once daily for 7 days)—competitively binds to androgen receptors, reduces 5-α-reductase, inhibits testosterone transport into prostate cells.
- Delmadinone acetate (3 mg/kg SC once)—antiandrogenic activity due to competitive binding to androgen receptors.
- Deslorelin acetate (subcutaneous implant administered every 6–12 months)—gonadotropin-releasing hormone (GnRH) agonist to inhibit hypothalamic–pituitary–gondal axis by negative feedback.

CONTRAINDICATIONS/POSSIBLE INTERACTIONS

- Potential for glucocorticoid insufficiency during stressful events for unspecified period after delmadinone acetate treatment.
- GnRH agonists contraindicated in breeding dogs as will inhibit fertility.

FOLLOW-UP

- Castration is treatment of choice for nonbreeding dogs, will result in 80% reduction in prostate volume within 12 weeks.
- Finasteride is treatment of choice for breeding males. Side effects in dogs reported. Prostate reduced 50–70% between 16 and 53 weeks of treatment. Testosterone preserved, thus finasteride not associated with decline in libido or semen quality. BPH will recur after withdrawal of finasteride; time until clinical signs recur is variable.

MISCELLANEOUS

Associated Conditions

Particularly in intact males.

Prostatitis/Prostatic Abscess

- Inflammation/infection of prostate.
- Acute or chronic bacterial infection, abscess usually secondary to chronic bacterial prostatitis.
- Also associated with benign prostatic hyperplasia (BPH) or retention cysts.
- Bacterial colonization is typically via ascending urinary tract pathogens, though concurrent URI not always noted in chronic cases; hematogenous spread possible.
- Common isolates include *Escherichia coli*, *Klebsiella*, *Pseudomonas*, *Pasteurella*, streptococci, and staphylococci species.

- *Brucella canis* may be associated with acute or chronic prostatitis and has zoonotic potential.
- Fungal prostatitis has been reported (*Blastomyces* and *Cryptococcus*).

■ Signs and findings
- Acute: systemic illness (vomiting, fever, inappetence); pyuria; stiff-legged gait.
  - Fever, dehydration, sepsis/shock; caudal abdominal pain; normal to enlarged, asymmetric, painful prostate.
  - Leukocytosis and neutrophilia (±immaturity and signs of toxicity); pyuria; bacteriuria; hematuria.
- Chronic: recurrent/chronic urinary tract infection; stiff gait; infertility
  - Symmetric, nonpainful, firm, normal size prostate; may have fluctuant areas (focal cysts) on palpation.
  - Occasionally leukocytosis; pyuria; bacteriuria; hematuria.
  - Prostatic fluid culture—culture third ejaculate fraction or fine-needle aspirate of prostate; positive growth supports bacterial prostatitis.
  - Paired seminal fluid and urethral culture—prostatitis is confirmed when seminal fluid bacterial growth (in colony-forming units) is $\geq$100 times corresponding urethral/urine growth.

■ Imaging—to differentiate prostatic diseases.
- Abdominal ultrasound—detects size, homogeneity of prostate. Identifies focal parenchymal abnormalities (cysts or abscesses); loss of tissue homogeneity (prostatitis or neoplasia); regional lymph nodes and paraprostatic structures (paraprostatic cysts).
- Ultrasound-guided fine-needle aspirate—cytologic evaluation may distinguish between BPH, prostatitis, and neoplasia; aspiration of active infections may seed periprostatic and subcutaneous tissues; aspiration of cysts rarely provides clinical resolution.

■ Treatment
- Antimicrobials (based on culture and sensitivity) and that penetrate blood–prostate barrier (e.g., veterinary fluoroquinolone for Gram-negative organisms and clindamycin or a macrolide for Gram-positive organisms). Chloramphenicol and trimethoprim–sulfonamide are additional options.
  - Antimicrobials with poor penetration through an intact blood–prostate barrier should not be used.
  - Antimicrobials should be administered for a minimum of 4 weeks in acute cases and up to 6 weeks for chronic cases.
  - Response to therapy should be monitored based on clinical signs, prostatic size and architecture, return of semen quality. Repeat cultures are not recommended unless poor initial response.
- Finasteride may be considered to treat underlying prostatic pathology in dogs with future breeding intent. Castration is advised for nonbreeding animals and those that respond poorly to appropriate therapy.
- Prostatic abscesses should be percutaneously drained with ultrasound guidance after administration of perioperative antimicrobials.

■ Chronic prostatitis more refractory to medical management; castration may be indicated.

Prostatic Cysts

- Coalescing glandular/cystic hyperplasia and ductular occlusion (retention cysts) caused by estrogen effects (e.g., from Sertoli cell tumor).
- Paraprostatic cysts are attached to prostate, lined by secretory epithelium, and variable in size; larger cysts may be transabdominally palpable; almost always sterile.
- Prostatic cysts—prevalence around 14%; 42% of these had evidence of bacterial infection
- Prostatic cysts—more common after 8 years of age.
- If mild, generally asymptomatic.
- If infected see signs associated with prostatitis.
- Signs and findings
  - Symmetric, enlarged prostate with fluctuant areas; large cysts may preclude rectal palpation, enlarged prostate may be transabdominally palpable.
  - External signs of feminization if cyst formation is due to estrogen exposure.
    - Anemia (if hyperestrogenism present).
- Treatment—castration is treatment of choice
  - Finasteride if associated with BPH.
  - Remove source of estrogen if squamous metaplasia.
  - Large solitary cysts—surgical marsupalization and castration.
  - Paraprostatic cysts—may be surgically excised.
  - Aspiration and drainage of cysts—not associated with resolution; fluid should be cultured.

Prostatic Neoplasia

- Prostatic adenocarcinoma (ACA) is most common; other tumor types include fibrosarcoma, leiomyosarcoma, and squamous cell carcinoma (SCC).
- Prostatic transitional cell carcinoma (TCC) arise from the prostatic urethra and invade the prostate gland.
- BPH is not a risk factor for prostatic neoplasia.
- Tumor development is androgen independent; castration is not protective.
- Tumors typically detected after metastatic spread as clinical signs occur late and early screening is unavailable.
- ACA bone metastasis is common, typically to spine or pelvis; intraprostatic fibrosis with some areas of ossification and hyperplasia is seen.
- Signalment
  - Prevalence 0.2–0.6% in general population, 5–7% of dogs with prostatic disease.
  - Mean age: 10 years.
- Signs and findings
  - Emaciation; dyschezia; rear limb locomotory disturbance; lumbosacral pain.
  - Large, asymmetric, irregular painful prostate.
  - Rectal, abdominal, lumbosacral pain.
  - Palpable abdominal mass.
  - Lymphadenopathy (sublumbar).
- Diagnostics
  - Leukocytosis and neutrophilia.
  - Elevated alkaline phosphatase.
  - Pyuria; hematuria; atypical cells may be noted in urine sediment.
  - Lack of prostatic mineralization in intact dogs with prostatomegaly has a negative predictive value of 96% for neoplasia.

- Treatment
    - Differentiation between ACA and TCC will determine appropriate treatment (see specific chapters).
    - Urine culture.
    - A piroxicam trial should always be offered with or without chemotherapy.

Abbreviations

- BPH = benign prostatic hyperplasia
- DHT = dihydrotestosterone.
- GnRH = gonadotropin-releasing hormone.

Suggested Reading—Benign Prostatic Hyperplasia

Christensen, BW. Canine prostate disease. *Vet Clinics North Am Small Anim Pract* 2018;48(4):701–719.
Smith J. Canine prostatic disease: a review of anatomy, pathology, diagnosis, and treatment. *Theriogenology* 2008;70:375–383.

Suggested Reading—Prostate Disease in the Breeding Male Dog

Weese J. Blondeau J, Boothe D, et al. International Society for Companion Animal Infectious Diseases (ISCAID) guidelines for the diagnosis and management of bacterial urinary tract infections in dogs and cats. *Vet J* 2019;247:8–25.

Author/editor: Heidi Lobprise
Topic adapted from Five Minute Veterinary Consultation, 7th edition, 2021
Original Topics: Benign Prostatic Hyperplasia; and Prostate Disease in the Breeding Male Dog

Author: Bruce Christensen
Consulting Editor: J.D. Foster

Chapter 87

Incontinence, Urinary

BASICS

DEFINITION

Loss of voluntary control of micturition, usually observed as involuntary urine leakage.

PATHOPHYSIOLOGY

Most commonly a disorder of the storage phase of micturition, resulting from impaired urethral sphincter mechanism, detrusor hyperreflexia, or poor bladder compliance. Congenital malformations such as ectopic ureters or urethral malformation can also cause incontinence. Overflow incontinence can result from partial or complete functional urethral obstruction or bladder atony.

SYSTEMS AFFECTED

- Renal/urogenital.
- Nervous.
- Skin—urine scald, perineal and ventral dermatitis.

INCIDENCE/PREVALENCE

Urinary incontinence may affect up to 20% of female spayed dogs and up to 30% of those weighing over 20 kg.

SIGNALMENT

- Dog and rarely cat.
- Most common in spayed female dogs.
- More common in dogs >20 kg.
- Overflow incontinence most common in young-to-middle-aged, large- to giant-breed male dogs.

Blackwell's Five-Minute Veterinary Consult Clinical Companion: Small Animal Senior Care, First Edition. Edited by Heidi B. Lobprise.

Companion website: www.wiley.com/go/lobprise/Senior

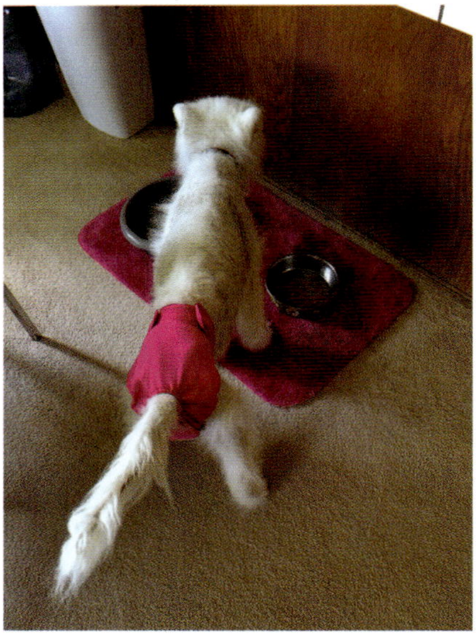

■ **Figure 87.1** This senior female has multiple conditions including hyperadrenocorticism, diabetes mellitus, and hip dysplasia, so using diapers helped manager her urinary incontinence issues. Source: Photo Courtesy of Dr. Mary Gardner.

CAUSES

Anatomic

- Congenital abnormality of the urethral sphincter mechanism.
- Ectopic ureters that terminate in the bladder neck, urethra, vestibule, or vagina.
- Shortened (hypoplastic) urethra.
- Ureterovaginal hypoplasia/aplasia (cats).
- Cystic hypoplasia.
- Patent urachal remnant.
- Intrapelvic bladder interfering with abdominal pressure transmission to the proximal urethra.
- Vestibular or vulvar conformational abnormalities contributing to urine pooling and leakage.

Neurologic

- Central or peripheral lower motor neuron injury to the sacral spinal cord and pudendal nerve leading to weak urethral closure and flaccid bladder.
- Overflow incontinence secondary to upper motor injury of the thoracolumbar spinal cord and loss of inhibitory signaling to the urethral sphincter.
- Dysautonomia leading to urine retention and overflow incontinence.
- Damage to local reflex arc allowing for relaxation of the urethral sphincter when the detrusor contracts.
- Lesions of the cerebellum or cerebral micturition center affecting inhibition and voluntary control of voiding, resulting in frequent involuntary urination or leakage of small amounts of urine.
- Feline leukemia virus–associated myelopathy leading to progressive paresis or paralysis.

Urinary Bladder Dysfunction

- Bladder atony leading to incomplete voiding and overflow incontinence.
- Bladder overdistension with loss of cellular tight junctions and incomplete contractile signal transmission.
- Bladder fibrosis leading to poor compliance and decreased storage capacity.
- Detrusor hyperreflexia (overactive bladder) and poor compliance.

Urethral Disorders

- Congenital or acquired urethral sphincter mechanism incompetence (most common).
- Functional outlet obstruction leading to overflow incontinence (detrusor urethral dyssynergia).
- Mechanical outflow obstruction from enlarged prostate, benign or malignant neoplasia, urolith, foreign body, or external compression.

Urine Retention

Overflow incontinence when intravesicular pressure exceeds outlet resistance.

Mixed Urinary Incontinence

Any combination of factors in dogs and cats leading to involuntary urine loss. Not typically defined in the way human mixed urinary incontinence is (overactive bladder and stress incontinence).

RISK FACTORS

- Large-breed (>20 kg) spayed female dog. (Figure 89.1)
- Early spay (<12 weeks).
- Breed predispositions are possible.
- Intrapelvic bladder.
- Urogenital conformational abnormalities affecting bladder neck, urethral length, or vestibule.
- Other possible risk factors include obesity, tail-docking, and polyuria.

DIAGNOSIS

DIFFERENTIAL DIAGNOSIS

- Voluntary inappropriate urination.
- Pollakiuria.
- Prostatic or vaginal discharge.
- Polyuria—may worsen minor incontinence because of increased pressure on already weakened urethral sphincter mechanism.

CBC/BIOCHEMISTRY/URINALYSIS

- Hematology and serum biochemistry are indicated in patients with polyuria and polydipsia.
- CBC and serum biochemistry are usually normal unless comorbidities exist.

- Urinalysis frequently normal.
- Urine sediment may indicate urinary tract infection or polyuria.

OTHER LABORATORY TESTS

- Urine culture may be indicated if clinical signs (straining to urinate, pollakiuria) and urine sediment (pyuria, bacteriuria, hematuria) are consistent with urinary tract infection.
- Cats should be tested for feline leukemia virus.
- Additional testing for causes of polyuria and polydipsia may be indicated based on serum biochemistry and urinalysis results.

IMAGING

Radiographic Findings

- Plain radiography may identify a pelvically placed bladder.
- Intravenous contrast excretory urography may identify dilated or ectopic ureters; however, careful attention must be paid to proper technique and the sensitivity of the imaging is inferior to other methods.
- Retrograde contrast vaginourethrography may reveal congenital abnormalities of the vagina, urethra, and vestibule, and occasionally ectopic ureters.
- Single- or double-contrast cystourethrography allows for accurate assessment of bladder position and urethral length.
- Imaging of the dog or cat with acquired urethral sphincter mechanism incompetence, the most common cause of acquired urinary incontinence, is usually normal.

Ultrasonographic Findings

- Ultrasound assessment may detect ureteral dilation or ectopic ureters; however, the sensitivity is very operator dependent.
- Allows for evaluation of kidneys, bladder, and prostate.

CT Findings

CT excretory urography is currently the imaging modality of choice to diagnose ectopic ureters.

DIAGNOSTIC PROCEDURES

- Neurologic examination—tail tone, anal tone, perineal reflexes and sensation, and bulbospongiosus reflexes.
- Orthopedic examination—determination of pain or difficulty posturing to urinate, which can lead to urine retention.
- Urethral catheterization—to determine patency of urethra and residual urine volume in patients with suspected urine retention and overflow incontinence.
- Cystoscopy—evaluates urethra and bladder as well as visualization of position and shape of ureteral openings.
- Urodynamic assessment—may document decreased urethral pressure or detrusor hyperreflexia; limited availability at some specialty clinics.

TREATMENT

APPROPRIATE HEALTH CARE

- Usually outpatient.
- Medical therapy is primary treatment for patients with urethral sphincter mechanism incompetence.
- Urinary tract infection should be treated appropriately if identified.
- Address partial urethral obstructive and neurologic disorders if identified.
- Ectopic ureters should be corrected either by cystoscopic laser ablation if intramural (common) or surgery if extramural (rare).
- Anatomic disorders should be identified and corrected if possible.
- Functional abnormalities of the bladder or urethra may require medical treatment.
- Bulking agents such as bovine cross-linked collagen may be injected into urethral submucosa, or surgical salvage procedures such as placement of urethral hydraulic occluder if urethral sphincter incompetence not responsive to medical therapy.

MEDICATIONS

DRUG(S) OF CHOICE

Urethral Sphincter Mechanism Incompetence

- Alpha-adrenergic agonist treatment (e.g., phenylpropanolamine)
  - 1–2 mg/kg PO q8–12h
  - Extended release 2–4 mg/kg once daily
- Estrogen compounds (e.g., estriol 2 mg/dog PO q24h for 2 weeks, then decrease dose q2 weeks to lowest effective dose; diethylstilbestrol 0.1–1 mg/dog PO q24h for 5–7 days, then 0.1–1 mg/dog q5–7 days PRN).
- Phenylpropanolamine and estrogens may be used in combination in spayed females and may have a synergistic effect.
- Imipramine (5–15 mg/dog PO q12h), a tricyclic antidepressant with cholinergic and alpha-agonist effects, may be of use if other medical therapy fails, especially if detrusor hyperreflexia is suspected as well.
- Testosterone cypionate (2.2 mg/kg IM q30–45 days) may be used in males with urethral sphincter mechanism incompetence; however, its efficacy is far below phenylpropanolamine.

Detrusor Hyperreflexia

Antimuscarinic agents (oxybutynin chloride 0.2–0.3 mg/kg PO q8–12h or 1.25–5 mg/dog PO q8–12h; imipramine 5–15 mg/dog PO q12h).

Functional Outflow Obstruction

See Urinary Tract Obstruction.

CONTRAINDICATIONS

- Do not use estrogens in males or intact females.
- Do not use alpha agonists in patients with hypertension, and use with caution in patients with conditions that predispose to hypertension.
- Do not use anticholinergics in patients with glaucoma or cardiac disease.

PRECAUTIONS

- Adrenergic agonists can cause hypertension, changes in appetite, and restlessness.
- Adverse effects of estrogen use include vulvar swelling, mammary development, and attractiveness to males; these are usually dose dependent and will subside with dose reduction; always use the lowest effective dose.
- Bone marrow suppression is extremely rare secondary to estrogen use at the recommended doses.
- Testosterone use can lead to signs of aggression and increased libido in males.
- Anticholinergic agents can cause nausea, vomiting, and constipation.

POSSIBLE INTERACTIONS

- Do not administer tricyclic antidepressants concurrently with monoamine oxidase inhibitors (e.g., amitriptyline, clomipramine, imipramine).
- Hypertensive risk increases with concurrent use of alpha agonists and tricyclic antidepressants.

FOLLOW-UP

PATIENT MONITORING

- Monitor blood pressure periodically in patients receiving alpha agonists.
- Monitor vulvar and mammary swelling in patients receiving estrogen treatment.
- Monitor prostate size in males receiving testosterone.
- Once continence is achieved, gradually reduce to lowest effective dose.
- Perform urine cultures to guide treatment and prevent resistance of symptomatic urinary tract infections.

POSSIBLE COMPLICATIONS

- Hypertension.
- Recurrent and resistant urinary tract infections.
- Urine scald and perineal (females) or ventral abdominal (males) dermatitis.
- Refractory incontinence.

MISCELLANEOUS

Associated Conditions

- Urinary tract infection.
- Hydroureter and hydronephrosis in some ectopic ureter patients, even after correction.

Pregnancy/Fertility/Breeding

Dogs with congenital anomalies such as ectopic ureters should be removed from the breeding population.

Synonyms

- Hormone-responsive incontinence.
- Enuresis.

Suggested Reading

Acierno M, Labato M. Canine incontinence. *Vet Clin North Am Small Anim Pract* 2019;49(2):125–140.
Byron J, Taylor K, Phillips G, Stahl M. Urethral sphincter mechanism incompetence in 163 neutered female dogs: diagnosis, treatment, and relationship of weight and age at neuter to development of disease. *J Vet Intern Med* 2017;31(2):442–448.

Author/editor: Heidi Lobprise
Topic adapted from Five Minute Veterinary Consultation, 7th edition, 2021
Original Topic: Incontinence

Author: Julie K. Byron
Consulting Editor: J.D. Foster

Chapter 88

Perineal Hernia

BASICS

OVERVIEW

- Perineal hernia (PH)—the pelvic diaphragm is weakened, with rupture or atrophy of the muscles. Rectal sacculation and dilation often occur; feces can become entrapped and can even lead to herniation of the pelvic and abdominal viscera.
- Hormonal influences and increased pressure secondary to enlargement of the prostate thought to contribute.

SIGNALMENT

Intact male dogs are at highest risk; rare in other dogs and cats.

SIGNS

- Constipation is the main feature, although some patients present with diarrhea as looser stool escapes around the firmer stool.
- Unilateral or bilateral perineal bulge due to fecal impaction and/or herniation, dynamic or static
    - May be more obvious during barking, coughing, defecation, and urination.
- Straining to urinate if bladder incarceration occurs.

CAUSES AND RISK FACTORS

- Intact status in older male dogs or cryptorchidism.
- Excessive straining due to prostatomegaly (male dogs); megacolon (cats)
- Caudal neuropathy, malformation, or injury such as tail traction or avulsion.
- Trauma (rare).

Blackwell's Five-Minute Veterinary Consult Clinical Companion: Small Animal Senior Care, First Edition. Edited by Heidi B. Lobprise.

Companion website: www.wiley.com/go/lobprise/Senior

DIAGNOSIS

CBC/BIOCHEMISTRY/URINALYSIS

No specific abnormalities. Azotemia if urinary obstruction occurs.

IMAGING

- Abdominal radiography—evaluate constipation or obstipation, prostatomegaly, sublumbar lymphadenomegaly, location of urinary bladder and prostate, and megacolon in cats.
- Pelvic radiography—evaluate pelvic fracture malunion, intrapelvic mass, caudal displacement of the prostate and bladder, entrapment of bladder or bowel in hernia.
- Abdominal ultrasonography—evaluate the size and consistency of the prostate, location of urinary bladder and prostate, intrapelvic or caudal abdominal masses, sublumbar lymphadenomegaly, presence of abdominal cryptorchid testicle.
- Perineal ultrasonography—evaluate presence of abdominal viscera or masses.

DIAGNOSTIC PROCEDURES

- Visual perianal examination:
  - With a weak perineal diaphragm, the anus migrates caudally. May be severe in bilateral PH.
  - Eliciting a cough reflex by gentle tracheal palpation will increase intra-abdominal pressure and aid evaluation of the position and movement of the anus.
- Rectal examination:
  - Confirm accumulation of feces in the dilated and sacculated rectum and perineal laxity.
  - If the integrity of the pelvic diaphragm has been compromised, it will be possible to pinch the rectal mucosa and skin together between the tip of the forefinger and thumb without palpating a muscle shelf in between.
  - Evaluate both sides; bilateral PH is common especially in intact male dogs.
- Endoscopy or percutaneous fine-needle aspiration biopsy may be indicated if a mass lesion is present extra- or intraluminally.

TREATMENT

- Surgical management required for definitive treatment; emergent if visceral entrapment.
- Conservative treatment may temporarily ameliorate clinical signs with low residue diet and stool softeners.

Nursing Care

- IV fluid therapy in the pre- and post-operative period.
- Incisional icing postoperatively.
- Elizabethan collar postoperatively.

Activity

Restrict for at least 3–4 weeks following surgical repair.

Diet

- Low-residue canned diet:
  - Part of conservative medical management.
  - Postoperatively.

Surgical Considerations

- Castration of male dogs should always be performed simultaneously with herniorrhaphy.
- In patients with bladder retroflexion and entrapment, the urethra should be catheterized, and the bladder decompressed if possible:
  - Percutaneous perineal cystocentesis may be required to decompress and reposition the bladder before a urethral catheter can be passed.
  - If the bladder is able to be decompressed, correction of biochemical abnormalities is preferred prior to anesthesia and surgery in the urinary obstruction patient with PH.
- Use an epidural with local anesthetic and/or morphine.
- Impacted feces should be gently removed from the rectum prior to surgery:
  - Enemas are not recommended as liquid feces may not be completely evacuated, leading to excessive contamination during surgery and postoperatively.
- Primary repair of the weakened muscles alone often leads to recurrence and is not recommended as the only form of repair.
- Repair with an internal obturator muscle flap combined with primary bolstering of the perineal musculature on both side, even if unilateral hernia.
- In large dogs with large bilateral hernias and bladder or visceral entrapment, reposition the bladder and rectum, and perform incisional colopexy and cystopexy via laparotomy.
  - Herniorrhaphy can be performed at a later time (2–7 days), when the patient's condition has stabilized and the perineal edema has resolved.
  - In patients with poor perineal muscle development and in patients with large defects, the repair is often bolstered with the use of secondary local muscle flaps.
  - Absorbable and nonabsorbable mesh implants are needed in some severe cases.
  - A superficial gluteal muscle flap is recommended in cats and very small dogs to bolster the internal obturator muscle flap and primary repair techniques.

MEDICATIONS

DRUG(S) OF CHOICE

- Stool softeners for conservative medical management or prior to surgery:
  - Lactulose 0.5–1 mL/kg PO q8–12h, adjusted to effect.
  - PEG 3350 (MiraLax®) ¼–1 tsp on food q12h, adjusted to effect.
  - Goal is 2–3 soft-formed stools per day.
- Intraoperative antibiotics may be given, but there is no indication to continue antibiotic treatment postoperatively unless significant contamination occurs during surgery.

CONTRAINDICATIONS/POSSIBLE INTERACTIONS

Avoid stool softeners postoperatively, as they may lead to diarrhea and fecal soiling in the first days after surgery, especially if a bilateral repair has been performed.

FOLLOW-UP

PATIENT MONITORING

- The patient should be evaluated frequently for the first 48 hours following surgery, with particular attention paid to urination and defecation regardless if bladder entrapment was present preoperatively.
- A rectal examination should be performed at the time of suture removal (10–14 days) if feasible.

PREVENTION/AVOIDANCE

- Castration.
- Address conditions causing straining during defecation and urination, if present.

POSSIBLE COMPLICATIONS

- Constipation, obstipation, and bladder retroflexion/obstruction, visceral entrapment, and strangulation.
- Postoperative complications include recurrence (greatly reduced by castration and use of internal obturator flap), and temporary or permanent dysfunction of the anal sphincter due to stretching following bilateral herniorrhaphy:
    - Fecal and urinary incontinence can occur if excessive dissection around the pudendal nerve, caudal rectal nerve, or peritoneal reflections are performed.

EXPECTED COURSE AND PROGNOSIS

- Excellent with surgery.
- There is a 10–50% risk of recurrence depending on presence of underlying conditions, surgical technique, and reproductive status of the dog.

Suggested Reading

Gill SS, Barstad RD. A review of the surgical management of perineal hernias in dogs. *J Am Anim Hosp Assoc* 2018;4:179–187.

Mann F. Serum testosterone and estradiol 17-beta concentrations in 15 dogs with perineal hernia. *J Am Vet Med Assoc* 1989;194:1578–1580.

Souza CH, Mann T. Perineal hernias. In: Monnet E (ed.) *Small Animal Soft Tissue Surgery*. Hoboken, NJ: Wiley Blackwell, 2013; pp. 286–296.

Szabo S, Wilkens B, Radasch, RM. Use of polypropylene mesh in addition to obturator transposition: a review of 59 cases (2000–2004). *J Am Anim Hosp Assoc* 2007;43:136–142.

Author/editor: Heidi Lobprise
Topic adapted from Five Minute Veterinary Consultation, 7th edition, 2021
Original Topic: Perineal Hernia

Author: Stephen Mehler
Consulting Editor: Mark P. Rondeau

Section 3

Management Strategies

Anesthesia; Pain Management Mobility

Chapter 89

Anesthesia for Senior Pets

BASICS

OVERVIEW

Although "age is not a disease," additional considerations must be made for senior pets undergoing general anesthesia (GA). Risks can be minimized with thorough patient evaluation, selection of customized analgesic and anesthetic protocols, and optimal patient care and management. The benefits of the procedures needed under GA will often outweigh the risks.

Terms Defined

- Elderly normal—a relatively health older patient but still with declines in organ function and reserve

ISSUES AND OPTIONS

Challenges with Senior Anesthesia

- Decreased physiological reserve capacity of organ systems.
- Decreased ability to compensate for altered physiology during anesthesia.
- The aging process varies among the organ systems within the individual.
- Subclassification[1]
    - Healthy patients with age-related changes—"elderly normal"
    - Those with subclinical organ dysfunction
    - Those with an overt condition or conditions

Physiological Considerations

- Cardiovascular
    - Myocardial atrophy and fibrosis—impair cardiac output (CO).
    - Left ventricular output—increased resistance.
    - Decreased ventricular compliance and cardiac reserve.
    - Less tolerant of acute changes in intravascular volume (fluid loss and fluid overload).
    - Autonomic responses slower—heart rate and blood pressure (BP)—can't compensate as quickly for hypotension.
        - Increases heart rate/CO instead of vasoconstriction but also fluid overload risk if fluids are increased to combat hypotension
        - Hypercapnea—sympathetic response with tachycardia, arrhythmias, hypertension

Blackwell's Five-Minute Veterinary Consult Clinical Companion: Small Animal Senior Care, First Edition. Edited by Heidi B. Lobprise.

Companion website: www.wiley.com/go/lobprise/Senior

- Pulmonary
  - Increased ventilation–perfusion mismatch can decrease gas exchange efficiency.
  - Decreased respiratory reserve; hypoxemia risk increased.
  - Decreased lung elasticity and thoracic compliance; additional effort to maintain perfusion.
  - May have decreased laryngeal and pharyngeal reflexes and increased gastro-esophageal reflux, increasing risk of aspiration pneumonia (especially in brachycephalic breeds and dogs with GOLPP).[2]
- Central nervous system (CNS)
  - Neurodegenerative changes and potential cognitive issues.
  - Decreased anesthetic requirements (including inhalant anesthetics) due to loss of functional neurons.[3]
  - Less effective response to challenges due to increase sympathetic and decreased parasympathetic activity.
  - Closely monitor to prevent anesthetic overdose.
- Renal
  - Decreased glomerular filtration rate (GFR) and renal blood flow (RBF); renal ischemia more likely to cause renal failure.
  - Impaired ability to excrete fluids and solutes; predisposed to volume overload.
  - Decreased metabolism and clearance of drugs.
  - Renal function may be well-compensated, but when stressed by anesthesia there can be a decline in post-operative renal function.
- Hepatic
  - Decreased metabolism and clearance of drugs.
  - Co-administered drugs that inhibit enzyme system cytochrome P450.
- Muscle/fat/water content
  - Decreased lean body mass, increased fat, decreased total body water content leads to increased plasma drug levels that can reach the CNS.
- Thermoregulation
  - Higher risk of hypothermia with poor thermoregulation, slower metabolism rate, body condition, and CNS aging.
- Anxiety—can lead to increased catecholamine release, cardiac arrhythmias, peripheral vasoconstriction, increased cardiac work, and decreased tissue perfusion.

APPLICATIONS IN PRACTICE

Patient Evaluation and Preparation

- Thorough physical examination, ausculate heart and lungs
- Exercise intolerance—predictor of outcome in geriatric anesthesia
- Correct significant pre-existing abnormalities
- Hydration status
- Diagnostics—CBC, serum biochemistry panel, electrocardiogram, urinalysis.

Pre-visit Protocols

- Anxiolytics
  - If the patient is on any medication for anxiety, such as Trazodone or gabapentin (among others), have the owner administer the medication the night before and the morning of the procedure.

   - If this is a new prescription for the patient, have the owner do a trial period of medication at least a week prior to the procedure. If there is any ataxia or excessive drowsiness, the dose may need to be decreased or stopped completely.
- Give all other medication with the exception of antihypertensive medications (for 1 day) and anti-coagulants (up to 2 weeks)
   - Diabetic patients should receive ½ dose insulin 2–4 hours prior to the procedure with ½ of a meal at the same time.
- Food and water restriction[4]
   - Most patients should have free access to water.
   - Only restrict water to those patients with a risk of regurgitation (then withhold 6–12 hours).
   - Withhold food in most healthy patients for only 4–6 hours, or 6–12 hours in regurgitant-risk patients.
      - On those patients, consider feeding 10–25% of a pate consistency food 4–6 hours prior to anesthesia.
- Patients with a risk of regurgitation should receive anti-emetic, antacid, and promotility medications.
   - Regurgitation and nausea are not biologically linked; regurgitation can still happen with excellent anti-emetic management.[5]
   - Brachycephalic dogs premedicated with an antiemetic and famotidine have a decreased incidence of post-operative regurgitation.[6]
- Maropitant—anti-emetic
   - In a study, maropitant decreased the anesthetic requirement.[7]

Preanesthetic Period

- Use appropriate analgesia and sedation protocols
- Choose drugs that are:
   - Reversible
   - Can be given "to effect"
   - Have a short duration of action.
- Opioids are potent analgesics that can be reversed (if hepatic function decreased)
   - They can provide sedation as well
   - Pure agonists have greater cardiovascular and respiratory depression (morphine, hydromorphone, oxymorphone)
   - Partial agonists (buprenorphine) and agonist-antagonist (butorphanol) have less analgesia but less depression
   - In dogs, they can be significantly anesthetic sparing, less so in cats.
- Local and regional blocks.
- NSAIDs—avoid or use with caution if renal impairments exist.
- Anticholinergics
   - Pre-emptive use may cause tachycardia, increased oxygen consumption
   - May consider in brachycephalic patients with high vagal tone
   - Only treat bradycardia if it occurs.
- Sedatives
   - Help alleviate stress
   - Benzodiazapines—reversible, combine with other sedatives or analgesics
      - Produce more reliable sedation in older patients than in young ones
      - Midazolam can be given IM
      - Midazolam 0.2 mg/kg IM or IV, or diazepam 0.2 mg/kg IV

- Alpha 2 adrenergic agonists (dexmedetomidine)—reversible
    - Judicious use of low doses (2 µg/kg medetomidine).
    - Closely monitor cardiovascular function.
    - Use when benefits outweigh risks—rapid onset of action, can be titrated to effect and are reversible.
- Acepromazine—possible hypotension and hypothermia, not reversible
    - Not contraindicated but dose requirements are markedly decreased.
    - Long duration of action and not reversible.
    - Vasodilation enhances heat loss.
    - Protects renal function despite decrease in blood pressure.
    - 0.01–0.02 mg/kg IM.

Anesthetic Period

- Anesthetic Induction
    - Pre-oxygenate for 5 minutes
    - Propofol—1–3 mg/kg
        - Initial apnea.
        - Titrate carefully to avoid respiratory and cardiovascular depression.
        - Older dogs require less due to pharmacokinetics and clearance is slower.[8]
        - Metabolized in liver but also cleared by the lungs.
        - No active metabolite—no "hang-over."
    - Alfaxalone—large doses given rapidly will cause cardiorespiratory depression
        - Can be given IM.
    - Etomidate—minimal cardiopulmonary effect, especially in cardiac patients.[9]
    - Ketamine with benzodiazepine
        - Use with caution due to tachycardia.
        - Mild respiratory depression, may improve cardiovascular function; does not impair tissue oxygenation.[10, 11]
        - Plays a role in preventing central plasticity (sensitization).
        - Requires hepatic metabolism or renal clearance.
    - Inhalant induction—only in sedated or debilitated patients with very close monitoring.
- Anesthetic maintenance
    - Inhalants—dose-dependent hypotension, hypoventilation, impaired cardiac contractility and hypothermia.
    - Use local and regional blocks to decrease inhalant need.
    - Supplemental analgesia if needed.
- Supportive care
    - Caution with aggressive fluid therapy
        - Difficulty excreting salt and water loads—volume overload.
    - Hypothermia (see Figure 89.1)
        - Increases incidence of adverse myocardial outcomes, surgical wound infections, affect immune defenses, increases thermal discomfort and delays recovery.
        - Shivering is not benign—increases oxygen consumption that may not be met.
    - Monitoring—during and after anesthesia.
- Recovery
    - Monitoring—The post-operative period is the highest risk period with a number of risk factors for mortality.[12]
        - Remote monitors can capture temperature, pulse and respiration and relay parameters to a remote device.

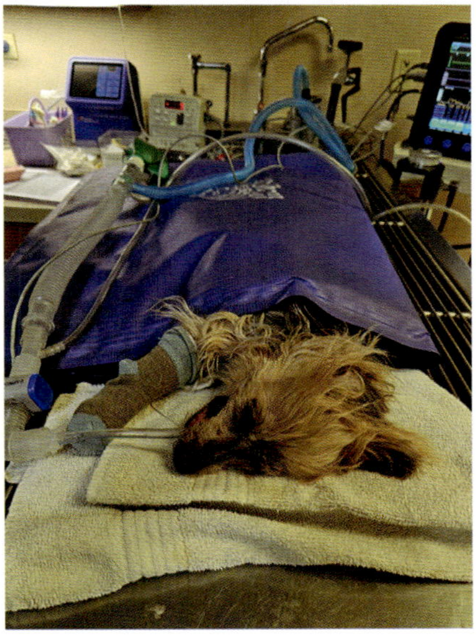

■ **Figure 89.1** A small, older dog undergoing general anesthesia with a warming device and socks. Source: Heidi Lobprise.

- Reverse any agents possible.
- Midazolam—reverse with flumazenil.
- Naloxone for opioid.
- Atipamazole for dexmedetomidine.
  - Full reversal may result in a more dysphoric recovery.
  - Either reverse one-half or be prepared to give a micro-dose if necessary.

Refining Your Protocols

- With your pre-anesthetic communication and admission forms, be sure to have reliable contact information.
  - Forms may also include a selection for DNR (do not resuscitate) or to approve levels of intervention if any complications arise.
- Pre-medication adjustments
  - Acepromazine should be avoided as a premedicant for animals receiving ACE inhibitors, calcium channel blockers or pimobendan for cardiac disease: acepromazine will potentiate vasodilation, causing severe hypotension.
  - Many older animals are receiving long-term non-steroidal anti-inflammatory drugs (NSAIDs) for arthritis. These animals should not receive the full post-operative dose of NSAID after surgery. NSAIDs should never be given concurrently with steroids. For further information on the use of NSAIDs for peri-operative analgesia see below.
- Pre-hydrate renal patients or if dehydrated.
- Pre-oxygenation with a face mask and 100% oxygen, or use "flow-by" technique if mask is not well-tolerated.
- Co-induction techniques—giving 1.0 mg/kg of propofol followed by midazolam (0.25 mg/kg), then titrating propofol until dogs could be intubated resulted in a total dose of 1.1 ± 0.2 mg/kg propofol compared to 3.2 ± 0.6 mg/kg when using propofol alone.[13]

- CRI—opioids and low doses of ketamine
  - Use a loading dose (0.25–0.5 mg/kg) then a lower dose for infusion.
  - For induction, up to 5 mg/kg is required.
- Decrease the speed of injection—lower cardiac output and slower circulation times; give sufficient time for drug to get to the brain.
- Keep them warm.
- Post-operative—monitors, fluids, warmth
  - Hypoxemia.
  - Shivering in the recovery period increases oxygen requirements and if this demand is not met, myocardial hypoxia and arrhythmias can develop.
- May respond poorly to environmental changes and have clinical signs of cognitive dysfunction, so minimize hospital stay.[14, 15]
- Avoid tachycardia—it increases cardiac work and myocardial oxygen demand.
- Caution with NSAIDs (being used for chronic pain or as perioperative analgesic)—they can block prostaglandins that are important for maintaining renal blood flow, so prevent, recognize, and treat hypotension.

Client Communication

- Good client communication and education can help relieve their concerns and fears about anesthesia by working with them to minimize their pet's risks, stress, and negative outcomes.
- Compliance with pre- and post-operative instructions can make the procedure and recovery smoother.
- Even with minimal issues, sedation and general anesthesia can always pose a risk with senior patients, even through the post-operative period. Have frank conversations with the owner if risks are applicable and be empathetic to their concerns.

Abbreviations

- ACE inhibitor = angiotensin-converting enzyme inhibitor
- BP = blood pressure
- CO = cardiac output
- CRI = constant rate infusion
- GA = general anesthesia
- GFR = glomerular filtration rate
- NSAID = non-steroidal anti-inflammatory drug
- RBF = renal blood flow

Internet Resources

Accessed 26 June 2024

- 2020 AAHA Anesthesia and Monitoring Guidelines for Dogs and Cats—AAHA
- Anesthesia Guidelines|American Association of Feline Practitioners (catvets.com)
- https://ivapm.org/professionals/cri-calculator/
- www.vasg.org

Additional Reading

Grimm KA, Tranquilli WJ, Lamont LA. *Essentials of Small Animal Anesthesia and Analgesia*, 2nd edn. Chichester: John Wiley & Sons, Inc. 2011.

References

1. Kukanich B. Geriatric veterinary pharmacology. *Vet Clin North Am Small Anim Pract* 2012 Jul;42(4):631–642, v. doi: https://doi.org/10.1016/j.cvsm.2012.04.007. Epub 2012 May 10. PMID: 22720805.
2. Hughes J. Anaesthesia for the geriatric dog and cat. *Ir Vet J* 2008 Jun 1;61(6):380–387. doi: https://doi.org/10.1186/2046-0481-61-6-380. PMID: 21851715; PMCID: PMC3113863.
3. Magnusson KR, Scanga C, Wagner AE, Dunlop C. Changes in anesthetic sensitivity and glutamate receptors in the aging canine brain. *J Gerontol A Biol Sci Med Sci* 2000 Sep;55(9):B448–B454. doi: https://doi.org/10.1093/gerona/55.9.b448. PMID: 10995042.
4. Grubb T, Sager J, Gaynor JS, Montgomery E, Parker JA, Shafford H, Tearney C. 2020 AAHA anesthesia and monitoring guidelines for dogs and cats. *J Am Anim Hosp Assoc* 2020 Mar/Apr;56(2):59–82. doi: https://doi.org/10.5326/JAAHA-MS-7055. PMID: 32078360.
5. Moyer AL, McKee TS, Bergman PJ, Vinayak A. Low incidence of postoperative nausea, vomiting, regurgitation, and aspiration pneumonia in geriatric dogs receiving maropitant, famotidine, and fentanyl as part of an anesthesia protocol. *J Am Vet Med Assoc* 2021 Dec 15;260(S1):S46–S51. doi: https://doi.org/10.2460/javma.21.05.0237. PMID: 34914625.
6. Costa RS, Abelson AL, Lindsey JC, et al. Postoperative regurgitation and respiratory complications in brachycephalic dogs undergoing airway surgery before and after implementation of a standardized perianesthetic protocol. *J Am Vet Med Assoc* 2020;256(8):899–905. doi:https://doi.org/10.2460/javma.256.8.899
7. Boscan P, Monnet E, Mama K, Twedt DC, Congdon J, Steffey EP. Effect of maropitant, a neurokinin 1 receptor antagonist, on anesthetic requirements during noxious visceral stimulation of the ovary in dogs. *Am J Vet Res* 2011 Dec;72(12):1576–1579. doi: https://doi.org/10.2460/ajvr.72.12.1576. PMID: 22126683.
8. Reid J, Nolan AM. Pharmacokinetics of propofol as an induction agent in geriatric dogs. *Res Vet Sci* 1996 Sep;61(2):169–171. doi: https://doi.org/10.1016/s0034-5288(96)90095-8. PMID: 8880990.
9. Pascoe PJ, Ilkiw JE, Haskins SC, Patz JD. Cardiopulmonary effects of etomidate in hypovolemic dogs. *Am J Vet Res* 1992 Nov;53(11):2178–2182. PMID: 1466517.
10. Pozzi A, Muir WW, Traverso F. Prevention of central sensitization and pain by N-methyl-d-aspartate receptor antagonists. *J Am Vet Med Assoc* 2006 Jan 1;228(1):53–60. doi: https://doi.org/10.2460/javma.228.1.53. PMID: 16426166.
11. Haskins SC, Patz JD. Ketamine in hypovolemic dogs. *Crit Care Med* 1990 Jun;18(6):625–629. doi: https://doi.org/10.1097/00003246-199006000-00010. PMID: 2111756.
12. Brodbelt D. Perioperative mortality in small animal anaesthesia. *Vet J* 2009 Nov;182(2):152–161. doi: https://doi.org/10.1016/j.tvjl.2008.06.011. Epub 2008 Jul 26. PMID: 18658000.
13. Sánchez A, Belda E, Escobar M, Agut A, Soler M, Laredo FG. Effects of altering the sequence of midazolam and propofol during co-induction of anaesthesia. *Vet Anaesth Analg* 2013 Jul;40(4):359–366. doi: https://doi.org/10.1111/vaa.12038. Epub 2013 Apr 9. PMID: 23570259.
14. Landsberg GM, Denenberg S, Araujo JA. Cognitive dysfunction in cats: a syndrome we used to dismiss as 'old age'. *J Feline Med Surg* 2010 Nov;12(11):837–848. doi: https://doi.org/10.1016/j.jfms.2010.09.004. PMID: 20974401.
15. Chapagain D, Range F, Huber L, Virányi Z. Cognitive aging in dogs. *Gerontology* 2018;64(2):165–171. doi: https://doi.org/10.1159/000481621. Epub 2017 Oct 25. PMID: 29065419; PMCID: PMC5841136.

Author: Heidi Lobprise
Thanks to: Sheilah Robertson for resources

Chapter 90

Pain Management for Senior Pets

BASICS

OVERVIEW

One of the major factors in maintaining a senior pet's quality of life is minimizing their pain and discomfort. Sometimes, the pain may be visceral, dental, or spinal, but the most common source of pain in senior pets is some form of osteoarthritis (OA) and/or degenerative joint disease (DJD). Being able to accurately diagnose, assess, and modulate pain is a critical part of gerontology. Acute pain (adaptive pain) may still be essential for an individual to respond to some noxious stimuli. Yet, when it extends beyond the short time needed to alleviate the cause, then chronic (maladaptive) pain becomes the primary problem.

Terms Defined

- Adaptive pain produces behavior that promotes healing and recovery. Nociceptive pain results from damage or potential damage to the body caused by harmful stimuli. It is termed inflammatory pain if that stimulus occurs during an inflammatory or immune response. Identifying the cause of adaptive pain is typically straightforward, and it is usually reversible or self-limiting if treated appropriately.
- Maladaptive pain is not protective and has no biological value. It is often experienced at a more significant proportion to the actual tissue damage and lasts long after the tissues have healed. It can be the cause of great suffering in humans and animals and should be considered a disease in itself. It results from changes in pain processing systems and can be separated into two types:
    - Neuropathic pain is a result of neural tissue damage, central or peripheral.
        - Somatosensory nervous system damage may be felt in places with no tissue damage.
    - Functional pain does not involve neural damage or inflammation that can be detected. Instead, it is caused by a malfunction or dysfunction in the nociceptive system.
- Central sensitization represents an enhancement in the function of neurons and circuits in nociceptive pathways caused by increased membrane excitability, synaptic efficacy, and reduced inhibition.
- Hyperalgesia—increased pain signaling from a stimulus that usually provokes pain.
- Allodynia—pain resulting from a stimulus that would not normally provoke pain.

Blackwell's Five-Minute Veterinary Consult Clinical Companion: Small Animal Senior Care, First Edition. Edited by Heidi B. Lobprise.

Companion website: www.wiley.com/go/lobprise/Senior

ISSUES AND OPTIONS

- Pharmacodynamics of medications in geriatrics may be different
  - Senior pets have changes in body composition (decreased lean body mass), drug receptors, and neurotransmitters.[1]
  - With slower recovery times and reduced resilience, therapy duration may be extended.
  - Concurrent comorbidities and associated treatments/medications/supplements can impact a senior pet's response to drugs.
- Most animals, particularly cats, can be very good at hiding pain until it is advanced.
  - Cats exhibit more behavioral changes of OA than clinical ones.[2,3]
  - Educate clients to watch for early signs of pain as educated owners are good at identifying behaviors instead of believing the sign is just "normal aging." [4,5]
- Pain should be ruled out for a patient with a sudden change in behavior.
  - Behavior change: 28–82% of cases referred to behaviorists have an underlying pain issue.[6]
  - Dogs that develop noise sensitivities later in life should be investigated thoroughly for musculoskeletal pain.[7]
- Osteoarthritis is very common in senior patients (see Osteoarthritis).
  - Dog—very common; up to 38% of dogs have some degree of OA.[8]
    - Signs become more prevalent or worsen in older pets.
  - Cat—Reports of OA range from affecting 22–90% of populations with higher prevalence in older study groups.[9]
    - 90% of cats over 12 years of age had evidence of OA or DJD on radiographs.[9]

Detection and Assessment

- Presenting signs (partial list).
  - Dogs—lameness, trouble rising from a sitting or lying down position, being unable to maintain a posture for elimination, hunched over, not eating.
  - Cats—less time spent grooming, or excessive grooming of one joint, not jumping up or down, unable to get into the litter box.
- Pain Assessment Tools—See Internet Resources below.
  - Chronic pain scales and assessments, dogs
    - ACVS Canine Orthopedic Index (COI)
      - ◇ Evaluates stiffness, gait, function, and quality of life for dogs with OA.
    - Canine Brief Pain Inventory (CPBI)
      - ◇ Evaluates pain severity and pain interference with function for dogs with OA and bone cancer.
    - Canine Osteoarthritis Staging Tool (COAST)
      - ◇ The joint and the dog are evaluated to assign a stage of OA.
    - Dog OA Checklist (Zoetis Petcare)
      - ◇ Lists signs of OA, grading of activity and behavior, and asks history questions that can be emailed or printed to provide to the veterinary team facilitating pain and OA discussions.
    - Liverpool Osteoarthritis in Dogs (LOAD)
      - ◇ Evaluates mobility in general and at exercise for use in dogs with OA.
  - Chronic pain scales and assessment, cats
    - Cat OA Checklist (Zoetis Petcare)
      - ◇ Lists signs of OA, grading of activity and comfort, and asks about behavior changes so that the answers can be emailed or printed to provide to the veterinary team facilitating pain and OA discussions.

- Montreal Instrument for Cat Arthritis Testing (Caretaker)—Version 2
  - Owner assessment of feline OA by assessing agility, social and play behaviors, and physical conditions.
- North Carolina State Translation Research in Pain (TRiP) Clinical Metrology Instruments:
  - Feline Musculoskeletal Pain Index (FMPI)
    - Evaluates mobility, ability to perform daily activities, and interaction with other pets and people.
  - Client-Specific Outcome Measure (CSOM)
    - Three home activities are selected and tracked over time to monitor the cat's response to treatment or level of impairment.
  - Subjective Nighttime Restlessness Evaluation (SNoRE)
    - Owner assessment of the severity of disturbed sleep due to chronic pain
  - Feline Joint Pain, Muscle Atrophy, and Sensitivity Scoring System
    - Clinician assessment of joint pain/crepitus/thickening, muscle mass, palpation sensitivity, and muscle atrophy.
- Feline Musculoskeletal Pain Screening Checklist (MiPSC)
    - Early OA screening tool/checklist for owners.
    - Developed to increase awareness of OA in cats.[10]

- Acute pain scales, dogs
  - Colorado State University Canine Acute Pain Scale
    - Observational and hands-on evaluation places the patient into one of five categories.
    - Not formally validated, yet a useful teaching tool for students.
  - Glasgow Composite Measure Pain Scale—Short Form (CMPS-SF)
    - Maximum score of 24, or 20 if mobility cannot be assessed.
    - Rescue analgesia is necessary when the score is ≥6/24 or 5/20.
- Acute pain scales and assessment, cats
  - Colorado State University Feline Acute Pain Scale
    - Observational and hands-on evaluation places the patient into one of five categories.
    - Reliability demonstrated; validity testing has not been evaluated.
  - Feline Grimace Scale (FGS) (see Figure 90.1)
    - Validated by veterinarians, technicians, students, and cat owners to score ear position, orbital tightening, muzzle tension, whisker position, and head position.
    - Maximum score of 10; rescue analgesia necessary when ≥4/10.
    - A free phone application is available for the user to select each position score.
    - Tably®: An owner's camera phone photo is evaluated using AI to score a cat as happy (FGS score ≤3) or unhappy (FGS score ≥4).
  - Glasgow Composite Measure Pain Scale—Feline (CMPS-Feline)
    - Validated; the maximum score is 20.
    - Rescue analgesia is necessary when the score is ≥5/20.
  - UNESP-Botucatu Multidimensional Feline Pain Assessment Scale (UFEPS)
    - Scoring of 10 observations including pre-surgical blood pressure; max score 30.
    - Validated, yet may be time-consuming and complex.[11]
  - UFEPS Short Form (UFEPS-SF)[11]

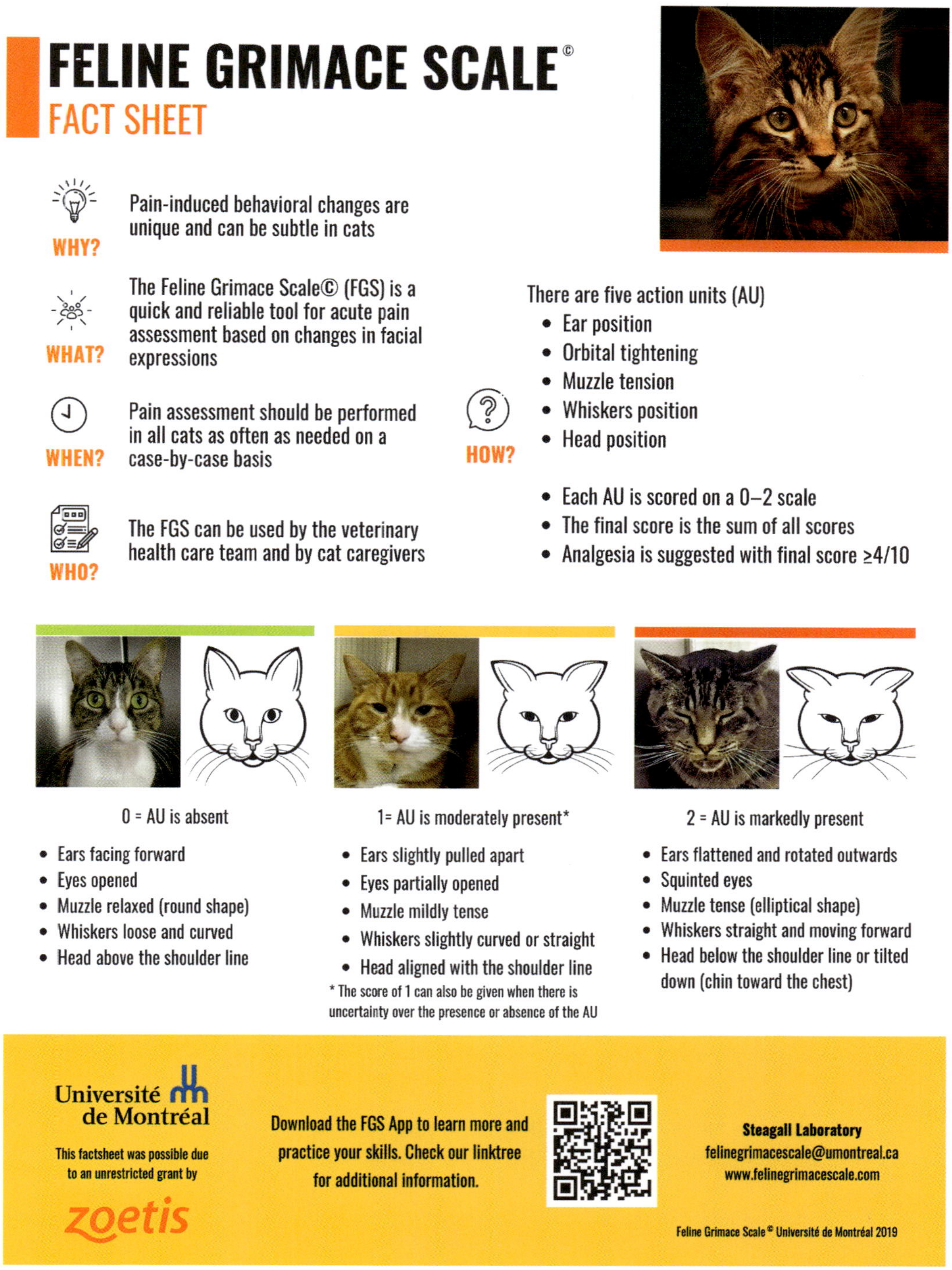

■ **Figure 90.1** Assessment of acute pain in cats based on changes in facial expressions. Pain assessment in cats | Feline Grimace Scale.

        - ◇ Score posture, activity, attitude, and reaction to palpation (0–3).
        - ◇ Validated and easy; maximum score of 12; rescue analgesia needed at ≥4.
    - Force plate and pressure-sensitive walkway with gait analysis.
    - A wearable monitor that can quantify both acute and chronic pain by measuring the biosignal response on the skin to stimuli sensor (pain).
    - Thermal imaging—areas with inflammation will have a higher temperature and increased blood flow than non-inflamed areas.
- Home videos
    - Pets often will not want to ambulate in the clinic or may not show signs of lameness.
    - Have pet owners take videos of their pet walking, rising from a sitting or lying-down position, going up or down stairs, jumping up and off chairs or counters (cats), or any other activity they feel has changed.

Treatment—Management

Most patients will benefit from a multi-modal approach to pain management (treatment with different modes of action and a clear rationale) instead of polypharmacy (multiple therapies that may work through the same pathway or lack rationale). By combining different classes of drugs and interventions, we can address pain at different levels of the pain pathway. Doing so allows us to use lower doses of each of these drugs to achieve a greater total effect. Lower doses translate to decreased adverse effects of each drug as well. A long-term management plan should include pharmaceutics and non-pharmaceutic therapies such as supplements, physical therapy, exercise, and weight loss. Each treatment plan should be individualized to the patient and condition, keeping the caregiver's capabilities in mind as well. While some approaches may have to take a trial-and-error approach to see what best fits that patient, starting with a well-considered plan based on evaluation and observation can optimally make a difference in that pet's comfort and mobility. With maladaptive or chronic pain, the owner needs to realize that there is likely no cure, so the goal will be a more comfortable pet with a reasonable quality of life (QoL).

Pharmaceutics

NSAIDs—COX inhibitors

- NSAIDs are typically the foundation of most pain management protocols, though they can have adverse effects in geriatrics as well as other age groups.
    - If there is concern with inappetence during NSAID administration, you need to find out if it is secondary to a gastric ulcer forming.
    - Don't administer an NSAID unless a pet has voluntarily eaten that day.
- It is not uncommon for cats with OA/DJD to have some degree of CKD. Long-term use of low-dose (0.02 mg/kg/day) meloxicam has shown less progression of renal disease in one large prospective study[12] and some incidence of increased proteinuria in another small study.[13] Caution should always be taken as acute kidney injury (AKI) has been documented post meloxicam injections in some cats.[14] Since there is an inflammatory component to renal disease in cats, careful administration and monitoring could be beneficial for pain management, provided no adverse effects occur.

Grapiprant

- Prostaglandin receptor agonist (PRA) targets canine OA pain and inflammation without COX inhibition, which can impact gastrointestinal, renal, and hepatic metabolism. (EP4 location of action).

Acetaminophen/paracetamol

- NEVER use in cats.
- Ineffective anti-inflammatory.
- Antagonizes COX3 to inhibit CNS prostaglandins (fever reduction).
- Serotonin agonist requiring intact cannabinoid receptors for action.
- Can sometimes be used in combination with opioids (monitor tramadol as it also serotonin effect).
- Rapidly absorbed in dogs, but has a very short half-life, and never use alone.
    - if patient can't tolerate NSAID, needs analgesia during NSAID washout period, or with NSAID (33 mg/kg q8h for 3–5 days, then 15–25 mg/kg BID or TID).[15]

Tramadol

- The M1 metabolite (O-desmethyltramadol) binds to the μ opioid receptor to provide analgesia. Cats produce O-desmethyltramadol whereas dogs do not produce M1 significantly. M1 half-life is 2 hours in dogs vs. 7 hours in people. (4–10 mg/kg PO q6h dogs; 2–4 mg/kg PO q6–12h cats)[16]
- Any benefit is through serotoninergic and noradrenergic effects for analgesia in dogs.
    - Serotonin toxicity clinical signs: increased neuromuscular activity, tachycardia, fever, tachypnea, and agitation.
- Never administer alone for pain management.
- Controlled substance with limited use; consider alternatives.

Opioids

- Opioids are poorly absorbed orally in dogs.
- They can provide extra pain relief for hospice care patients, ideally through the utilization of a CRI.
- Buprenorphine, a partial μ agonist, in the transdermal form (Zorbium®) can provide analgesia for up to four days in cats. There is a greater μ receptor affinity with buprenorphine, so administration of full μ agonists in nearby time periods may not have the desired effect.[17]
- Opioids can impact hepatic, renal, and GI function at high doses.

Amantadine—N-methyl-D-aspartate (NMDA) receptor antagonist

- NDMA—a glutamate receptor in the dorsal horn of spinal cord that plays a role in the development of hyperalgesia and allodynia.
- Amantadine can decrease the activation of NMDA receptors and is best combined with NSAIDs.
- 3–5 mg/kg SID—improved activity after 21 days used in combination with an NSAID.[18]

Ketamine—NMDA antagonist—"reset button for chronic pain"

- Hospitalized on a CRI to provide a "pain vacation"
    - IV loading dose 0.25–0.5 mg/kg.
    - 75 mg ketamine added to 500 mL of fluids running at 2 mL/kg/h provides 0.3 mg/kg/h.
    - CRI can be administered up to 72 hours.[19]
- Anecdotal, low-dose regular injections 0.5 mg/kg subcutaneously.[20]

Gabapentin/Pregabalin

- Mode of action for pain is unknown; has been shown to reduce hyperalgesia in several animal models.
- Gabapentin is eliminated unchanged in urine (non-metabolized).
    - Poor renal function may result in reduced elimination, increased duration, and plasma concentration; monitor renal function.
- 5–10 mg/kg PO q8–12h.[19]
- Start at 3–5 mg/kg once daily for 5–14 days and gradually increase to the intended dose. The gradual introduction minimizes the sedation and ataxia side effects as the body acclimates to the drug.

- Make sure mobility is not impaired; reduce dose if necessary.
- If you need to discontinue, do it gradually with a tapering dose; don't stop precipitously, as it can cause rebound pain.

Maropitant

- Not consistent in the control of pain.[19]
- The anti-vomiting effect is important, and this may help with visceral pain.
- Not for nausea—use ondansetron.

Anti-Nerve Growth Factor (NGF) monoclonal antibody (mAb)

- Species-specific biological therapies.
- NGF—is released in the peripheral tissues like cartilage and is involved in peripheral inflammation. NGF also plays a role in central sensitization.[21]
- Dogs – Bedinvetmab: Canine anti-NGF antibody—decreased OA pain in as little as 7 days. At least two injections, one month apart, are needed to reach steady-state levels.
- Cats—Frunevetmab: Felinized anti-NGF antibody injection—effect noticed typically within 3 weeks and lasted up to 6 weeks.
- Anecdotally beneficial for cats with idiopathic cystitis or FCGS.

Nonpharmacologic Therapies

- Oral omega 3 fatty acids—EPA + DHA—As a supplement or functional food.
  - Have the most consistent evidence of efficacy over other nutraceuticals.[22]
  - 50–60 mg EPA + DHA per kg for cats (don't overdose).
  - Starting dose dogs: 100 mg EPA + DHA/kg lean body weight.
    - Recommended mg is 310 × (kg body weight)$^{0.75}$
    - Do not exceed the safe upper limit of 370 × (kg body weight)$^{0.75}$
- PSGAG—polysulfated glycosaminoglycan and pentosan polysulfate sodium intramuscular injections.
  - PSGAG administered twice weekly can inhibit catabolic enzymes that contribute to cartilage loss.
    - Begin early in the disease process to slow progression of cartilage damage
    - Label dose high; use 5 mg/kg once weekly for 4–6 weeks, then once monthly in dogs
    - Cats—same for 4 weeks, then every other week, then monthly
  - Pentosan polysulfate sodium—1 mL/33 kg once weekly for 4 weeks, then once monthly (Canada, Europe, Australia).
- Cannabinoids
  - Two primary receptors: CB1 (psychoactive mediator) & CB2 (anti-inflammatory and immunosuppressive actions).
  - Endocannabinoids, phytocannabinoids (plant based), and synthetic cannabinoids
  - Cannabidiol (CBD) had analgesia and immune-modulating effects at CB2 receptors with minimal sedating and psychotropic effects.
  - THC (delta-9-tetrahydrocannabinol) is a strong agonist of CB1. Effects are psychoactive with anxiety, tachycardia, and peripheral vasodilation.
  - Small amounts of THC can increase efficacy when administered with CBD.[23]
  - Recommendations are challenging as laws vary widely in regions.
  - Caution when used with other drugs, especially calcium channel drugs such as gabapentin.
  - OA—start low at 2 mg/kg CBD oil twice daily; monitor hepatic function.
- Nutritional Supplements—See Nutritional Supplements topic
  - Glucosamine/chondroitin, avocado-soybean unsaponifiables, undenatured collagen type II, green-lipped mussel, microlactin, curcumin: additional evidence needed, variability in efficacy, variability in quality of products.[22]

Regenerative Medicine

- To grow, repair, replace injured or diseases cells, organs, or tissues.
- Progenitor cells are present in every tissue; they are self-renewing, can differentiate and signal other cells to repair tissue.
- Stem cell therapy: Adipose-derived and bone-marrow-derived mesenchymal stem cells (unspecialized adult cells)
  - These have immunomodulatory and anti-inflammatory effects that can migrate to the sites of tissue injury.
  - Benefits are likely due to growth factors.
- Platelet-rich plasma (PRP)
  - See Intra-articular injections below.

Intra-Articular (IA) Injections

- Hyaluronic acid (HA) is injected IA or given orally. It is a natural component of joint fluid and cartilage.
- Platelet-rich plasma (PRP) contains growth factors and proteins with anti-inflammatory properties.
  - The patient's own blood is collected and processed, then injected into affected joints.
- Collagen–Elastin Hydrogel Microparticles (CEHM^s) are injected creating a sponge-like, insoluble matrix which simulates cartilage. A single injection can last months to years.
- Tin colloid delivered with IA injection of a radioisotope. This requires a license for radioactive medical therapies. May provide analgesia for up to 1 year.[19]
- Transient receptor potential vanilloid 1 (TRPV1) agonist.
  - Expressed in nociceptive sensory neurons.
  - Target for pain management with capsaicin and resiniferatoxin but not yet available.

Physical Therapies

Rehabilitation

- Aims to restore, maintain, and promote optimal function and QOL as related to mobility disorders.
- Senior patients can have sarcopenia, an anticipated loss of muscle mass.
- They can also have disuse atrophy with DJD, and this can become a vicious cycle with decreased mobility.
- Types of rehabilitation
  - Manual therapies—joint mobilization, traction, myofacial release, assisted range of motion
  - Therapeutic and proprioceptive exercise—physioballs, therapy bands, rocker/wobble boards, cavaletti poles, land treadmills
  - Hydrotherapy—pools, resistance pools, underwater treadmills.
  - Therapeutic exercises—
    - Produces exercise-induced hypoalgesia: activates the opioid system with endorphin release.
    - Stretching, strengthening, balance, proprioception, flexibility, endurance, and muscle reeducation.

Acupuncture

- Defined locations in the body are rich in neurovascular or myofascial structures (neuroanatomic points).
- Acupuncture methods stimulate an endogenous response to promote analgesia, healing, and immune modulation.

- It can be used in combination with other modalities as an adjunct and even as a stand-alone therapy.
- It can help decrease the use of medications in the presence of organ dysfunction.
- Dry needling can be combined with electrical stimulation (electroacupuncture) for added benefit.
- Inexpensive but requires training.

Massage and Fascial Tissue Mobilization

- Can cause release of growth factor, proteins, and neurotransmitters.
- Can provide relief of myofascial pain, neuromuscular stimulation, and a feeling of well-being.
- It can increase blood flow and improve lymphatic drainage.
- Massage or trigger point therapy with acupuncture needles can help relieve myofascial pain.
  - When a muscle is held in contraction for a period of time, a taut band is formed.
  - If formed across a joint with DJD, this is painful and causes further damage to the joint.

Weight Loss

- Excess adipose tissue can increase the levels of circulating inflammatory agents.
  - It places extra demands on cardiovascular and respiratory systems, and the musculoskeletal system.
- Moderate weight loss (just over 6%) has shown a positive impact on lameness and gait analysis in dogs.[24]

Cryotherapy and Thermotherapy

- Cold therapy can help reduce pain, inflammation, and swelling in acute pain or acute-on-chronic pain, but only to a shallow depth.
- Heat therapy can reduce pain, improve joint mobility, and increase blood flow for chronic or sub-acute situations.

Electrical Stimulation

- Can promote wound healing, provide pain control/relief, result in reduction of inflammation, muscle reeducation, and strengthening and reversal of atrophy.
- Works at cellular level to cause excitation of nerves, change in membrane permeability, stimulate protein synthesis, osteosynthesis and fibroblast formation.
- At a tissue level there is skeletal and smooth muscle contraction.
- Segmental-level action results in muscle-pumping action to improve joint mobility and improve circulatory and lymphatic drainage.
- Transcutaneous Electrical Nerve Stimulation (TENS).
- Neuromuscular Electric Stimulation (NMES).

Shock Wave (Sound) Therapy

- Extracorporeal shock wave therapy (ESWT) results in increased serotonin activity in dorsal horn and descending inhibition of pain signals.
- A sudden high-powered shock wave is released producing tissue modulation in a very focused depth of tissue.
- Immediate pain relief lasting days to weeks.
- Common areas treated: hip and elbow dysplasia, supraspinatus tendinopathy.
- Newer devices seldom need patient sedation.

Laser—Photobiomodulation

- For pain management, control of inflammation and tissue healing.
- Penetration of laser energy determined by wavelength (patented).
- Accelerated cell division via mitochondrial stimulation, increased leukocyte phagocytosis, stimulation of fibroblast production, enhanced synthesis of ATP and angiogenesis.

tPEMF—Targeted Pulsed Electromagnetic Field

- Reduction of inflammation and pain[25] (see Figure 90.2)
- Cell proliferation (i.e., multiplication) and collagen formation
- Increase in circulation and oxygenation of tissue

Surgical Interventions

- Limb amputation—failed fracture repair, osteosarcoma
- Total joint replacement
- Excision arthroplasty—femoral head and neck excision
- Arthrodesis—permanently eliminates movement of a joint and minimizes pain
- Sensory denervation—(hip, elbow) when other medical, surgical, and adjunctive therapy has failed

Environmental Adaptation and Mobility Assist (See Mobility and Environment Enrichment and Adaptation)

- Raising food and water dishes
- Yoga mats or rugs to reduce slipping
- Ramps
- Baby gaits to limit access
- Orthopedic bed
- Harnesses, slings

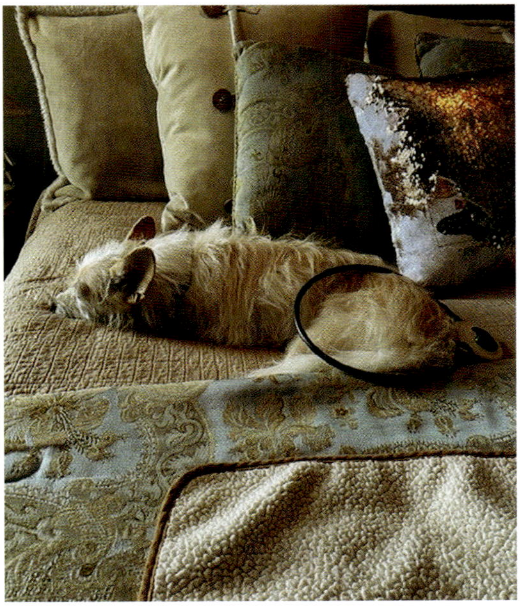

■ **Figure 90.2** Sixteen-year-old Hazel resting during her Assisi Loop™ tPEMF (pulsed electromagnetic field) therapy for osteoarthritis pain. Source: Image courtesy of Steve Dale.

- Booties, power socks, toe grips
- Carts and wheelchairs
- Bedding and positioning
- Movement and gentle exercise

APPLICATION IN PRACTICE

- Evaluate each patient and determine the analgesic protocol that will often be multimodal.
  - Consider overall drug burden—how many drugs and how often? How to prioritize the most critical.
  - The patient's tolerance to prescribed drugs and their administration.
- Evaluate the ease of administration—palatability, owner skills, pet's likes and dislikes.
- Access to non-drug therapies (physical therapy, acupuncture, etc.) and the patient's likely tolerance of that therapy.

Team Roles And Training

- Team communication
  - Every person in the practice should be aware of FAS and pain scoring to aid in observations as to patient improvements and the need for pain management
- Front office staff
  - When a client calls for an appointment to evaluate a pet's lameness, instruct them to record videos.
  - Instruct clients to use osteoarthritis checklists (see Internet Resources below).
- Veterinary technicians and assistants
  - Obtain a history of any discomfort or lameness; if checklists have been submitted, review answers with the owner.
  - Technicians and assistants can implement veterinary-prescribed laser and some other physical therapies and instruct clients on tPEMF, environmental modifications, home manual therapies, and exercise.
- Veterinarians
  - Pain score on every visit and at frequent intervals with in-hospital administered treatments.
  - Thorough physical examination with evaluation of limb/joint palpation, abdominal palpation, gait, range of motion, goniometry, and behaviors. COAST and other pain assessments can be utilized to provide baselines and aid in treatment planning as well as response to therapy.

Client Communication

- Since owners might not be aware of or may underestimate chronic pain, educating and engaging clients is essential for identifying and understanding the necessity of chronic pain treatment and improving outcomes after implementing treatments.
- Setting and communicating achievable goals with the owner prior to the initiation of treatment is crucial for the effective implementation of a pain management and osteoarthritis treatment plan. This helps ensure that the owner's expectations are realistic and the selected therapies are more likely to gain compliance in the home environment.
- It's important to set realistic expectations, emphasizing that outcomes are not usually instant and that the condition is expected to be permanent and requires lifelong management.
- Prior to initiating any treatment, obtain informed consent.

FURTHER PAIN TYPES AND THERAPIES

Neuropathic pain

- Gabapentin/pregabalin
- NSAIDs
- Amantadine
- Ketamine (sub-anesthetic dose as a CRI or possibly subcutaneous)
- Anti-NGF mAbs
- Physical modalities—cold/heat therapy, acupuncture/electroacupuncture, stretching, and massage
- Avoid opioids (see Cautions)

Severe Acute-on-Chronic Hyperalgesia and Allodynia

- Neuro-modifying techniques in the hospital
  - Locoregional blocks
  - Intravenous analgesics—lidocaine 1 mg/kg bolus with 30 µg/kg/min CRI (cautious use in cats)
  - Ketamine as above or IV bolus 0.5–1 mg/kg then CRI of 2–10 µg/kg/min CRI
  - Acupuncture/electroacupuncture

Cancer Pain

- Vary—duration, location, type of cancer
- Inflammation, tissue infiltration, organ distension, nerve infiltration or compression, and factors released by tumor
- Bone tumors—invasion of tissues and release of chemical mediators—neuropathic-like signs
- Chemotherapy and radiation therapy can also be associated with significant pain
- Other pain may promote cancer progression
- Multi-modal: NSAIDs, opioids, and adjunctive drugs (gabapentin); bisphosphonates.

Cautions

- Avoid opioids in cases of neuropathic pain—may exacerbate via neuroinflammation and glial amplification.[26]
- Switching NSAIDs or transitioning from an NSAID to steroids—a minimum of a 5–7 days washout is needed, longer if the pet experienced an adverse event.
- See Gabapentin dosing above: work up to the desired dose to minimize the appearance of weakness; slowly withdraw when ending so as to avoid rebound pain.
- Set realistic expectations with the client; attempt to underpromise and overdeliver; set achievable goals with the client reminding them this is usually a lifelong condition.

Abbreviations

- AKI = acute kidney injury
- CPBI = Canine Pain B Index
- COAST = Canine Osteoarthritis Staging Tool
- COX = cyclooxygenase
- CKD = chronic kidney disease
- CB1 & 2 = cannabinoid receptors 1 & 2

- CBD = cannabinoid
- DHA = docosahexaenoic acid
- EPA = eicosapentaenoic acid
- DJD = degenerative joint disease
- FMPI = Feline Musculoskeletal Pain Index
- HA = hyaluronic acid
- mAbs = monoclonal antibodies
- MiPSC = Musculoskeletal Pain Score Checklist
- NGF = nerve growth factor
- NMDA = N-methyl-D-aspartate
- NMES = neuromuscular electric stimulation
- NSAID = non-steroidal anti-inflammatory drug
- OA = osteoarthritis
- PEMF = Pulsed electromagnetic field
- PSGAG = PSGAG = polysulfated glycosaminoglycan and pentosan polysulfate sodium
- PRP = platelet-rich protein
- PRA = prostaglandin receptor agonist
- QOL = Quality of life
- TENS = transcutaneous electrical nerve stimulation
- THC = delta-9-tetrahydrocannabinol
- TPRV1 = transient receptor potential vanilloid 1

Internet Resources

Pain Assessment Tools:

- Overview, by species: https://www.thinkanesthesia.education/sites/default/files/2021-12/Veterinary%20Pain%20Assessment%20Tool%20-%20v2.1.pdf
- Chronic pain scales and assessments
  - ACVS Canine Orthopedic Index (COI)
    - https://www.vet.upenn.edu/research/clinical-trials-vcic/our-services/pennchart/canine-orthopedic-index
  - Canine Brief Pain Inventory (CPBI)
    - https://www.vet.upenn.edu/research/clinical-trials-vcic/our-services/pennchart/cbpi-tool
  - Canine Osteoarthritis Staging Tool (COAST)
    - https://assets.elanco.com/0cec44ed-3eaa-0009-2029-666567e7e4de/b2d5f58c-2645-46ad-b5e5-65906b491bf3/COAST%20Printable%20PDF.pdf
    - https://www.frontiersin.org/articles/10.3389/fvets.2023.1137888
  - Liverpool Osteoarthritis in Dogs (LOAD)
    - https://dspace.uevora.pt/rdpc/bitstream/10174/19611/2/liverpoolOAindogs-load.pdf
  - Montreal Instrument for Cat Arthritis Testing (Caretaker)—Version 2
    - https://ars.els-cdn.com/content/image/1-s2.0-S0168159117303271-mmc2.pdf
  - NC State TRiP Clinical Metrology Instruments: (FMPI, CSOM, SNoRE, MiPSC, etc.)
    - https://cvm.ncsu.edu/research/labs/clinical-sciences/comparative-pain-research/clinical-metrology-instruments/
  - Zoetis questionnaire for owners
    - Canine: https://www.zoetispetcare.com/checklist/osteoarthritis-checklist
    - Feline: https://www.zoetispetcare.com/checklist/osteoarthritis-checklist-cat

- Acute pain scales and assessment
  - Colorado State University Acute Pain Scale
    - Canine: https://vetmedbiosci.colostate.edu/vth/wp-content/uploads/sites/7/2020/12/canine-pain-scale.pdf
    - Feline: https://vetmedbiosci.colostate.edu/vth/wp-content/uploads/sites/7/2020/12/feline-pain-scale.pdf
  - Feline Grimace Scale (FGS)
    - https://www.felinegrimacescale.com/
    - https://www.sylvester.ai/how-tably-works
  - Glasgow Composite Measure Pain Scale (Canine short form and Feline)
    - https://www.newmetrica.com/acute-pain-measurement/
  - UNESP- Botucatu Multidimensional Composite Pain Scale
    - UFEPS: http://www.animalpain.com.br/assets/upload/escala-en-us.pdf
    - UFEPS short form: https://www.ncbi.nlm.nih.gov/pmc/articles/PMC8048399/
- Pain Trace wearable monitor: https://paintrace.com/clinical-use/
- Canine EPA+DHA Dosing Chart: https://vetmedbiosci.colostate.edu/vth/services/orthopedic-medicine/fish-oil-dosing/
- CEHM, Spryng™ Osteocushion: https://www.sprynghealth.com/small-animal-how-it-works

Additional Resources and Organizations

- 2022 AAHA Pain Management Guidelines: https://www.aaha.org/resources/2022-aaha-pain-management-guidelines-for-dogs-and-cats/
- 2022 ISFM Consensus Guidelines on the Management of Acute Pain in Cats: https://journals.sagepub.com/doi/epdf/10.1177/1098612X211066268
- 2024 ISFM/AAFP Consensus Guidelines on the Long-term Use of NSAIDs in Cats: https://catvets.com/guidelines/practice-guidelines/nsaids-consensus-guidelines
- Review of NSAID Induced Adverse Effects in Dogs: https://doi.org/10.1111/jvim.12127
- CARE: Canine Arthritis Resources and Education: https://caninearthritis.org/
- 2022 WSAVA Pain Guidelines: https://onlinelibrary.wiley.com/doi/10.1111/jsap.13566
- WSAVA Global Nutrition Guidelines: https://wsava.org/global-guidelines/global-nutrition-guidelines/
- International Veterinary Academy of Pain Management (IVAPM): https://www.ivapm.org/pain-guidelines
- Veterinary Anesthesia and Analgesia Support Group (VASG): https://vasg.org/
- Zero Pain Philosophy: https://www.zeropainphilosophy.com/vet-professionals

References

1. Hughes J. Anaesthesia for the geriatric dog and cat. *Ir Vet J* 2008 Jun 1;61(6):380–387. doi: https://doi.org/10.1186/2046-0481-61-6-380. PMID: 21851715; PMCID: PMC3113863.
2. Jaffe M. Diagnosis and management of feline osteoarthritis. *Today's Veterinary Practice* 2023 Mar/Apr:80–90. Accessed 9 June 2024: https://todaysveterinarypractice.com/orthopedics/diagnosis-and-management-of-feline-osteoarthritis/.
3. Merola I, Mills DS. Behavioural signs of pain in cats: an expert consensus. *PLoS One* 2016 Feb 24;11(2):e0150040. doi: https://doi.org/10.1371/journal.pone.0150040. PMID: 26909809; PMCID: PMC4765852.
4. Lascelles BD, Hansen BD, Roe S, DePuy V, Thomson A, Pierce CC, Smith ES, Rowinski E. Evaluation of client-specific outcome measures and activity monitoring to measure pain relief in cats with osteoarthritis. *J Vet Intern Med* 2007 May–Jun;21(3):410–416. doi: https://doi.org/10.1892/0891-6640(2007)21[410:eocoma]2.0.co;2. PMID: 17552444.

5. Kerwin SC. Osteoarthritis in cats. *Top Companion Anim Med* 2010 Nov;25(4):218–223. doi: https://doi.org/10.1053/j.tcam.2010.09.004. PMID: 21147475.
6. Mills DS, Demontigny-Bédard I, Gruen M, et al. Pain and problem behavior in cats and dogs. Animals 2020;10(2). doi: https://doi.org/10.3390/ani10020318
7. Lopes Fagundes AL, Hewison L, McPeake KJ, Zulch H, Mills DS. Noise Sensitivities in Dogs: An Exploration of Signs in Dogs with and without Musculoskeletal Pain Using Qualitative Content Analysis. *Front Vet Sci* 2018 Feb 13;5:17. doi: https://doi.org/10.3389/fvets.2018.00017. PMID: 29487858; PMCID: PMC5816950.
8. Wright A, Amodie DM, Cernicchiaro N, Lascelles BDX, Pavlock AM, Roberts C, Bartram DJ. Identification of canine osteoarthritis using an owner-reported questionnaire and treatment monitoring using functional mobility tests. J Small Anim Pract. 2022 Aug;63(8):609–618. doi: https://doi.org/10.1111/jsap.13500. Epub 2022 Apr 6. PMID: 35385129; PMCID: PMC9543207.
9. Lascelles BD, Henry JB 3rd, Brown J, Robertson I, Sumrell AT, Simpson W, Wheeler S, Hansen BD, Zamprogno H, Freire M, Pease A. Cross-sectional study of the prevalence of radiographic degenerative joint disease in domesticated cats. *Vet Surg* 2010 Jul;39(5):535–544. doi: https://doi.org/10.1111/j.1532-950X.2010.00708.x. Epub 2010 Jun 18. PMID: 20561321.
10. Enomoto M, Lascelles BDX, Gruen ME. Development of a checklist for the detection of degenerative joint disease-associated pain in cats. *J Feline Med Surg* 2020 Dec;22(12):1137–1147. doi: https://doi.org/10.1177/1098612X20907424. Epub 2020 Mar 3. PMID: 32122226; PMCID: PMC7736399.
11. Belli M, de Oliveira AR, de Lima MT, Trindade PHE, Steagall PV, Luna SPL. Clinical validation of the short and long UNESP-Botucatu scales for feline pain assessment. *PeerJ* 2021 Apr 12;9:e11225. doi: https://doi.org/10.7717/peerj.11225. PMID: 33954046; PMCID: PMC8048399.
12. Gowan RA, Lingard AE, Johnston L, Stansen W, Brown SA, Malik R. Retrospective case-control study of the effects of long-term dosing with meloxicam on renal function in aged cats with degenerative joint disease. *J Feline Med Surg* 2011 Oct;13(10):752–761. doi: https://doi.org/10.1016/j.jfms.2011.06.008. Epub 2011 Sep 9. PMID: 21906984.
13. KuKanich K, George C, Roush JK, Sharp S, Farace G, Yerramilli M, Peterson S, Grauer GF. Effects of low-dose meloxicam in cats with chronic kidney disease. *J Feline Med Surg* 2021 Feb;23(2):138–148. doi: https://doi.org/10.1177/1098612X20935750. Epub 2020 Jun 29. PMID: 32594827; PMCID: PMC10741344.
14. Wun MK, Leister E, King T, Korman R, Malik R. Acute kidney injury in 18 cats after subcutaneous meloxicam and an update on non-steroidal anti-inflammatory drug usage in feline patients in Australia. *Aust Vet J.* 2023 Mar; 101(3):90–98. doi: https://doi.org/10.1111/avj.13222 Epub 2022 Dec 5. PMID: 36470590.
15. Gurney M. Paracetamol for long term use. *Zero Pain Philosophy* 2024. Accessed 30 June 2024: https://www.zeropainphilosophy.com/post/paracetamol-for-long-term-use.
16. Ruel HLM, Steagall PV. Adjuvant analgesics in acute pain management. *Vet Clin North Am Small Anim Pract* 2019 Nov;49(6):1127–1141. doi: https://doi.org/10.1016/j.cvsm.2019.07.005. Epub 2019 Aug 30. PMID: 31474414.
17. Mathis JR. Oral pain management. In Lobprise HB (ed.) *Blackwell's Five-Minute Veterinary Consult Clinical Companion: Small Animal Dentistry*, 3rd edn. Hoboken, NJ: John Wiley & Sons, Inc., 2021; pp 84-96 doi: https://doi.org/10.1002/9781119584414.ch8
18. Lascelles BD, Gaynor JS, Smith ES, Roe SC, Marcellin-Little DJ, Davidson G, Boland E, Carr J. Amantadine in a multimodal analgesic regimen for alleviation of refractory osteoarthritis pain in dogs. *J Vet Intern Med* 2008 Jan–Feb;22(1):53–59. doi: https://doi.org/10.1111/j.1939-1676.2007.0014.x. PMID: 18289289.
19. Monteiro BP, Lascelles BDX, Murrell J, Robertson S, Steagall PVM, Wright B. 2022 WSAVA guidelines for the recognition, assessment, and treatment of pain. *J Small Anim Pract* 2023 April; 64(4):177–254. doi: https://doi.org/10.1111/jsap.13566
20. Gurney M. Subcutaneous ketamine for analgesia. *Zero Pain Philosophy* 2024. Accessed 30 June 2024: https://www.zeropainphilosophy.com/post/subcutaneous-ketamine-for-analgesia.
21. Enomoto M, Mantyh PW, Murrell J, Innes JF, Lascelles BDX. Anti-nerve growth factor monoclonal antibodies for the control of pain in dogs and cats. *Vet Rec* 2019 Jan 5;184(1):23. doi: https://doi.org/10.1136/vr.104590. Epub 2018 Oct 27. PMID: 30368458; PMCID: PMC6326241.

22. Cachon T, Frykman O, Innes JF, Lascelles BDX, Okumura M, Sousa P, Staffieri F, Steagall PV, Van Ryssen B. COAST Development Group's international consensus guidelines for the treatment of canine osteoarthritis. *Front Vet Sci* 2023 Aug 3;10:1137888. doi: https://doi.org/10.3389/fvets.2023.1137888. PMID: 37601753; PMCID: PMC10436090.
23. Vaughn D, Kulpa J, Paulionis L. Preliminary investigation of the safety of escalating cannabinoid doses in healthy dogs. *Front Vet Sci* 2020 Feb 11;7:51. doi: https://doi.org/10.3389/fvets.2020.00051. PMID: 32118071; PMCID: PMC7029731.
24. Marshall WG, Hazewinkel HA, Mullen D, De Meyer G, Baert K, Carmichael S. The effect of weight loss on lameness in obese dogs with osteoarthritis. *Vet Res Commun* 2010 Mar;34(3):241–253. doi: https://doi.org/10.1007/s11259-010-9348-7. Epub 2010 Mar 17. PMID: 20237844; PMCID: PMC2855019.
25. Pinna S, Landucci F, Tribuiani AM, Carli F, Venturini A. The effects of pulsed electromagnetic field in the treatment of osteoarthritis in dogs: clinical study. *Pak Vet J* 2013;33(1):96–100.
26. Salvemini D, Doyle TM. Targeting neuroinflammation in neuropathic pain and opioid use. *J Exp Med* 2023 Feb 6;220(2):e20221244. doi: https://doi.org/10.1084/jem.20221244. Epub 2022 Dec 23. PMID: 36562735; PMCID: PMC9793426.

Authors: Heidi Lobprise and Jennifer Mathis

Chapter 91

Mobility in Senior Pets

BASICS

OVERVIEW

Mobility is a key factor in maintaining the quality of life of senior and geriatric pets. From frailty and muscle weakness to neurological issues, a decline in mobility can impact their—and their owners'—lives. Osteoarthritis is one of the most common issues with senior pets, so early detection and appropriate management is critical. Other neurological and skeletal issues may affect these special patients as well. Standard therapies using NSAIDS and supplements, weight management, and exercise can be augmented by physical modalities from laser therapy, pulsed electromagnetic fields, and shock (acoustic) wave therapy. Environmental management with non-slid runners, ramps for furniture and vehicles, elevated food bowls, and orthopedic bedding can also help.

Terms Defined

- Mobility—the ability to move freely and easily.
- Functional mobility—the physiological ability to move around their environment to carry out activities of daily living (ADL).[1]
- Static posturography—measuring the center of pressure excursions in a standing dog to determine changes in postural sway.[2]

ISSUES AND OPTIONS

- Normal function requires strength, balance, and energy.
- Biological aging processes can impact function.
    - Loss of muscle strength, cardiorespiratory function decrease, chronic inflammation, and age-related diseases.
    - Adverse effects of medical treatment can also impact function.
    - In humans, there are well-supported interventions to preserve and restore function.[3]
- Loss of function and mobility can impact health span, quality of life, and time to death.[4]
- Frailty—loss of strength and function, increased risk of disability, disease, and death.[5]
- In contrast, vigor looks at retaining strength, speed, and energy.
- Osteoarthritis (OA) and degenerative joint disease (DJD) (see Osteoarthritis).
    - In dogs, OA is not just an old dog disease, though its incidence does increase as age advances, due to the long-term impact of underlying issues, and up to 20% of older dogs suffer from it.

Blackwell's Five-Minute Veterinary Consult Clinical Companion: Small Animal Senior Care,
First Edition. Edited by Heidi B. Lobprise.

Companion website: www.wiley.com/go/lobprise/Senior

    - Conformational issues such as hip or elbow dysplasia can be the primary problem, or injuries such as articular fractures or cranial cruciate ligament problems.
    - For evaluation, determine if the patient has a primary problem and has or will develop OA, or had the primary problem in the past and now suffers from "typical" OA.
    - Management should be multimodal, including weight control, pain medication, anti-inflammatory efforts, exercise, and rehabilitation (see Osteoarthritis).
  - In cats, DJD is a primary condition and less understood.
    - 90% of older cats exhibit some level of radiographic changes; clinical impact is variable.
    - Weight control and medications are used for management, as in dogs.
    - Exercise may not be as successful, but environmental adjustments (lower sides on litter box, easier-to-use cat towers, benches to access higher perches or windows) can help (Figure 91.1).
    - Anti-NGF (nerve growth factor) monoclonal antibody therapies are now available for cats and dogs in many regions.
- Neuromuscular—musculoskeletal disorders.
  - Intervertebral disc disease can occur at any age, but progression during aging can exacerbate discomfort and impact mobility.
  - Degenerative myelopathy affects white matter of the spinal cord and results in a slowly progressive hind limb weakness and paralysis.
    - Intense directed physical therapy has been shown to prolong the quality of life and preserve muscle mass.
    - While not painful, since this often impacts larger dogs, caregiver impact must be considered.
  - GOLPP—Geriatric Onset Laryngeal Paralysis and Paresis.
    - Middle-aged to older, medium, and large breeds are more likely to develop this condition that initially presents as laryngeal paralysis (see GOLPP).

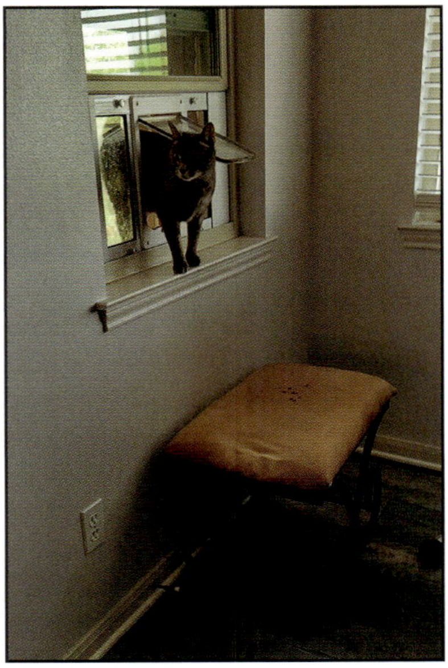

Figure 91.1 Placement of a stool to ease access to a cat door placed in the window.

    - This progressive neuromuscular disease can also affect the esophageal function and leads to progressive weakness of the hind limb muscles.
  - Assess any signs of ataxia, paresis, or abnormal vestibular function to correlate with mobility issues.

APPLICATIONS IN PRACTICE

- A complete history from owners about the pet's daily functions can help assess mobility issues.
  - Getting up from sitting or lying down—any indication of pain, is the pet slower than before?
  - Climbing up and down stairs—any impairment or slowing down.
  - Jumping up and down off surfaces (especially cats).
  - Difficulties getting across slick floors.
  - Posturing during elimination—do they complete the process of urination/defecation?

Mobility Assessments

- Static posturography—measuring the center of pressure excursions in the standing dog to determine age-related changes in postural sway.[2]
  - Two center-of-pressure (COP) measures discriminated between healthy adults and senior dogs.
    - Root mean square overall
    - Acceleration in the craniocaudal direction variable
  - Postural sway increases with age and joint pain.
- Low-technology methods for morphology and mobility trial measurement.[6]
  - Measured height, forelimb length, torso length, left and right thigh circumferences
  - Timed mobility trials
    - Flat surface—on-leach with owner, then investigator; off-leash
    - On stairs
  - Age was a weak but significant predictor of decreased dog speed.
  - Stair ascent—more complex assortment of components.
- Geriatric assessments in rehabilitation.[4]
  - BADIM—basic activity for daily independent mobility
    - Rising from a down position
    - Ambulating in and out of the home
    - Posturing to eliminate
    - Posturing to eat and drink
  - Instrumental activity for daily quality of life (IADQOL)
    - Ascending/descending a flight of stairs
    - Moving in and out of a vehicle
    - Walking short distances outside
    - Exploring the home environment
    - Interacting in play
    - Ability to navigate place of rest (see Figure 91.2)
    - Maintain control of urination and defection for 6–8 hours
  - Canine geriatric functional score (CGFL)
    - TUG—timed up and go (rise from sternal and travel 10 body lengths)

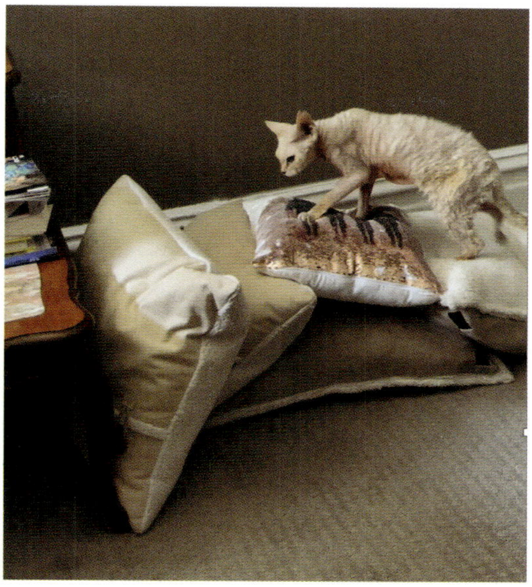

Figure 91.2 Pillows have been placed to help this senior cat with access to the bed. Rearranging the pillows on occasion provides enrichment as well. Source: Photo Courtesy of Steve Dale.

    - Cavaletti—stepping over Cavaletti rail obstacles
    - Walking Figure 8—balance and proprioception
    - Down—number of times sternal to rise in 60 seconds (assist allowed to reposition into down
  - Follow up with professional assessment to reset goals, with weight and body condition score (BCS) every 4–6 weeks.
    - Objective assessments—muscle girth, kinematic gait, weight-bearing, goniometry; canine digital health monitors
    - Subjective assessments
      - CSOM—client-specific outcome measures—assess pain and QOL
      - A task-dependent movement scale can help
  - BADIM and IADQOL need justification and validation.[1]
  - CGFL—artificial nature of tasks, may be unrepresentative of ADL.[1]
- GenPup-M—early detection of mobility changes at time points.[7]
  - Assessed with Liverpool Osteoarthritis in Dogs (LOAD), kinetic and kinematic gait analysis.
  - Even early onset mobility impairments correlated with all three objective measurements.[7]
- Assessment of pain
  - Owner input
  - Clinical evaluation
    - Radiographs
    - Musculoskeletal examination
      - Palpate for discomfort
      - Evaluate joint range of motion
      - Evaluate lean body mass—sarcopenia
  - Chronic pain scales include mobility assessment.

Management to Maximize Mobility

- Pain management
    - If any medication results in drowsiness or decrease in coordination, the dose may need to be reduced or the drug stopped altogether.
- Inflammation management—antioxidants, omega-3 fatty acids.
- Manual therapies
    - Joint mobilization—passive movements of joints using manual techniques, within the joint's range of motion (ROM). This can help address the need for normal movement and stresses to maintain tissue integrity, as well as decrease pain, reduce muscle inhibition, and improve function.[8]
    - Soft tissue mobilization may include massage, stretching, and myofascial release. Soft tissue are extended through stretching during most joint manipulation techniques. Massage can be provided by a variety of techniques and intensities to manipulate the tissues for therapy or relaxation. This can reduce pain, stress, and muscle tension and increase circulation and elasticity.[9]
    - Thermotherapy—the therapeutic use of superficial heat and cold.[10]
        - Cryotherapy, applied soon after the injury or insult (including surgical procedures), can help reduce inflammation, edema, muscle spasm, pain, and hemorrhage.
        - Applying superficial heat too early during healing can increase inflammation and enzymatic activity.
        - Once acute inflammation is resolved, superficial heat increases vasodilation, tissue oxygenation, and the enzymatic activity that can help tissue healing.
        - Superficial heat is also beneficial prior to joint or soft tissue mobilization to increase soft tissue extensibility and decrease joint stiffness.
    - When owners are trained in these therapies, they can be performed in the pet's home.
- Environmental adjustments (see Environmental Enrichment and Adaptation)
    - Non-skid rug runners, yoga mats for slick floors
        - Trimming hair on feet, booties, or application of toe-grips (see Figure 91.3)
    - Exercise balls to assist when standing for feeding or elimination
    - Harness assists (see Figure 91.4)

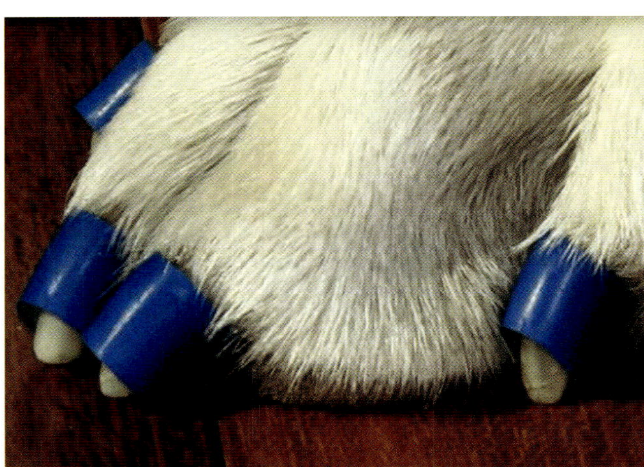

Figure 91.3 Dr.Buzby's ToeGrips(R) can assist in mobility. Courtesy of Dr. Julie Buzby.

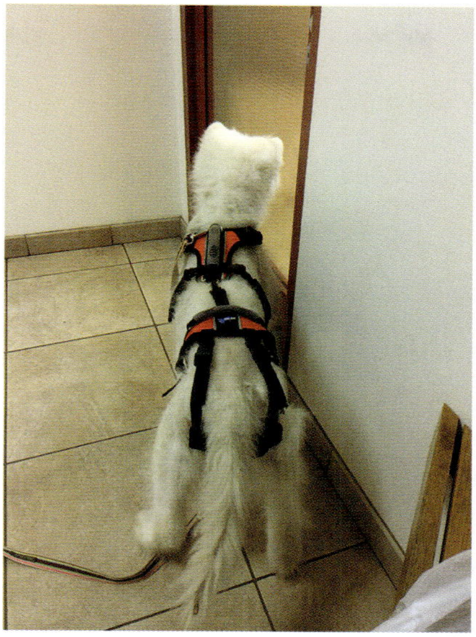

■ **Figure 91.4** Use of a supportive harness and be beneficial to senior dogs with mobility issues. courtesy of Dr. Mary Gardner. Source: Photo Courtesy of Dr. Julie Buzby.

- Elevating food and water bowls when indicated
- Enhance access to places of elimination
  - Make sure there are no physical mobility or other impediments to using a doggy door
  - Low sides on litter boxes
- Use ramps for stairs or doorways if needed

■ Wearable sensors to detect activity and any changes from baseline

Client Communication

■ Help owners understand that a decrease in mobility may not just be part of the aging process.
- Early detection of any declines in mobility can allow potential identification of contributing diseases or processes.
  - Have them keep a video library of basic functions—walking, climbing stairs, getting up from lying down, and posturing for elimination.
- If there is pain or inflammation—multimodal approach to manage.

■ Diet and exercise adjustments may help increase functional abilities and improve quality of life and health span.

■ If mobility is a significant issue for the pet, review what environmental adjustments may be helpful.
- Be empathetic for any caregiving issues that might be challenging for the owner to provide.

See Also

■ GOLPP—Geriatric Onset Laryngeal Paralysis and Paresis
■ Osteoarthritis
■ Quality of Life

Abbreviations

- ADL = activities of daily life
- BADIM = basic activity for daily independent mobility
- BCS = body condition score
- CGFL = Canine Geriatric Functional Score
- COP = center of pressure
- DJD = degenerative joint disease
- GOLPP = geriatric onset laryngeal paralysis and paresis
- IADQOL = Instrumental activity for daily quality of life
- LOAD = Liverpool Osteoarthritis in Dogs
- NGF = nerve growth factor
- NSAID = nonsteroidal anti-inflammatory drug
- OA = osteoarthritis
- QoL = quality of life

Internet Resources

Accessed June 26, 2024

- AARV—American Association of Rehabilitation Veterinarians
  - https://www.rehabvets.org/
- Canine Arthritis Resources and Education
  - Canine Arthritis Resources & Education | Dog arthritis tips and resources

Additional Reading

McKenzie BA, Chen FL. Assessment and management of declining physical function in aging dogs. *Top Companion Anim Med* 2022 Nov–Dec;51:100732. doi: https://doi.org/10.1016/j.tcam.2022.100732. Epub 2022 Oct 21. PMID: 36273752.

References

1. Wells GM, Young K, Haskell MJ, Carter AJ, Clements DN. Mobility, functionality and functional mobility: a review and application for canine veterinary patients. *Vet J* 2024 Jun;305:106123. doi: https://doi.org/10.1016/j.tvjl.2024.106123. Epub 2024 Apr 19. PMID: 38642699.
2. Mondino A, Wagner G, Russell K, Lobaton E, Griffith E, Gruen M, Lascelles BDX, Olby NJ. Static posturography as a novel measure of the effects of aging on postural control in dogs. *PLoS One* 2022 Jul 8;17(7):e0268390. doi: https://doi.org/10.1371/journal.pone.0268390. PMID: 35802714; PMCID: PMC9269968.
3. McKenzie BA, Chen FL. Assessment and management of declining physical function in aging dogs. *Top Companion Anim Med* 2022 Nov–Dec;51:100732. doi: https://doi.org/10.1016/j.tcam.2022.100732. Epub 2022 Oct 21. PMID: 36273752.
4. Frye C, Carr BJ, Lenfest M, Miller A. Canine geriatric rehabilitation: considerations and strategies for assessment, functional scoring, and follow up. *Front Vet Sci* 2022 Feb 25;9:842458. doi: https://doi.org/10.3389/fvets.2022.842458. PMID: 35280131; PMCID: PMC8914307.
5. Hua J, Hoummady S, Muller C, Pouchelon J-L, Blondot M, Gilbert C, Desquilbet L. Assessment of frailty in aged dogs. *Am J Vet Res* 2016;77:1357. doi: https://doi.org/10.2460/AJVR.77.12.1357.
6. Morgan EM, Heseltine JC, Levine GJ, Promislow DEL, Creevy KE. Evaluation of a low-technology system to obtain morphological and mobility trial measurements in dogs and investigation of potential predictors of canine mobility. *Am J Vet Res* 2019 80:670–679. doi: https://doi.org/10.2460/ajvr.80.7.670.
7. Clark NL, Bates KT, Harris LK, Tomlinson AW, Murray JK, Comerford EJ. GenPup-M: a novel validated owner-reported clinical metrology instrument for detecting early mobility changes in dogs. *PLoS One* 2023 Dec 27;18(12):e0291035. doi: https://doi.org/10.1371/journal.pone.0291035. PMID: 38150469; PMCID: PMC10752556.

8. Saunders DG, Walker JR, Levine D. Joint mobilization. *Vet Clin North Am Small Anim Pract* 2005 Nov;35(6):1287–1316, vii–viii. doi: https://doi.org/10.1016/j.cvsm.2005.07.003. PMID: 16260314.
9. Bergh A, Asplund K, Lund I, Boström A, Hyytiäinen H. A systematic review of complementary and alternative veterinary medicine in sport and companion animals: soft tissue mobilization. *Animals (Basel)* 2022 Jun 2;12(11):1440. doi: https://doi.org/10.3390/ani12111440. PMID: 35681903; PMCID: PMC9179335.
10. Dragone L, Heinrichs K, Levine D, Tucker T, Millis D. Superficial thermal modalities In: Millis D, Levine D (eds) *Canine Rehabilitation and Physical Therapy*, 2nd edn. Philadelphia: W.B. Saunders, 2014; pp. 312–327, ISBN 9781437703092, doi: https://doi.org/10.1016/B978-1-4377-0309-2.00018-1.

Author: Heidi Lobprise

Nutrition

Chapter 92

Nutrition for Senior Pets

BASICS

Nutritional assessment is now considered the fifth vital sign in the evaluation of veterinary patients. With all the changes of "normal aging" and age-related diseases, nutrition plays a key role in the management of senior pets, potentially contributing to longevity and a healthy life.

As there are no specific feeding guidelines from AAFCO, the task of determining appropriate diets for senior patients belongs to the veterinary team. On a basic level, considerations of the energy density of the diet, intake of protein, phosphorus, sodium, and other nutrients start the process. From there, specific nutrients and nutraceuticals may be considered to ameliorate or manage typical aging conditions, with focused recommendations for specific disease states such as CKD, obesity, and OA.

ISSUES AND OPTIONS

Nutrient Needs of the Senior Pet

- Energy needs—
    - Dogs have overall decreased energy needs, but some may be underweight
        - Lifetime caloric restriction (25% less than control)—1.8 years longer median lifespan, delayed onset of age-related diseases.[1]
    - Cats—
        - Cats 5–11 years of age often have issues with being overweight, higher BCS—decreased MER from 7 to 11 years.[2]
        - Cats older than 11 years are more likely to be underweight and may need caloric density increased.[2, 3]
        - Highest MER increase after 13 years of age (LaFlamme 2014).
- Protein
    - Dogs may need increased protein due to increased protein turnover, unless protein restriction is needed for disease management (renal disease).
    - Cats—decreased ability to digest protein and altered protein metabolism; may have increased protein requirements in order to maintain lean body mass.[4]
        - One study showed no significant change, possibly due to low number of older cats in the study.[5]
- Fat
    - Dogs—while there is no alteration in digestibility, may need to be altered to affect energy density (increase or decrease as needed).
    - Cats—digestibility is reduced in at least 1/3 of cats over 13 years of age.[6]
        - Linoleic acid—essential FA—minimum 1 g/1000 kcal

Blackwell's Five-Minute Veterinary Consult Clinical Companion: Small Animal Senior Care,
First Edition. Edited by Heidi B. Lobprise.

Companion website: www.wiley.com/go/lobprise/Senior

- Fiber
  - To dilute caloric density to limit weight gain.
  - While often added to "support gastrointestinal health," excess amounts may impact digestibility.[7]
- Polyunsaturated fatty acids (PUFA)
  - Dogs—no alteration needed; while evidence is not conclusive, they may delay aging changes and progression of age-related diseases.
- Antioxidants
  - Dogs—no alteration needed; while evidence is not conclusive, studies show they may improve cognitive function.

Nutrient Digestion and Absorption

- Structural and physiological changes
  - Senior dogs have greater colonic crypt depth and young dogs have greater jejunal villus height.[8]
    - Diminished hydrochloric acid and bile acids, changes in salivary glands, small intestine, liver and pancreas, but these may not be clinically relevant.
- In dogs, most studies report no changes in absorption of nutrients.[9]

Aging Changes

- Gastrointestinal microbiota—Variable changes in different studies with concentrations of different strains increased, decreased or with no change in small intestine and gastric contents.
  - Fecal bacterial populations show no significant difference, but lower concentrations of bacterial metabolites, so may indicate a difference in intestinal absorption or degradation of metabolites.
- Brain health—oxidative stress with high ROS production and limited regenerative capacity; glucose metabolism is less efficient.
- Alterations in gene expression are more pronounced in dogs fed a higher-fat and higher-protein diet compared to lower-fat, lower-protein plant-based diet.[10]
- Decreased sensory abilities may contribute to a decrease in cephalic stage of feeding.[11]
- The decreased ability to respond to dehydration may also be present in dog.[8]
- Normal insulin responses changes with age.[12]
- Reduced response to ghrelin present in older dogs.[13]

Nutritional Management in Healthy Senior Pets

- Energy requirements
  - Dogs—decreased up to 50% in dogs[14, 15]
    - Lower lean body mass (driver of resting energy) and concurrent increase in body fat mass.
    - Lower activity levels with risk of obesity.
    - Many senior diets have higher fiber and lower energy density.
    - While caloric restrictions may increase longevity, geriatric dogs can have unintentional weight loss due to underlying disease that is undiagnosed or uncontrolled.
  - Cats show an increase in energy requirements despite progressive weight loss.[15]
    - In last 2 years of life, LBM and fat mass decline.
    - In older cats, fat digestibility declines.[16]
    - In cats—extreme leanness is detrimental.[3]

- Protein turnover is increased, with increased nitrogen excretion, but a decline in synthesis.
  - In dogs, no decreased digestibility.
  - Cat—obligate carnivores and will catabolize lean tissue if inadequate dietary protein. Digestibility can be decreased in some cats.
  - Unless medically indicated, don't restrict protein.
  - The proportion of energy from protein should be increased if caloric intake is decreased.
- Phosphorus—
  - Stimulates FGF-23 (fibroblast growth factor phosphatonin) that can affect CKD mineral and bone disorder (CKD-MBD).
  - Dogs—unless chronic kidney disease is present, there is no evidence that phosphorus should be restricted.
    - AAFCO minimum of 1.4 g phosphorus/1000 kcal
      - Some senior diets have up to three times that.
  - Cats—restrict phosphorus if IRIS (International Renal Interest Society) stages 2–4
    - <1.6 g/1000 kcal/ME
  - Calcium levels should be closely monitored for both hypocalcemia and hypercalcemia
    - Dietary phosphorus restrictions in cats with low baseline potassium and phosphate are risk factors for hypercalcemia that is associated with increasing renal disease, so adjustments to moderate phosphate restriction may be needed.[17]
- Sodium

  Healthy dogs with unrestricted access to water can tolerate a wide range of sodium
    - Sodium restriction has minimal effect on dogs with primary hypertension.
    - Sodium restriction may activate RAAS (renin–angiotensin–aldosterone–system), influencing hypertension.
    - Avoid excessive amount—safe upper limit of 3.76 g/1000 kcal
- Antioxidants—scavenge toxic free radicals to help manage oxidative stress
  - Cellular antioxidants
    - Vitamin E—lipid soluble, protects plasma membranes from oxidative damage
    - Vitamin C—water soluble, helps replenish cellular concentrations of Vitamin E
    - Carotenoids and flavonoids from fruits and vegetables have additional antioxidant activity
  - Mitochondrial co-factors
    - L-Carnitine—precursor to acetyl-L-carnitine, mitochondrial lipid metabolism.
    - Alpha lipoic acid—reduction–oxidation of other antioxidants and increasing glutathione.
    - Glutathione—the primary intracellular and water-soluble antioxidant.
    - Co-enzyme Q.
  - Vits C, E, and beta carotene reduce oxidative stress and DNA damage in lymphocytes in cats with renal insufficiency.[18]
- Prebiotics—Probiotics
  - Prebiotic fibers fermented in the colon stimulate growth of *Bifidobacteria* and *lactobacilli* species that are usually reduced in older animals.[19]
  - Inulin in chicory—source of fructo-oligosaccharide (FOS) prebiotic.
  - Study in 90 cats—base diet1; diet2 with antioxidants; diet3 with antioxidants and pre-biotic.[19]
    - Diet 3 group—39% the hazard of dying compared to group 1, decreased thyroid hyperplasia, gastrointestinal pathology, overall improvement of fecal flora profile and serum levels of vitamin E, beta-carotene, and linoleic acid all increased.
    - Body weight and BCS all decreased, but less in group 3.

- Polyunsaturated fatty acids (PUFA)—omega n-3 and n-6—requirements may change with age.
  - Anti-inflammatory effects have a role in the immune system.
  - If essential FAs are deficient in diet, skin and hair coat changes and increase of water through skin.[20]

Nutritional Management for Age-related Diseases

- Cognitive dysfunction
  - Antioxidants
    - Cellular antioxidants—Vitamins C, E, polyphenols.
    - Mitochondrial co-factors—carnitine, lipoic acid, CoQ-10.
  - Long-chain omega 3 PUFA (polyunsaturated fatty acids)
    - High concentrations in brain; anti-inflammatory.
  - Lactate and ketones as alternate energy sources for the brain
    - MCT—medium-chain triglycerides increase ketone production that cross the blood brain barrier and can spare glucose up to 20%.[21]
  - Glutathione protection—cysteine, methionine, SAMe
- Immunosenescence—vulnerable to oxidative stress
  - Antioxidants and mitochondrial co-factors—increase neutrophil phagocytosis
    - While vitamin C is not an essential nutrient in dogs and cats, with aging, synthesis capacity can be decreased.
      - One study showed no effect on antioxidant status.[22]
    - Vitamin E—enhance cellular immunity, not humoral immunity.[23]
    - Vitamin A—increased CD4+/CD8+ ratio, increased peripheral blood mononuclear cells, increased delayed-type immunity.
      - Supplemental with lutein to enhance cell-mediated and humoral response.[24]
    - Lipoic acid—in WBC, favorable ratio of oxidized glutathione.[25]
      - Do NOT use in cats.
- Degenerative Joint Disease/Osteoarthritis
  - Weight and body condition control
    - Weight loss has been shown to improve lameness in dogs with osteoarthritis.[26]
    - Adipose tissue—proinflammatory, increased oxidative stress.
    - Maintain lean body mass, slow or prevent sarcopenia with adequate protein and exercise.
  - Long-chain omega-3 PUFAs from marine oils have the most scientific evidence for efficacy.[27]
    - 2.5 g/1000 kcal.
    - Excess amounts can increase measures of lipid peroxidation and suppress cell-mediated immunity if Vitamin E intake is inadequate.[28]
  - Green-lipped mussel extract—varying studies
  - Glucosamine and chondroitin—conflicting veterinary data
    - Variability in formulation.
  - Other supplements—turmeric effect (wide bioavailability), Boswellia, microlactin, elk velvet antler, avocado, and soy unsaponifiables.
- Chronic Kidney Disease
  - In cats, weight loss may precede CKD by 3 years, and body weights under 4.2 kg have shorter survival times.[29]
  - Maintaining lean body mass and caloric intake is imperative.
    - Appetite dysregulation (dysrexia) is seen in up to 92% of CKD cats.[29]

- In early IRIS 1, cats fed a diet to promote healthy aging—stable renal function compared to owner-choice diet.[30]
- Dogs and cats with earlier stages of CKD will likely tolerate higher protein levels than those with severe azotemia.
- Nutrient modification:
    - Phosphorus—the essential mineral—used by the body in the form of inorganic phosphate (Pi).
        - Decreased intake in dogs slowed CKD progression and prolonged survival times.[31]
        - Hyperphosphatemia reduces survival times in cats.
        - Dietary phosphorus:calcium and serum levels of both are important.
        - IRIS recommendation of maintaining levels at 2.7–4.6 mg/dL.
    - Protein
        - Controversial to restrict in cats; adequate essential amino acids (AA) are critical.
        - Protein requirements in cats
            - Previous determination by nitrogen balance—1.5 g/kg BW.
            - To maintain lean body mass—5.2 g/kg BW (park 49).
        - Protein requirements in dogs—>5.1 g/100 kcal to[49] maintain body condition (park[50] 50)
        - Cats—IRIS recommends diets with decreased protein and restricted phosphorus in stages 2–4.
            - If dysrexia, alternative of senior diet for cats.[32]
        - EXCEPT in protein-losing nephropathy (PLN)—usually glomerular disease with urine:creatinine ratio of 2.0 or more
            - Decrease protein enough to decrease proteinuria but not contribute to LBM loss.
            - Renal diet, avoid high protein treats, strategically supplement essential AAs.
            - Supplement keto acids to stimulate protein synthesis while inhibiting protein breakdown.[33]
    - Potassium—hypokalemia in 20–30% of cats
        - Dogs—RAAS may contribute to hyperkalemia
    - Sodium—avoid high intake; excessive restriction can activate RAAS.
    - Vitamin D derangements
        - Dietary intake is essential in dogs and cats (no skin synthesis)
        - Dogs can use both animal- and plant-based vitamin D, cats can only utilize Vit D3 (cholecalciferol) well.
        - Hypovitaminosis can be an issue in CKD.
        - Calcitriol is costly, needs monitoring and can have toxicity.
        - Secondary hyperparathyroidism and increasing FGF-23 (fibroblast growth factor) are negatively associated with Vit D levels and survival duration.[34]
    - Calcium
        - Reduced phosphorus diet may contribute to hypercalcemia, if lower baseline potassium and phosphate.
        - Optimal dietary management is challenging, using a moderately phosphate-restricted diet helped normalize iCa levels.[35]
    - Omega-3 fatty acids—anti-inflammatory, no optimal dose, may be in diet
        - Dogs—50–75 mg/kg or up to 140 mg/kg EPA (eicosopentaenoic acid) and DHA (docosahexaenoic acid)

Senior Diets

- Senior cat foods formulated for cats >7 years or cats >11 years.[7]
  - All met AAFCO recommendations for adult maintenance.
  - Highly variable in caloric density and nutrients (protein, fat, phosphorus).
    - Slight increase in caloric density in diets for 11+ compared to diets for >7 years of age.
  - Many moderately decreased in protein.
  - Only 3 diets restricted phosphorus to <1.6 g/1000 kcal.
    - For IRIS stage 2–4 CKD cats if they won't eat renal diets, senior diets with low phosphorus may be acceptable.
  - Crude fiber—increased in all, possibly for support of gastrointestinal health but may impact digestibility.

Studies

- Diet effects on metabolic markers and gut microbiota in the cat.[36]
  - Beta-glucan source (oat groats, brown rice) for colon fermentation.
  - Fiber blend broccoli and tomato pomace—natural antioxidant poly phenols.[37]
  - Control diet had twice as much fish oil and was higher in fiber digestibility.
  - Test diet—lower uremic toxins, slightly higher true protein digestibility, and favorable gut microbiota.
    - Favored saccharolysis instead of proteolysis in the control diet.
- Diet for cats with CKD.[38]
  - Supplement with betaine (beets, spinach, whole grains) and prebiotics.
    - Betaine—osmoprotective effects on the kidney and decreases homocysteine concentrations in mice.[39]
      - Acts as a chaperone to stabilize protein structure.[40]
    - Prebiotics favor the growth of sacchrolytic bacteria that produce beneficial short-chain fatty acids (fructo-oligosaccharides—scFOS)
  - Indole compounds decreased.
- Study from data of dogs fed an antioxidant diet with and without behavioral enrichment (BE), evaluated over 2.8 years.[41]
  - Cellular antioxidants—vitamins E, C, fruits and vegetables.
  - Mitochrondrial co-factors—lipoid acid and carnitine.
  - Published data:
    - Group with anti-oxidant diet and group with BE showed increased brain-derived neurotrophic factor (BDNF) mRNA.[42]
    - Diet improved mitochondrial parameters (decreased ROS [reactive oxygen species] production and increased NADH-linked respiration [nicotinamide adenine dinucleotide-hydrogen), while BE alone did not.[41]
    - Diet group had cognitive improvements at 2 weeks and with subsequent testing; also benefited from BE, superior to either treatment alone.[43]
- Dogs and cats fed a supplement (brain protection blend—BPB Improvement in cognitive testing categories Pan Pan.[44]
- Study of diet with MCT (6.5% or 9%) and BPB versus control.[44]
  - Significantly improve in all six categories with 6.5% MCT and BPB.
  - Diet with 9% MCT and BPB had higher dropout rates, smaller group.
  - Control diet dogs had some improvement.
- Study with client-owned dogs—fed an enriched diet and lifelong training factors.[46]

  - Antioxidants (Vitamin C, Vitamin E, polyphenols), DHA, phosphatidylserine, and tryptophan.
  - Lifelong training had no effect, training scores low.[45]
  - Lack of diet effect—either the diet was ineffective or study limitations.
- Therapeutic Diet Study for feline DJD.[46]
  - EPA, DHA, green-lipped mussels and glucosamine/chondroitin sulfate.
  - Improved objective measures of mobility in the treated group and activity declined in the control group.

APPLICATIONS IN PRACTICE

- Approach to nutrition care—two aspects:
  - Screen for and address physiologic changes caused by aging
  - Screen for and address age-related diseases
- Nutritional assessment
  - Evaluation of the patient
    - Assessment of BCS and MCS should be done at every visit, with changes noted
  - Evaluation of the diet (Figure 92.1)
    - What are the components?
    - Are they eating appropriate amounts for their energy and nutrient needs?
    - Are they able to prehend, masticate, and swallow the food?
  - Feeding management—making adjustment for the individual
    - Dogs fed once daily had decreased cognitive dysfunction scoring, lower odds of gastrointestinal, dental, orthopedic, kidney/urinary and liver/pancreas disorders[47]
      - Intermittent fasting and time-restricted feeding benefits
    - With sensory declines—is the diet palatable? Can you warm it up?
    - With mobility issues—are they able to access the food source easily?
  - Enrichment—regular exercise can help maintain ideal BCS, manage OA, and positively impact sarcopenic changes

Abbreviations

- AAFCO = Association of American Feed Control Officials
- BCS = body condition score
- BDNF = brain-derived neurotropic factor
- BE = behavioral enrichment
- BPB = brain protection blend
- BW = body weight.
- CKD = chronic kidney disease
- CKD-MBD = CKD = mineral and bone disorder
- DEXA = dual energy X-ray absorptiometry
- DHA = docosahexaenoic acid
- EPA = eicosapentaenoic acid
- FA = fatty acid
- FGF = fibroblast growth factor
- IRIS = International Renal Interest Society
- LBM = lean body mass

WSAVA
Global Nutrition Committee

Short Diet History Form

Please answer the following questions about your pet

Pet's name: ____________ Species/breed: ____________ Age: ____________

Owner's name: ____________

Date form completed: ____________

Gender male ☐ female ☐ Neutered/spayed **No** ☐ **Yes** ☐

1. How active is your pet? **Very active** ☐ **Moderately active** ☐ **Not very active** ☐
2. How would you describe your pet's weight? **Overweight** ☐ **Ideal weight** ☐ **Underweight** ☐
3. Where does your pet spend most of the time? **Indoors** ☐ **Outdoors** ☐ **Indoors and outdoors** ☐

Please list below the brands and product names (if applicable) and the amount of ALL foods, treats, snacks, dental hygiene product, rawhides and any other foods that your pet currently eats, including foods used to administer medications:

Food	Form	*Amount	Number	Fed since
Examples:				
• *Purina Dog Chow*	*dry*	*1 ½ cups*	*2x/day*	*Jan 2010*
• *Science Diet Adult Gourmet Beef Entrée*	*moist*	*½ can*	*2x/day*	*Jan 2010*
• *90% lean hamburger*	*pan-fried*	*3 oz (85 grams)*	*1x/week*	*May 2011*
• *Milk Bone medium*	*dry*	*2*	*3/day*	*Aug 2012*

*If you feed by volume, what size measuring device do you use? ____________

*If you feed tinned/canned food, what size tins/cans? ____________

4. Do you give any dietary supplements to your pet (for example: vitamins, glucosamine, fatty acids, or any other supplements)? **No** ☐ **Yes** ☐

   If yes, please list brands and amounts: ____________

Information below to be completed by the veterinarian:

Current body weight: ____________ Ideal body weight: ____________

Current body condition score* ____/9 or ____/5 *Refer to the body condition scoring chart

Muscle Condition Score: normal ☐ mild wasting ☐ moderate wasting ☐ severe wasting ☐

wsava.org

■ **Figure 92.1** WSAVA Global Nutrition Committee—Short diet history form. Source: Diet-History-Form.pdf (wsava.org).

- LE = life expectancy
- MCT = medium-chain triglyceride
- MER = maintenance energy requirement
- MCS = muscle condition score
- NADH = Nicotinamide adenine dinucleotide—hydrogen
- OA = osteoarthritis
- Pi = inorganic phosphate
- PUFA = polyunsaturated fatty acids
- RAAS = renin–angiotensin–aldosterone system
- ROS = radical oxygen species
- SAMe = S-Adenosyl-Methionine
- scFOS = short-chain fructo-oligosaccharides

INTERNET RESOURCES

Accessed June 29, 2024

- https://wsava.org/Global-Guidelines/Global-Nutrition-Guidelines/
- https://www.aaha.org/resources/2021-aaha-nutrition-and-weight-management-guidelines/
- https://petnutritionalliance.org/

Additional Reading

Larsen JA, Farcas A. Nutrition of aging dogs. *Vet Clin North Am Small Anim Pract* 2014 Jul;44(4):741–759, vi. doi: https://doi.org/10.1016/j.cvsm.2014.03.003. Epub 2014 May 6. PMID: 24951344.

Laflamme D, Gunn-Moore D. Nutrition of aging cats. *Vet Clin North Am Small Anim Pract* 2014 Jul;44(4):761–774, vi. doi: https://doi.org/10.1016/j.cvsm.2014.03.001. PMID: 24951345

Laflamme DP. Nutritional care for aging cats and dogs. *Vet Clin North Am Small Anim Pract* 2012 Jul;42(4):769–791, vii. doi: https://doi.org/10.1016/j.cvsm.2012.04.002. Epub 2012 May 8. PMID: 22720813.

Parker VJ. Nutritional management for dogs and cats with chronic kidney disease. *Vet Clin North Am Small Anim Pract* 2021 May;51(3):685–710. doi: https://doi.org/10.1016/j.cvsm.2021.01.007. Erratum in: *Vet Clin North Am Small Anim Pract* 2021 Sep;51(5):ix. doi: https://doi.org/10.1016/j.cvsm.2021.07.014. PMID: 33773648.

References

1. Lawler DF, Larson BT, Ballam JM, Smith GK, Biery DN, Evans RH, Greeley EH, Segre M, Stowe HD, Kealy RD. Diet restriction and ageing in the dog: major observations over two decades. *Br J Nutr* 2008 Apr;99(4):793–805. doi: https://doi.org/10.1017/S0007114507871686. Epub 2007 Dec 6. Erratum in: *Br J Nutr* 2009 Apr;101(7):1112. PMID: 18062831.
2. Lund EM, Armstrong PJ, Kirk CA, et al. Prevalence and risk factors for obesity in adult cats from private US veterinary practices. *Intern J Appl Res Vet Med* 2005;3(2):88–96.
3. Montoya M, Morrison JA, Arrignon F, Spofford N, Charles H, Hours MA, Biourge V. Life expectancy tables for dogs and cats derived from clinical data. *Front Vet Sci* 2023 Feb 21;10:1082102 doi: https://doi.org/10.3389/fvets.2023.1082102. PMID: 36896289; PMCID: PMC9989186.
4. Teshima E, Brunetto MA, Vasconcellos RS, Gonçalves KN, De-Oliveira LD, Valério AG, Carciofi AC. Nutrient digestibility, but not mineral absorption, is age-dependent in cats. *J Anim Physiol Anim Nutr (Berl)* 2010 Dec;94(6):e251–e258. doi: https://doi.org/10.1111/j.1439-0396.2009.00964.x. PMID: 20455969.
5. Schauf S, Stockman J, Haydock R, Eyre R, Fortener L, Park JS, Bakke AM, Watson P. Healthy ageing is associated with preserved or enhanced nutrient and mineral apparent digestibility in dogs and cats fed commercially relevant extruded diets. *Animals (Basel)* 2021 Jul 17;11(7):2127. doi: https://doi.org/10.3390/ani11072127. PMID: 34359256; PMCID: PMC8300295.Schauf.

6. Patil A, Cupp C, Perez-Camargo G: Incidence of impaired nutrient digestibility in aging cats. *Compend Contin Educ Pract Vet Suppl* 2004;26(Suppl 2A):72.
7. Summers SC, Stockman J, Larsen JA, Sanchez Rodriguez A, Zhang L. Evaluation of nutrient content and caloric density in commercially available foods formulated for senior cats. *J Vet Intern Med* 2020 Sep;34(5):2029–2035. doi: https://doi.org/10.1111/jvim.15858. Epub 2020 Jul 10. PMID: 33463789; PMCID: PMC7517497.
8. Kuzmuk KN, Swanson KS, Tappenden KA, Schook LB, Fahey GC Jr. Diet and age affect intestinal morphology and large bowel fermentative end-product concentrations in senior and young adult dogs. *J Nutr* 2005 Aug;135(8):1940–1945. doi: https://doi.org/10.1093/jn/135.8.1940. PMID: 16046720.
9. Sheffy BE, Williams AJ, Zimmer JF, Ryan GD. Nutrition and metabolism of the geriatric dog. *Cornell Vet* 1985 Apr;75(2):324–347. PMID: 2985334.
10. Kil DY, Vester Boler BM, Apanavicius CJ, Schook LB, Swanson KS. Age and diet affect gene expression profiles in canine liver tissue. *PLoS One* 2010 Oct 12;5(10):e13319. doi: https://doi.org/10.1371/journal.pone.0013319. PMID: 20967283; PMCID: PMC2953517.
11. Fahey GC Jr, Barry KA, Swanson KS. Age-related changes in nutrient utilization by companion animals. *Annu Rev Nutr* 2008;28:425–445. doi: https://doi.org/10.1146/annurev.nutr.28.061807.155325. PMID: 18598137.
12. Larson BT, Lawler DF, Spitznagel EL Jr, et al. Improved glucose tolerance with lifetime diet restriction favorably affects disease and survival in dogs. *J Nutr* 2003;133:2887–2892.
13. Bhatti SF, Duchateau L, Van Ham LM, De Vliegher SP, Mol JA, Rijnberk A, Kooistra HS. Effects of growth hormone secretagogues on the release of adenohypophyseal hormones in young and old healthy dogs. *Vet J* 2006 Nov;172(3):515–525. doi: https://doi.org/10.1016/j.tvjl.2005.04.025. Epub 2005 Jun 13. PMID: 15951209.
14. Speakman JR, van Acker A, Harper EJ. Age-related changes in the metabolism and body composition of three dog breeds and their relationship to life expectancy. *Aging Cell* 2003 Oct;2(5):265–275. doi: https://doi.org/10.1046/j.1474-9728.2003.00061.x. PMID: 14570234.
15 Harper EJ. Changing perspectives on aging and energy requirements: aging and energy intakes in humans, dogs and cats. *J Nutr* 1998 Dec;128(12 Suppl):2623S–2626S. doi: https://doi.org/10.1093/jn/128.12.2623S. PMID: 9868222.
16. Peachey SE, Dawson JM, Harper EJ. The effect of ageing on nutrient digestibility by cats fed beef tallow-, sunflower oil- or olive oil-enriched diets. *Growth Dev Aging* 1999 Spring–Summer;63(1–2):61–70. PMID: 10885858.
17. Tang PK, Geddes RF, Chang YM, Jepson RE, Bijsmans E, Elliott J. Risk factors associated with disturbances of calcium homeostasis after initiation of a phosphate-restricted diet in cats with chronic kidney disease. *J Vet Intern Med* 2021 Jan;35(1):321–332. doi: https://doi.org/10.1111/jvim.15996. Epub 2020 Dec 24. PMID: 33368694; PMCID: PMC7848342.
18 Yu S, Paetau-Robinson I. Dietary supplements of vitamins E and C and beta-carotene reduce oxidative stress in cats with renal insufficiency. *Vet Res Commun* 2006 May;30(4):403–413. doi: https://doi.org/10.1007/s11259-006-3269-5. PMID: 16502108.
19. Cupp CJ, Jean-Philippe C, Kerr, WW, Patil AR, Perez-Camargo G. Effect of nutritional interventions on longevity of senior cats. *Intern J Appl Res Vet Med* 2007;5(3):133.
20. MacDonald ML, Anderson BC, Rogers QR, Buffington CA, Morris JG. Essential fatty acid requirements of cats: pathology of essential fatty acid deficiency. *Am J Vet Res* 1984 Jul;45(7):1310–1317. PMID: 24049889.
21. Taha AY, Henderson ST, Burnham WM. Dietary enrichment with medium chain triglycerides (AC-1203) elevates polyunsaturated fatty acids in the parietal cortex of aged dogs: implications for treating age-related cognitive decline. *Neurochem Res* 2009 Sep;34(9):1619–1625. doi: https://doi.org/10.1007/s11064-009-9952-5. Epub 2009 Mar 20. PMID: 19301124.
22. Hesta M, Ottermans C, Krammer-Lukas S, Zentek J, Hellweg P, Buyse J, Janssens GP. The effect of vitamin C supplementation in healthy dogs on antioxidative capacity and immune parameters. *J Anim Physiol Anim Nutr (Berl)* 2009 Feb;93(1):26–34. doi: https://doi.org/10.1111/j.1439-0396.2007.00774.x. PMID: 19386005.

23 Hall JA, Tooley KA, Gradin JL, Jewell DE, Wander RC. Effects of dietary n-6 and n-3 fatty acids and vitamin E on the immune response of healthy geriatric dogs. *Am J Vet Res* 2003 Jun;64(6):762–772. doi: https://doi.org/10.2460/ajvr.2003.64.762. PMID: 12828263.

24 Kearns RJ, Hayek MG, Turek JJ, Meydani M, Burr JR, Greene RJ, Marshall CA, Adams SM, Borgert RC, Reinhart GA. Effect of age, breed and dietary omega-6 (n-6): omega-3 (n-3) fatty acid ratio on immune function, eicosanoid production, and lipid peroxidation in young and aged dogs. *Vet Immunol Immunopathol* 1999 Aug 2;69(2-4):165–183. doi: https://doi.org/10.1016/s0165-2427(99)00052-5. PMID: 10507303.

25 Zicker SC, Hagen TM, Joisher N, Golder C, Joshi DK, Miller EP. Safety of long-term feeding of dl-alpha-lipoic acid and its effect on reduced glutathione : oxidized glutathione ratios in beagles. *Vet Ther* 2002 Summer;3(2):167–176. PMID: 19750748.

26 Impellizeri JA, Tetrick MA, Muir P. Effect of weight reduction on clinical signs of lameness in dogs with hip osteoarthritis. *J Am Vet Med Assoc* 2000 Apr 1;216(7):1089–1091. doi: https://doi.org/10.2460/javma.2000.216.1089. PMID: 10754668.Far 98

27 Barbeau-Grégoire M, Otis C, Cournoyer A, Moreau M, Lussier B, Troncy E. A 2022 systematic review and meta-analysis of enriched therapeutic diets and nutraceuticals in canine and feline osteoarthritis. *Int J Mol Sci* 2022 Sep 8;23(18):10384. doi: https://doi.org/10.3390/ijms231810384. PMID: 36142319; PMCID: PMC9499673.

28 Wander RC, Hall JA, Gradin JL, Du SH, Jewell DE. The ratio of dietary (n-6) to (n-3) fatty acids influences immune system function, eicosanoid metabolism, lipid peroxidation and vitamin E status in aged dogs. *J Nutr* 1997 Jun;127(6):1198–1205. doi: https://doi.org/10.1093/jn/127.6.1198. PMID: 9187636.

29 Freeman LM, Lachaud MP, Matthews S, Rhodes L, Zollers B. Evaluation of weight loss over time in cats with chronic kidney disease. *J Vet Intern Med* 2016 Sep;30(5):1661–1666. doi: https://doi.org/10.1111/jvim.14561. Epub 2016 Aug 16. PMID: 27527534; PMCID: PMC5032880.

30 Hall JA, MacLeay J, Yerramilli M, Obare E, Yerramilli M, Schiefelbein H, Paetau-Robinson I, Jewell DE. Positive impact of nutritional interventions on serum symmetric dimethylarginine and creatinine concentrations in client-owned geriatric cats. *PLoS One* 2016 Apr 14;11(4):e0153654. doi: https://doi.org/10.1371/journal.pone.0153654. PMID: 27078852; PMCID: PMC4831797.

31 Finco DR, Brown SA, Crowell WA, Duncan RJ, Barsanti JA, Bennett SE. Effects of dietary phosphorus and protein in dogs with chronic renal failure. *Am J Vet Res* 1992 Dec;53(12):2264–2271. PMID: 1476305.

32 Sparkes AH, Caney S, Chalhoub S, Elliott J, Finch N, Gajanayake I, Langston C, Lefebvre HP, White J, Quimby J. ISFM consensus guidelines on the diagnosis and management of feline chronic kidney disease. *J Feline Med Surg* 2016 Mar;18(3):219–239. doi: https://doi.org/10.1177/1098612X16631234. PMID: 26936494.

33 Aparicio M, Bellizzi V, Chauveau P, Cupisti A, Ecder T, Fouque D, Garneata L, Lin S, Mitch WE, Teplan V, Zakar G, Yu X. Protein-restricted diets plus keto/amino acids—a valid therapeutic approach for chronic kidney disease patients. *J Ren Nutr* 2012 Mar;22(2 Suppl):S1–S21. doi: https://doi.org/10.1053/j.jrn.2011.09.005. PMID: 22365371.

34 Geddes RF, Elliott J, Syme HM. Relationship between plasma fibroblast growth factor-23 concentration and survival time in cats with chronic kidney disease. *J Vet Intern Med* 2015 Nov–Dec;29(6):1494–1501. doi: https://doi.org/10.1111/jvim.13625. Epub 2015 Sep 25. PMID: 26403212; PMCID: PMC4895675.

35 Geddes RF, van den Broek DHN, Chang YM, Biourge V, Elliott J, Jepson RE. The effect of attenuating dietary phosphate restriction on blood ionized calcium concentrations in cats with chronic kidney disease and ionized hypercalcemia. *J Vet Intern Med* 2021 Mar;35(2):997–1007. doi: https://doi.org/10.1111/jvim.16050. Epub 2021 Feb 1. PMID: 33527601; PMCID: PMC7995425.

36 Ephraim E, Jewell DE. Effect of nutrition on age-related metabolic markers and the gut microbiota in cats. *Microorganisms* 2021 Nov 25;9(12):2430. doi: https://doi.org/10.3390/microorganisms9122430. PMID: 34946032; PMCID: PMC8706506.

37 Baroni L, Sarni AR, Zuliani C. Plant foods rich in antioxidants and human cognition: a systematic review. *Antioxidants (Basel)* 2021 Apr 30;10(5):714. doi: https://doi.org/10.3390/antiox10050714. PMID: 33946461; PMCID: PMC8147117.

38. Hall JA, Jewell DE, Ephraim E. Feeding cats with chronic kidney disease food supplemented with betaine and prebiotics increases total body mass and reduces uremic toxins. *PLoS One* 2022 May 24;17(5):e0268624. doi: https://doi.org/10.1371/journal.pone.0268624. PMID: 35609046; PMCID: PMC9129019.
39. Liu YL, Pan Y, Wang X, Fan CY, Zhu Q, Li JM, Wang S-J, Kong LD. Betaine reduces serum uric acid levels and improves kidney function in hyperuricemic mice. *Planta Med* 2014;80(1):39–47. doi: https://doi.org/10.1055/s-0033-1360127. PMID: 24338552.
40. Ueland PM, Holm PI, Hustad S. Betaine: a key modulator of one-carbon metabolism and homocysteine status. *Clin Chem Lab Med* 2005;43(10):1069–1075. doi: https://doi.org/10.1515/CCLM.2005.187. PMID: 16197300.
41. Head E, Nukala VN, Fenoglio KA, Muggenburg BA, Cotman CW, Sullivan PG. Effects of age, dietary, and behavioral enrichment on brain mitochondria in a canine model of human aging. *Exp Neurol* 2009 Nov;220(1):171–176. doi: https://doi.org/10.1016/j.expneurol.2009.08.014. Epub 2009 Aug 22. PMID: 19703441; PMCID: PMC2761532.
42. Fahnestock M, Marchese M, Head E, Pop V, Michalski B, Milgram WN, Cotman CW. BDNF increases with behavioral enrichment and an antioxidant diet in the aged dog. *Neurobiol Aging* 2012 Mar;33(3):546–554. doi: https://doi.org/10.1016/j.neurobiolaging.2010.03.019. Epub 2010 May 5. PMID: 20447733; PMCID: PMC2935515.
43. Dowling AL, Head E. Antioxidants in the canine model of human aging. *Biochim Biophys Acta* 2012 May;1822(5):685–689. doi: https://doi.org/10.1016/j.bbadis.2011.09.020. Epub 2011 Oct 8. PMID: 22005070; PMCID: PMC3291812.
44. Pan Y, Landsberg G, Mougeot I, Kelly S, Xu H, Bhatnagar S, Gardner CL, Milgram NW. Efficacy of a therapeutic diet on dogs with signs of cognitive dysfunction syndrome (CDS): a prospective double blinded placebo controlled clinical study. *Front Nutr* 2018 Dec 12;5:127. doi: https://doi.org/10.3389/fnut.2018.00127. PMID: 30619873; PMCID: PMC6299068.
45. Chapagain D, Wallis LJ, Range F, Affenzeller N, Serra J, Virányi Z. Behavioural and cognitive changes in aged pet dogs: No effects of an enriched diet and lifelong training. *PLoS One* 2020 Sep 16;15(9):e0238517. doi: https://doi.org/10.1371/journal.pone.0238517. PMID: 32936808; PMCID: PMC7494100.
46. Lascelles BD, DePuy V, Thomson A, Hansen B, Marcellin-Little DJ, Biourge V, Bauer JE. Evaluation of a therapeutic diet for feline degenerative joint disease. *J Vet Intern Med* 2010 May–Jun;24(3):487–495. doi: https://doi.org/10.1111/j.1939-1676.2010.0495.x. Epub 2010 Mar 22. PMID: 20337921.
47. Bray EE, Zheng Z, Tolbert MK, McCoy BM, Dog Aging Project Consortium, Kaeberlein M, Kerr KF. Once-daily feeding is associated with better health in companion dogs: results from the Dog Aging Project. *Geroscience* 2022 Jun;44(3):1779–1790. doi: https://doi.org/10.1007/s11357-022-00575-7. Epub 2022 Apr 28. PMID: 35484470; PMCID: PMC9213604.
48. Laflamme DP. Nutrition for aging cats and dogs and the importance of body condition. *Vet Clin North Am Small Anim Pract.* 2005 May;35(3):713–42. doi: https://doi.org/10.1016/j.cvsm.2004.12.011. PMID: 15833567.
49. Laflamme DP, Hannah SS. Discrepancy between use of lean body mass or nitrogen balance to determine protein requirements for adult cats. *J Feline Med Surg* 2013;15(8):691–7.
50. Sanderson SL, Tetrick M, Brown SA, et al. Effect of dietary approach on clinical outcome measures in dogs with naturally occurring chronic kidney disease (abstract). *J Anim Physiol Anim Nutr* 2013;97:1198–9.

Author: Heidi Lobprise

Chapter 93

Obesity

BASICS

DEFINITION

Obesity is the unhealthy accumulation of body fat. Precise definitions are debated, but it is widely accepted that dogs or cats with body condition score (BCS) 6 or 7 on a 9-point scale are overweight, and those with BCS 8 or 9 are obese. With as many as 65% of dogs and 25% cats being overweight or obese, the impact on aging can be considered widespread.

Meta-inflammation—low-grade inflammation throughout the body induced by chronic over-nutrition and obesity.

ISSUES AND OPTIONS

Pathophysiology

- Animals gain weight when energy intake from food chronically exceeds energy expended to maintain basic homeostatic processes and during exercise.
- Homeostatic neuroendocrine responses ensure food intake meets energy requirements and establishes modest energy reserves in case of a period of fasting.
- Energy homeostasis may be disrupted by: ready availability of highly palatable energy-dense food (which elicits hedonic responses that override homeostatic satiation); genetic variation in appetite; neutering; and limits to a pet's ability to exercise.

Systems Effected

- Endocrine—insulin resistance develops secondary to obesity and can lead to diabetes mellitus (DM) in cats.
- Overweight BCS or obesity is the most recognized factor for type 2 DM with insulin resistance, decreased sensitivity of insulin.
- Body weight gain a more likely risk factor than dry diets and carbohydrates.[1]
- Immune—adipose tissue dysfunction in obesity causes a proinflammatory state.
- Other organ systems may be affected by the mechanical effect of increased body fat and/or endocrine and metabolic disruption, including dermatologic, musculoskeletal, respiratory, and urinary.[2]

Blackwell's Five-Minute Veterinary Consult Clinical Companion: Small Animal Senior Care, First Edition. Edited by Heidi B. Lobprise.

Companion website: www.wiley.com/go/lobprise/Senior

Genetics

- Breed variation in obesity predisposition suggests obesity susceptibility is in part heritable with a polygenic mode of inheritance.
- Mutations in the genes *POMC* (Labrador and flatcoat retrievers) and *MC4R* (beagles) are associated with obesity and/or food motivation.

Meta-inflammation

- mRNA data suggest either an increased population of macrophages or increased inflammatory nature of adipocytes in adipose tissue of aged dogs compared to young adult dogs.[3]
  - This change in adipogenic potential can impact stress response, inflammation, insulin sensitivity, and lipid metabolism
- After weight loss in dogs there is reduction in inflammatory adipokines and improvement in insulin resistance.[4]

Impact on Longevity

- In a large cohort study on Life Expectancy (LE), obese dogs had significantly lower LE at birth than overweight and ideal weight dogs.[5]
  - LE at birth of cats with BCS 4/5 was significantly higher than cats with BCS 5/5 or 3/5.[5]
- Another study compared normal BCS to overweight dogs in 12 breeds.[6]
  - Median life span shorter in the overweight dogs; the greatest difference was in Yorkshire terriers (12.7 years vs. 16.2 years) and the least difference was in German Shepherd dogs (12.1 years vs. 12.5 years)
- In looking at potential determinants for successful aging in Labrador retrievers, life-long maintenance of lean body mass and attenuated accumulation of body fat are key factors in longer lifespan.[7]
- Recent data showed that communication about life expectancy related to obesity to be the most important factor when considering vet recommendations to cat and dog owners.[8,9]

APPLICATIONS IN PRACTICE

Evaluation of Body Condition Score and Body Fat Mass

- Ultrasound, MRI, or dual-energy x-ray absorptiometry can measure body fat more accurately.
- BCS is a semi-quantitative, ordinal measure of body composition. Observation and palpation are used to assign a score based on how findings best match a series of descriptors. The best validated 9-point scale assigns BCS 4–5 as ideal, 6–7 as overweight, and 8–9 as obese (Figure 93.1).
- Serial measurement of body weight is more sensitive for monitoring.

Appropriate Health Care

- Calorie restriction is the mainstay of successful weight loss.
- Changes in owner management behavior are critical to success.
- Energy requirements for maintenance are lower after weight loss, so long-term vigilance and food restriction are required to prevent recurrence.

ACTIVITY

- Increasing exercise is ineffective to induce weight loss alone, so if owners are reluctant to make management changes, focus should be on food restriction.
- However, exercise is encouraged because it promotes retention of lean mass (muscle) during weight loss.

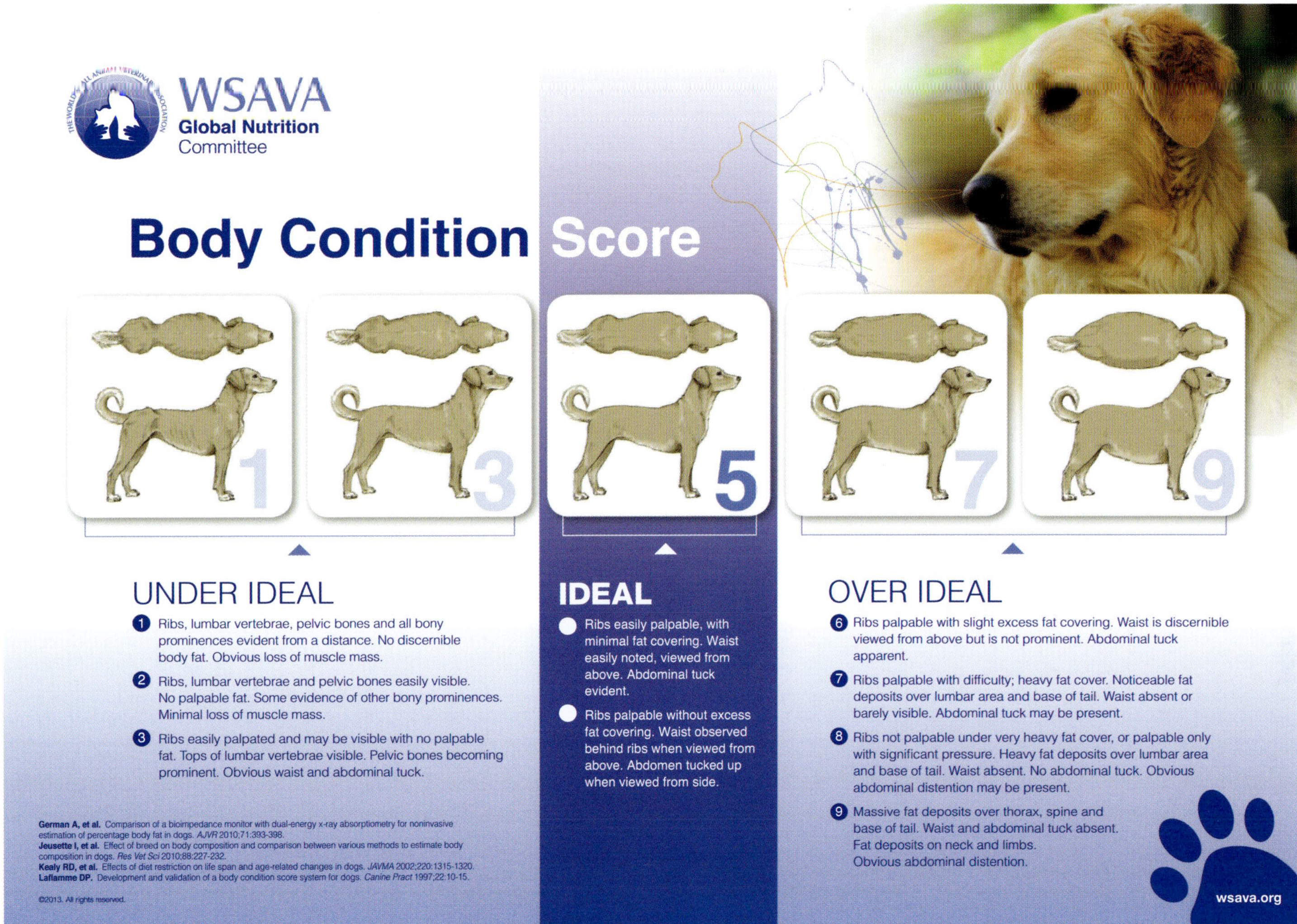
WSAVA
Global Nutrition
Committee
Body Condition Score
1
3
5
7
9
UNDER IDEAL
1 Ribs, lumbar vertebrae, pelvic bones and all bony prominences evident from a distance. No discernible body fat. Obvious loss of muscle mass.
2 Ribs, lumbar vertebrae and pelvic bones easily visible. No palpable fat. Some evidence of other bony prominences. Minimal loss of muscle mass.
3 Ribs easily palpated and may be visible with no palpable fat. Tops of lumbar vertebrae visible. Pelvic bones becoming prominent. Obvious waist and abdominal tuck.
IDEAL
Ribs easily palpable, with minimal fat covering. Waist easily noted, viewed from above. Abdominal tuck evident.
Ribs palpable without excess fat covering. Waist observed behind ribs when viewed from above. Abdomen tucked up when viewed from side.
OVER IDEAL
6 Ribs palpable with slight excess fat covering. Waist is discernible viewed from above but is not prominent. Abdominal tuck apparent.
7 Ribs palpable with difficulty; heavy fat cover. Noticeable fat deposits over lumbar area and base of tail. Waist absent or barely visible. Abdominal tuck may be present.
8 Ribs not palpable under very heavy fat cover, or palpable only with significant pressure. Heavy fat deposits over lumbar area and base of tail. Waist absent. No abdominal tuck. Obvious abdominal distention may be present.
9 Massive fat deposits over thorax, spine and base of tail. Waist and abdominal tuck absent. Fat deposits on neck and limbs. Obvious abdominal distention.
German A, et al. Comparison of a bioimpedance monitor with dual-energy x-ray absorptiometry for noninvasive estimation of percentage body fat in dogs. AJVR 2010;71:393-398.
Jeusette I, et al. Effect of breed on body composition and comparison between various methods to estimate body composition in dogs. Res Vet Sci 2010;88:227-232.
Kealy RD, et al. Effects of diet restriction on life span and age-related changes in dogs. JAVMA 2002;220:1315-1320.
Laflamme DP. Development and validation of a body condition score system for dogs. Canine Pract 1997;22:10-15.
©2013. All rights reserved.
wsava.org

Figure 93.1 Body Condition Score for dogs—WSAVA Global Nutrition Committee with a 9-point scale to determine body condition. Source: Body-Condition-Score-Dog.pdf (wsava.org).

DIET

- Reducing daily energy intake in food to below maintenance requirements is essential.
- Target weight is estimated from current weight and BCS—every 1 unit increase over BCS 5/9 equates to 10% excess body mass; e.g., to calculate the target weight of a dog in BCS 7, divide current weight by 1.2.
- The amount of food required to promote weight loss can be estimated from calculated maintenance energy requirements (MER) or by reducing current food intake by 10–20%.
- To calculate MER, use estimated target weight (MER (kJ) = $440 \times$ body weight $[BW]_{kg}^{0.75}$) and feed 50–65% of MER as a starting point.
- Feeding recommendations should be altered from baseline to maintain weight loss at 0.5–1%/week until target weight is reached.
- For weight loss of <20% (i.e., starting BCS <6), food restriction is moderate and a conventional diet is adequate, although specialized diets may be advantageous. Where energy restriction is greater (starting BCS >7), the density of essential nutrients in maintenance diets may be inadequate, so a specialized diet is recommended.
- Specialized diets improve the success of weight loss programs and improve satiety, which itself may improve compliance because owners are subjected to less begging behavior.
- Specialized diets are commonly formulated to provide: high essential nutrient density; low energy density (added water in canned food or air in kibble); high protein (improves satiety and promotes lean mass retention); and high fiber (promotes satiety). Canned (compared to dry) food may improve weight loss in cats.
- Accurate feeding using weighed portions is important. Treats are ideally excluded but if owners feel they are essential, factor them into the diet plan.

CLIENT EDUCATION

- Owners of obese pets often do not follow advice to reduce their pets' weight because they do not recognize obesity, do not see it as a problem, or struggle to follow the advice. By definition, they have already failed to make the small adjustments needed to keep their dog slim; it follows that they are likely to find making the major changes required to reduce their dog's weight difficult.
- Although it might sound simple to "feed less and exercise more," the reality is that owners are being asked to change established habits, spend more time caring for their pets, and perhaps work to motivate other family members.
- Promoting those behavioral changes requires us to motivate owners, to understand their barriers to change, and to offer practical and simple advice on how to overcome those barriers. Information does not automatically lead to motivation; it is more likely if the actions required are consistent with their existing values and beliefs.
- Owners may not recognize obesity. Being overweight is regarded as the norm for some breeds. Regular recording of body weight and BCS can objectively identify a problem early ("I see she's gained a pound—it would be good to cut the food down before that becomes a problem").
- Owners may not appreciate that obesity causes health problems. Positive motivation ("slimming him down could really improve his mobility") is more effective than negative ("if he doesn't lose weight, he'll never walk properly again").
- Lack of motivation may be difficult to modify ("his breeder says his weight is fine") or challenge ("everyone in our family carries a little extra weight—it's cuddly").

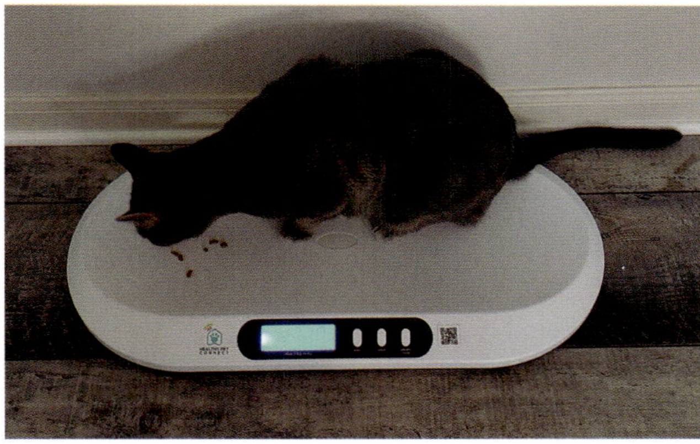

Figure 93.2 Particularly for small dogs and cats, it is simple to have the owner get a small scale for regular "weigh-ins." This system from Healthy Pet Connect was originally designed to assist owners in weight loss for their cats, but can also be used to track unintended weight loss. It include a Pet Parent App that communicates with their Vet Dashboard. Source: Home Health Data From Pet to Vet (healthypetconnect.com)/Bug Ventures, Inc.

- Owners often find food restriction difficult. Reducing intake in highly food-motivated animals may require constant vigilance to reduce scavenging, stealing, or hunting. Ignoring begging requires a strong will because of the importance of food-giving in maintaining the human–animal bond. Owners may not feel confident in how or what to feed. Practical problems may limit the exercise they offer their pet.
- Practical advice to overcome those barriers should ideally be tailored to each owner. If owners complain their pets are always hungry, a satiety-promoting diet or trickle feeding using toys or frequent small meals may help. If owners insist on treat feeding, suggest low-calorie treats or factor planned treats into the daily ration. If owner mobility restricts dog walks, suggest ball play or longer time in the yard to increase activity.
- Human behavior change is also improved by goal-setting, action planning, and monitoring. For instance, the aim for a weight loss consultation could be that owners leave with written plans formulated in the session: "my goal is to slim her down to 18 kg"; "I have chosen to make these three management changes from the list of suggestions . . ."; and "I will bring her back once a month to be weighed." (see Figure 93.2).
- Fostering a nonjudgmental and supportive veterinary practice culture regarding pet obesity should encourage owners to seek support and act early.

FOLLOW-UP

PATIENT MONITORING

- Monitoring progress is important. After initiating a diet change, check progress after 2 weeks and alter food ration to aim for 0.5–1% body weight loss/week. Regular monthly visits promote owner compliance and allow ration changes to maintain progress.
- Once target weight is achieved, ongoing monitoring is essential to minimize rebound weight gain. Weighing at veterinary visits is ideally supplemented by owners becoming more adept at noticing weight gain and acting to reverse it.

PREVENTION/AVOIDANCE

- Prevention should be a central aim of routine vet visits. Veterinary teams should work to empower owners to recognize a healthy weight and to intervene effectively when obesity occurs.
- Weight and BCS should be recorded at every practice visit.
- Incorporating weight management advice into waiting room displays will establish the importance of maintaining a healthy weight to the client population.

EXPECTED COURSE AND PROGNOSIS

- Food restriction leads to weight loss in research settings but in client-owned dogs has lower success rates. Compliance is frequently poor and total weight loss often falls short of the target. Rebound weight gain is common.
- Encouragingly, however, even modest weight loss (of approximately 10%) can produce clinically significant improvement.

Miscellaneous

Age-associated obesity and muscle atrophy (sarcopenia) are intimately connected and are reciprocally regulated by adipose tissue and skeletal muscle dysfunction. During aging, adipose inflammation leads to the redistribution of fat to the intra-abdominal area (visceral fat) and fatty infiltrations in skeletal muscles, resulting in decreased overall strength and functionality. Lipids and their derivatives accumulate both within and between muscle cells, inducing mitochondrial dysfunction, disturbing β-oxidation of fatty acids, and enhancing reactive oxygen species (ROS) production, leading to lipotoxicity and insulin resistance, as well as enhanced secretion of some pro-inflammatory cytokines. In turn, these muscle-secreted cytokines may exacerbate adipose tissue atrophy, support chronic low-grade inflammation, and establish a vicious cycle of local hyperlipidemia, insulin resistance, and inflammation that spreads systemically, thus promoting the development of sarcopenic obesity (SO). We call this the metabaging cycle. Patients with SO show an increased risk of systemic insulin resistance, systemic inflammation, associated chronic diseases, and the subsequent progression to full-blown sarcopenia and even cachexia. Meanwhile in many cardiometabolic diseases, the ostensibly protective effect of obesity in extremely elderly subjects, also known as the "obesity paradox," could possibly be explained by our theory that many elderly subjects with normal body mass index might actually harbor SO to various degrees, before it progresses to full-blown severe sarcopenia. Our review outlines current knowledge concerning the possible chain of causation between sarcopenia and obesity, proposes a solution to the obesity paradox, and the role of fat mass in aging.

See Also

Diabetes Mellitus.

Abbreviations

- BCS = body condition score
- DM = Diabetes mellitus
- LE = Life expectancy
- MER = maintenance energy requirement.
- mRNA = mitochondrial RNA

INTERNET RESOURCES

Accessed 29 June 2024

- Nutrition Guidelines—WSAVA
- https://petnutritionalliance.org/

Suggested Reading

Flanagan J, Bissot T, Hours M-A, et al. Success of a weight loss plan for overweight dogs: the results of an international weight loss study. *PLoS One* 2017;12(9):e0184199.

Laflamme DP. Development and validation of a body condition score system for cats: a clinical tool. *Feline Pract* 1997;25:13–18.

Laflamme DP. Development and validation of a body condition score system for dogs: a clinical tool. *Canine Pract* 1997;22:10–15.

Linder DE, Parker VJ. Dietary aspects of weight management in cats and dogs. *Vet Clin North Am Small Anim Pract* 2016;46:869–882.

Raffan E, Dennis RJ, O'Donovan CJ, et al. A deletion in the canine POMC gene is associated with weight and appetite in obesity-prone Labrador retriever dogs. *Cell Metab* 2016;23(5):893–900.

References

1. Slingerland LI, Fazilova VV, Plantinga EA, Kooistra HS, Beynen AC. Indoor confinement and physical inactivity rather than the proportion of dry food are risk factors in the development of feline type 2 diabetes mellitus. *Vet J* 2009 Feb;179(2):247–253. doi: 10.1016/j.tvjl.2007.08.035. Epub 2007 Oct 26. PMID: 17964833.
2. Teng KT, McGreevy PD, Toribio JL, Raubenheimer D, Kendall K, Dhand NK. Strong associations of nine-point body condition scoring with survival and lifespan in cats. *J Feline Med Surg* 2018 Dec;20(12):1110–1118. doi: 10.1177/1098612X17752198. Epub 2018 Feb 2. PMID: 29393723; PMCID: PMC11104206.
3. Swanson KS, Belsito KR, Vester BM, Schook LB. Adipose tissue gene expression profiles of healthy young adult and geriatric dogs. Arch Anim Nutr. 2009 Apr;63(2):160–171. doi: 10.1080/17450390902733934. PMID: 19489458.
4. German AJ, Hervera M, Hunter L, Holden SL, Morris PJ, Biourge V, et al. Improvement in insulin resistance and reduction in plasma inflammatory adipokines after weight loss in obese dogs. *Domest Anim Endocrinol* (2009) 37:214–26. doi: 10.1016/j.domaniend.2009.07.001.
5. Montoya M, Morrison JA, Arrignon F, Spofford N, Charles H, Hours MA, Biourge V. Life expectancy tables for dogs and cats derived from clinical data. *Front Vet Sci* 2023 Feb 21;10:1082102. doi: 10.3389/fvets.2023.1082102. PMID: 36896289; PMCID: PMC9989186.
6. Salt C, Morris PJ, Wilson D, Lund EM, German AJ. Association between life span and body condition in neutered client-owned dogs. *J Vet Intern Med* 2019 Jan;33(1):89–99. doi: 10.1111/jvim.15367. Epub 2018 Dec 11. PMID: 30548336; PMCID: PMC6335446.
7. Adams VJ, Watson P, Carmichael S, Gerry S, Penell J, Morgan DM. Exceptional longevity and potential determinants of successful ageing in a cohort of 39 Labrador retrievers: results of a prospective longitudinal study. *Acta Vet Scand* 2016 May 11;58(1):29. doi: 10.1186/s13028-016-0206-7. PMID: 27169845; PMCID: PMC4863359.
8. Sutherland KA, Coe JB, Groves CNH, Shepherd ML, Grant LE. Information about life expectancy related to obesity is most important to cat owners when deciding whether to act on a veterinarian's weight loss recommendation. *J Am Vet Med Assoc* 2024 Mar 13;262(6):798–807. doi: 10.2460/javma.23.12.0703. PMID: 38513353.
9. Davies AR, Sutherland KA, Groves CNH, Grant LE, Shepherd ML, Coe JB. Impact on life expectancy was the most important information to clients when considering whether to take action for an overweight or obese dog. *J Am Vet Med Assoc* 2024 Mar 19;262(6):808–817. doi: 10.2460/javma.23.12.0697. PMID: 38513358.

10. Lo JH, U KP, Yiu T, Ong MT, Lee WY. Sarcopenia: Current treatments and new regenerative therapeutic approaches. *J Orthop Translat* 2020 Apr 30;23:38–52. doi: 10.1016/j.jot.2020.04.002. PMID: 32489859; PMCID: PMC7256062.

Author/editor: Heidi Lobprise
Topic adapted from Five Minute Veterinary Consultation, 7th edition, 2021
Original Topic: Obesity

Author: Eleanor Raffan
Consulting Editor: Mark P. Rondeau

Chapter 94

Weight Loss, Sarcopenia, and Cachexia

BASICS

OVERVIEW

Unplanned weight loss, particularly that of lean muscle mass, is a critical factor in evaluating and managing senior pet health care. A body condition score (BCS) of 3–4 on a 9-point scale may be considered underweight, and those with a BCS of 1–2 can be considered emaciated (Figure 94.1).

Further evaluation of lean body mass by determining a muscle condition score (MCS) can be even more essential in senior pets. Once muscle loss occurs (mild, moderate, or severe), it can be challenging to manage, so regular examination and early detection is important.

Terms Defined

- Sarcopenia—the progressive decrease of skeletal muscle mass, strength, and function with age, in the absence of disease.
- Cachexia is an unintended loss of more than 5% of body weight over 12 months or less, in a patient with a known illness.
    - Several other criteria include loss of muscle strength, decreased appetite, fatigue, and inflammation.
    - Precachexia is defined as a loss of up to 5% of body weight while having a known illness or disease, accompanied by appetite loss, inflammation, and changes in metabolism.
    - Refractory cachexia applies to individuals with cancer, with weight loss, muscle loss, loss of function, plus a failure to respond to cancer treatment.
- Sarcopenia Obesity (SO)—Age-associated obesity and muscle atrophy (sarcopenia) that are intimately connected.
- Overcoat syndrome—when a patient has excessive adipose tissue with a seemingly high BCS but moderate-to-severe muscle loss.

ISSUES AND OPTIONS

- Sarcopenia is a normal part of the aging process (see Figure 94.2).
    - It can result in diminished strength and mobility.
    - Various reasons include deficient nutritional intake, digestive issues, increased cytokine production, decreased concentrations of growth hormone and testosterone, insulin resistance, and physical inactivity.

Blackwell's Five-Minute Veterinary Consult Clinical Companion: Small Animal Senior Care, First Edition. Edited by Heidi B. Lobprise.

Companion website: www.wiley.com/go/lobprise/Senior

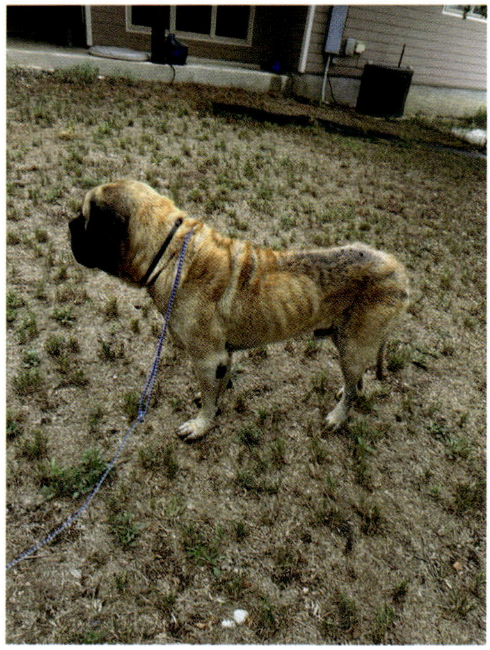

■ **Figure 94.1** An older rescue dog has a very low BCS and MCS score, so complete health evaluation, medical and nutritional management is critical.

Weight history (in lbs)	
05-24-24	9.47
04-08-24	9.60
08-26-16	11.80
05-21-15	12.60
07-23-14	13.00
02-17-14	12.00
01-03-14	11.60
10-17-13	10.80
05-08-13	11.00
01-15-13	11.40
10-17-12	12.00
06-06-12	10.60
08-29-11	8.80
06-06-11	8.80
04-06-11	9.00
03-07-11	8.40
11-22-10	8.40
11-01-10	8.00
09-27-10	7.40
07-29-10	4.80
07-01-10	3.60
05-28-10	2.00
05-24-10	1.80

■ **Figure 94.2** Records of a senior cat show the progression of weight gain through the growth period, some mature weights that are slightly elevated. There is a gap from 6 years of age to 14 years of age with a decrease in weight that likely started around 11 years of age. This also indicates a lack of veterinary care that can be common in older cats, until they show signs of disease.

- Regular exercise and a protein-rich diet can help reduce the consequences of sarcopenia and preserve muscular health as one matures.
  - Animals with chronic inflammatory conditions have improved survival if weight is maintained.[1]
- Cellular changes in sarcopenic muscle are characterized by the decrease in the size and number of type II muscle fibers with intramuscular and intermuscular fat infiltration.
  - Lipids and their derivatives impact mitochondrial dysfunction, disturbing β-oxidation of fatty acids, and enhancing reactive oxygen species (ROS) production, leading to lipotoxicity and insulin resistance, as well as enhanced secretion of some pro-inflammatory cytokines.
- The upregulation of autophagy to recycle cellular components will increase markers of autophagy Beclin 1 and LC3 with an increase in lipofuscins (due to ROS-induced damage and mitochondrial dysfunction).[2]
- In patients with chronic kidney failure, low lean body mass can reduce serum creatinine concentrations, so SDMA can provide a more accurate estimation of GFR (glomerular filtration rate).
- Hyperthyroidism in cats—increased metabolic rates.

- Cachexia—Involuntary loss of weight and muscle mass.
  - Accompanied by:
    - Upregulation of inflammatory cytokines (e.g., interleukin-6 [IL-6], tumor necrosis factor-α [TNF-α]), catecholamines, neurohormones, and cortisol.
    - Increases in oxidative stress; activation of catabolic pathways (e.g., ubiquitin–proteasome system).
    - Decreases in anabolic factors (e.g., growth hormone [GH], insulin-like growth factor I [IGF-1]).
  - Decreased nutrition due to the patient eating less or digestive issues.
  - Changes in metabolism cause the body to break down too much muscle.
    - Response to fighting disease to get fuel for the brain.
  - Both inflammation and substances created by tumors can affect appetite and cause the body to burn calories more quickly than usual.
  - Increases weakness and frailty, vulnerability to infections, and increases morbidity and mortality.
  - Getting more nutrition or calories isn't enough to reverse cachexia.

Evaluation of Lean Body Mass (LBM)

- Muscle condition score—MCS.
- Ultrasound and computed tomography were able to detect reduced epaxial muscle height (EMH).[3]
  - Inflammatory markers were not significantly different in young vs. old dogs.
  - With adequate training, can be part of annual wellness evaluation.
- DEXA—Dual-Energy X-Ray Absorptiometry: not readily available in most practice settings.

Weight Loss in Disease

- Congestive heart failure (CHF)—42.5% of dogs; 34% of cats.
- Cancer—5.5–69% of dogs; 60% of cats.
- Chronic kidney disease (CKD)—28.9–55% of dogs; 36–81% of cats.

Cachexia in Disease

- CHF—48.3–54% of dogs; unknown in cats.
- Cancer—35% of dogs; 91% of cats.
- CKD—28.9% of dogs (weight loss/cachexia); 81% of cats.

APPLICATIONS IN PRACTICE

- Train veterinary team to regularly assess muscle condition score (MCS) on all patients, but seniors in particular. (WSAVA Nutrition Guidelines) (Figure 94.3)
  - This should be part of a brief nutrition screening along with diet history and BCS.
  - Assign an MCS score to all senior patients, similar to BCS.

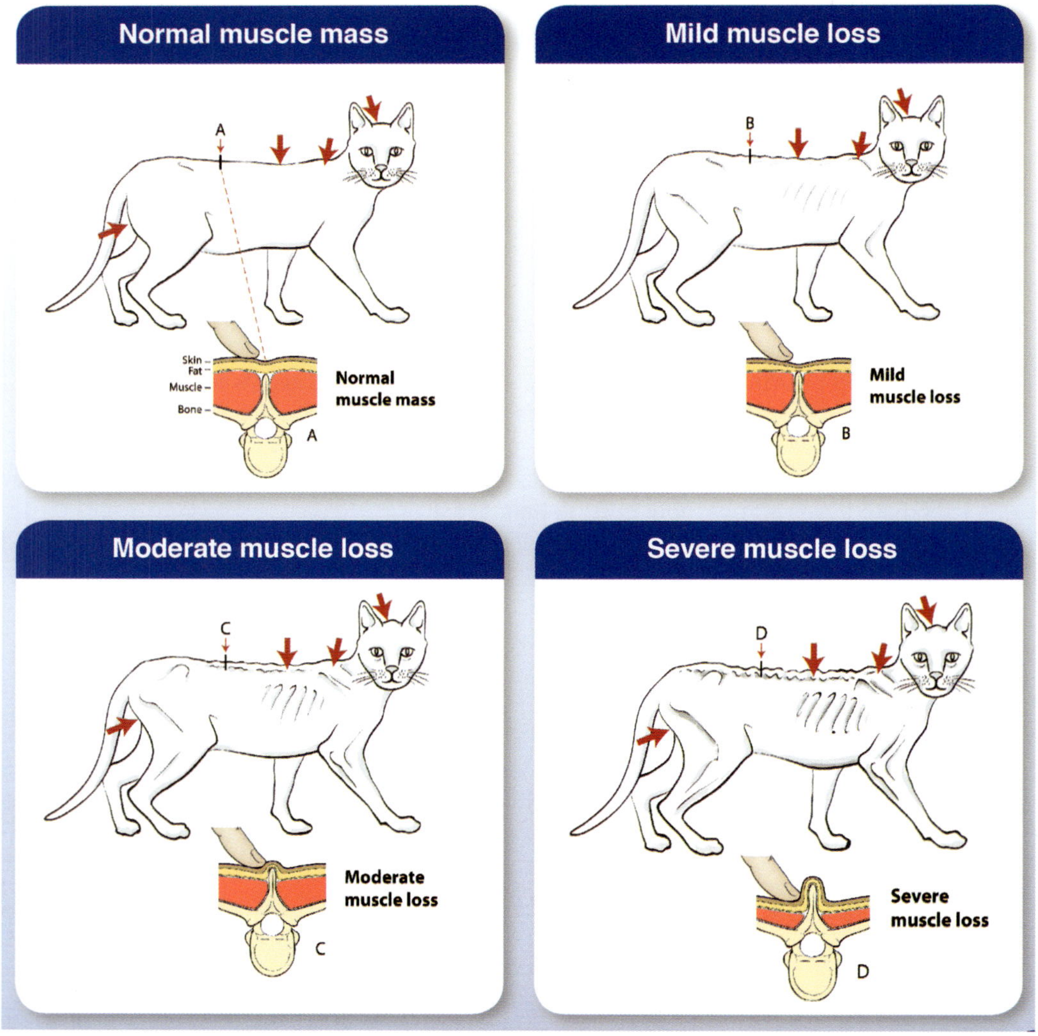

■ **Figure 94.3** Muscle Condition Score in Cats—WSAVA Global Nutrition Committee—determining the amount of lean muscle mass by palpating the epaxial muscle height to assess normal versus mild, moderate-to-severe muscle loss. Full chart available in resources online. Source: With permission of World Small Animal Veterinary Association.

- Simply palpating the spine can alert staff to evaluate MCS more fully.
- Ultrasound evaluation of epaxial muscle height can also be done (training required).

- Current Practice Information Management Systems do not have a field to record MCS
  - Contact your PIMS provider to customize your system to add the field.
- If decreases in MCS are found, perform further diagnostics to determine if any underlying disease or condition could be contributing:
  - Gastrointestinal—inadequate diet, digestion, or absorption.
  - Presence of neoplasia, cardiac disease, renal disease, or chronic inflammation.
- If sarcopenia with mild levels of muscle loss is present, discuss nutrition and exercise with client (see DIET below).
- Dietary protein
  - Evaluate actual diet that is consumed, amount of protein, quality of protein.
  - Meat- and dairy-based protein provide essential amino acids compared to soy proteins.[1]
  - Older pets can benefit from smaller, more frequent feedings, even warmed.
- Exercise
  - While it can be challenging in frail patients, those with mobility issues and nearly every cat, encouraging some degree of activity can have benefits for the patient.
  - In people, resistance exercise may be more beneficial than aerobic exercise.
  - Restores mitochondrial homeostasis and produces exercise-induced cytokine that are anti-inflammatory.[4]

DIET

- Resting energy requirements (RER)—70 kcal × kg $BW^{0.75}$; may need to exceed RER in cachectic patients, if tolerated:
  - Maintenance energy requirement [MER] for neutered adult dog: 1.6 × RER but may exceed 2.0–3.0 × RER in individual patients.
  - MER for neutered adult cat: 1.2 × RER but may be higher in individual patients.
- Unless contraindicated, exceed Association of American Feed Control Officials (AAFCO) protein minimum in cachectic patients:
  - Dogs—4.5 g/100 kcal; cats—instead of: 6.5 g/100 kcal.
  - Most critical care, performance, and growth diets are high in protein and fat.
  - Kitten foods may be suitable for adult cats; cat foods may be suitable for dogs.
- Prolonged anorexia—deliver 25–33% of RER on day 1; gradually increase to 100% RER over 3–5 days, if tolerated:
  - Monitor serum potassium, phosphorus, and magnesium during refeeding; supplement if needed.

Oral Nutrition

- Preferred if patient is physically able to ingest, digest, and absorb nutrients.
- To increase voluntary food intake, offer palatable food several times daily; offer the patient's usual food; offer moist food unless dry is preferred; offer food warmed to body temperature.
- Consider diets enriched with eicosapentaenoic acid (EPA) and docosahexaenoic acid (DHA) for cachectic patients or those with inflammatory conditions (e.g., therapeutic diets for arthritis or dermatologic conditions):
  - Most diets provide less than recommended EPA/DHA amounts (see below); additional supplementation may be beneficial.

- If underweight patients refuse therapeutic diets (e.g., renal diet), try alternate brand or texture, add broth or other palatability enhancer:
    - Adequate intake of a maintenance diet is typically preferable to inadequate intake of a therapeutic diet.
- Consider appetite stimulants (see Medications).
- Forced feeding is rarely effective and is not recommended due to high risk of aspiration.

Enteral Nutrition

- Preferred if patient is anorexic/pseudoanorexic but can digest and absorb nutrients.
- Place feeding tubes as far proximal in the GI tract as tolerated.
- Nasoesophageal or nasogastric tubes (5–12Fr) can be used temporarily. Due to small tube size, only liquid diets can be used.
- Esophagostomy (12–18Fr) or gastrostomy tubes (16–24Fr) are semi-permanent:
    - Preferred over nasogastric tubes for outpatient management.
    - Allow higher caloric-density slurry diets, therapeutic diets, medication, and oral water administration.
- Liquid/slurry feedings q6–8h; initial feedings <10 mL/kg/feeding.
- Jejunostomy or gastro-jejunostomy tubes (5–8Fr) are more difficult to place and manage, and require liquid diets fed via chronic infusion:
    - Rarely indicated.

Parenteral Nutrition

- Only if enteral feeding is contraindicated.
- If required, recommend referral to an appropriate tertiary facility.

Appetite Stimulants

- Adjust selection and dosage based on underlying disease.
- Mirtazapine: 7.5 and 15 mg tablets; 2% transdermal suspension (cats):
    - Cats: 1.88 mg/cat PO q24–48h; 2 mg/cat transdermally q24–48h.
    - Dogs: 1–30 mg/dog PO q8–24h; recommend 1 mg/kg PO q8–12h.
- Capromorelin: 30 mg/mL oral suspension:
    - Dogs: 3 mg/kg PO q24h.
    - Cats: 2 mg/kg PO q24h.
    - Also increases IGF-1 secretion.

Omega-3 Fatty Acids

- Fish oil, krill oil, omega-3 supplements:
    - Vary widely in EPA and DHA content; check each supplement individually.
- Dogs and cats—40 mg/kg/day EPA + 25 mg/kg/day DHA:
    - Avoid fish oil supplements with vitamins A and D if using at this dose.
- Plant-based fatty acid sources (flaxseed, canola, etc. with alpha linoleic acid ALA) should not be used due to inefficient conversion to long chain PUFAs in mammals (Free 131).
- In dogs, linoleic acid is considered an essential nutrient and is converted to arachidonic acid (AA).
- Cats have a dietary need for arachidonic acid.
- While there can be a focus on omega ratios (6 : 3), it is more important to use the total intake, type, and amounts in considerations.

- There are potential side effects of omega-3 fatty acids including platelet function, wound healing, gastrointestinal issues, lipid peroxidation, and hypervitaminosis A and D (cod liver oil), but these are typically dose dependent.[5]
- Note: both alpha linoleic acid and alpha lipoic acid have the same acronym (ALA), and while lipoic acid does have its indications, it can be toxic, especially in cats.

Targets for Intervention

- Decreased energy intake
    - Altered neural control of appetite in cachexia; satiety factors are increased or not appropriately decreased.
        - Ghrelin—increase food intake if no resistance; also increases growth hormone
    - Enhanced inflammatory state.[6]
- Metabolic alterations
    - Inflammatory cytokines—TNF-α (Tumor Necrosis Factor) and IL-6 (Interleukin-6) and impact on nuclear factor ƘB (NF-ƘB) (neurohormonal activation).
        - Altered protein flux
        - Anti-TNF studies
        - Omega 3 Fatty acids—decrease inflammatory cytokines
    - Ubiquitin–Proteosome pathways—pro-cachexia—NF-ƘB is a common pathway.
        - Myostatin—negatively regulates skeletal muscle mass
            - Levels are decreased by exercise training, allowing muscles increase in size.[7]
            - Angiotensin II increases myostatin expression, and it is increased in people with chronic heart failure.
            - A proteo-lipid myostatin antagonist from fertilized egg yolk (Fortetropin) to inhibit myostatin has been shown to reverse muscle atrophy in rodent models.[8, 9]
                - Prevented a rise in myostain post-surgery with exercise restriction in dogs.[10]
                - Demonstrated no benefit in dogs with cardiac cachexia, likely due to the timing of intervention.[11]
    - Catecholamines and RAAS increase metabolism,[12] so there is a benefit of beta-blockers, ACE-inhibitors.
    - Adipokines—leptin, resistin, and adiponectin.
        - Adiponectin—highest concentration in adipocytes
            - Anti-inflammatory effect.[13]
    - Anabolic agents.
        - IGF-1—independent predictor of survival in dogs with CHF.[14]
        - Testosterone is anabolic but has unwanted side effects.
- Stem cell considerations
    - Research on what type of stem cell, safety issues, and quality control.
    - Secretome of stem cells are the main anti-inflammatory component.[4]
    - Extracellular vesicles and factors for growth, cytoskeletal remodeling, and immunomodulatory are being investigated (mouse model).[15]
        - Increased lean body mass, decreased fat mass
        - Increased myofiber cross-sectional area
        - Reduced lipid content in adipocytes and improved insulin sensitivity.

- STEM—combination of potent immunomodulatory and cytoskeletal factors.[16]
  - Mixture of molecules to recruit immune cells, deliver growth factors and mediators of collagen turnover.
  - Mitigate muscle atrophy due to disuse and during recovery.

Client Communication

- If communication and demonstration about determining BCS has been done in the past, add in the discussion of MCS with pet owners as the pet ages, or as MCS is discovered.
  - Instruct them how to evaluate the pet's lean body mass. (WSAVA)
  - Have them monitor body weight, activity levels and diet at home.
- If cachexia is already present, impress upon the owner the need for full diagnostics to determine what disease process is impacting the patient's health.
  - With frailty and weakness, discuss supporting mobility in the house (See Senior-Friendly Homes).
  - Nutritional support is critical for these patients. Determine the level of intervention that will best "fit" the patient–client relationship. Keep in mind the level of caregiver burden supplement feeding may entail.

Abbreviations

- AAFCO = Association of American Feed Control Officials
- ACTH = adrenocorticotropic hormone
- AA = amino acid
- ALA = Alpha linoleic acid (or Alpha lipoic acid)
- BCS = body condition score
- BW = body weight
- CHF = congestive heart failure
- CKD = chronic kidney disease
- DEXA = dual-energy X-ray absorptiometry
- DHA = docosahexaenoic acid
- EMH = apaxial muscle height
- EPA = eicosapentaenoic acid.
- GFR- glomerular filtration rate
- GH = growth hormone
- GI = gastrointestinal
- IGF-1 = insulin-like growth factor I
- IL-6 = interleukin-6
- LBM = lean body mass
- LE = life expectancy
- MER = maintenance energy requirement
- MCS = muscle condition score
- MRI = magnetic resonance imaging
- NF-kB = necrosis factor ƙ Beta
- PIMS = practice information management system
- PUFA = polyunsaturated fatty acids
- RER = resting energy requirements
- SDMA = symmetric dimethylarginine
- SO = sarcopenic obesity

- TLI = trypsin-like immunoreactivity
- TNF-α = tumor necrosis factor-α
- WSAVA = World Small Animal Veterinary Association

Internet Resources

Accessed 29 June 2024

- To find a veterinary nutritionist qualified to assist in formulating homemade therapeutic or maintenance diets: http://www.ACVN.org
- To find a certified veterinary rehabilitation professional: https://rehabvets.org/directory.lasso
- Information on small animal nutrition guidelines, body condition scoring, and muscle condition scoring: https://wsava.org/global-guidelines/global-nutrition-guidelines/

Additional Reading (From Original Topic)

Eirmann L. Esophagostomy feeding tubes in dogs and cats. In: Chan DL (ed.) *Nutritional Management of Hospitalized Small Animals*. Chichester: John Wiley & Sons, 2015; pp. 29–40.

Freeman LM. Cachexia and sarcopenia. In: Ettinger SJ, Feldman EC, Côté E (eds) *Textbook of Veterinary Internal Medicine*, 8th edn. St. Louis, MO: Elsevier, 2017; pp. 739–744.

Freeman LM. Cachexia and sarcopenia: emerging syndromes of importance in dogs and cats. *J Vet Intern Med* 2012;26:3–17.

Johnson LN. Recognizing, describing, and managing reduced food intake in dogs and cats. *J Am Vet Med Assoc* 2017;251:1260–1266.

Larsen JA. Enteral nutrition and tube feeding. In: Fascetti AJ, Delaney SJ (eds) *Applied Veterinary Clinical Nutrition*. Ames, IA: Wiley-Blackwell, 2012; pp. 329–352.

References

1 Parker VJ. Sarcopenia of ageing and cachexia in dogs and cats. *Hills Global Symposium*, 2018, Lisbon.

2 Pagano TB, Wojcik S, Costagliola A, De Biase D, Iovino S, Iovane V, Russo V, Papparella S, Paciello O. Age related skeletal muscle atrophy and upregulation of autophagy in dogs. *Vet J* 2015 Oct;206(1):54–60. doi: 10.1016/j.tvjl.2015.07.005. Epub 2015 Jul 6. PMID: 26257260.

3 Hutchinson D, Sutherland-Smith J, Watson AL, Freeman LM. Assessment of methods of evaluating sarcopenia in old dogs. *Am J Vet Res* 2012 Nov;73(11):1794–1800. doi: 10.2460/ajvr.73.11.1794. PMID: 23106466.

4 Lo JH, U KP, Yiu T, Ong MT, Lee WY. Sarcopenia: Current treatments and new regenerative therapeutic approaches. *J Orthop Translat* 2020 Apr 30;23:38–52. doi: 10.1016/j.jot.2020.04.002. PMID: 32489859; PMCID: PMC7256062.

5 Lenox CE, Bauer JE. Potential adverse effects of omega-3 Fatty acids in dogs and cats. *J Vet Intern Med* 2013 Mar–Apr;27(2):217–226. doi: 10.1111/jvim.12033. Epub 2013 Jan 16. PMID: 23323770.

6 Laviano A, Inui A, Marks DL, et al. Neural control of the anorexia-cachexia syndrome. *Am J Physiol Endocrinol Metab* 2008;295:E1000–E1008.

7 Lenk K, Schur R, Linke A, et al. Impact of exercise training on myostatin expression in the myocardium and skeletal muscle in a chronic heart failure model. *Eur J Heart Fail* 2009;11:342–348

8 Hetrick K, Harkin KR, Roush JK. Evaluation of Fortetropin in geriatric and senior dogs with reduced mobility. *Can Vet J* 2022 Oct;63(10):1057–1060. PMID: 36185794; PMCID: PMC9484193.

9 Freeman LM, Rush JE, Cunningham SM, Yang VK, Bulmer BJ. Pilot study of a myostatin antagonist in dogs with cardiac cachexia. *J Vet Cardiol* 2015 Sep;17(3):210–215. doi: 10.1016/j.jvc.2015.06.004. Epub 2015 Sep 26. PMID: 26412784.—Abstract only.

10 White DA, Harkin KR, Roush JK, Renberg WC, Biller D. Fortetropin inhibits disuse muscle atrophy in dogs after tibial plateau leveling osteotomy. *PLoS One* 2020 Apr 9;15(4):e0231306. doi: 10.1371/journal.pone.0231306. PMID: 32271840; PMCID: PMC7144988.

11. Freeman LM, Rush JE, Cunningham SM, Yang VK, Bulmer BJ. Pilot study of a myostatin antagonist in dogs with cardiac cachexia. *J Vet Cardiol* 2015 Sep;17(3):210–215. doi: 10.1016/j.jvc.2015.06.004. Epub 2015 Sep 26. PMID: 26412784.
12. Doehner W, Anker SD. Cardiac cachexia in early literature: a review of research prior to Medline. *Int J Cardiol* 2002;85:7–14.
13. Fonfara S, Hetzel U, Tew SR, et al. Leptin expression in dogs with cardiac disease and congestive heart failure. *J Vet Intern Med* 2011;25:1017–1024.
14. Freeman LM, Rush JE, Kehayias JJ, Ross JN Jr, Meydani SN, Brown DJ, Dolnikowski GG, Marmor BN, White ME, Dinarello CA, Roubenoff R. Nutritional alterations and the effect of fish oil supplementation in dogs with heart failure. *J Vet Intern Med* 1998 Nov–Dec;12(6):440–448. doi: 10.1111/j.1939-1676.1998.tb02148.x. PMID: 9857337.
15. Fennel ZJ, Bourrant PE, Kurian AS, et al. Stem cell secretome treatment improves whole-body metabolism, reduces adiposity, and promotes skeletal muscle function in aged mice. *Aging Cell* 2024 Jun;23(6):e14144. doi: 10.1111/acel.14144. Epub 2024 Mar 18. PMID: 38500398
16. Fix DK, Mahmassani ZS, Petrocelli JJ, de Hart NMMP, Ferrara PJ, Painter JS, Nistor G, Lane TE, Keirstead HS, Drummond MJ. Reversal of deficits in aged skeletal muscle during disuse and recovery in response to treatment with a secrotome product derived from partially differentiated human pluripotent stem cells. *Geroscience* 2021 Dec;43(6):2635–2652. doi: 10.1007/s11357-021-00423-0. Epub 2021 Aug 24. PMID: 34427856; PMCID: PMC8602548.

Author: Heidi Lobprise
Topic adapted from Five Minute Veterinary Consultation, 7th edition, 2021
Original Topic: Weight Loss and Cachexia

Authors: Laura Rayhel and Valerie J. Parker
Consulting Editor: Mark P. Rondeau

Miscellaneous

Chapter 95

Senior-Friendly Practice

BASICS

OVERVIEW

Older pets are part of a growing demographic within our patient population; estimates of up to 4[illegible]% are considered senior.[1]

Most practices have a general appreciation for the added extent of care a senior pet may need, including more regular examination, continuation of preventive care including vaccines, parasite control and dental care, and optimally early detection of any disease process.

Paying special attention to senior-specific issues by creating a senior-friendly practice can help clients appreciate the efforts you make for these family members. And that, in turn, optimizes the care you can provide them (see Figure 95.1).

Terms Defined

- Senior:
    - Dogs: The 2019 AAHA Canine Life Stage Guidelines define senior as "the last 25% of estimated lifespan through end of life."[1]
    - Cats: The 2021 AAHA/AAFP Feline Life Stage Guidelines and the 2021 AAFP Feline Senior Care Guidelines define senior as cats greater than 10 years of age.[2, 3]
- Geriatric: This term is sometimes used interchangeably with "senior" but may be used to include patients that have exceeded their anticipated lifespan or a senior with extensive health issues.
- Healthspan: An individual's years lived in good health, without disease, chronic illness, and disability.
- Mobility: The ability of an animal to move without restriction or pain.
- Anxiety: The anticipation of future danger that may be unknown, imagined, or real. It can result in physiologic responses similar to those associated with fear.

ISSUES AND OPTIONS

Identifying and Recording Senior Lifestage Status

- One of the biggest challenges in developing your senior-friendly practice is to have a simple way to determine and record this lifestage for dogs.
    - Life expectancy and aging for dogs depends on the size and breed, as well as individual variations.
- This is one area where cats are "simpler" than dogs—they are senior at 11 years of age.

Blackwell's Five-Minute Veterinary Consult Clinical Companion: Small Animal Senior Care, First Edition. Edited by Heidi B. Lobprise.

Companion website: www.wiley.com/go/lobprise/Senior

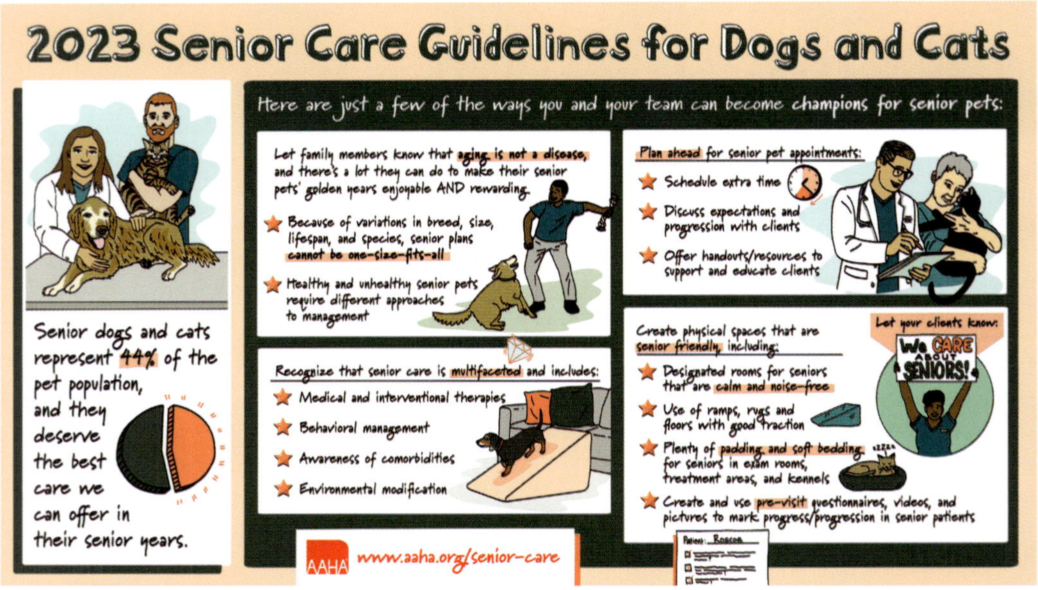
2023 Senior Care Guidelines for Dogs and Cats
Senior dogs and cats represent 44% of the pet population, and they deserve the best care we can offer in their senior years.
Here are just a few of the ways you and your team can become champions for senior pets:
Let family members know that aging is not a disease, and there's a lot they can do to make their senior pets' golden years enjoyable AND rewarding.
Because of variations in breed, size, lifespan, and species, senior plans cannot be one-size-fits-all
Healthy and unhealthy senior pets require different approaches to management
Recognize that senior care is multifaceted and includes:
Medical and interventional therapies
Behavioral management
Awareness of comorbidities
Environmental modification
Plan ahead for senior pet appointments:
Schedule extra time
Discuss expectations and progression with clients
Offer handouts/resources to support and educate clients
Create physical spaces that are senior friendly, including:
Designated rooms for seniors that are calm and noise-free
Use of ramps, rugs and floors with good traction
Plenty of padding and soft bedding for seniors in exam rooms, treatment areas, and kennels
Create and use pre-visit questionnaires, videos, and pictures to mark progress/progression in senior patients
Let your clients know:
We CARE ABOUT SENIORS!
Patient: Roscoe
AAHA
www.aaha.org/senior-care

■ **Figure 95.1** 2023 AAHA Senior Care Guidelines for Dogs and Cats graphic highlights for practices.

- Most practice information management systems (PIMS) do not have a specific field for a pet's lifestage, though some systems can be customized to have a field added. This may require a manual update when a pet reaches that status, but hopefully in the future, this will automatically be calculated based on age for cats, and age and weight for dogs.
- Until lifestage is a common designation with PIMS, measurement and marketing to this demographic would be very difficult to implement.

Senior Pets Are Not Coming into the Practice

- Data was evaluated from more than 817,000 pets who were euthanized in clinics and uncovered that 55% of cats and 40% of dogs did not see their veterinarian in the 18 months before they were euthanized.[4]
- Cat visits to veterinarians can be reduced due to increased intervals between vaccinations, challenges to bring cats into the practice, and economic factors.
  - Since cats can hide early signs well, they can have significant levels of disease before they are brought into the clinic, often with weight loss already apparent.

APPLICATION TO PRACTICE

- As with any protocol or procedure, creating a senior-friendly practice takes agreement and commitment from all team members for optimal application.
- Having the group's input in implementing changes in client communication and education, facility updates and even social media can engage everyone.
- Part of making a practice more senior-friendly involves physical adjustments or additions to a current facility. Some suggestions may be challenging if space is limited, but even small improvements can be helpful to those patients and clients.
- The key is to look at ways to facilitate senior pet visits from the start to discharge.

Pre-appointment Preparation

- Have your staff be on the lookout for any special needs a patient might have, particularly when it comes to their mobility. If there is a history of previous injury or osteoarthritis, have an alert recorded for that pet.
- For any new pet joining your practice, particularly if they are in the senior lifestage, ask about any mobility issues or other special needs.
- Once you have the information, be ready to assist the owner as the pet arrives for the appointment or procedure:
  - Special signage can be used for a parking space or two, similar to handicapped parking for people. In fact, if there is a space near a curb-cut, utilize that one.
    - The signs that were used during COVID for curb-side service can be re-purposed for this.
  - Curb ramps can help if a curb-cut is not available (see Figure 95.2).
  - Ramps can be obtained for use to help patients in and out of vehicles with assistance from staff (see Figure 95.3).
  - A supply of washable vinyl harnesses or slings can be on hand to provide additional mobility support (see Figure 95.4).
- If anxiety is an issue (and it is a common senior problem), consider the use of pre-visit pharmaceuticals as appropriate and other Fear Free® methods.

Entrance and Check-in

- Slick floors can be scary and uncomfortable for patients with pain or mobility issues. Non-slippery flooring can be easily provided by putting down washable yoga mats. Sticky socks can also be provided for senior pets for better footing (see Figure 95.5).

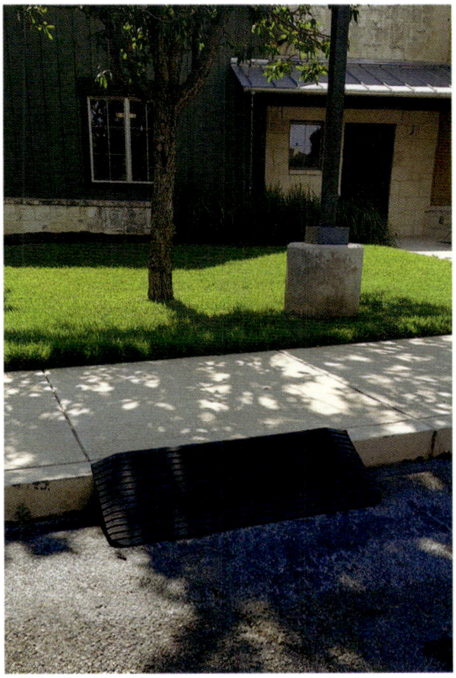

Figure 95.2 A ramp can be used to facilitate dogs with mobility issues over the curb at the clinic.

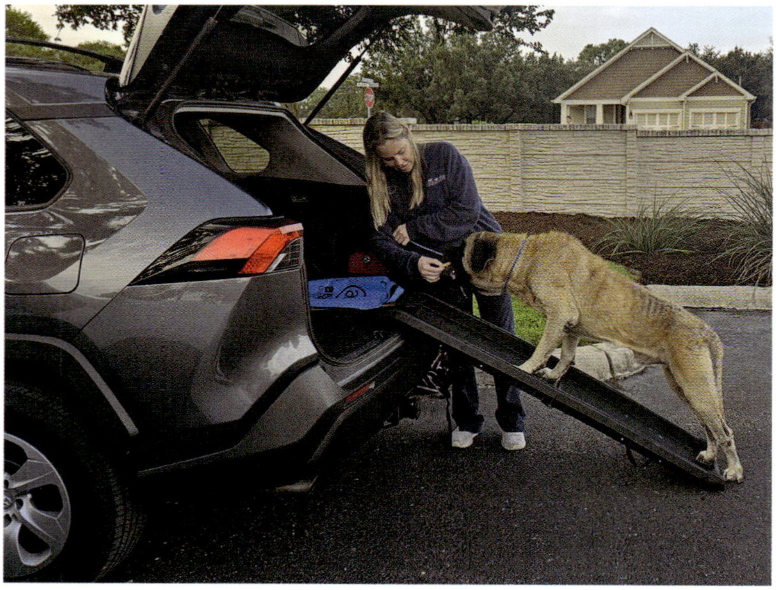

■ **Figure 95.3** Ramps made for cars can assist patients getting into and out of vehicles, with a little training (and treats!).

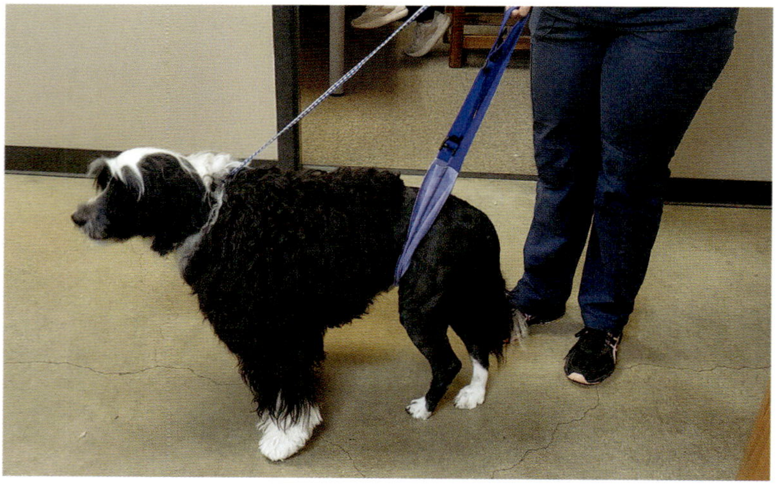

■ **Figure 95.4** The use of a sling or harness can help the pet navigate around the clinic.

- Starting or continuing harness usage can help with mobility. In fact, the use of collars is not recommended in older patients, particularly in those with tracheal issues, laryngeal paralysis (LarPar; geriatric-onset laryngeal paralysis and polyneuropathy), and they can even increase intraocular pressure.[5]
- Have a comfort area set up with orthopedic bedding (washable covers) for dogs, providing water if needed, and even a small fan for overheated dogs, or those with LarPar/GOLPP. This area should be positioned near the anticipated examination room to be used (see Figure 95.6).
- Keep senior cats in a quiet area, if possible, covering the cage with a towel or blanket.

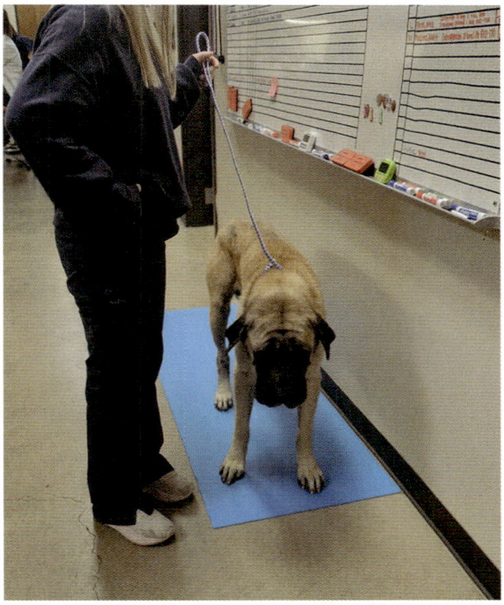

Figure 95.5 Yoga mats can be placed to assist with examination or multiple ones placed to help with gait assessment.

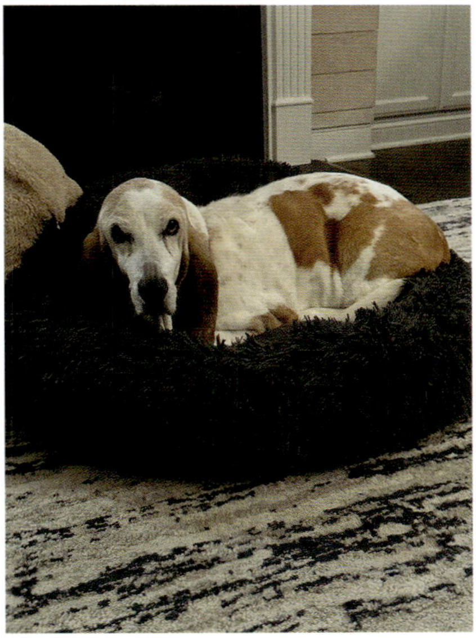

Figure 95.6 Orthopedic bedding provided for older dogs in the reception area and examination room can make them more comfortable.

- Seniors can be more prone to anxiety, so utilize any of the Fear Free® methods your clinic implements, including pre-visit pharmaceuticals.
    - Use pheromones on towels for cats and on bandanas for dogs (spray the bandana 15 minutes prior to putting on dog; or keep treated ones in a plastic bag). Diffusers for both species can be kept in rooms.
    - Use considerate approach, gentle control, and touch gradient.

Examination Room

- Keep rooms close to the reception designated as "Senior Sites."
    - Provide a yoga matt pathway from their reception area and use rubber mats in the room, as well as moving their orthopedic bedding into the room with them.
- Position them in the room for optimal examination without having to move them frequently. Use patient holding techniques designed for comfort and stability.
    - For larger dogs, this will most likely be on the floor as trying to move them and keeping them on an elevated table may cause anxiety.
    - To keep staff more comfortable, provide garden kneeling pads.
- Many cats prefer elevated surfaces.
    - Provide a comfortable towel, blanket, or pad infused with pheromones. For cats and small dogs the use of baby changing pads with washable covers and two raised sides can be helpful if your tables are long enough. Rubber strips on the bottom will help keep it from sliding on the table (see Figure 95.7).
- Reduce noise if possible, as seniors can be sensitive, especially if painful, some even to the level of hyperalgesia and central plasticity.
    - Use quiet clippers.
    - Providing analgesics, behavior modification, and anxiolytics might be warranted.

Diagnostics and Procedures

- In restraint or adjusting their position for a procedure such as intravenous catheter placement, take any painful conditions (osteoarthritis) into consideration.
    - Cats may be more comfortable on their sides and limb selection can be helpful.
    - Topical anesthetic (lidocaine/prilocaine) application can provide additional comfort and decrease stress.
- Lifting and positioning large pets should be done with balanced support and cushioning to avoid post-operative nerve and pressure point injuries.

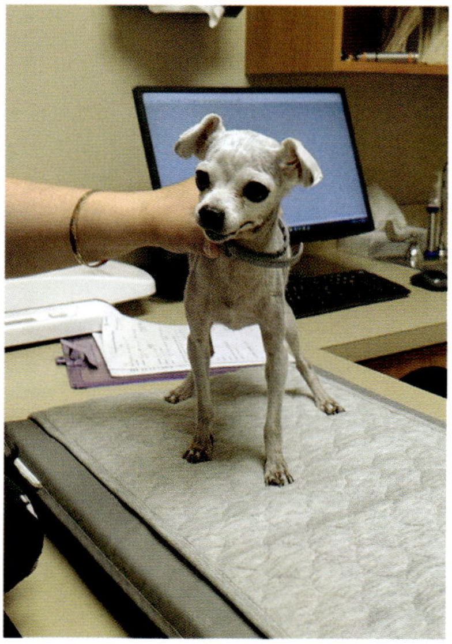

Figure 95.7 16-year-old Riley has a soft, washable cover to make him comfortable during his pre-operative examination for a dental procedure, especially with his mom close by.

- Restraining the limbs in stressful position with tie-downs should be avoided.
- V-shaped tables and memory foam pads or baby changing pads can be helpful, but watch v-trough placement if it does not support the entire body.
- Placing the patient in a lateral/neutral position is preferred, as dorsal positioning can put excessive flexion and extension pressures on the neck.
    - Provide sufficient padding and support if dorsal positioning is necessary.

- Going into recovery, replace the harness to help transport and support patients initially and then as they return to mobility.
- Since a senior pet has decreased thermoregulation, continue any supportive care during recovery.

Discharge

- Continue the use of any mobility assistance, even loaning or selling a harness for the pet, and the vehicle ramp, if the pet will use it.
- Have the owner pre-warm or pre-cool the car before the pet leaves and help the pet with a last elimination before the trip.
- Provide potty pads just in case they have an accident on the way home.

Post-Visit and at Home

- If there has been any kind of procedure, especially with sedation or anesthesia, call the owner the next day to see how the pet is returning to function, including appetite, mobility, and even cognition.
- In people with cognitive issues, there can be some declines after surgery or hospitalization; pets with similar should be monitored.

TEAM TRAINING/TEAM ROLES

- In addition to engaging the entire team in creating your Senior-Friendly Practice, review areas where regular room preparation or maintenance may be required:
    - Remember that seniors can be noise sensitive, have mobility issues and even issues with thermoregulation.
    - With orthopedic bedding, yoga mats, and baby changing pads for cats, these items should be clean and ready for use, just like prepping the room with thermometers and ear cones. Collection and cleaning of items should be done after the appointment.
- Have Client Service Representatives (as well as all team members) well versed in determining the senior status of a pet:
    - For cats—11 years and older.
    - For dogs—a "Relative Age" chart can be used to determine "human years" and lifestage.
    - If there are any pertinent questionnaires or check lists available on your website, have them inform the owner to review those prior to the appointment, or have an email sent with the links.
    - When calling to confirm an appointment, ask if there are any special needs and inform the owner of available assistance, such as the parking spot, vehicle ramp, or harnesses.
        - When the owner arrives, they can call in to the front desk and ask for assistance.
- For technician/nurses and assistants
    - With the initial assessment of history and vital signs, have a general checklist of common senior issues such as mobility, weight (loss or gain), diet, elimination issues, and behavior/cognition.

    - If the patient has not started senior level care, start the discussion about more frequent examinations (at least twice yearly) and diagnostics, as well as continuing preventive care. A senior care bundle with 2–4 visits can encourage regular checkups.
- Veterinarian—collaborate with team to identify those pets as seniors and pay close attention to potential issues to provide optimal care.

Senior Care Programs

- Your clinic may have a "senior care program," and it likely includes recommendations for at least two clinic visits per year, diagnostics such as blood work and urinalysis, EKG, and even screening radiographs.
    - While screening diagnostics may uncover hidden problems (and early detection is optimal), even "normal" results help provide a good baseline and a starting point to track any trends or gradual changes.
- Having the program in place is a good start, but it must be used regularly and effectively.
    - Tracking the number of senior pets in your practice and compliance with recommendations will be challenging until the senior lifestage can be easily determined.
- Pet owners need to be made aware of the comprehensive assistance you can offer.
    - They may have anxiety or denial about their pet getting old and suddenly hearing about the need for more visits and diagnostics can be worrisome.
    - They may start connecting senior care with end-of-life (EOL) care, and you have to educate them about maximizing their pet's healthspan.
- Form a senior pet advocates team made of a client service representative, 1 or 2 technicians/nurses and 1 veterinarian; have them:
    - Review current senior programs to make any updates necessary.
    - Coordinate an outreach program to disseminate information to senior patient owners about the level of care you can provide.
    - Collect or develop senior care topics:
        - Handouts for owners on particular conditions their pet may have.
        - Questionnaires on general senior health, and for specific conditions such as osteoarthritis.
        - For newsletters, blogs, and vlogs.
    - Build a senior section in your clinic's website.
        - Images of clinic members working with senior pets, especially when using some of the supplies and equipment that help seniors (harnesses, ramps, mats on the floor and tables).
        - Post photos of older pets, especially on their birthdays and list their "relative age."
        - Feature clinic team members' own senior pets and their stories.
    - Post these photos on a bulletin board.
    - Make a portion of your social media posts about senior pets.
    - In all of these communications—CELEBRATE those pets with their "upgraded" status to senior.
- Until lifestage becomes a field in PIMS, sending out information to a senior pet demographic may be challenging.
    - Except in cats: information, articles, and questionnaires can be sent to owners of cats that are 11 years of age and older.
        - If your clinic sends out birthday emails, this would be a good time to reach out to individual cats; maybe send something at 10 years of age to prep them.

- Sending out information to owners of dogs 7 years and older will "miss" some senior patients, but it would be an opportunity to call attention to the fact that in dogs, "7 is senior" or "dog's age times 7" are not correct.
    - Send out the relative age chart with questions about senior issues to that group. Those with pets that fit the senior lifestage can start evaluating their pet. Those with pets that are still mature adults can be informed and be ready when their pet's time comes to be a senior. (PRN sheet in resources)
    - Again, if your clinic sends out birthday emails, this would also be a good time to start the conversation.
- If the senior care is pressed upon the owner all of a sudden, they could be suspicious that you are just trying to drum up business.
- Providing good education through a continuum of care throughout the lifestages can show the clients that this is the next phase with a different set of considerations.
    - Just as people get older, various assessments are recommended, so they may be able to relate to the added level of care needed.
    - These aging changes in their pets can change quickly, so having the client help in monitoring for early signs can be critical.
    - With the proper information, they will help you determine when an issue need intervention, not "just getting older."
- The key is to show how your team can help that pet age as gracefully as possible, expanding that healthspan throughout the golden years.
- Don't forget about the clients: develop materials about caregiver burden to help the pet owners themselves.
    - A caregiver assessment chart is available from Lap of Love:
        - Dogs owners: bit.ly/dogcgqol
        - Cat owners: bit/ly/catcgqol
    - Share the website for pet caregivers and their burdens.
        - Petcaregiverburden.com
    - Let them know there are Facebook support groups for various pet ailments.
    - When needed there are pet loss support resources as well
        - Lapoflove.com/our-services/pet-loss-support

Client Communication

- Working together with clients as senior pet advocates can increase their awareness of common health issues, early identification of any problems, and proactive care to enhance the pets' healthspan.
    - Have appropriate senior care-based handouts, questionnaires and reading material available.
- Keeping a health journal for their pet can provide a framework for items they should be monitoring and even help to drive discussions on care (see Additional Reading for Clients below).
- Encourage owners to get photos and videos of their pets on a regular basis.
    - Mobility—walking, playing, getting up from a down position, going up and down stairs.
    - Tumor map—photos of masses or skin issues, with an object (coin) to show any changes in size.
    - Body condition score images—side, skyline view, and face.
- Especially in cats and small dogs, have them get a pet or baby scale to weigh their pet on a regular basis.
- When they understand aging in pets and relative life stages, they can often empathize with senior care issues similar to those experienced in humans.

Abbreviations

- GOLPP = Geriatric onset laryngeal paralysis and polyneuropathy
- LarPar = laryngeal paralysis
- PIMS = practice information management systems

Internet Resources

Accessed 29 June 2024

- amazon.com/shop/drmarygardner/
- A caregiver assessment chart is available from Lap of Love:
- Dogs owners: dog_caregiver_QOL.pdf (drmarygardner.com)
- Cat owners: geriatric cat journal tables for web.indd (drmarygardner.com)
- Fear Free Pets—Taking the "Pet" Out of "Petrified" for All Animals
- HOME|GOLPP (allaboutgolpp.com)

Additional Reading for Clients

By Mary Gardner:

- It's Never Long Enough: A Practical Guide to Caring for Your Geriatric Dog
- Nine Lives Are Not Enough: A Practical Guide to Caring for Your Geriatric Cat
- Geriatric Dog Health & Care Journal: A Complete Toolkit for the Geriatric Dog Caregiver
- Geriatric Cat Health & Care Journal: A Complete Toolkit for the Geriatric Cat Caregiver

References

1. Dhaliwal R, Boynton E, Carrera-Justiz S, Cruise N, Gardner M, Huntingford J, Lobprise H, Rozanski E. 2023 AAHA senior care guidelines for dogs and cats. *J Am Anim Hosp Assoc* 2023 Jan 1;59(1):1–21. doi: https://doi.org/10.5326/JAAHA-MS-7343. PMID: 36584321.
2. Quimby J, Gowland S, Carney HC, DePorter T, Plummer P, Westropp J. 2021 AAHA/AAFP Feline life stage guidelines. *J Feline Med Surg* 2021 Mar;23(3):211–233. doi: https://doi.org/10.1177/1098612X21993657. Erratum in: *J Feline Med Surg* 2021 Aug;23(8):NP3. doi: https://doi.org/10.1177/1098612X211024041. PMID: 33627003; PMCID: PMC10812130.
3. Ray M, Carney HC, Boynton B, Quimby J, Robertson S, St Denis K, Tuzio H, Wright B. 2021 AAFP Feline senior care guidelines. *J Feline Med Surg* 2021 Jul;23(7):613–638. doi: https://doi.org/10.1177/1098612X211021538. Erratum in: *J Feline Med Surg* 2021 Oct;23(10):NP4. doi: https://doi.org/10.1177/1098612X211040404. PMID: 34167339; PMCID: PMC10812122.
4. Data from Dr. Mary Gardner—Lap of Love, Inc.
5. Pauli AM, Bentley E, Diehl KA, Miller PE. Effects of the application of neck pressure by a collar or harness on intraocular pressure in dogs. *J Am Anim Hosp Assoc* 2006 May–Jun;42(3):207–211. doi: https://doi.org/10.5326/0420207. PMID: 16611932.

Author: Heidi Lobprise

Thanks to: Mary Gardner and Sheilah Robertson for resources

Chapter 96

Senior-Friendly Homes

BASICS

OVERVIEW

Just as modifications in a practice can make the space more comfortable and safer for senior patients, alterations at their homes can optimize their experiences there. Each senior patient may have specific issues and needs for which the owner can address and provide solutions.

ISSUES AND OPTIONS

Mobility

- As discussed in Senior Pet Comfort and Mobility, if the patient has any pain or hurdles to getting around, daily functions can be impacted.
- First and foremost, a complete medical examination and diagnostics should be done to identify a source of pain or reason for mobility impairment.
    - Emphasis should be placed on compliance with medical, supplement, and physical management recommendations.
    - Alleviation of pain and discomfort can potentially remove the challenge of some of these barriers.
    - Weight management may be beneficial.
- Have the owner evaluate any potential obstacles to easy maneuverability around the house for daily functions.
    - If the cat or dog needs to go up or down stairs to access food, water, or a place to eliminate, see if other options are available.
        - Limit accessibility to stairs if they pose a danger to the pet.
    - Doggy doors:
        - Evaluate if the pet can easily access the outdoors and return inside.
        - Teach them to ring "potty bells."
        - Determine if cognitive issues have impacted their learning and memory.
    - Litter boxes
        - Get larger ones with low edges—under-bed shoe storage box. (see Figure 96.1).
    - Elimination
        - Can they maintain an elimination posture until bowel/bladder is empty?
        - May drip or leak if not complete.
        - May need to assist with harness or physio balls.
- Eating and Drinking

Blackwell's Five-Minute Veterinary Consult Clinical Companion: Small Animal Senior Care, First Edition. Edited by Heidi B. Lobprise.

Companion website: www.wiley.com/go/lobprise/Senior

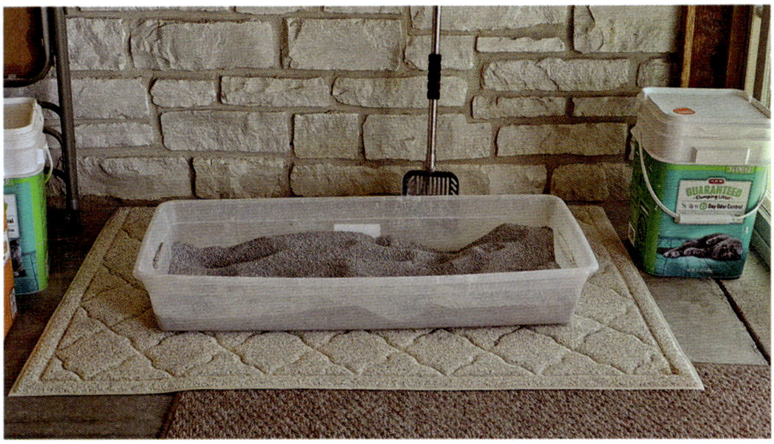

■ **Figure 96.1** Under-bed storage box used as a cat litter box with low sides. Source: Image—Heidi Lobprise.

- Jumping up on furniture, beds, counters (when appropriate)
  - Control pain
  - Provide stairs or ramps
  - Assist on and off.
- In and out of cars
- Maintain activity
  - Control pain
  - Don't overdo it
  - Encourage some level of activity or up to PT (physical therapy) levels as prescribed.
- Management
  - Pain, comprehensive
  - Mobility assistance
    - Non-slick flooring or mats
    - Dr. Buzby's toe grips
    - Sticky socks
    - Trim nails and hair on feet
    - Ramps for stairs (see Figure 96.2)
    - Harnesses, basic or help-em-up.
  - Raised food bowls—painful neck
  - Stability assistance
    - Peanut or PT balls—when eating, being groomed or cleaned.

Cognition (See "Cognitive Dysfunction Syndrome")

- Complete medical/behavioral evaluation and management
- Decrease in cognition is emotional
- Logistical for eating, eliminating, sleeping
  - Sleep disruption affect owners, other pets?
    - Ear plugs
    - Find separate space
  - Help them find food bowls, doggie doors, take them out more frequently (PU/PD [polyuric/polydipsic], don't fully eliminate)

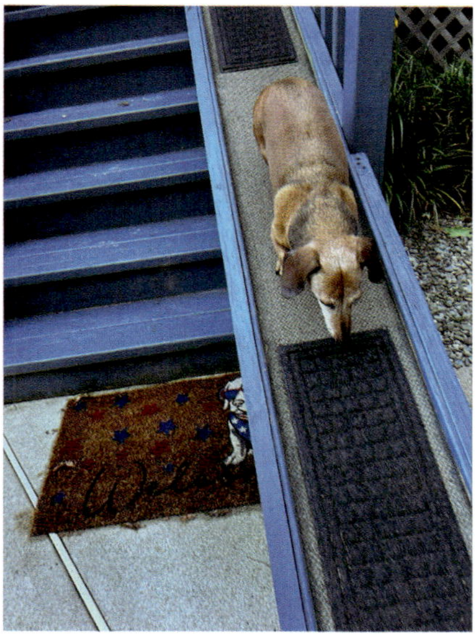

Figure 96.2 Ramp on stairs leading into the house helps with mobility issues. Source: Photo Courtesy of Dr. Adam Christman.

- Limit their accessibility—make their space special
  - Less injury
  - Less getting lost
  - Decrease potential adverse interaction with other pets
  - Quiet space—helps anxiety
- Anxiety—
  - Very common in older pets
  - Complete medical/behavioral evaluation and management
    - Appropriate medications, diets, supplements, activities
    - Pain can make a patient more anxious, even more noise sensitive, so control pain
    - Separation anxiety
  - Fear Free™ modalities
    - Pheromones
    - Don't make many changes and never abruptly
    - May need limited accessibility—their own special space
  - Provide structure and predictability—older animals don't adapt to change well.

Blindness/Hearing—Sensory Deficits

- Blindness
- Finding their food and water
  - Don't move the bowls
  - Make sure the pathway is free from obstacles
  - Feed at specific times—assist pet to bowl
- Access to elimination locations
  - Teach to ring potty bells
  - Leash walks for dogs—more consistent schedule
  - Do NOT move litter boxes; take cat to it 3–4 times daily

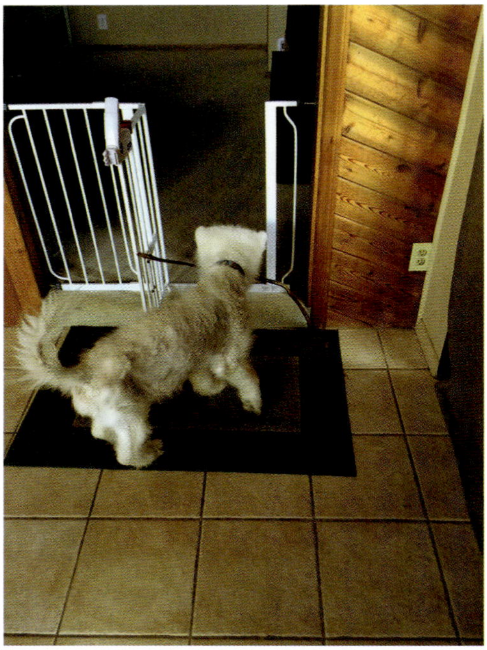

■ **Figure 96.3** Baby gates used to restrict access to unsafe areas for this senior dog; her optimism in fetching this large stick did present an issue. Source: Photo Courtesy of Dr. Mary Gardner.

- Safety on stairs or climbing apparatuses
  - Block access—baby gates
  - Motion activated noise maker
  - Climbing towers—block access or use shorter ones with soft landing spots
- General safety—bumping into or knocking over things
  - Restrict access—child proof, gates (see Figure 96.3)
  - Bumpers on corners and points
  - Bumper collars/halos for pet
- Increased anxiety
  - See above, evaluate and manage, provide structure and predictability
- Intraspecies communication—nonverbal
  - Fighting can increase as ability for low-level communication is lost
  - Bells on collars of other pets
  - Careful monitoring of interactions
  - Separation may be necessary, especially during feeding time
- Hearing
  - Training—hand signals from a young age
  - Leashed at all time
  - Emergency attention with a vibration collar—must be trained positively
  - Sleep startle aggression—approach with foot stomps, treats under nose, then gentle touch at ear
  - Separation anxiety challenging

Pet Interactions—Safe Space, Quality Time, Supervised

- Interspecies communication can be diminished with sensory deficits and cognitive issues
  - Early communication or warning signs may be ignored or not provided

  - Aggression can escalate quickly
  - Senior pet not as quick, slower to recover
- Supervision, especially at mealtimes
- May need separation with all resources available
- If separated, make sure to provide quality time for enrichment

Diet and Water

- Nutritional needs—the veterinary team needs to be the resource for dietary management
  - Appropriate diet
    - Components
      - Individual medical needs
    - Avoid raw, be aware of grain-free and boutique diets
  - Weight management—mobility, OA, diabetes, inflammaging
  - Keep constants—don't move bowls or make quick changes, regular schedule if possible
  - Some seniors do better with smaller, more frequent meals, more savory
  - May have to provide separate feeding units
    - Smart feeders (see Figure 96.4)
    - Auto feeders with specific amounts
  - Feeding toys—enrichment
  - May need to elevate bowls
  - Need to be able to measure what has been eaten, by whom
- Water
  - Multiple sources of fresh water available daily
    - Cats—are fountains preferred?
  - Challenging to monitor intake with multiple pets, multiple sources
    - Water source with chip reader to measure consumption of multiple pets

Elimination—See Mobility

- Incontinence issues
  - Urinary—up to 20% of spayed females have urinary incontinence (see Incontinence—Urinary)
    - Waterproof sheets under bedding may be necessary

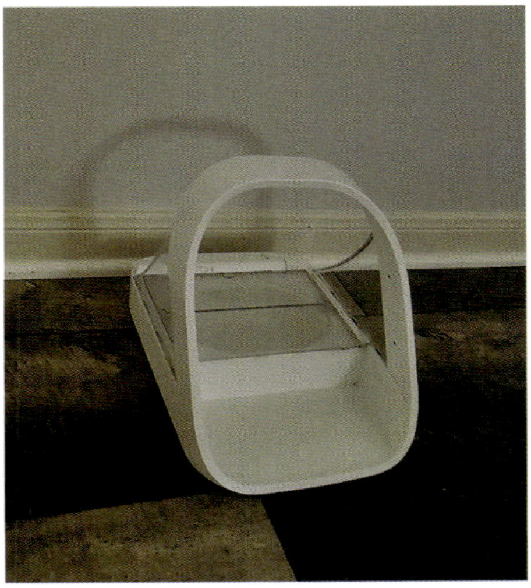

Figure 96.4 Surefeed® Microchip pet feeder with sensor in the arch that only opens for the pet with the appropriate microchip. Source: Image—Heidi Lobprise.

- Fecal—(see Incontinence—Fecal)
    - This is usually seen with neurological decline, so can be a significant change
    - Sanitary clips may help with cleanup
    - Some clients learn how to evacuate the bowel

Bedding and Sleep

- Ease of access—stairs or ramps to a bed or couch
    - Remove obstacles if sight is impaired
- Comfort—orthopedic bed (see Figures 96.4 and 96.5)
    - Don't forget the cats! (see Figure 96.6)
- Try to maintain a regular schedule for sleep as much as possible.
    - Dim lighting, sound and monitor temperature.
- If the senior pet has sleep cycle disturbances, it can disrupt the owner's sleep patterns
    - For some, keeping the pet in a separate space may be necessary, if not too stressful.

Client Communication

- Clients are our best resource for daily pet information and the pet's best advocate if appropriate measures are taken for making the home senior-friendly.
- Journals for recording and monitoring pet details help your practice in their health care, and their awareness of issues that may arise with senior pets.

See Also

- Cognitive Dysfunction syndrome
- Environmental Enrichment and Adjustment
- Incontinence—Fecal
- Incontinence—Urinary
- Mobility in Senior Pets

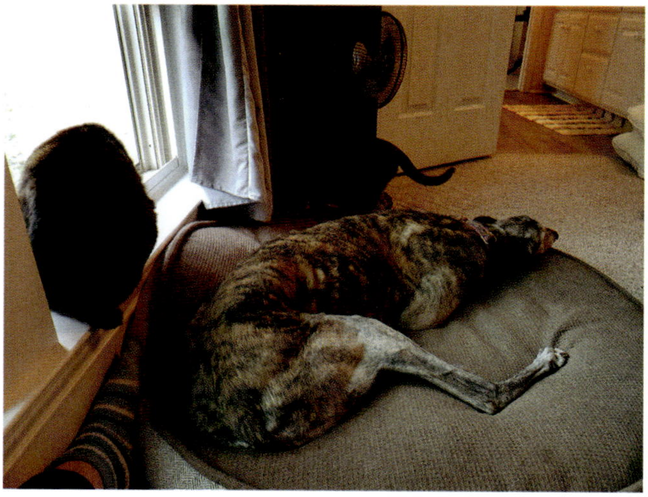

Figure 96.5 Orthopedic bedding is important for older pets with osteoarthritis pain . . .. Source: Image— Heidi Lobprise.

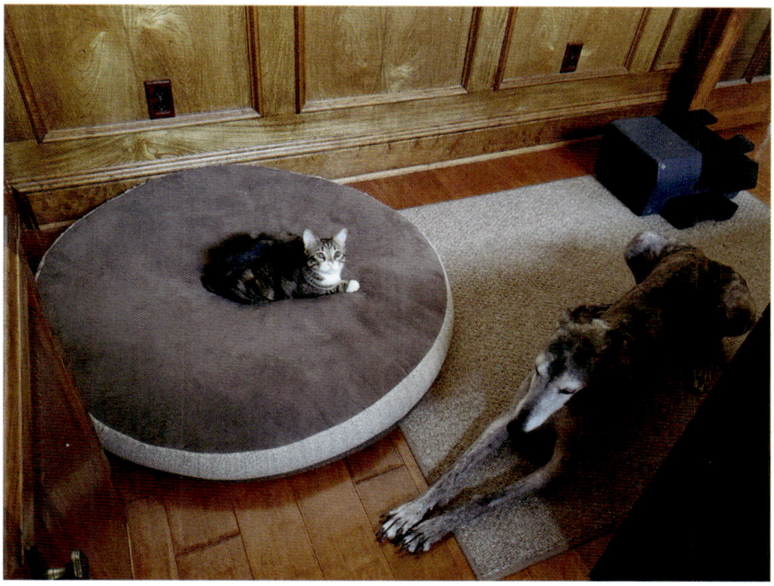

Figure 96.6 . . . if their housemate lets them use it.

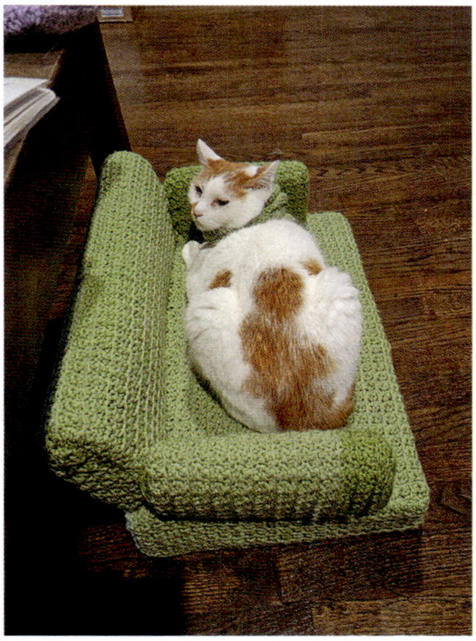

Figure 96.7 Mowgli is enjoying his cat couch crocheted by his grandmother. Source: Image—Heidi Lobprise.

Abbreviations

- OA = osteoarthritis
- PT = physical therapy
- PU/PD = polyuric/polydipsic

Internet Resources

Accessed June 29, 2024

- amazon.com/shop/drmarygardner – a variety of products for senior pets
- Dr. Buzby's ToeGrips for Dogs | Stop Your Dog from Slipping
- Sure Petcare | Award Winning Microchip Cat Doors & Feeders

Additional Reading for Clients

By Mary Gardner:

- It's Never Long Enough: A Practical Guide to Caring for Your Geriatric Dog
- Nine Lives Are Not Enough: A Practical Guide to Caring for Your Geriatric Cat
- Geriatric Dog Health & Care Journal: A Complete Toolkit for the Geriatric Dog Caregiver
- Geriatric Cat Health & Care Journal: A Complete Toolkit for the Geriatric Cat Caregiver

Author: Heidi Lobprise
Thanks to: Mary Gardner, Sheilah Robertson and Amy Pike for resources

Chapter 97

Environmental Enrichment and Adaptation

BASICS

OVERVIEW

Zoos have been working toward enriching the environment of their residents for decades, providing living spaces that attempt to recreate a portion of their natural habitats and activities that support their natural instincts and behaviors. Recent efforts to reduce the stresses a shelter environment has on dogs may include olfactory (pheromones, lavender, etc.) and music stimuli to help them show more resting behaviors.[1] The Dog Aging Project has identified components of the social environment and show that more social companions and better household stability predicted better health outcomes.[2]

Environmental Enrichment (EE) is a dynamic process in which changes to structures and care practices are made with the goal of increasing the behavioral choice available to animals and drawing out their species-appropriate behaviors and abilities, thus enhancing their welfare.

Terms Defined

- Environmental enrichment is a process for improving or enhancing animal environments and care within the context of their inhabitants' behavioral biology and natural history.
- Animate strategies—introduction or increased interaction with others of its species (intraspecific) or humans and other animals (interspecific).[3]
- Inanimate strategies—use of toys, feeding, physical adjustments in flooring or objects, or sensory (visual, auditory, olfactory, pheromones).

ISSUES AND OPTIONS

- Environmental Enrichment (EE) should be addressed at every life stage, but efforts to provide support for senior pets can enhance their behavioral, physical, and emotional stability.
- Cats are born with a hard-wired prey drive, and they continue to have the need to chase, pounce, and "kill" even as they age.
- Most dogs were bred for a purpose, from retrieving waterfowl to herding sheep to guarding property, and having a purpose in life seems to be healthful in dogs as it is in people.
- Without EE, "pampered" pets may not have as much activity, gain weight, and be more anxious with more stress, and that weight gain may cause and/or contribute to health and behavioral problems.

Blackwell's Five-Minute Veterinary Consult Clinical Companion: Small Animal Senior Care, First Edition. Edited by Heidi B. Lobprise.

Companion website: www.wiley.com/go/lobprise/Senior

- A small study looking at a variety of EE activities showed the highest behavioral changes with conspecific play (supervised interaction for 15 minutes with a known conspecific).[4]
  - Other impactful activities included the playhouse (tunnels, slides, and platforms with 15 minutes of exploration and handler encouragement when needed) and a bubble machine that emits bacon-flavored bubbles for 15 minutes.
  - Food-based activities had the least changes (interactive toy and stuffed food toy).
  - A variety of EE activities, providing new ones and rotating them at random can maximize benefits.[4]
- EE adjustments (quiet rooms with white noise and classical music, pheromones, positive human interactions, and food toys) post-surgically reduced analgesic needs and increased return to eating function.[5]

APPLICATIONS IN PRACTICE AND AT HOME

- Feeding options—a combination of EE and weight management strategies:
  - Food toys and puzzles (See Figure 97.1).
  - Place food at various places to simulate hunting.
  - Pets may have mobility and sensory decline that can limit typical options.
  - High-value treats or foods, especially with appealing odors may be needed to stimulate appetite.
  - In cats, toys that simulate the chase and pounce help trigger the motion response.[3]
  - Interactive play and games with cats with "fishing rod toys."
    - These toys should be removed after play to maintain their EE value.[3]
  - Appropriate chew toys/items for dogs.
    - Not hard enough to break teeth; they need to be compressible or bendable or small enough.
    - Monitor first time use; make sure they don't break off large portions and swallow them.

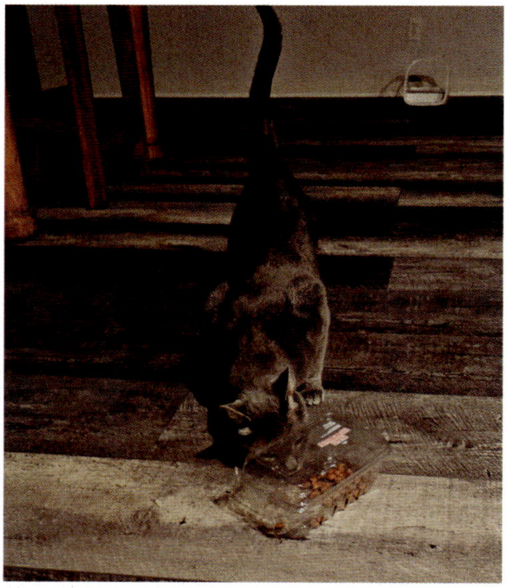

Figure 97.1 Make a simple food toy placing a portion of their daily kibble in a produce container with holes. Source: Image—Heidi Lobprise.

    - Reasonable vertical spaces for cats—cat trees, shelves, ropes, boxes, and there are now manufactured products specifically made with easy step for older cats. Even geriatric cats appreciate and benefit from vertical space.
- Cognitive enrichment
    - It is optimal to encourage a continuum of learning throughout life.
        - Regular interaction with pet
        - Introduce new items, textures, and odors. Note: Too many new introductions or "the wrong kinds of novelty" may frighten some cats.
    - Cognitive enrichment with an antioxidant diet showed increased levels of brain-derived neurotrophic factor (BDNF), one of the factors underlying improvements in learning and memory.[6]
    - Computer touchscreen learning in the future?[7]
- Visual enrichment
    - Providing window access to look outside.
    - TV or videos—birds and small mammals for cats.[3]
        - As long as it doesn't frustrate them since they can't reach the objects.
- Olfactory enrichment
    - Many older pets have sight and hearing deficits, but it is more challenging to assess olfactory abilities.
    - Provide appetite-stimulating foods and treats—warmed up.
    - Exchange soft toys with a friend's dog.
    - Scent training (at-home nose work) and exercise can be beneficial.
    - Toys with catnip (and other compounds) may provide enrichment for some cats.[7]
    - Pheromones to ease anxiety.
- Auditory management
    - Having quieter spaces may be helpful with some pets, as loud noises can affect those with maladaptive pain and anxiety. Provide a place or places (with easy access from other pets) to hide and rest.
    - Animals appear less stressed or anxious when exposed to classical music, though more study is needed.[8]
- Social enrichment—interaction
    - Take a stroll—appropriate length for pet, not too fast.
        - Greet friendly walkers and pets.
        - Smell the roses.
        - Use a carrier or wagon if the pet isn't mobile. (Figure 97.2)
    - Adding a new pet
        - May be beneficial.
        - Too much change can be stressful, especially if the senior pet is ill.
        - Older cats need very gradual introductions, if any.

SPECIAL SITUATIONS

With aging, declines in mobility, cognition, sight and hearing can limit the pet's ability to perform everyday tasks, or cause sufficient anxiety to make them less likely to complete those tasks. For various disabilities, steps can be taken to make the environment safer and easier to navigate. (Note, thanks to Dr. Amy Pike for sharing important information on these situations.)

Loss of Sight

- Challenges with finding food and water, access to elimination locations, safety on stairs or cat towers, general safety, access to other pets.

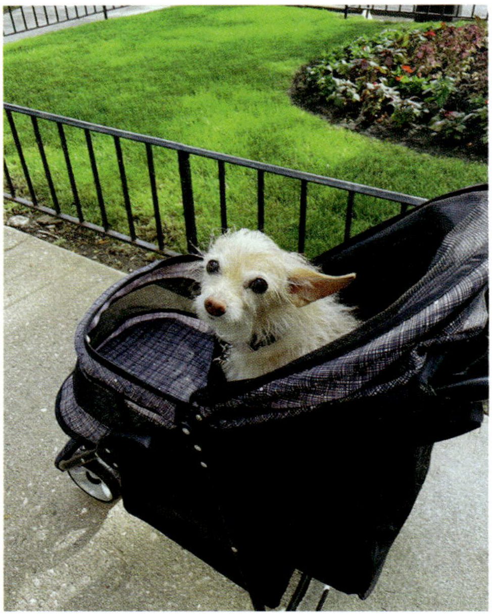

■ **Figure 97.2** While Hazel at 16 can still get around fairly well, one of her favorite activities is taking a "stroll" around the park—PSBO (power supplied by owner). Source: Photo Courtesy of Steve Dale—Steve Dale.

- Food and water—don't move it and make sure the path is clear.
  - Specific times for feeding—a regular schedule may benefit some pets; sometimes older animals may refuse food one time and inexplicably be eager to eat the same thing 30 minutes or a few hours later. Your flexibility is key.
  - Stable or lifted bowls.
- Access for elimination—may have to confine to area that is easily cleaned.
  - Dogs—Take them on regularly scheduled walks, especially after a meal.
    - Teach to ring potty bells. Reward dogs (and even geriatric cats) for doing their business as you might a puppy or kitten.
  - Cats—don't move litter box; take cat to the litter box several times a day.
    - Sides—since nearly 90% of cats show radiographic signs of degenerative joint disease, lower sides on the litter box may be beneficial.
- Safety on stairs or cat towers
  - May need to limit access—use baby gates or other barriers.
  - Warning treads with different texture or motion activated noise maker at stairs.
  - Cat-climbing towers—limit access, use a shorter tower, and have soft-landing spots.
- General safety—child-proof house; bumpers on corners; halo or bumper collars.
- Anxiety—avoid change, keep a schedule.
  - Pharmaceuticals, pheromones, supplements.
- Other pets and people
  - Intraspecies communication is mostly nonverbal, so the ability to avoid another pet is decreased.
  - Place bell on other pets' collars.
  - Approach pet slowly, use heavy footsteps when approaching.

Hearing Loss

- Training should include hand signals from a young age if possible and use high-value rewards.
  - Attention cue—double touch on rear.
  - Tap on the side for dog to turn.
- Must be leashed at all times.
- Emergency attention with a vibration collar; use high-value treats, gradual introduction and training.
- Sleep startle aggression: use foot stomps to awaken, then a treat under nose.
  - Gentle touch on rear if other action does not waken them.
- Separation Anxiety
  - Gradual training to accustom the dog to when you leave with high-value treats.

Cognitive Decline

- See topic—Cognitive Dysfunction Syndrome.
- No changes—feeding, sleeping, eliminating.
- May need to keep in a confined, familiar space.

Mobility

- See topic—Mobility in Senior Pets.
- Environmental adjustments are usually necessary.
  - Slick floors, stairs
  - Comfortable bedding
  - Ease of elimination access and completion

Client Communication

Throughout the life stages, client education and pet training can be started with senior care in mind.

- Environmental enrichment with appropriate feeding toys, interactions and learning; give them "jobs."
- Appropriate early training with both verbal and visual directions in case of sensory loss.
- Regular exercise, adjusted to pet's ability, no matter how old. Studies in humans demonstrate movement is excellent for heart health, circulation and brain health, as well as "loosening up" arthritic joints.
- When special situations arise (mobility, sight, hearing, cognition), prepare the client to make the spatial adjustments for optimal patient experience (see Senior-Friendly Homes).

See Also

- Cognitive Dysfunction Syndrome
- Mobility in Senior Pets

Abbreviations

- BDNF = brain-derived neurotrophic factor
- EE = Environmental Enrichment

Additional Reading

Dodman N, Lidner L (eds). *Good Old Dog: Expert Advice for Keeping Your Aging Dog Happy, Healthy and Comfortable*. Boston, MA: Mariner Books, 2012.

Landsberg G, Hunthausen W, Ackerman L. *Behavior Problems of the Dog and Cat*, 3rd edn.St Louis, MO: Elsevier Saunders, 2013.

Milgram NW, Siwak-Tapp CT, Araujo J, Head E. Neuroprotective effects of cognitive enrichment aging research. *Aging Res Rev* 2006;5(3):354–369.

References

1. Amaya V, Paterson MBA, Phillips CJC. Effects of olfactory and auditory enrichment on the behaviour of shelter dogs. *Animals (Basel)* 2020 Mar 30;10(4):581. doi: https://doi.org/10.3390/ani10040581. PMID: 32235593; PMCID: PMC7222336.
2. McCoy BM, Brassington L, Jin K, Dolby GA, Shrager S, Collins D, Dunbar M, Dog Aging Project Consortium, Ruple A, Snyder-Mackler N. Social determinants of health and disease in companion dogs: a cohort study from the Dog Aging Project *Evol Med Public Health* 2023 May 13;11(1):187–201. doi: https://doi.org/10.1093/emph/eoad011. PMID: 37388194; PMCID: PMC10306367.
3. Ellis SL. Environmental enrichment: practical strategies for improving feline welfare. *J Feline Med Surg* 2009 Nov;11(11):901–912. doi: https://doi.org/10.1016/j.jfms.2009.09.011. PMID: 19857853.
4. Hunt RL, Whiteside H, Prankel S. Effects of environmental enrichment on dog behaviour: pilot study. *Animals (Basel)* 2022 Jan 7;12(2):141. doi: https://doi.org/10.3390/ani12020141. PMID: 35049764; PMCID: PMC8772568.
5. Pennington E, Springer C, Albright J, Castel A. Evaluation of different methods of environmental enrichment to control anxiety in dogs undergoing hemilaminectomy after acute intervertebral disc extrusion: a randomized double-blinded study. *Front Vet Sci* 2023 May 30;10:1124982. doi: https://doi.org/10.3389/fvets.2023.1124982. PMID: 37323840; PMCID: PMC10267703.
6. Fahnestock M, Marchese M, Head E, Pop V, Michalski B, Milgram WN, Cotman CW. BDNF increases with behavioral enrichment and an antioxidant diet in the aged dog. *Neurobiol Aging* 2012 Mar;33(3):546–554. doi: https://doi.org/10.1016/j.neurobiolaging.2010.03.019. Epub 2010 May 5. PMID: 20447733; PMCID: PMC2935515
7. Wallis LJ, Range F, Kubinyi E, Chapagain D, Serra J, Huber L. Utilising dog-computer interactions to provide mental stimulation in dogs especially during ageing. *ACI 2017 Improv Relat* 2017;2017:1. doi: https://doi.org/10.1145/3152130.3152146. PMID: 30283918; PMCID: PMC6166787.
8. Bol S, Caspers J, Buckingham L, Anderson-Shelton GD, Ridgway C, Buffington CA, Schulz S, Bunnik EM. Responsiveness of cats (*Felidae*) to silver vine (*Actinidia polygama*), Tatarian honeysuckle (*Lonicera tatarica*), valerian (*Valeriana officinalis*) and catnip (*Nepeta cataria*). *BMC Vet Res* 2017 Mar 16;13(1):70. doi: https://doi.org/10.1186/s12917-017-0987-6. PMID: 28302120; PMCID: PMC5356310.
9. Lindig AM, McGreevy PD, Crean AJ. Musical dogs: a review of the influence of auditory enrichment on canine health and behavior. *Animals (Basel)* 2020 Jan 13;10(1):127. doi: https://doi.org/10.3390/ani10010127. PMID: 31941064; PMCID: PMC7022433.

Authors: Heidi Lobprise and Steve Dale
Thanks to: Steve Dale and Amy Pike for resources

Chapter 98

Quality of Life

BASICS

OVERVIEW

According to the World Health Organization, quality of life (QoL) refers to "an individual's perception of their position in life in the context of the culture and value systems in which they live and in relation to their goals, expectations, standards and concerns." For our small-animal patients, that perception is based on their present situation, without concern about the future, goals, or expectations, except for maybe when their next meal arrives. In general, a QoL assessment refers to how well a pet is doing, often in the context of having a disease impacting health. We typically look at HRQOL—Health-related quality of life measurements, as health care is a primary goal of veterinary medicine. The AVMA Veterinarian's Oath goes on to include "the protection of animal health and welfare, the prevention and relief of animal suffering," so aspects of welfare and suffering are also critical features of our jobs.

All of these aspects can be evaluated by assessing how the patients are functioning on a basic level—eating, drinking, breathing, walking, eliminating, grooming, and sleeping, as well as comfort, mobility, and pain levels. By using these assessment tools beyond individual disease impact, we can evaluate the welfare of our patients and help the owners make decisions as to health care options (Fulmer).

Terms Defined

- Quality of Life (QoL)—an individual's perception of their position in life; welfare
- Sentience—the ability to have feelings that matter

ISSUES AND OPTIONS

- Historically, veterinary medicine has focused on physical health, but mental and emotional health can have an impact on the animal's overall enjoyment of life (see Figure 98.1).
    - Optimal QoL is not just good health and avoidance of suffering, but the promotion of positive emotions.
    - Physical suffering from pain, nausea, pruritis, respiratory distress, thirst, and hunger can impact their QoL.
    - Mental or emotional suffering from anxiety, phobias, fear, isolation and loneliness, boredom or frustration, and stress can impact it as well.
- Sentience (the ability to have feelings that matter) and consciousness are the prerequisites for suffering, which our patients can have.

Blackwell's Five-Minute Veterinary Consult Clinical Companion: Small Animal Senior Care,
First Edition. Edited by Heidi B. Lobprise.

Companion website: www.wiley.com/go/lobprise/Senior

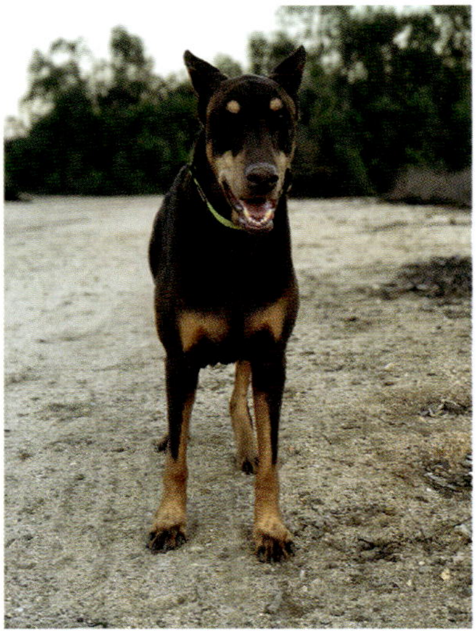

■ **Figure 98.1** Mental and emotional health of pets can be enhanced by sharing in their favorite activities. Source: Photo Courtesy of Dr. Mary Gardner.

- QoL is a balance between positive and negative inputs.
- For our assessments, the patient cannot tell us directly, so we have to rely on proxy input—observer-related outcomes (ORO)—as assessed by owner or veterinary team.
- As humans, we can make personal decisions to accept temporary suffering during therapy with the understanding that we will feel better later.
    - Animals are only in the present and only know what they are experiencing at that time point.
- We need to keep all of these facets in mind when advocating for the pet and providing our professional input to help owners make appropriate health care decisions.
- While we now have amazing abilities to offer advanced diagnostics, procedures, and therapies, we have to ask—at what cost?
- Will QoL be put at risk just to increase longevity?

APPLICATIONS IN PRACTICE

Quality-of-Life Assessment Tools

- QoL assessment tools
    - Quantitative guidelines to assist both in treatment and euthanasia decisions.[1]
    - Can be used for terminally ill patients near their end of life, or for palliative care decisions.
    - Screening for medical conditions.
    - Identify health issues or a decline in well-being early on.[2]
    - Monitor changes over time, including response to medical intervention.
        - QoL showed demonstrable improvement after weight loss in obese dogs.[3]
    - To raise awareness of welfare and to help owners understand the severity of illness in pet dogs.[4]
    - By asking a global, open-ended question, it can allow pet owners to reflect on their pet's QoL.
    - 81% of pet owners expressed an interest in learning about QoLs.[5]
    - QoL of the caregiver is very important as well.[6] (See Caregiver Burden.)

- Disease-specific tools—the majority of available QoL tools.
    - Dogs—atopy, cancer, pain, cardiac disease, obesity, osteoarthritis.
    - Cats—diabetes mellitus, cardiac disease, degenerative joint disease.
    - Not suitable for all animals or for those with co-morbidities such as geriatric pets.
- Generic QoL review
    - Nine tools reviewed with similar aspects of dog and cat QoL—activity level, desire for interaction, and appetite.
        - Cats also had aspects for mood and grooming.
        - Only 5 of the 9 included at least one item relevant to pain. Clinically, pain is likely a very important consideration for QoL.
    - Villalobos[1]
        - HHHHHMM—guideline for caregivers of terminally ill pets.
        - Seven domains—hurt, hunger, hydration, hygiene, happiness, mobility, and more good days than bad days (see Figure 98.2).
        - https://vetsocialwork.utk.edu/wp-content/uploads/2016/03/Quality-of-Life.pdf
    - Freeman[7]
        - Cat Health and Well-Being (CHEW)
        - Eight domains—mobility, emotion, energy, engagement, eyes, coats, appetite, fitness (see Figure 98.3).
        - Two broad questions—overall QoL and overall health
        - https://journals.sagepub.com/doi/suppl/10.1177/1098612X16657386/suppl_file/Supplementary_Material_Qol_Questionnaire_FINAL.pdf
    - Mullan[4]
        - To raise awareness regarding welfare of pet dogs visiting a clinic—four parts:
            - Personality and history
            - Comfort, exercise, diet, mental stimulation, and companionship
            - Behavior
            - Owners to list three important changes they would make to improve their dog's QoL

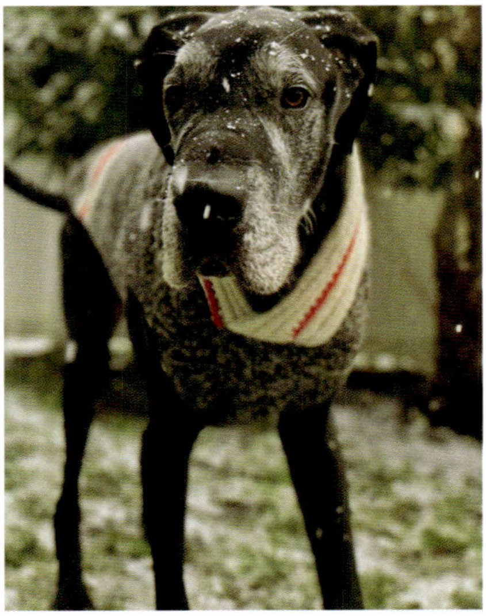

■ **Figure 98.2** A quality-of-life assessment may include the caregiver assessing a level of happiness, which is positive in this older Great Dane's excursion into the snow, on a very good day! Source: Photo Courtesy of Kitty Nicole Doenges.

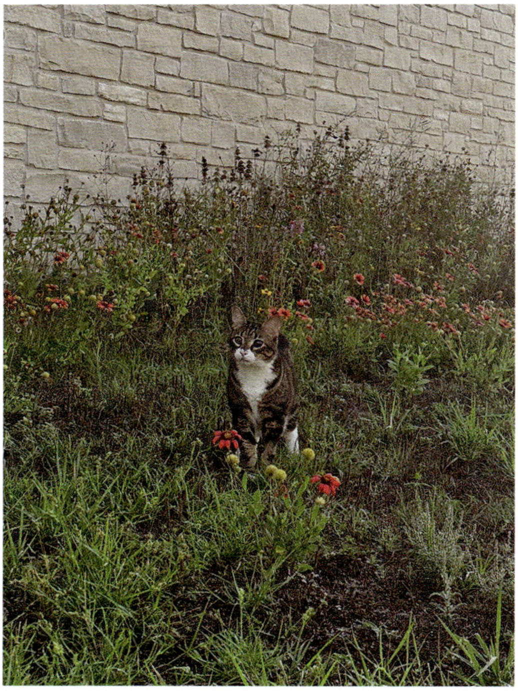

■ **Figure 98.3** George's walk in the garden can impact many domains evaluated by CHEW.[7] Source: Heidi Lobprise.

- Bijsmans[8]
    - General QoL for cats—but also to compare to CKD CatQoL
        - Four domains—general health, eating, behavior, and management
        - One broad question—general QoL
- Wojciechowska[9]
    - Discriminative questionnaire for assessment of non-physical aspect of QoL in dogs
        - Welfare and behavior
        - Five domains—satisfaction of telos needs, opportunities for pleasure, minimal fear and distress, distressing events, being outdoors
- Yeates[10]
    - Tool to encourage discussions and decisions about dogs Qol
        - Seven items—food, exercise, comfort, company of humans, company of other dogs, route vet care, and care of illnesses
- Lavan[11]
    - Generic QoL dogs for use in clinical and research settings
        - Canine Health-related QoL (CHQLS-21, 15)
        - Four domains—happiness, physical functioning, hygiene, mental status
        - Two open ended—general health; direct QoL assessment
    - Later revised with eight domains of mobility, energy and vitality, physical health, appetite and hydration, emotional functioning, cognitive functions, social functioning and general health.[12]—HRQoL
        - Many items have common elements seen in aging dogs
    - Also helped developed HCBQ—Human canine animal bond questionnaire
        - Four domains—trust and security, communication, spending quality time/companionship and general bonding

        - Two global concept items—caretaker's bond to dog; attachment of caretaker to dog
        - Correlations between physical attributes (mobility, E/V, and physical) and behavioral attributes were moderately strong, underscoring the relationship between physical health and behavior
  - Noble[13]
    - Generic Qol for cats
      - Healthy and sick cats; 39 items online survey; narrowed to 20 items
      - Three domains—vitality, comfort, emotional well-being
      - Available through NewMetrica and is fee-based
  - Tatlock[14]
    - QoL for cats in general practice
      - Sixteen items
      - Domains—healthy behaviors and clinical signs
- Glasgow based development—web-based questionnaire
  - Validation and reliability.[15]—4 domains, 46 items
    - Energetic/Enthusiastic (E/E)
    - Happy/Content (H/C)
    - Active/Comfortable (A/C)
    - Calm/Relaxed (C/R)
  - Shortening of the instrument (22 items) to provide a superior assessment that can be accessed on a mobile phone; likely to increase acceptability with dog owners.[16]
  - Early-warning system for owners and use in a large cohort of dogs[17] (see Figure 98.4).
    - Preventive measure to provide early detection of disease
    - Provides an alert to pet owner that a significant deterioration in health status has occurred
    - 27% of pets thought to be "in perfect health" by owners had alert triggers, informed to seek veterinary care.

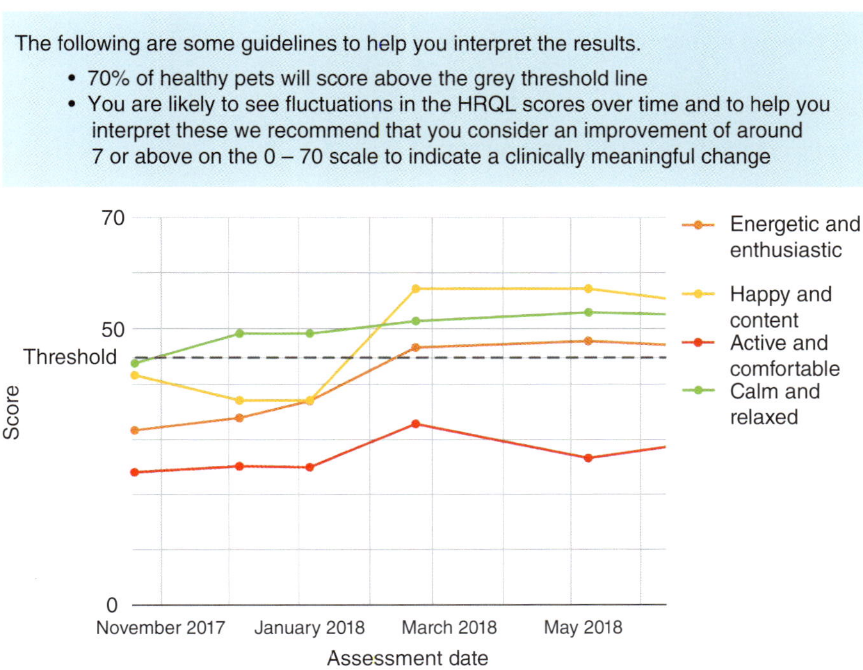

■ **Figure 98.4** Example of a histogram readout from a simulated owner-reported health-related quality of life web-based assessment instrument. Source: Courtesy of Dr. Jacky Reid.[15]

- Can show declines in dogs with advancing age (E/E, H/C, A/C)
- Can also highlight the risks in relying on owner impression of health status.[18]
  - Veterinary records of 152; 63 had signs of chronic disease
  - Disagreement between owner impression and veterinary assessment was as high as 43% in older dogs.

■ Another dog QoL instrument developed five daytime domains (energetic, mobile, relaxed, happy, and sociable) as well as three mealtime domains (relaxed, interested, and satisfied).[19]

Team Roles/Engagement

■ In the UK, a Pet Wellbeing Task Force (PWTF) helped develop hospital-based Champions for animal welfare and ethics to help implement new policies and campaigns.[20]
- While not specifically targeting senior patients, facets such as providing frequent QoL assessments, pain-scoring hospitalized patients, and promoting standardized analgesic protocols certainly can benefit that demographic.

■ In the US—Fear Free™ concepts, Cat-Friendly hospital programs and pain management enhancements continue to improve the welfare of our patients.
- The development of a Senior-Friendly Hospital program would also be of benefit.

■ Utilizing QoL instruments in the practice
- A survey of veterinary professionals in the UK evaluated the use of canine QoL instruments.[21]
  - 29% were aware of their existence, less than 4% were using them.
  - 55% were willing to use them but stated a lack of time or resistance from pet owners as potential barriers.
- In another UK Survey[22]
  - Almost all dog owners (95.8%) were comfortable discussing their dog's QoL with their veterinarians, but only 32% reported this topic was raised.
  - 70.8% of owners were interested in QoL tools, but very few had these provided by their veterinarians.
- 81% of pet owners expressed an interest in learning about QoLs[5] (see Figure 98.5).

Client Communication

■ As part of a comprehensive patient care regimen, the use of QoL tools can be used throughout their lifestages.
- Discussing welfare and QoL can educate the owners about all critical aspects of their pets' lives, not just the health aspects.
- In senior pets, many of these facets are significantly impacted.
- As the QoL declines, this information gives the owner a more complete awareness of their pet's over-all wellbeing (see Figure 98.6).

Abbreviations

■ CHEW = Cat Health and Well-Being
■ CHQLS = canine health-related quality of life survey
■ CKD = chronic kidney disease
■ HCBQ = human–canine animal bond questionnaire
■ HRQOL = health-related quality of life
■ ORO = observer-related outcomes
■ PWTF = Pet Wellbeing Task Force

Lap of Love Pet
Quality-of-Life Scale

When evaluating the quality of life of your pet, personalized patient and family information is important when reaching an educated, informed, and supported choice that fits not only your pet's medical condition, but also your wishes and expectations. In short, quality of life applies not only to the pet, it also applies to you!

Your Name: ______________________________

Pet's Name: ______________________________

Date & Time: ______________________________

SCORE EACH SUBSECTION ON A SCALE OF 0-2:

0 = agree with statement (describes my pet)
1 = some changes seen
2 = disagree with statement (does not describe my pet)

SOCIAL FUNCTIONS

_____ Desire to be with the family has not changed

_____ Interacts normally with family or other pets (i.e., no increased aggression or other changes)

HEALTH

_____ No changes in breathing or panting patterns

_____ No outward signs of pain (excessive panting, pacing, and whining are most commonly seen)

_____ No pacing around the house

_____ My pet's overall condition has not changed recently

MENTAL HEALTH

_____ Enjoys normal play activities

_____ Still dislikes the same thing (i.e., still hates the mailman = 0, or doesn't bark at the mailman anymore = 2)

_____ No outward signs of stress or anxiety

_____ Does not seem confused or apathetic

_____ Nighttime activity is normal, no changes seen

NATURAL FUNCTIONS

_____ Appetite has stayed the same

_____ Drinking has stayed the same

_____ Normal urination habits

_____ Normal bowel movement habits

_____ Ability to ambulate (walk around) has stayed the same

RESULTS

_____ Total score added from each section

0-8: Quality of life is most likely adequate. No medical intervention required yet, but guidance from your veterinarian may help you identify signs to look for in the future.

9–16: Quality of life is questionable and medical intervention is suggested. Your pet would certainly benefit from veterinary oversight and guidance to evaluate the disease process he/she is experiencing.

17-32: Quality of life is a definite concern. Changes will likely become more progressive and more severe in the near future. Veterinary guidance will help you better understand the end stages of your pet's disease process in order to make a more informed decision of whether to continue hospice care or elect peaceful euthanasia.

Lap of Love
Veterinary Hospice & In-Home Euthanasia

■ **Figure 98.5** A Quality Life Scale (developed by Lap of Love Pet) engages the owner in observing their pet's Quality of Life, building awareness of potential issues. Source: lap-of-love-quality-of-life-scale.pdf (lapoflove.com).

Good days vs Bad days – Quality of Life

Use a similar calendar to mark down how your pet's day was:

- Good day – interactive, comfortable, eating
  - Mark it green
- So-so day – not as active or interested in playing, appetite not great, may be a little painful
  - Mark it yellow
- Bad day – not eating, painful, not getting around or interacting with others
  - Mark it red

Sunday	Monday	Tuesday	Wednesday	Thursday	Friday	Saturday

Keep track from week to week or month to month, and use trends in color changes to help you assess your pet's quality of life

	This week/ this month	Last week/ last month	2 weeks ago, 2 months ago	3 weeks ago, 3 months ago	4 weeks ago, 3 months ago
Green/Good days					
Yellow/so-so days					
Red/bad days					

Figure 98.6 Pet Quality of Life Calendar. Source: Lap of Love.

Internet Resources

Accessed 26 June 2024

- Quality-of-Life Assessment|Lap of Love
- interactive-quality-of-life-assessment-and-diary.pdf (lapoflove.com)
- Quality of Life Scale for Pets online calculator (journeyspet.com)
- https://journals.sagepub.com/doi/suppl/10.1177/1098612X16657386/suppl_file/Supplementary_Material_Qol_Questionnaire_FINAL.pdf
- https://vetsocialwork.utk.edu/wp-content/uploads/2016/03/Quality-of-Life.pdf

Additional Reading

Fulmer AE, Laven LJ, Hill KE. Quality of life measurement in dogs and cats: a scoping review of generic tools. *Animals (Basel)* 2022 Feb 8;12(3):400. doi: https://doi.org/10.3390/ani12030400. PMID: 35158723; PMCID: PMC8833627.

References

1. Villalobos AE. Quality-of-life assessment techniques for veterinarians. *Vet Clin North Am Small Anim Pract* 2011 May;41(3):519–529. doi: https://doi.org/10.1016/j.cvsm.2011.03.013. PMID: 21601744.
2. Spofford N, Lefebvre SL, McCune S, Niel L. Should the veterinary profession invest in developing methods to assess quality of life in healthy dogs and cats? *J Am Vet Med Assoc* 2013 Oct 1;243(7):952–956. doi: https://doi.org/10.2460/javma.243.7.952. PMID: 24050560.
3. German AJ, Holden SL, Wiseman-Orr ML, Reid J, Nolan AM, Biourge V, Morris PJ, Scott EM. Quality of life is reduced in obese dogs but improves after successful weight loss. *Vet J* 2012 Jun;192(3):428–434. doi: https://doi.org/10.1016/j.tvjl.2011.09.015. Epub 2011 Nov 9. PMID: 22075257.
4. Mullan S, Main D. Preliminary evaluation of a quality-of-life screening programme for pet dogs. *J Small Anim Pract* 2007 Jun;48(6):314–322. doi: https://doi.org/10.1111/j.1748-5827.2007.00322.x. Epub 2007 May 8. PMID: 17490443.
5. Mwacalimba KK, Contadini FM, Spofford N, Lopez K, Hunt A, Wright A, Lund EM, Minicucci L. Owner and veterinarian perceptions about use of a canine quality of life survey in primary care settings. *Front Vet Sci* 2020;7:1–11. [CrossRef] [PubMed]
6. Niessen SJ. Quality-of-life assessment: honouring our oath in practice and research. *J Small Anim Pract* 2011 Sep;52(9):453–454. doi: https://doi.org/10.1111/j.1748-5827.2011.01121.x. PMID: 21896017.
7. Freeman LM, Rodenberg C, Narayanan A, Olding J, Gooding MA, Koochaki PE. Development and initial validation of the Cat HEalth and Wellbeing (CHEW) Questionnaire: a generic health-related quality of life instrument for cats. *J Feline Med Surg* 2016 Sep;18(9):689–701. doi: https://doi.org/10.1177/1098612X16657386. PMID: 27562979.
8. Bijsmans ES, Jepson RE, Syme HM, Elliott J, Niessen SJ. Psychometric validation of a general health quality of life tool for cats used to compare healthy cats and cats with chronic kidney disease. *J Vet Intern Med* 2016 Jan-Feb;30(1):183–191. doi: https://doi.org/10.1111/jvim.13656. Epub 2015 Nov 14. PMID: 26567089; PMCID: PMC4913638.
9. Wojciechowska JI, Hewson CJ, Stryhn H, Guy NC, Patronek GJ, Timmons V. Development of a discriminative questionnaire to assess nonphysical aspects of quality of life of dogs. *Am J Vet Res* 2005 Aug;66(8):1453–1460. doi: https://doi.org/10.2460/ajvr.2005.66.1453. PMID: 16173493.
10. Yeates JW, Mullan S, Stone M, Main DC. Promoting discussions and decisions about dogs' quality-of-life. *J Small Anim Pract* 2011 Sep;52(9):459–463. doi: https://doi.org/10.1111/j.1748-5827.2011.01094.x. PMID: 21896019.
11. Lavan RP. Development and validation of a survey for quality of life assessment by owners of healthy dogs. *Vet J* 2013 Sep;197(3):578–582. doi: https://doi.org/10.1016/j.tvjl.2013.03.021. Epub 2013 Apr 29. PMID: 23639368.
12. Lavan RP, Tahir M, O'Donnell C, Bellenger A, de Bock E, Koochaki P. Development and Validation of a Canine Health-Related Quality of Life Questionnaire and a Human-Canine Bond Questionnaire for Use in Veterinary Practice. *Animals (Basel)* 2023 Oct 18;13(20):3255. doi: https://doi.org/10.3390/ani13203255. PMID: 37893979; PMCID: PMC10603719.
13. Noble CE, Wiseman-Orr LM, Scott ME, Nolan AM, Reid J. Development, initial validation and reliability testing of a web-based, generic feline health-related quality-of-life instrument. *J Feline Med Surg* 2019 Feb;21(2):84–94. doi: https://doi.org/10.1177/1098612X18758176. Epub 2018 Feb 21. PMID: 29463202; PMCID: PMC10814614.
14. Tatlock S, Gober M, Williamson N, Arbuckle R. Development and preliminary psychometric evaluation of an owner-completed measure of feline quality of life. *Vet J* 2017 Oct;228:22–32. doi: https://doi.org/10.1016/j.tvjl.2017.10.005. Epub 2017 Oct 16. PMID: 29153104.

15. Reid J, Wiseman-Orr ML, Scott EM, Nolan AM. Development, validation and reliability of a web-based questionnaire to measure health-related quality of life in dogs. *J Small Anim Pract* 2013 May;54(5):227–233. doi: https://doi.org/10.1111/jsap.12059. Epub 2013 Apr 5. PMID: 23557412.
16. Reid J, Wiseman-Orr L, Scott M. Shortening of an existing generic online health-related quality of life instrument for dogs. *J Small Anim Pract* 2018 Jun;59(6):334–342. doi: https://doi.org/10.1111/jsap.12772. Epub 2017 Oct 11. PMID: 29023735.
17. Davies V, Scott EM, Wiseman-Orr ML, Wright AK, Reid J. Development of an early warning system for owners using a validated health-related quality of life (HRQL) instrument for companion animals and its use in a large cohort of dogs. *Front Vet Sci* 2020 Sep 24;7:575795. doi: https://doi.org/10.3389/fvets.2020.575795. Erratum in: *Front Vet Sci* 2021 Apr 15;8:676049. doi: https://doi.org/10.3389/fvets.2021.676049. PMID: 33195573; PMCID: PMC7541963
18. Rodger S, Scott EM, Nolan A, Wright AK, Reid J. Effect of age, breed, and sex on the health-related quality of life of owner assessed healthy dogs. *Front Vet Sci* 2021 Feb 5;8:603139. doi: https://doi.org/10.3389/fvets.2021.603139. PMID: 33614760; PMCID: PMC7892584.
19. Schmutz A, Spofford N, Burghardt W, De Meyer G. Development and initial validation of a dog quality of life instrument. *Sci Rep* 2022 Jul 28;12(1):12225. doi: https://doi.org/10.1038/s41598-022-16315-y. PMID: 35902606; PMCID: PMC9334304
20. Wensley S, Betton V, Martin N, Tipton E. Advancing animal welfare and ethics in veterinary practice through a national pet wellbeing task force, practice-based champions and clinical audit. *Vet Rec* 2020 Oct 17;187(8):316. doi: https://doi.org/10.1136/vr.105484. Epub 2020 Jun 12. PMID: 32532843; PMCID: PMC7606500.
21. Roberts C, Blackwell EJ, Roe E, Murrell JC, Mullan S. Awareness and use of canine quality of life assessment tools in UK veterinary practice. *Animals (Basel)* 2023 Mar 20;13(6):1105. doi: https://doi.org/10.3390/ani13061105. PMID: 36978644; PMCID: PMC10044674.
22. Hale H, Blackwell E, Roberts C, Roe E, Mullan S. Broadening the veterinary consultation: dog owners want to talk about more than physical health. *Animals (Basel)* 2023 Jan 24;13(3):392. doi: https://doi.org/10.3390/ani13030392. PMID: 36766281; PMCID: PMC9913647.MWAS.

Author Heidi Lobprise
Thanks to: Mary Gardner and Sheilah Robertson for resources

Chapter 99

Caregiver Burden

BASICS

OVERVIEW

When a senior pet has health issues that need medical, physical, and emotional attention, the bulk of care is taken on by the pet owner. Depending on the extent of the condition and even the size of the pet, this care puts a burden on the caregiver that can impact their own physical and emotional health. Understanding the demands this care can place on the owner is an important aspect in providing instructions for at-home management of the patient.

Terms Defined

- Caregiver burden results from the multiple physical, psychological, social, and financial stressors associated with caregiving.
- Anticipatory grief (AG) is worrying or grieving before the loss occurs.
- Grief is a bereavement response characterized by emotional reactions like sadness, anger, guilt, and despair, as well as physical effects like reduced sleep.
- Quality of Life "an individual's perception of their position in life in the context of the culture and value systems in which they live and in relation to their goals, expectations, standards and concerns."

ISSUES AND OPTIONS

- Caregiver burden (CB) is the #2 reason for euthanasia, after pet quality of life.
- It can be present in the earliest stages of a disease.[1]
- Slightly lower CB for cat owners than most dog owners, though the CB for ill cats is significantly greater than for healthy cats.[2]
- The strain on caregivers of senior pets is highly variable, subjective, and personal.
    - Greater depression, anxiety and stress, poorer psychosocial function, and greater veterinary care use with high CB.
    - Burden transfer—greater demand on veterinary teams for non-billable attention and support.[1]
- Emotions, physical ability, finances, work, and leisure schedules can all be impacted—the "wallets" with resources of each category.
- Factors include changes in care routines, perception that compliance with new routines was challenging, and difficulty adhering to medication routines.[1]
- This is an important concept in human medicine and caregivers of the elderly.[3]

Blackwell's Five-Minute Veterinary Consult Clinical Companion: Small Animal Senior Care, First Edition. Edited by Heidi B. Lobprise.

Companion website: www.wiley.com/go/lobprise/Senior

APPLICATION IN PRACTICE

Caregiver Burden Assessment Tool[4]

- Modified from a human assessment tool (Zarit Burden Interview)[3]
- Three factors, seven items
  - General factors
    - Do you feel that because of the time you spend with your pet that you don't have enough time for yourself?
    - Do you feel stressed between caring for your pet and trying to meet other responsibilities for your family or work?
    - Do you feel you have lost control of your life since your pet's illness?
  - Affect/relational discomfort
    - Do you feel angry when you are around your pet?
    - Do you feel embarrassed over your pet's behavior?
  - Guilt/uncertainty
    - Do you feel you should be doing more for your pet?
    - Do you feel you could do a better job in caring for your pet?

Understanding Caregiver Burden, Anticipatory Grief, and the Owner's QoL[5]

- These are not interchangeable but may be correlated, and all can impact owner decision and behavior.
- Influenced by their pet's QoL, the nature of the illness, and the owner's attachment.
- Clients with high CB may need collaborative problem solving.
- Clients with high AG may need empathetic responses.
- Four owner profiles identified:
  - Distressed—the distress pervades their life
    - Highest CB and AG, lowest QoL, have taken more steps to euthanize.
    - How to respond: they seem more dependent or prone to complain, so try to understand the source of their behavior and set boundaries.
  - Resilient—compartmentalize their distress
    - Second highest CB and AG, but better QoL.
    - They will work through EOL (end-of-life) issues in a compartmentalized manner.
    - How to respond: while they have high CB they may show less obvious signs of stress; proactively ask about concerns.
  - Non-distressed—relatively unafflicted
    - Low CB (below a clinically meaningful level).
    - Pet more likely to have a chronic illness as compared to a terminal disease; they also may have lower levels of attachment to their pet.
    - How to respond: they may have compliance issues, so provide clear rationale for recommendations; work with the client's economic and lifestyle parameters.
  - Experiencing strain due to other influences—challenging to fully assess
    - Great impact on QoL, but borderline CB and lower AG; better pet QoL.
    - How to respond: pet's care might be lower on their priority list; focus to meet pet's needs as pragmatically as possible.
    - If there are concerning indications, reach out to other professionals—veterinary social workers.

Help the Owner to Assess the Burdens—In Greater Detail (See Figure 99.1)

- Sleeping—does the owner have to wake up for pets' vocalization, excessive elimination or clean-up (including vomiting), or to comfort their pet?
- Owners' mentation/thoughts
  - Do they worry about their pet when they are gone or about pets' suffering?
  - Do they have to constantly monitor the pets' whereabouts?
  - It's challenging to manage their pets' cognitive disorders
    - This can impact the human–companion animal bond
  - Unsure how to evaluate pet's happiness and comfort
  - Loud vocalization of cats
- Pet's appetite, thirst, medication, and treatment
  - Are they eating and drinking enough?
  - Does a special diet take more time or cost?
  - Is there a struggle giving medication, fluids, oxygen, or physical therapy?
    - Does this impact compliance?
- Cleanliness and appearance
  - Cleaning up after accidents, vomiting
  - Challenge to brush, groom; odors
  - Restricting access to parts of the house
- Mobility (see Figure 99.2)
  - Challenging to get dog up, up and down stairs or into car
  - Dog—can't go on walks or play anymore

Impact on the "Wallets"

- Emotional
  - Seeing their pet age can trigger emotions from experiencing similar issues with elderly family members, or their own issues.
  - All the caregiver stressors can negatively impact the human–companion animal bond.
  - Thinking about having to make end-of-life decisions can be very stressful: how, when?
- Physical
  - Especially caring for larger dogs, having to assist with mobility and normal activity can be very difficult.
- Financial
  - Extensive costs for medical care and management can put a burden on everyday living expenses.
  - Having to decide between the pets' care and their own family's care can be very challenging and even cause guilty feelings for deciding one way or another.
- Schedules—work and leisure
  - Older pets with extensive health issues may require regular veterinary visits and time-consuming care at home.
  - Families may decrease, forego, or cancel plans for leisure and travel if a senior pet requires extensive daily medication or care.
    - Options for boarding the pet or pet sitters may be challenging or expensive.

Team Training/Team Roles

- It can be challenging for all team members to appreciate the level of care a patient may require at home, and the capabilities of a pet owner to provide that care.

Lap of Love
Pet Family Concerns

SCORE EACH ITEM ON A SCALE OF 0-2:	0 = I am not concerned at this time 1 = There is some concern 2 = I am concerned about this

I AM CONCERNED ABOUT THE FOLLOWING THINGS:

_____ Pet suffering

_____ Pet dying alone

_____ Not knowing the right time to euthanize

_____ Concern for other household animals

_____ Desire to perform nursing care for your pet

_____ Ability to perform nursing care for your pet

_____ Coping with loss

_____ Concern for other members of the family (i.e. children)

RESULTS

_____ Total score added from each section

0-4: Your concerns are minimal at this time. You have either accepted the inevitable loss of your pet and understand what lies ahead, or have not yet given it much thought. If you have not considered these things, now is the time to begin evaluating your own concerns and limitations.

5–9: Your concerns are mounting. Begin your search for information by educating yourself on your pet's condition; it's the best way to ensure you are prepared for the emotional changes ahead.

10-16: Although you may not place much value on your own quality of life, your concerns about the changes in your pet are valid. Now is the time to prepare yourself and to build a support system around you. Veterinary guidance will help you prepare for the medical changes in your pet while counselors and other health professionals can begin helping you with anticipatory grief.

DISCUSS THE QUESTIONS BELOW, AND THE ENTIRE QUALITY-OF-LIFE SCALE, WITH YOUR VETERINARIAN

Below are some open-ended questions that assist gauge your family's time, emotional, and (when appropriate, financial) budgets:

1. Have you ever been through the loss of a pet before? If so, what was your experience (good or bad, and why)?
2. What do you hope the life expectancy of your pet will be? What do you think it will be?
3. What is the ideal situation you wish for your pet's end of life experience? (at home, pass away in her sleep, etc.)

Suggestions on using this quality-of-life scale:

1. Complete the scale at different times of the day, note circadian fluctuations in well-being. (We find most pets tend to do worse at night and better during the day.)
2. Request multiple members of the family complete the scale; compare observations.
3. Take periodic photos of your pet to help you remember their physical appearance.

Resources:

1. AAHA/AAFP Pain Management Guidelines for Dogs and Cats, www.aahanet.org/Library/PainMgmt.aspx

Lap of Love
Veterinary Hospice & In-Home Euthanasia

Figure 99.1 An assessment of Pet Family concerns (developed by Lap of Love Pet) can help the caregivers clarify their concerns about caring for their aging pet. Source: lap-of-love-quality-of-life-scale.pdf (lapoflove.com).

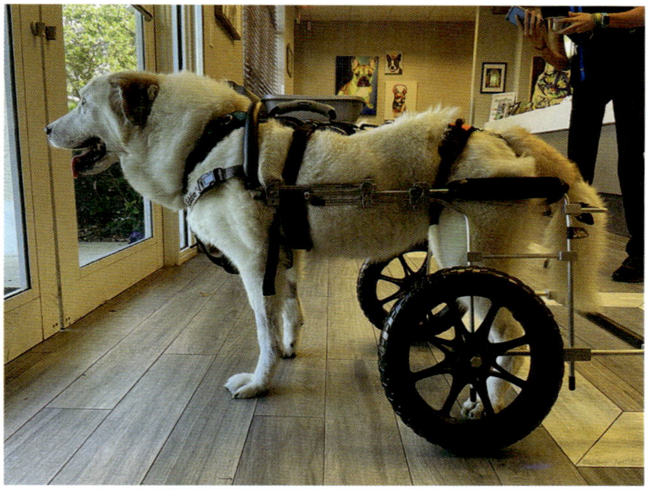

Figure 99.2 While many resources can be used to help pets with mobility and paresis issues, such as this wheelchair for Sam, it is important to fully explain any additional care needed, for elimination and grooming. Source: Photo Courtesy of Dr. Mary Gardner.

- Some team members can be judgmental if a pet owner is too burdened to provide or continue appropriate levels of care.
  - Team members likely have better capabilities than most pet owners and may find it hard to understand why care is not given optimally. Especially in a multi-pet household.
- Team discussion or training on being empathetic with clients, understanding the potential limits the client might have (see Assess the Burden and "Wallets" above).

Client Communication

- As stated above, caregiver burden is the second most common driver of euthanasia.
- Any instructions for health management should be explained in full when extensive care is needed.
  - Medications—if multiple prescriptions are recommended, help the owner set up a schedule or spreadsheet for administration (take a photo of the medications).
    - Assess their ability to administer whatever care is needed; provide options if appropriate (Figure 99.3).
    - Discuss which ones are the most critical, if a pet decides it doesn't want to take all of them (polypharmacy), prioritize the list.
    - If timing of medication is important, make sure the owner knows that, and any contraindications with feeding or other supplements/medications.
  - Prognosis—be honest about what to expect with the progression of a disease if that is known.
    - Discuss potential issues with mobility and the pet's self-care, including nutrition and elimination.
  - Set up a regular re-examination schedule to see how the pet is progressing, if there is compliance issues with any management, and to see how the client is handling things.
- Educate them about aspects of caregiver burden; let them know that this can be a real issue for pet owners; it is understandable if they experience the same matters. You can ask:
  - Are they stressed or overwhelmed by the amount of care?
  - Do they no longer want to be the caregiver?

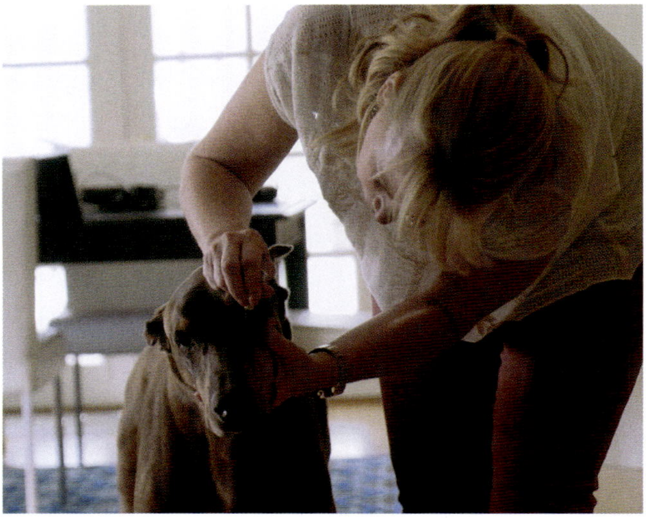

■ **Figure 99.3** Caregiver duties, such as administering medication, should be discussed thoroughly, even helping them set up a schedule for everything needed. Source: Photo Courtesy of Dr. Mary Gardner.

  - Do they have their own health or financial issues that should be a stronger priority?
  - Would like more emotional and physical support from others?
  - Do they feel anticipatory grief—how much time is left?
  - Do they feel anger for having to provide all the care?
  - Do they feel guilty for not being able to provide all the care?
  - Are they worried they will let pet suffer if they are unable to provide the care?
  - Do they need help to tell when it is time?
- If there are other family members that can help provide some of the care, involve them in the discussions and see if the tasks can be shared.
- Let them know that you and your team understand the burden that caregivers can experience, and that each situation is unique.
  - While we can provide extraordinary care and even advanced diagnostics and procedures with specialty referrals, we need to acknowledge that the pet-family situation is critical in making any decisions for care.
    - What level of care and how long would that care be needed?
    - Would heroic efforts just increase the lifespan and not necessarily the healthspan of the pet?
  - What is right for that pet and family, is right for that pet and family, without judgment.
  - If they are having trouble making big decisions immediately, provide options for care and palliation, allow them to meet with family members for discussion and generation of any questions, and agree to meet again for further assessment.

See Also

- Quality of Life

Abbreviations

- AG = anticipatory grief
- CB = caregiver burden
- EOL = end of life
- QoL = Quality of Life

Internet Resources

Accessed on 29 June 2024

- Pet Loss Support|Lap of Love
- Sick Pet | Petcaregiverburden.com
- dog_caregiver_QOL.pdf (drmarygardner.com)
- geriatric cat journal tables for web.indd (drmarygardner.com)

Additional Reading

Gardner M, McVety D. *Treatment and Care of the Geriatric Veterinary Patient*. Hoboken, NJ: John Wiley & Sons, 2017.

Additional Reading For Clients

By Mary Gardner:

- It's Never Long Enough: A Practical Guide to Caring for Your Geriatric Dog
- Nine Lives Are Not Enough: A Practical Guide to Caring for Your Geriatric Cat
- Geriatric Dog Health & Care Journal: A Complete Toolkit for the Geriatric Dog Caregiver
- Geriatric Cat Health & Care Journal: A Complete Toolkit for the Geriatric Cat Caregiver

References

1. Shaevitz MH, Tullius JA, Callahan RT, Fulkerson CM, Spitznagel MB. Early caregiver burden in owners of pets with suspected cancer: owner psychosocial outcomes, communication behavior, and treatment factors. *J Vet Intern Med* 2020 Nov;34(6):2636–2644. doi: https://doi.org/10.1111/jvim.15905. Epub 2020 Sep 24. PMID: 32969546; PMCID: PMC7694845.
2. Spitznagel MB, Gober MW, Patrick K. Caregiver burden in cat owners: a cross-sectional observational study. *J Feline Med Surg* 2023 Jan;25(1):1098612X221145835. doi: https://doi.org/10.1177/1098612X221145835. PMID: 36705958; PMCID: PMC10812038.
3. Zarit SH, Reever KE, Bach-Peterson J. Relatives of the impaired elderly: correlates of feelings of burden. *Gerontologist* 1980 Dec;20(6):649–655. doi: https://doi.org/10.1093/geront/20.6.649. PMID: 7203086. (Historical reference).
4. Spitznagel MB, Mueller MK, Fraychak T, Hoffman AM, Carlson MD. Validation of an abbreviated instrument to assess veterinary client caregiver burden. *J Vet Intern Med* 2019 May;33(3):1251–1259. doi: https://doi.org/10.1111/jvim.15508. Epub 2019 Apr 29. PMID: 31033026; PMCID: PMC6524077.
5. Spitznagel MB, Anderson JR, Marchitelli B, Sislak MD, Bibbo J, Carlson MD. Owner quality of life, caregiver burden and anticipatory grief: how they differ, why it matters. *Vet Rec* 2021 May;188(9):e74. doi: https://doi.org/10.1002/vetr.74. Epub 2021 Feb 2. PMID: 33960467.

Authors: Heidi Lobprise and Mary Gardner

Thanks to: Mary Gardner for resources

Small Animal Senior Care: Senior Pet Care-Affiliated Groups: Senior Pet Care Research

Senior Pet Advocates
Senior Pet Advocates—A resource library for veterinary professionals

The Grey Muzzle Organization
Home | The Grey Muzzle Organization

Senior and Geriatric Dog Society
Home | Senior and Geriatric Dog Society (seniordogvets.com)

The Dog Aging Project and
Home—Dog Aging Project
Dog Aging Institute

Morris Animal Foundation Golden Retriever Lifetime Study https://dogaginginstitute.org/
Golden Retriever Lifetime Study (morrisanimalfoundation.org)

Loyal—Research to increase the lifespan of pets
Helping dogs live longer, healthier lives | Loyal

Blackwell's Five-Minute Veterinary Consult Clinical Companion: Small Animal Senior Care,
First Edition. Edited by Heidi B. Lobprise.

Companion website: www.wiley.com/go/lobprise/Senior

Small Animal Senior Care—Online Resources for Veterinary Clients

Note: Other clinic materials available in "Toolkits" listed in veterinary resources

AAFP RESOURCES FOR CLIENTS

- Treating Chronic pain with NSAIDS
    - https://catvets.com/public/PDFs/ClientBrochures/AAFP-ClientBroch-Guideline_ChronicPainwNSAIDs_Web.pdf
- Hospice and Palliative Care for Your Cat
    - https://catvets.com/public/PDFs/ClientBrochures/AAFP_HPC_Client_Broch_Web.pdf
- Getting your Cat to the Veterinary Practice
    - https://catvets.com/public/PDFs/ClientBrochures/AAFPGettingCatToVetWeb.pdf
- Senior Cat Have Special Needs
    - https://catvets.com/public/PDFs/ClientBrochures/AAFPSeniorCareBrochureWeb.pdf
- Your Cat's Life Stages
    - https://catvets.com/public/PDFs/ClientBrochures/AAFPLifeStageGuidelineBrochureWeb.pdf
- Feline Diabetes
    - https://catvets.com/public/PDFs/ClientBrochures/AAFP-Diabetes-Brochure-Web.pdf
- Feline Anesthesia
    - https://catvets.com/public/PDFs/ClientBrochures/AAFP-Anesthesia-Client-Broch-Web.pdf
- How Do I Know if my Cat is in Pain?
    - https://catvets.com/public/PDFs/ClientBrochures/PainManagement-WebView.pdf
- Degenerative Joint Disease in Cats
    - https://catvets.com/public/PDFs/ClientBrochures/DJD-Webview.pdf
- Feline Hyperthyroidism
    - https://catvets.com/public/PDFs/ClientBrochures/Hyperthyroidism-WebView.pdf
- Your Cat's Environmental Needs
    - https://catvets.com/public/PDFs/ClientBrochures/Environmental%20GuidelinesEViewFinal.pdf
- Friends for Life—Caring for your older cat
    - 077966_AAFP_SeniorCare_Brochure_HR (catfriendly.com)

Blackwell's Five-Minute Veterinary Consult Clinical Companion: Small Animal Senior Care, First Edition. Edited by Heidi B. Lobprise.

Companion website: www.wiley.com/go/lobprise/Senior

AVMA CLIENT RESOURCES

- Pet Loss and Grief
  - AVMA Store—Product
- AVMA Pet Euthanasia
  - AVMA Store—Product

CARE—CANINE ARTHRITIS RESOURCES AND EDUCATION

- 5 Reasons Pet Obesity is a Serious Problem
  - Consequences Of Pet Obesity—Pet Obesity Prevention | CARE (caninearthritis.org)
- EOL decisions in dogs with mobility concerns
  - End-of-life decision-making in dogs with mobility concerns | Canine Arthritis Resources and Education

CARDIAC EDUCATION GROUP—

- Cardiac Diseases and Cardiac Drugs
  - For Your Clients—Cardiac Education Group

ZOETIS

- Solensia owner brochure
  - Solensia-Branded-Pet-Owner-Resources-Digital-Brochure.pdf (solensiavetteam.com)
- Librela
  - Librela-Pet-Owner-Resources-Brochure.pdf (zoetisus.com)

Online Resources for Small Animal Senior Care

SENIOR CARE AND LIFE-STAGE GUIDELINES AND TOOL KITS

- AAHA Senior Care Guidelines and toolkit
  - 2023 AAHA Senior Care Guidelines for Dogs and Cats—AAHA
  - AAHA Senior Care Guidelines Toolkit—AAHA
- AAFP Senior Care Guidelines
  - Senior Care Guidelines | American Association of Feline Practitioners (catvets.com)
- AAFP Life Stage Guidelines
  - Life Stage Guidelines | American Association of Feline Practitioners (catvets.com)

QUALITY OF LIFE AND END OF LIFE RESOURCES

- Lap of Love QoL resources
  - quality-of-life-calendar.pdf (lapoflove.com)
  - lap-of-love-quality-of-life-scale.pdf (lapoflove.com)
  - interactive-quality-of-life-assessment-and-diary.pdf (lapoflove.com)
- AAFP Hospice and Palliative Care Guidelines and EOL toolkit
  - Feline Hospice and Palliative Care Guidelines|American Association of Feline Practitioners (catvets.com)
  - End of Life Toolkit|American Association of Feline Practitioners (catvets.com)
- AVMA End of Life Care Policy
  - Veterinary end-of-life care | American Veterinary Medical Association (avma.org)
- CHeW—Cat Health and Wellbeing Questionnaire
  - https://journals.sagepub.com/doi/suppl/10.1177/1098612X16657386/suppl_file/Supplementary_Material_Qol_Questionnaire_FINAL.pdf

CAREGIVER BURDEN

- Lap of Love resources
  - Pet Loss Support|Lap of Love—support group
  - dog_caregiver_QOL.pdf (drmarygardner.com)
  - geriatric cat journal tables for web.indd (drmarygardner.com) (Cat caregiver QoL)
- Pet Caregiver Burden website
- Sick Pet|Petcaregiverburden.com

Blackwell's Five-Minute Veterinary Consult Clinical Companion: Small Animal Senior Care, First Edition. Edited by Heidi B. Lobprise.

Companion website: www.wiley.com/go/lobprise/Senior

ANESTHESIA RESOURCES

- AAHA Anesthesia and Monitoring Guidelines
  - 2020 AAHA Anesthesia and Monitoring Guidelines for Dogs and Cats—AAHA
- AAFP Anesthesia Guidelines
  - Anesthesia Guidelines|American Association of Feline Practitioners (catvets.com)
- Veterinary Anesthesia and Analgesia Support Group
  - www.vasg.org
- Zoetis anesthesia CE
  - https://www.thinkanesthesia.education/sites/default/files/2021-12/Veterinary%20Pain%20Assessment%20Tool%20-%20v2.1.pdf

PAIN MANAGEMENT RESOURCES

- 2022 AAHA Pain Management Guidelines and toolkit
  - https://www.aaha.org/resources/2022-aaha-pain-management-guidelines-for-dogs-and-cats/
  - aaha-pain-management-toolkit.pdf
- AAFP Chronic Pain Education Toolkit
  - Chronic Pain Educational Toolkit | American Association of Feline Practitioners (catvets.com)
- 2022 ISFM Consensus Guidelines on the Management of Acute Pain in Cats:
  - https://journals.sagepub.com/doi/epdf/10.1177/1098612X211066268
- 2022 WSAVA Pain Guidelines:
  - https://onlinelibrary.wiley.com/doi/10.1111/jsap.13566
- IVAPM – International Academy of Pain Management
  - https://www.ivapm.org/pain-guidelines
  - https://ivapm.org/professionals/cri-calculator/
- Zero Pain Philosophy:
  - https://www.zeropainphilosophy.com/vet-professionals
- Chronic pain scales and assessments
  - ACVS Canine Orthopedic Index (COI)
    - https://www.vet.upenn.edu/research/clinical-trials-vcic/our-services/pennchart/canine-orthopedic-index
  - Canine Brief Pain Inventory (CPBI)
    - https://www.vet.upenn.edu/research/clinical-trials-vcic/our-services/pennchart/cbpi-tool
  - Canine Osteoarthritis Staging Tool (COAST)
    - https://assets.elanco.com/0cec44ed-3eaa-0009-2029-666567e7e4de/b2d5f58c-2645-46ad-b5e5-65906b491bf3/COAST%20Printable%20PDF.pdf
    - https://www.frontiersin.org/articles/10.3389/fvets.2023.1137888
  - Liverpool Osteoarthritis in Dogs (LOAD)
    - https://dspace.uevora.pt/rdpc/bitstream/10174/19611/2/liverpool OA in dogs - load.pdf
  - Montreal Instrument for Cat Arthritis Testing (Caretaker)—Version 2
    - https://ars.els-cdn.com/content/image/1-s2.0-S0168159117303271-mmc2.pdf
  - NC State TRiP Clinical Metrology Instruments: (FMPI, CSOM, SNoRE, MiPSC, etc)
    - https://cvm.ncsu.edu/research/labs/clinical-sciences/comparative-pain-research/clinical-metrology-instruments/

  - Zoetis questionnaire for owners
    - Canine: https://www.zoetispetcare.com/checklist/osteoarthritis-checklist
    - Feline: https://www.zoetispetcare.com/checklist/osteoarthritis-checklist-cat
- Acute pain scales and assessment
  - Colorado State University Acute Pain Scale
    - Canine: https://vetmedbiosci.colostate.edu/vth/wp-content/uploads/sites/7/2020/12/canine-pain-scale.pdf
    - Feline: https://vetmedbiosci.colostate.edu/vth/wp-content/uploads/sites/7/2020/12/feline-pain-scale.pdf
  - Feline Grimace Scale (FGS)
    - https://www.felinegrimacescale.com/
    - https://www.sylvester.ai/how-tably-works
  - Glasgow Composite Measure Pain Scale (Canine short form and Feline)
    - https://www.newmetrica.com/acute-pain-measurement/
  - UNESP- Botucatu Multidimensional Composite Pain Scale
    - UFEPS: http://www.animalpain.com.br/assets/upload/escala-en-us.pdf
    - UFEPS short form: https://www.ncbi.nlm.nih.gov/pmc/articles/PMC8048399/
- Pain Trace wearable monitor: https://paintrace.com/clinical-use/
- Canine EPA+DHA Dosing Chart: https://vetmedbiosci.colostate.edu/vth/services/orthopedic-medicine/fish-oil-dosing/
- CEHM, Spryng™ Osteocushion: https://www.sprynghealth.com/small-animal-how-it-works

ADDITIONAL RESOURCES AND ORGANIZATIONS

- 2024 ISFM/AAFP Consensus Guidelines on the Long-term Use of NSAIDs in Cats:
  - https://catvets.com/guidelines/practice-guidelines/nsaids-consensus-guidelines
- Review of NSAID Induced Adverse Effects in Dogs:
  - https://doi.org/10.1111/jvim.12127
- CARE: Canine Arthritis Resources and Education:
  - https://caninearthritis.org/

MOBILITY RESOURCES

- AARV—American Association of Rehabilitation Veterinarians
  - https://www.rehabvets.org/
- Geriatric Onset Laryngeal Paralysis and Polyneuropathy
  - HOME|GOLPP (allaboutgolpp.com)
- Dr. Buzby's ToeGrips
  - Dr. Buzby's ToeGrips for Dogs|Stop Your Dog from Slipping

NUTRITION RESOURCES

- WSAVA Global Nutrition Guidelines:
  - https://wsava.org/global-guidelines/global-nutrition-guidelines/
  - Diet-History-Form.pdf (wsava.org)
  - Body-Condition-Score-cat-updated-August-2020.pdf (wsava.org)
  - Body-Condition-Score-Dog.pdf (wsava.org)
  - Muscle condition score chart-01.jpg (wsava.org)
  - Muscle-Condition-Score-Chart-for-Dogs.pdf (wsava.org)

- ACVN—American College of Veterinary Nutritionists—consultation
  - http://www.ACVN.org
- AAHA Nutrition and Weight management guidelines
  - https://www.aaha.org/resources/2021-aaha-nutrition-and-weight-management-guidelines/
- Pet Nutrition Alliance
  - https://petnutritionalliance.org/
- SureFeed pet feeders
  - Sure Petcare | Award Winning Microchip Cat Doors & Feeders

RESOURCES ON SPECIFIC DISEASES

- Cognitive Dysfunction assessment
  - DISHAA-Assessment-Tool.pdf (purinainstitute.com)
- Renal—International Renal Interest Society
  - IRIS Kidney - Guidelines (iris-kidney.com)
- Cardiology—C
  - Cardiac Education Group – Cardiac Education Group

ACVIM (AMERICAN COLLEGE OF VETERINARY INTERNAL MEDICINE) CONSENSUS STATEMENTS

ACVIM consensus statement on diagnosis and management of urinary incontinence in dogs - Kendall - 2024 - Journal of Veterinary Internal Medicine - Wiley Online Library

ACVIM consensus statement on the treatment of immune thrombocytopenia in dogs and cats - LeVine - Journal of Veterinary Internal Medicine - Wiley Online Library

ACVIM consensus statement on diagnosis and management of acute canine thoracolumbar intervertebral disc extrusion - Olby - 2022 - Journal of Veterinary Internal Medicine - Wiley Online Library

ACVIM consensus statement on pancreatitis in cats - Forman - 2021 - Journal of Veterinary Internal Medicine - Wiley Online Library

ACVIM consensus statement guidelines for the classification, diagnosis, and management of cardiomyopathies in cats - Luis Fuentes - 2020 - Journal of Veterinary Internal Medicine - Wiley Online Library

ACVIM consensus statement guidelines for the diagnosis, classification, treatment, and monitoring of pulmonary hypertension in dogs - Reinero - 2020 - Journal of Veterinary Internal Medicine - Wiley Online Library

ACVIM consensus statement on the treatment of immune-mediated hemolytic anemia in dogs - Swann - 2019 - Journal of Veterinary Internal Medicine - Wiley Online Library

ACVIM consensus statement on the diagnosis and treatment of chronic hepatitis in dogs - Webster - 2019 - Journal of Veterinary Internal Medicine - Wiley Online Library

ACVIM consensus guidelines for the diagnosis and treatment of myxomatous mitral valve disease in dogs - Keene - 2019 - Journal of Veterinary Internal Medicine - Wiley Online Library

ACVIM consensus statement: Guidelines for the identification, evaluation, and management of systemic hypertension in dogs and cats - Acierno - 2018 - Journal of Veterinary Internal Medicine - Wiley Online Library

ACVIM Small Animal Consensus Recommendations on the Treatment and Prevention of Uroliths in Dogs and Cats - Lulich - 2016 - Journal of Veterinary Internal Medicine - Wiley Online Library

Index

Note: page numbers in *italics* refer to *figures*; those in **bold** to **tables**

Blackwell's Five-Minute Veterinary Consult Clinical Companion: Small Animal Senior Care, First Edition. Edited by Heidi B. Lobprise.

Companion website: www.wiley.com/go/lobprise/Senior